Neurodevelopmental Diseases – Laboratory and Clinical Research Series

HANDBOOK OF DOWN SYNDROME RESEARCH

Neurodevelopmental Diseases – Laboratory and Clinical Research Series

Handbook of Down Syndrome Research
Dominicus Jelinek and Gijs Dvorak (Editors)
2009. ISBN: 978-1-60741-690-6

Neurodevelopmental Diseases – Laboratory and Clinical Research Series

HANDBOOK OF DOWN SYNDROME RESEARCH

DOMINICUS JELINEK
AND
GIJS DVORAK
EDITORS

Nova Biomedical Books
New York

For permission to use material from this book please contact us:
Telephone 631-231-7269; Fax 631-231-8175
Web Site: http://www.novapublishers.com

Library of Congress Cataloging-in-Publication Data

Handbook of Down syndrome research / [edited by] Dominicus Jelinek and Gijs Dvorak.
p. ; cm.
Includes bibliographical references and index.
ISBN 978-1-60741-690-6 (hardcover)
1. Down syndrome--Handbooks, manuals, etc. I. Jelinek, Dominicus. II. Dvorak, Gijs.
[DNLM: 1. Down Syndrome. WS 107 H2355 2009]
RC571.H36 2009
616.85'8842--dc22

2009021230

Published by Nova Science Publishers, Inc. ✢ New York

Contents

Preface

Down syndrome is a condition in which extra genetic material causes delays in the way a child develops, both mentally and physically. It affects about 1 in every 800 babies. The physical features and medical problems associated with Down syndrome can vary widely from child to child. In most cases, the child has short and squat body, big neck, macroglossia, hypotonia and handheld fold. While some kids with DS need a lot of medical attention, others lead healthy lives. Though Down syndrome cannot be prevented, it can be detected before a child is born. Furthermore, while some kids with DS have no significant health problems, others may experience a host of medical issues that require extra care. For example, almost half of all children born with DS will have a congenital heart defect. Kids with Down syndrome are also at an increased risk of developing pulmonary hypertension. This book examines this genetic disorder, the detection of possible causes and treatment options for the complications of the disease.

Chapter 1 - Down syndrome (DS) is one of the best known diseases caused by an anomaly in autosomal chromosomes. The name derives from John Langdon Down who described the disease in 1862, using the term "mongoloidism" because of somatic features of the face of the patients who draw those of Eastern Asian populations, such as the Mongols. Another term almost synonymous is "trisomy 21".

DS is caused by the presence of a total or partial supernumerary chromosome 21. In approximately 95% of cases, the cause of this genetic anomaly is the non-disjunction of chromosomes that occurs during one of the meiotic divisions leading to the formation of a parent's gametes. It follows that the zygote will have a set of 47 chromosomes, with a supernumerary chromosome 21 in all cells of the affected person, instead of the normal diploid number of 46 chromosomes typical of the human species. That is why this disease is also called trisomy 21.

The syndrome may be caused by another type of mutation: a Robertsonian translocation, in which an arm of the chromosome 21 merges with another acrocentric chromosome (usually chromosome 14). Individuals with such a translocation are phenotypically normal, but have a high probability of having children with DS (familial).

DS involves different situations of slow development, but generally does not preclude the possibility of a successful integration and coexistence, given the particular learning ability that characterizes the Down individual. In most cases, the subject has short and squat body, big neck, macroglossia, hypotonia, and handheld fold. Mental retardation (MR) varies from the most serious forms to minor defects in genetic mosaics. The patient has increased susceptibility to infections and often malfunction of the heart and other organs; it is primarily for this reason that the average life, without intervention, is no more than 30-40 years. But now it has raised up to 60 years, because of the progress of surgical techniques, so that many cardiac anatomical abnormalities can be successfully treated. An Alzheimer-like amiloidosis is associated with downism.

When studying cases of DS due to translocation, there is usually a parent, even if phenotypically normal, who has a karyotype of 45 chromosomes. One of these chromosomes is formed by the long arm of chromosome 21 joined to the long arm of another acrocentric chromosome (usually chromosome 14), while the remaining short arms unite to form a small acentric chromosome which is usually mitotically unstable and gets lost. But since they do not contain essential genes, there are not clinical consequences. So, parents of a child suffering from DS due to Robertsonian translocation imbalance should proceed to the determination of their karyotype: if one or the other parent are carriers of a translocation, they are warned that there is an increased probability of having another child suffering from DS.

From a long time it is thought that DS, and a number of other adverse effects associated with non-disjunction, is more likely in children born from aged women. The reasons for this are unclear but it was noticed that they are related to the time of permanence of the ovocyte in the ovary in the diplotene of profase of the first meiosis, in which there is exchange of fragments between two non-brothers chromatids of omologous chromosomes. The permanence in this stage of the exchange would amplify errors in the disjunction of chromosomes during the anafase. The age of the mother is strongly correlated to the likelihood of having a person suffering from DS. It has been noted that, on average, the probability for women aged between 20 and 24 years is much lower than that of women aged 45 years or more. But the fact that the probability is so different in relation to the mother must not let us think that most women who bore a son who suffers from trisomy 21 are relatively of advanced age. In fact, few women around 45 years of age choose to have a child. Thus, children born with trisomy 21 are more likely to involve relatively young mothers who conceive more than women of old age. However, we can say that the age of the mother is very influential to the likelihood that a child could suffer or not from trisomy 21. Recent studies have also shown that in about 5% of cases with DS due to non-disjunction the supernumerary chromosome derives from the father rather than from the mother.

Treatment can be indicated only for the complications of the disease, which can be, among the most frequent, deafness, cardio-vascular diseases, leukemia, premature aging, and diabetes. We can work individually on the single problems. The problem of language can be exceeded bringing regularly and diligently the subject to a speech specialist. The trend to become fat should be countered with a balanced diet and a regular physical activity. Finally, the issue of MR is the most important to be addressed and the general council is to stimulate the intellectual activity of the subject from an early age, without claiming great results. An important role is entrusted to the first educators, parents and close family members, who must never stop teaching things even more obvious. The patients suffering from this syndrome have a distinct, almost irrepressible, sociality. It is therefore recommended and meaningful to use this item as a stimulus for learning: when we talk about educational facilities, the isolation from the class of membership is often counterproductive, because it demots the boy and makes arduous the maintenance of the attention. Another very strong stimulus can be received from a pet (dog, cat, horse) with which he can establish a deep friendship, which allows the child affected by DS to overcome some difficulties in the relationship field. Also the possibility to develop a responsibility for an animal definitely contributes to the formation and maturation of his autonomy. The use of electronic tools is productive. Like all syndromes associated with MR, in fact, the boy suffering from DS is particularly sensitive to the ritual of actions and commands. This also implies a certain rigidity in learning that must arouse the attention of the educators, as if the boy has learned a wrong behaviour it becomes hard for him to learn a more appropriate one. For this, we should be very careful in teaching actions, phrases, and behaviours which may show him all possible ways and actions to be done so that the child should learn and then immediately use the one he thinks is easier.

While in the past the main problem regarding DS was its treatment, in recent times it has become a major issue of debate and research its prenatal diagnosis (PD). After the demonstration by Jérôme Lejeune of the presence of 3 chromosomes 21 in patients with DS (1958), the possibility of seeking this anomaly in the human fetus has been studied. The first results were collected with amniocentesis performed in 1969 in England and in 1973 in France. As known, this technique implies a possibility of fetal losses. It was then proposed a cut-off of 5% of the population which is the age group 35-38 years where the estimated risk to have a pregnancy with fetal trisomy was assumed to be 1/250. This method can detect 25-30% of trisomies 21. In an effort to expand the diagnostic possibilities, based on observations on the role of alpha-fetoprotein (AFP) in neural tube defects (NTD), in 1984 the observations of Mercatz allowed to propose the use of the level of this protein as a marker for the diagnosis of chromosomal pathology (assumed that the values of that protein decrease in patients with fetal trisomy). Later, in 1987 Bogar showed an increase of human chorionic gonadotrophin (hCG) in cases of trisomy 21 and in 1988 Canico has also shown a decrease in the rate of unconjugated estriol (uE3). Consequently, Wald proposed on that basis a calculation of risk of trisomy involving maternal age rates and the three serum markers above mentioned. This diagnostic approach (tri-test) gives a sensitivity of 60%. From the late 1980s, after the measuring of fetal nuchal thickness in the second trimester by Benaceraff but especially after the description of Szabo and Gellen in 1990 of the "accumulation of nuchal fluid" in trisomy 21 embryos, with the multicenter study published by Snijers about the assessment of nuchal translucency (NT) which with the help of Nicolaides and Cucile brings the diagnostic sensitivity to 70%.

The interest of the PD of trisomy 21 implies a possible option for patients with fetal affection to appeal to voluntary termination of pregnancy. Naturally, for this purpose gestational age must coincide with the dictates of legislation and therefore it should be diagnosed as early as possible (first trimester). The increase in the value of fetal NT is the main sign of alarm for a trisomy 21 in the first trimester of pregnancy. There is no value threshold so the calculation of the risk of trisomy 21 will be given by a formula or tables which will consider the measure of NT, the size of the fetus, and the age of the patient. This result can be changed including in this formula the tri-test or better the biological markers of the first trimester.

There are numerous warning signs that the ultrasound operator must seize out in an examination of patients at risk:

- the absence of the nasal bone;
- the measure of the frontal-jaw angle on a certain profile (the average is 83 degrees at 11 weeks and 76 degrees at 14 weeks but in trisomic fetuses the angle opening is more important, +7 degrees);
- the anomaly of the Doppler flow in the venous duct (channel of Aranzio);
- tricuspidal regurgitation;
- right succlavia aberrant artery: prevalence of 1% in the healthy population but of 30% in trisomy;
- lymphatic jugular bag, often associated with "nuchal edema";
- rarely present signs: amniotic sac not perfectly adherent to the uterine cavity, increased density and thus hyper-reflection of the umbilical vesicle, early ossification of the bone point of the heel (this sign in normal fetuses can be seen only after 22 weeks).

Based on the above, it is recommended a screening in the first trimester of pregnancy that is within the 14th week of amenorrhea (i.e., from day 11^{+0} to day 13^{+6} of amenorrhea), combining for calculating the extent of the risk NT, crown-rump length (CRL), and maternal serum markers (MSM) (pregnancy-associated plasma protein-A [PAPP-A] and free beta-hCG) with the age of the mother. If the criteria for calculating the risk are not satisfied, other parameters can be used such as MSM in the second trimester combined to the measure of NT.

Recently, a simple blood test to find out if a fetus is affected by DS has been proposed. The test, which opens new horizons in medicine, was developed by a group of Californian researchers at Stanford University leaded by Stephen Quake. Just a small sample of the mother's blood is need to see if there is the disease. The test, which within 2 to 3 years could be available in hospitals worldwide, was successfully conducted on a sample of 18 women. To all of them blood was taken to verify the presence of DS and in 9 cases the test defined clearly and correctly the fetal abnormality. All this without having to resort to traditional techniques of PD, based above all on amniocentesis or chorionic villous sampling (CVS), much more invasive methodologies. Indeed in 1% of cases is reported the risk of miscarriage according to the statistics of the British Royal College of Obstetrics and Gynecology (RCOG). The danger increases with the CVS and passes from 1% to 2% of cases.

The Californian test is able to identify and count the pieces of DNA and is able to intercept even the smallest increment of chromosome 21. So that the test, once developed, will allow to discover other potentially fatal defects of the fetus such as Edwards and Patau syndromes. Now researchers are being organized to assess the validity of the test on a large scale with a more numerous sample of women. The test, which could mark a turning point in the history of PD, is therefore safer than traditional methods; in addition it can be made at the 10th week and not at the 15th as in case of amniocentesis. Moreover, the results are available after 2 days against the 3 weeks necessary for the previous examination. Making this test earlier also allows to ensure much more time to a mother to decide what to do when faced with a possible anomaly. Nevertheless, the blood test has put in alarm the International

Association that deals with DS. Nobody questions the importance of this non-invasive examination, they say, but it is equally important to give accurate information to parents on what is this disease. Even if someone does not consider DS a reason for abortion, he should recognize that a blood test that can detect the anomaly earlier gives parents more time to reflect and decide.

Chapter 2 - Trisomy of human chromosome 21 (HSA21) is the most frequent genetic cause of mental retardation and other phenotypic abnormalities, including developmental defects, hematological and solid tissue malignancies, heart and cranio-facial abnormalities, cognitive impairment and Alzheimer's disease, collectively known as Down syndrome. The expression of these characteristic features is due to the dosage imbalance of HSA21 genes.

DNA sequencing of HSA21 and gene annotation improve identification of the gene products. These sequencing data and the development of molecular analysis tools allow large-scale application of gene expression analysis. Genotype/phenotype correlation, transcriptome, proteome and functional genomics studies have shown genetic program perturbation by gene-dosage effects caused by trisomy of HSA21. The elevated gene expression, that is especially critical in Down syndrome, is a product of genetic effects on different cells, structures, and functions throughout development, many of which may have cascading effects to produce clinically observed phenotypic end points in a given individual with trisomy 21. The developmental regulated expression of trisomic genes and their downstream effects, direct and indirect, on the expression of other genes is linked to phenotypic consequences, not only in fully differentiated cells, but also at all stages where euploid and trisomic developmental processes diverge.

The important contribution of the molecular biology of understanding the molecular mechanisms underlying Down syndrome becomes of the most interest in the molecular medicine and provides potential directions for clinical therapeutics.

Chapter 3 - The recent significant increase of cases with Down syndrome in Hungary (1.1/1000 total births between 1973 and 1988, 1.57/1000 between 1989 and 1999 and 1.71/1000 between 2000 and 2006) is explained mainly by the higher proportion of prenatally diagnosed cases. Less important segment of this increase is a somewhat higher proportion of mothers with advanced maternal age and the more complete ascertainment due to the extra effort to reveal all cases in the study.

The data of the Hungarian Surveillance of Germinal Mutations based on the Hungarian Congenital Abnormality Registry did not show significant increase in the two forms (pure trisomy 21 as indicator of genom mutations and Robertsonian translocation due to chromosomal mutations) of Down syndrome after the fall-out deposition from Chernobyl in Hungary. In addition the rate of sentinel anomalies (new mutations of autosomal dominant disorders) and unclassified multiple congenital abnormalities (as the most sensitive indicator of environmental hazards) did also not indicate any increase in germinal mutations in Hungary after 1986.

The Hungarian Congenital Abnormality Registry detected a very obvious spatial cluster of Down syndrome and other congenital abnormalities in a small Hungarian village, 1989 and 1990. The number of inhabitants in this village was 456 and they had 15 livebirths in 1989 and 1990, and out of these 15 babies, 11 (73.3%) were affected with congenital abnormalities, 4 were affected with Down syndrome. The case-control field study identified trichlorfon used in the fishfarms of the village, as an environmental agent that can induce Down syndrome in very large doses. This observation was confirmed in animal investigations. Thus our finding is an important argument for the necessity and importance of population-based registries of congenital abnormalities.

We studied the association between the use of nutritional supplements during the first gestational month and the origin of Down syndrome, and we found a significant protective effect of large doses (about 6 mg/day) of folic acid and iron (150-300 mg/day of ferrous sulfate) for the occurrence of cases with Down syndrome. In general, folic acid and iron were used together, therefore it was difficult to separate these effects due to the limited number of cases and controls. However, the main message of our study is that a pharmacological dose of folic acid and iron supplement appears to have a primary preventive effect for Down syndrome.

Chapter 4 - This chapter will commence with an overview of the literature on social functioning in Down syndrome (DS). The overview is structured according to Tager-Flusberg and Sullivan's (2000) model of social functioning, which differentiates social perceptual and social cognitive skills. Compared to the literature available for other developmental syndromes, there has been very little research exploring social abilities in DS, and studies have produced mixed findings. Following the overview, research limitations are discussed, then a research study is introduced which addresses some of the limitations and assesses social attribution in DS (N=17), Williams-Beuren syndrome (WBS, N=17), and in typically developing mental age matched controls (N=17, MAC) and chronological age matched controls (N=17, CAC). The research study compares individuals with DS, individuals with WBS, and MAC and CAC on the Social Attribution Task (SAT, Klin, 2000), which uses the Heider and Simmel (1944) silent cartoon animation in which geometric shapes enact a social plot. The SAT measures social abilities which are a fundamental basis of human social interaction (Klin, 2000). Findings indicated a comparable performance between DS, WBS, and MAC on all social cognitive indices from the SAT, but the DS group displayed reduced paralinguistic skills compared to MAC. All groups performed significantly below the level of CAC, except for their ability to attribute cognitive and affective mental states, which was comparable across the four groups. Findings are discussed in relation to Tager-Flusberg and Sullivan's model of social functioning and in relation to amygdala and frontal lobe brain impairments in DS.

Chapter 5 - Down syndrome (DS) is associated with a number of associated additional clinical problems, in addition to its classical neurological and skeletal features [viz: decreased muscle tone (floppy baby), short stature, decreased intellectual capacity and brachycephaly and congenital heart disease]. Of these, gastro-intestinal tract (GIT) malfunction remains one of the most significant, but congenital hearing deficits are also not infrequent and there is an increased risk of certain tumours (i.e. Leukemia, retro-peritoneal teratomas). On the other hand, certain other solid tumours have a decreased prevalence in DS (eg neuroblastoma, nephroblastoma, hepatoblastoma and medulloblastoma).

GI malfunction has been reported in as many as 77% of DS affected individuals but the true prevalence of functional GI disturbances in DS adults has been difficult to assess, as many DS individuals do not have access to regular healthcare checks.

From a genetic point of view, the genetic basis of DS is mostly either a Trisomy or a translocation of chromosome 21, and rarely involves a mosaic (often referred to as Partial trisomy). Essentially, this means that there is an extra copy of chromosome 21 is present in the majority of cases. It is currently thought that the resulting genetic imbalance plays a role in many of the debilitating Central Nervous system (CNS) associations of DS resulting in interest in the potential role of the 200-400 Chromosome 21 genes which may contribute to the phenotypic features of DS.

Chapter 6 - Infectious diseases of respiratory system frequently complicate pregnancy. This review is to evaluate the possible association between maternal infectious diseases of respiratory system during pregnancy and preterm birth or structural birth defects, i.e. congenital abnormalities (CAs), in addition their pregnancy complications based on the data set of the Hungarian Case-Control Surveillance of Congenital Abnormalities.

At the evaluation of *common cold*, it is necessary to differentiate the usual common cold (with short duration and without fever) and common cold with secondary complications (i.e. with longer duration and frequently high fever). Pregnant women with common cold mainly with secondary complications had not a higher incidence of pregnancy complications. The gestational age at delivery was 0.1 week shorter with a somewhat higher rate of preterm birth, but these differences had no real clinical importance. However, an association of common cold (mainly with secondary complications) in the second and/or third gestational month of pregnancy with a higher rate of newborns with congenital cataract, cleft lip ± palate and possible some other specific congenital abnormalities was found and these association was preventable with antifever drug treatments.

Acute infectious diseases of respiratory system cover a wide spectrum of diseases from sinusitis to pneumonia. These diseases during pregnancy have no obvious effect for pregnancy complications. Severe lower category of these infectious respiratory diseases associated with a higher risk for preterm birth, but their mild upper category seems to reduce indirectly the rate of preterm birth. Acute infectious diseases of respiratory system during the second and third gestational months of pregnancy did not associate with a higher risk for the total group or any specific group/entity of congenital abnormalities. However, the frequently high fever related tonsillitis in pregnant women associated with a higher risk for congenital cataract, neural-tube defects, cleft lip ± palate and unclassified multiple congenital abnormalities. We may suppose that the association between these fever sensitive defect groups and tonsillitis may be caused by high fever, because the parallel antifever treatment was able to prevent this risk.

Finally the *influenza* during pregnancy was evaluated. The short duration of influenza in pregnant women did not increase the risk for pregnancy complications. Our study showed that the appropriately treated pregnant women affected with influenza in the first and second trimester of pregnancy have no higher risk for preterm birth. However, the high fever related influenza in the second and/or third gestational month of pregnancy may associate with a higher risk of some - hyperthermia sensitive – CAs such as neural-tube defects, congenital cataract, cleft lip ± palate, cleft palate only, cardiovascular CAs, and unclassified multiple CAs. The main finding of our study is that this higher risk for these major CA can be prevented by the parallel use of antifever drugs.

Chapter 7 - This chapter guides readers through mitochondrial physiology, mitochondrial medicine and possible adjunctive therapy in Down syndrome (DS), and generally in neurodegenerative diseases. DS is an inherited disease with an extra copy of chromosome 21, and the onset of Alzheimer's disease by middle age. Mitochondrial dysfunction and oxidative damage have been implicated in the pathogenesis of DS, ageing and generally in neurodegenerative diseases.

Brain mitochondrial coenzyme "Q-CLOCK" as well as circadian cascade of oxidative phosphorylation presented in this chapter can contribute to the explanation of brain mitochondrial diseases.

Documented bioavailability of liposomal coenzyme Q_{10} in rats brain nuclei, tissue and mitochondria could be beneficial for the adjunctive therapy at the condition of damaged brain mitochondrial energy production and oxidative stress in patients with Down syndrome.

Chapter 8 - The importance of making an informed choice in a medical field depends on the specific clinical context. When patients refer minor everyday problems to health care professionals and there is a routine and simple treatment or benefit there is no need to initiate a process of informed decision making. In this case informed consent is enough. However, several of choices in pregnancy, such as how to give birth and whether or not to undergo screening test for Down's syndrome, have important implications for women and her family and thus informed choice has fundamental importance. Screening doesn't have only benefits but also has risks. Harms from screening arising mainly from the false negative and false positive results because of their medical, psychological and legal consequences. Therefore, the choice to undergo screening for Down's syndrome should be based on a full understanding of the likely benefits, harms and limitations. Many definitions have been given for informed choice but all these definitions have two core characteristics: a) relevant, good quality information and b) consistency between attitudes and behaviour. "An informed decision could be defined as a reasoned choice which is made by a reasonable individual using relevant information about the advantages and disadvantages of all possible courses of action in accord with the individual's belief". The conclusions that have been drawn from this chapter mainly concern the measurement, the determinants and the factors that may impact on informed choice. In general, there is a lack of standardized measures that assess the multidimensionality of informed choice, as the majority of the existent measures are either single dimensioned or measures of self report. According to the findings of relevant original studies, the majority of women have a relatively poor level of knowledge and understanding about the Down's syndrome screening and the vast majority of women have a positive attitude towards screening for Down's syndrome. In general, the rates of informed choice about screening for Down' syndrome have been found low. Since informed choice is determined by knowledge and by attitude-behaviour consistency of participants, the factors that may influence the knowledge and the attitudes of women could impact on informed choice rate. The factors that may impact on the informed choice of women by affecting their level of knowledge and their degree of understanding of information given, could be the way of presentation of information (special leaflets, video, computer systems), and the level of knowledge and the communication skills of health care professionals. Factors that may influence women's attitudes could be the attitudes of health care professionals, social influences and organizational factors such as the way of offering screening. Health care professionals (midwives and obstetricians) should dedicate more time to discussing with women and should provide information which is understandable and suitable to their learning ability. Moreover, it could be concluded that attitude is a stronger predictor of informed choice than level of knowledge since the majority of women who attend screening for Down syndrome have positive attitude and not good level of knowledge. Therefore, the attempt to increase attitude-behavior consistency could be more successful in increasing informed choice in screening for Down syndrome than increasing the level of knowledge.

Chapter 9 - Healthy parent-child interaction is as essential to the early development of children with Down Syndrome as it is for typically developing children. In early childhood, this transaction is largely regulated by reciprocal emotional exchanges between partners. Through their caregiving, parents supply their children with the experiences they need for both physical and psychological growth. Contemporary opinion is that positive emotional sharing is an indispensable frame to effective caregiving of children with an intellectual disability, but at the same time specific cognitive and/or motor impairments may short-circuit the child's ability to understand and exchange emotions.

In this chapter we first outline the current findings about parent-child interaction in children with Down Syndrome. Then we report in details the results of two studies about children with Down Syndrome in which we compared mother-child and father-child dyads with respect to some pivotal aspects of parent-child interaction, namely affective quality and play behaviours; for each study, the differences and similarities between mothers and fathers as well as the children's contribution to relationship functioning are presented. The discussion of the findings refer to the theoretical perspective according to which dyadic interactions based on emotional involvement may lead to enhanced cognitive functioning in children with Down Syndrome. Finally, the clinical implications of this framework are discussed.

Chapter 10 - The introduction of the ultrasound imaging technology in the second half of the 20th century has revolutionized prenatal care. The ultrasound-based diagnostic medical imaging technique is now an indispensable component of the screening system of every pregnant woman. It is used to confirm the gestational age of the fetus and detect problems of serious medical nature, such as blockage of the small intestine, heart defects and chromosomal abnormalities. Knowing about the existence of these fatal anomalies as early in pregnancy as possible helps parents in decision-making regarding the future of the fetus.

Studies in the mid-1990s have shown a strong association between the size of the collection of fluid at the back of the fetal neck, called nuchal transluceny (NT), and the risk of Down syndrome. Early attempts to use measurement of NT thickness were limited by a wide variety in measurement discrepancies. Ultrasound NT measurement is usually done between 10 and 14 weeks gestation. It is highly dependent on the experience of the ultrasonographer. Small differences -- less than one tenth of a millimeter -- in NT measurements can make the designation of "normal" or "abnormal" result. Recognizing the potential importance of the problem that would arise from the performance of NT measurement by untrained ultrasonographers, many authoritative organizations have recommended that first trimester screening not be made widely available until a national program of quality review and oversight is established for the United States. Thus, NT measurements should only be offered in the setting of an accredited sonography center.

Recently, standardized guidelines on measuring NT thickness along with specific training and certification have been instituted, making this ultrasound measurement a useful marker as part of first trimester screening. Correct performance of NT measurement is critical to the accuracy, safety, and effectiveness of the non-invasive prenatal screening system.

Chapter 11 - Down syndrome (DS) occurs in decorrence of a chromosomic abnormality and is characterized by physical and mental alterations. Individuals with DS are known to have a great predisposition to periodontal disease in early age, due to alterations in their immune system. This study was approved by the Ethics Committee of the Irmandade da Santa Casa de Misericórdia de São Paulo (Brazil). This case-control study aims at evaluating some behavioral characteristics related to dental hygiene, Gingival Modified Index (GMI) and Simplified Oral Hygiene Index (OHIS) in deciduous dentition of DS children. The study group (DS) was composed by 69 DS children, which were compared with 69 children without congenital abnormalities (control group). The oral hygiene habits were obtained by means of a questionnaire, the GMI used was the one proposed by Löe and Silness (1963) and modified by Lobene et al. (1986). The OHI-S was proposed by Greene e Vermillion (1964). Statistical comparisons between the groups were done using Chi-Squared and Fisher's Exact Test or "t" test. The data were analyzed with the aid of MINITAB® statistical software, 14.2 version. The results demonstrated that the study group (DS) had professional follow-up dental care more frequently ($p=0,010$) and higher frequency of daily dental brushing ($p<0,001$). The use of dental floss was, however, rare ($p<0,001$). A statistically significant difference between the groups related to GMI and OHI-S was observed ($p < 0,001$). GMI was found to be greater and OHI-S smaller in the study group (DS). Children from the study group (DS) presented better oral hygiene habits and attended regular dental check-ups more often than children from the control group.

Chapter 12 - Disorders of eating, drinking and swallowing (also known as ‘dysphagia’) commonly affect people with Down’s syndrome (DS) across the lifespan. This is due to the influence of several factors, including the abnormal oral-facial features that are characteristic of the syndrome, as well as comorbid health conditions that impact on the safety and integrity of the swallowing process. The relevant literature is consulted to explore aspects of the eating, drinking and swallowing process in people with Down’s syndrome from birth onwards, and examine how this process differs from that in the general population. Discussion focuses on how the typical eating, drinking and swallowing process in DS individuals is frequently associated with abnormal functioning of the swallowing mechanism at various levels, and how it can very often lead to dysphagia and its potentially life-threatening sequelae. Finally, this paper considers the role of healthcare practitioners in the identification and management of dysphagia in individuals with DS, including implications for treatment planning and health service delivery.

Chapter 13 - Prenatal screening is based on maternal serum biochemistry and ultrasound examination which are non invasive and are used as a first line for investigation. In the 2nd trimester of gestation, the multiple marker combination with the highest screening performance currently available is alpha-fetoprotein (AFP), unconjugated estriol (uE3), human chorionic gonadotropin (hCG), and inhibin A, in combination with maternal age. With this combination, a detection rate of 80% at a 5% false positive rate is achieved. First trimester screening tests combining maternal age, fetal nuchal translucency (NT) thickness and maternal serum free beta-hCG and PAPP-A are at least as accurate as traditional 2nd trimester testing and provide results earlier in pregnancy.

In this chapter, the various options for prenatal screening for DS are outlined. Current research efforts made to improve non invasive prenatal diagnosis based on fetal cells, cell free fetal DNA and proteins present in maternal circulation are also discussed.

Chapter 14 - This chapter presents a new methodology to detect Down's syndrome during the second-trimester of gestation. We propose a Fuzzy Logic based classification method that is able of both improving the classification accuracy of the existing screening methods and extracting a set of intelligible rules that explain the system found. The accuracy is improved by reducing the False Positive rate up to 3%-4%, with a 60% of True Positive rate. Never before a screening method could reduce the FP rate below 5%, with a 60% of TP. The intelligibility is obtained by getting a reduced set of rules, expressed in a fuzzy way, which helps to explain the knowledge contained in the classification system found. Finally, conclude that the medical staff was able to understand the system expressed in the Fuzzy rules found, where its number of rules is just 10.

Chapter 15 - Cerebral palsy (CP) describes a group of movement and posture development disorders attributed to non-progressive disturbances in the developing fetal or infant brain, causing activity limitations and being the most common cause of severe physical disability in childhood. The motor disorders of CP are often accompanied by disturbances of sensation, cognition, communication, perception, behavior, and seizure disorders.

Oromotor dysfunction and oral-ingestive problems, as uncoordinated control mechanisms of orofacial and palatolingual musculatures, are often observed in CP individuals, and varies from mild to severe. These disabilities are expressed by drooling, coughing, choking, rejection of solid food, food loss, and spillage during eating. Difficulties in spoon-feeding, biting, chewing, cup drinking, straw drinking, swallowing and clearing are also observed.

Another nutritional issue to be considered is the common inability of severely oromotor impaired CP individuals to ingest solid food, which often leads to an exclusively liquid or semi-solid diet. In spite of contributing to some degree to growth and nutritional disturbances, especially at an early age, food consistency may also cause a significant impact on oral health. Therefore, a timely nutritional rehabilitation and preventive measures in oral health may significantly improve the quality of life of these individuals, as well as prevent deleterious and noxious habits such as bottle feeding. Performing an adequate oral hygiene on CP individuals however, can be a very difficult task for the caregivers, due to the patient's persistent pathological biting reflex.

Food consistency, sugared beverages, and long term oral medicines, associated with oromotor dysfunction and oral hygiene difficulties, may explain the high incidence of caries and periodontal diseases exhibited by the CP population.

The influence of oromotor impairment in CP individuals as a risk factor in caries experience was not studied yet. Therefore, this study aimed at evaluating the influence of oral motricity and diet consistency on caries experience and growth rate in CP individuals.

Chapter 16 - The purpose of this paper is to analyze the changes brought about by growth in the craniofacial area in individuals with Down syndrome and compare them to the growth that occurs in the general population. In order to do so, the authors have carried out a longitudinal study on a sample of genetically diagnosed subjects with Down syndrome, recording craniofacial growth taken from cephalometric radiographs at yearly intervals. They will discuss all of the morphological aspects related to craniofacial growth found in our study, contrasting our findings with those published by other authors. By way of clarity, they will divide the discussion section into three main parts: cranial base growth, maxillary growth and mandibular growth in Down syndrome.

Chapter 17 - Evidence has been well-documented that persons with Down syndrome are particularly susceptible to hearing loss and middle ear pathology. Hearing loss associated with Down syndrome is usually late-onset and progressive in nature, deeming the regular practices of universal newborn hearing screening insufficient. The authors have carried out hearing screening and diagnostic assessment on schoolchildren with Down syndrome, in both special schools and mainstream schools, in two different nations in the past few years. The prevalence of hearing loss in these school-age populations, as well as the common degree, nature and underlying pathology of hearing loss/middle ear disorders, were investigated. This chapter presents discussion of the developmental implications of such hearing impairment for schoolchildren with Down syndrome, in addition to its influence on learning. Technological options for hearing and middle ear screening are explored, culminating in feasible and practical screening and surveillance protocols for this population. Finally, the authors discuss medical and audiological treatment options and outline recommendations for meeting the audiological rehabilitation needs of children with Down syndrome.

Chapter 18 - Down Syndrome (DS) (Trisomy 21) is a relatively common anomaly occurring in one in every 600-700 live births and characterized by impaired growth and development and early senescence. Signs of abnormal development have been observed on ultrasound as early as the first trimester. They include abnormal flow velocity patterns in the ductus venosus and hypoplasia of the nasal bone in addition to increased fetal nuchal translucency. By the second trimester additional signs are evident on ultrasound, affecting skeletal growth as well as other organ systems. Dental anomalies include reduced tooth size and number, thin enamel and abnormal crown form as well as taurodont roots and a high frequency of missing teeth. The severity of the dental defects varies along the tooth row with later developing teeth most severely affected. Recent studies carried out on exfoliated (shed) deciduous teeth using a combination of serial microCT scans and SEM have enabled us to reconstruct the chronology and extent of intrauterine and infant growth insults in DS infants, expressed in growth and differentiation of the developing teeth. Our results for the deciduous teeth show that in DS, there is accelerated dental development in the first trimester followed by progressive growth retardation associated with impaired differentiation of the dental tissues. These changes appear to primarily affect cells derived from ectoderm and affect cell division and differentiation. This results in a smaller modified tooth germ with impaired enamel matrix formation and bio-mineralization. The resulting enamel is thin and hypomineralized and this may contribute to the severe abrasion seen in the teeth of DS children despite the associated lack of muscle tone.

Chapter 19 - Down syndrome (DS) represents both the most common trisomy in newborns and the most frequent genetic cause of mental retardation. It is mainly due to the presence of all or a part of a complete extra-chromosome 21 that approximately in 95% of cases is caused by an abnormal segregation during meiosis. Maternal non-disjunction is responsible of about 90% of those cases. A risk of 0,5-1% is generally given after a DS affected pregnancy. Thus, the chromosomal type of DS must be extensively studied, as the assessment of the recurrence risk depends on different cytogenetic causes. James et Al. suggested a link between impaired folate metabolism and the risk of DS as the primary biological function of folate is to provide co-factors that carry one-carbon groups that play a pivotal role in DNA synthesis and methylation. Folate deficiency has been associated with abnormal chromosome segregation, supporting the possibility that low maternal folate status might be associated with the risk of non-disjunction. It is reported a significant association between frequency of C→T mutation at nucleotide 677 in the enzyme methylenetetrahydrofolate reductased and the risk of DS. Also the methionine synthase reductase A66G mutation was associated with DS risk. Both genes code for enzymes that control crucial key points in the folate pathway. In 2003 Barkai et Al. noted a significantly high frequency of DS in pregnancies with risk for neural tube defects, a condition often associated with impaired folate metabolism, enforcing a link between those two pathological conditions on the common base of abnormal folate status. A periconceptional folic acid supplementation at 5 mg/die was suggested to reduce both the occurrence and recurrence risk of DS pregnancies and of neural tube defects. Moreover, maternal plasma homocysteine/methionine ratio level was higher in DS related-mothers than in controls, suggesting that folic acid supplementation could reduce the risk of trisomy 21 conceptuses. However, the cause on non-disjunction in trisomy 21 is still almost entirely unknown. Given the link between impaired folate metabolism DS occurrence and recurrence risk, those considerations further support the need of more extensive research on the use of folic acid to prevent non-disjunction events leading to free trisomy 21.

Chapter 20 - DYRK1A kinase, the gene located within triplicated region on chromosome 21 in Down syndrome (DS), has been found to be associated with neuronal cytoskeleton. In pathological brains of DS and Alzheimer's disease (AD) patients the levels of major cytoskeleton proteins forming complexes with DYRK1A were greatly reduced. The changes were specific for AD dementia and present in young DS individuals whose brains were free of pathological burden, suggesting that early dysfunction of cytoskeleton may be at the root of neurodegenerative processes responsible for AD. Any malfunction of cytoskeleton during brain development may result in sculpting of the memory system with significantly reduced memory capacity, which late in life can become saturated incapacitating brain to acquire a constant input of new epigenetic information. This triggers a compensatory response, which up-regulates neuronal plasticity and through activation of dedifferentiation program forces post-mitotic neurons back into the cell cycle. Re-entering the cell cycle and high plasticity burden imposed on neurons of the memory system lead to its gradual degeneration resulting in dementia. Down syndrome patients with their developmentally impaired neuronal networking, caused by abnormal expression of DYRK1A and other genes from the region critical for DS, lend a lot of support for the proposed cascade of events leading to dementia.

In: Handbook of Down Syndrome Research
Editors: Dominicus Jelinek and Gijs Dvorak
ISBN 978-1-60741- 690-6

Chapter 1

Down Syndrome: Genetics, Screening, and Health

Ciro Comparetto[1] and Franco Borruto[2]
[1]Division of Obstetrics and Gynecology, City Hospital, Prato, Italy
[2]Department of Obstetrics and Gynecology, University of Verona, Italy

Abstract

Down syndrome (DS) is one of the best known diseases caused by an anomaly in autosomal chromosomes. The name derives from John Langdon Down who described the disease in 1862, using the term "mongoloidism" because of somatic features of the face of the patients who draw those of Eastern Asian populations, such as the Mongols. Another term almost synonymous is "trisomy 21".

DS is caused by the presence of a total or partial supernumerary chromosome 21. In approximately 95% of cases, the cause of this genetic anomaly is the non-disjunction of chromosomes that occurs during one of the meiotic divisions leading to the formation of a parent's gametes. It follows that the zygote will have a set of 47 chromosomes, with a supernumerary chromosome 21 in all cells of the affected person, instead of the normal diploid number of 46 chromosomes typical of the human species. That is why this disease is also called trisomy 21.

The syndrome may be caused by another type of mutation: a Robertsonian translocation, in which an arm of the chromosome 21 merges with another acrocentric chromosome (usually chromosome 14). Individuals with such a translocation are phenotypically normal, but have a high probability of having children with DS (familial).

DS involves different situations of slow development, but generally does not preclude the possibility of a successful integration and coexistence, given the particular learning ability that characterizes the Down individual. In most cases, the subject has short and squat body, big neck, macroglossia, hypotonia, and handheld fold. Mental retardation (MR) varies from the most serious forms to minor defects in genetic mosaics. The patient has increased susceptibility to infections and often malfunction of the heart and other organs; it is primarily for this reason that the average life, without intervention, is no more than 30-40 years. But now it has raised up to 60 years, because of the progress of surgical techniques, so that many cardiac anatomical abnormalities can be successfully treated. An Alzheimer-like amiloidosis is associated with downism.

When studying cases of DS due to translocation, there is usually a parent, even if phenotypically normal, who has a karyotype of 45 chromosomes. One of these chromosomes is formed by the long arm of chromosome 21 joined to the long arm of another acrocentric chromosome (usually chromosome 14), while the remaining short arms unite to form a small acentric chromosome which is usually mitotically unstable and gets lost. But since they do not contain essential genes, there are not clinical consequences. So, parents of a child suffering from DS due to Robertsonian translocation imbalance should proceed to the determination of their karyotype: if one or the other parent are carriers of a translocation, they are warned that there is an increased probability of having another child suffering from DS.

From a long time it is thought that DS, and a number of other adverse effects associated with non-disjunction, is more likely in children born from aged women. The reasons for this are unclear but it was noticed that they are related to the time of permanence of the ovocyte in the ovary in the diplotene of profase of the first meiosis, in which there is exchange of fragments between two non-brothers chromatids of omologous chromosomes. The permanence in this stage of the exchange would amplify errors in the disjunction of chromosomes during the anafase. The age of the mother is strongly correlated to the likelihood of having a person suffering from DS. It has been noted that, on average, the probability for women aged between 20 and 24 years is much lower than that of women aged 45 years or more. But the fact that the probability is so different in relation to the mother must not let us think that most women who bore a son who suffers from trisomy 21 are relatively of advanced age. In fact, few women around 45 years of age choose to have a child. Thus, children born with trisomy 21 are more likely to involve relatively young mothers who conceive more than women of old age. However, we can say that the age of the mother is very influential to the likelihood that a child could suffer or not from trisomy 21. Recent studies have also shown that in about 5% of cases with DS due to non-disjunction the supernumerary chromosome derives from the father rather than from the mother.

Treatment can be indicated only for the complications of the disease, which can be, among the most frequent, deafness, cardio-vascular diseases, leukemia, premature aging, and diabetes. We can work individually on the single problems. The problem of language can be exceeded bringing regularly and diligently the subject to a speech specialist. The trend to become fat should be countered with a balanced diet and a regular physical activity. Finally, the issue of MR is the most important to be addressed and the general council is to stimulate the intellectual activity of the subject from an early age, without claiming great results. An important role is entrusted to the first educators, parents and close family members, who must never stop teaching things even more obvious. The patients suffering from this syndrome have a distinct, almost irrepressible, sociality. It is therefore recommended and meaningful to use this item as a stimulus for learning: when we talk about educational facilities, the isolation from the class of membership is often counterproductive, because it demots the boy and makes arduous the maintenance of the attention. Another very strong stimulus can be received from a pet (dog, cat, horse) with which he can establish a deep friendship, which allows the child affected by DS to overcome some difficulties in the relationship field. Also the possibility to develop a responsibility for an animal definitely contributes to the formation and maturation of his autonomy. The use of electronic tools is productive. Like all syndromes associated with MR, in fact, the boy suffering from DS is particularly sensitive to the ritual of actions and commands. This also implies a certain rigidity in learning that must arouse the attention of the educators, as if the boy has learned a wrong behaviour it becomes hard for him to learn a more appropriate one. For this, we should be very careful in teaching actions, phrases, and behaviours which may show him all possible ways and actions to be done so that the child should learn and then immediately use the one he thinks is easier.

While in the past the main problem regarding DS was its treatment, in recent times it has become a major issue of debate and research its prenatal diagnosis (PD). After the demonstration by Jérôme Lejeune of the presence of 3 chromosomes 21 in patients with DS (1958), the possibility of seeking this anomaly in the human fetus has been studied. The first results were collected with amniocentesis performed in 1969 in England and in 1973 in France. As known, this technique implies a possibility of fetal losses. It was then proposed a cut-off of 5% of the population which is the age group 35-38 years where the estimated risk to have a pregnancy with fetal trisomy was assumed to be 1/250. This method can detect 25-30% of trisomies 21. In an effort to expand the diagnostic possibilities, based on observations on the role of alpha-fetoprotein (AFP) in neural tube defects (NTD), in 1984 the observations of Mercatz allowed to propose the use of the level of this protein as a marker for the diagnosis of chromosomal pathology (assumed that the values of that protein decrease in patients with fetal trisomy). Later, in 1987 Bogar showed an increase of human chorionic gonadotrophin (hCG) in cases of trisomy 21 and in 1988 Canico has also shown a decrease in the rate of unconjugated estriol (uE3). Consequently, Wald proposed on that basis a calculation of risk of trisomy involving maternal age rates and the three serum markers above mentioned. This diagnostic approach (tri-test) gives a sensitivity of 60%. From the late 1980s, after the measuring of fetal nuchal thickness in the second trimester by Benaceraff but especially after the description of Szabo and Gellen in 1990 of the "accumulation of nuchal fluid" in trisomy 21 embryos, with the multicenter study published by Snijers about the assessment of nuchal translucency (NT) which with the help of Nicolaides and Cucile brings the diagnostic sensitivity to 70%.

The interest of the PD of trisomy 21 implies a possible option for patients with fetal affection to appeal to voluntary termination of pregnancy. Naturally, for this purpose gestational age must coincide with the dictates of legislation and therefore it should be diagnosed as early as possible (first trimester). The increase in the value of fetal NT is the main sign of alarm for a trisomy 21 in the first trimester of pregnancy. There is no value threshold so the calculation of the risk of trisomy 21 will be given by a formula or tables which will consider the measure of NT, the size of the fetus, and the age of the patient. This result can be changed including in this formula the tri-test or better the biological markers of the first trimester.

There are numerous warning signs that the ultrasound operator must seize out in an examination of patients at risk:

1) the absence of the nasal bone;
2) the measure of the frontal-jaw angle on a certain profile (the average is 83 degrees at 11 weeks and 76 degrees at 14 weeks but in trisomic fetuses the angle opening is more important, +7 degrees);
3) the anomaly of the Doppler flow in the venous duct (channel of Aranzio);
4) tricuspidal regurgitation;
5) right succlavia aberrant artery: prevalence of 1% in the healthy population but of 30% in trisomy;
6) lymphatic jugular bag, often associated with "nuchal edema";
7) rarely present signs: amniotic sac not perfectly adherent to the uterine cavity, increased density and thus hyper-reflection of the umbilical vesicle, early

ossification of the bone point of the heel (this sign in normal fetuses can be seen only after 22 weeks).

Based on the above, it is recommended a screening in the first trimester of pregnancy that is within the 14th week of amenorrhea (i.e., from day 11^{+0} to day 13^{+6} of amenorrhea), combining for calculating the extent of the risk NT, crown-rump length (CRL), and maternal serum markers (MSM) (pregnancy-associated plasma protein-A [PAPP-A] and free beta-hCG) with the age of the mother. If the criteria for calculating the risk are not satisfied, other parameters can be used such as MSM in the second trimester combined to the measure of NT.

Recently, a simple blood test to find out if a fetus is affected by DS has been proposed. The test, which opens new horizons in medicine, was developed by a group of Californian researchers at Stanford University leaded by Stephen Quake. Just a small sample of the mother's blood is need to see if there is the disease. The test, which within 2 to 3 years could be available in hospitals worldwide, was successfully conducted on a sample of 18 women. To all of them blood was taken to verify the presence of DS and in 9 cases the test defined clearly and correctly the fetal abnormality. All this without having to resort to traditional techniques of PD, based above all on amniocentesis or chorionic villous sampling (CVS), much more invasive methodologies. Indeed in 1% of cases is reported the risk of miscarriage according to the statistics of the British Royal College of Obstetrics and Gynecology (RCOG). The danger increases with the CVS and passes from 1% to 2% of cases.

The Californian test is able to identify and count the pieces of DNA and is able to intercept even the smallest increment of chromosome 21. So that the test, once developed, will allow to discover other potentially fatal defects of the fetus such as Edwards and Patau syndromes. Now researchers are being organized to assess the validity of the test on a large scale with a more numerous sample of women. The test, which could mark a turning point in the history of PD, is therefore safer than traditional methods; in addition it can be made at the 10th week and not at the 15th as in case of amniocentesis. Moreover, the results are available after 2 days against the 3 weeks necessary for the previous examination. Making this test earlier also allows to ensure much more time to a mother to decide what to do when faced with a possible anomaly. Nevertheless, the blood test has put in alarm the International Association that deals with DS. Nobody questions the importance of this non-invasive examination, they say, but it is equally important to give accurate information to parents on what is this disease. Even if someone does not consider DS a reason for abortion, he should recognize that a blood test that can detect the anomaly earlier gives parents more time to reflect and decide.

Introduction

The first descriptions of the trisomy 21 phenotype were by Jean-Etienne-Dominique Esquirol (1838), Edouard Séguin (1846), and later by John Langdon Down in 1862. It took more than a century to Jérôme Lejeune's discovery of the first genetic substrate for mental retardation (MR) and to discover the extra-chromosomal origin of the syndrome commonly called "Down syndrome" (DS) and which should be referred to as "trisomy 21". The sequencing of human chromosome 21 (HSA21) was a new starting point which generated transcriptome studies and studies of gene over-expression have provided the impetus for discovering the HSA21 genes associated with trisomy 21 cognitive impairment [1].

Genetic disorders account for a significant number of the health care problems in our society. Advances in therapy and educational opportunities for the handicapped have increased both the life span and quality of life for many of those affected by genetic disorders. Recent developments in clinical and laboratory genetics have made possible the better delineation of certain malformation and/or MR syndromes so that their mode of inheritance can be understood. This information enables the genetic counselor to predict the risk for occurrence of a large number of genetic disorders. Often genetic counseling is done, however, only after the birth of at least one affected individual has alerted the family to their predilection for having children with a genetic disorder. The carrier state of a certain number of genetic disorders can now be detected, so that even before the birth of their first child a family can be forewarned that they are at increased risk. Previously this knowledge often influenced couples to decide against having any children. The advent of prenatal diagnosis (PD) of genetic disease, however, which was pioneered in the 1960s, allows specific diagnoses of inherited disorders in the fetus; parents no longer have only a mathematical risk figure for guidance. The techniques which permit a preview of the genotype of the fetus with respect to a certain disorder constitute an exciting field of medicine. They are now available for use in routine pregnancies, but in high-risk situations the collaboration of the primary care physician and the medical geneticist can contribute significantly to the prevention of certain severely handicapping genetic disorders. The field promises to offer much more in the future as more of the inherited disorders are biochemically characterized and become subject to PD [2].

Of particular concern to the human geneticist are the effects of genetic abnormalities on development. To gain an understanding of these effects it is necessary to engage in a reciprocal process of using knowledge of normal developmental events to elucidate the mechanisms operative in abnormal situations and then of using what is learned about these abnormal situations to expand our understanding of the normal. Many developmental abnormalities are ascribable to mutations in genes coding for enzymes and structural proteins. Some of these even produce multiple malformation syndromes with dysmorphic features. Not only monogenic developmental abnormalities, but also abnormalities resulting from chromosome imbalance must ultimately be explicable in molecular terms. However, the major problem confronted by the investigator interested in the pathogenesis of any of the chromosome anomaly syndromes is to understand how the presence of an extra set of normal genes or the loss of one of two sets of genes has an adverse effect on development. Several molecular mechanisms for which limited precedents exist may be considered on theoretical grounds. Because of the difficulties in studying developmental disorders in man, a variety of experimental systems have been employed. Particularly useful has been the mouse, which provides models for both monogenic and aneuploidy produced abnormalities of development. All whole arm trisomies and monosomies of the mouse can be produced experimentally and of special interest is mouse trisomy 16 which has been developed as an animal model of human trisomy 21. The most direct approach to elucidating the genetic problems of human development involves not only the study of man himself but also of the appropriate experimental models in other species [3].

Chromosomal abnormalities account for a significant percentage of congenital malformations in the neonate. While some of the syndromes can be suspected on clinical grounds, the clinician will need to have a high index of suspicion based on the presence of multiple abnormalities that cannot be accounted for by other causes. Chromosome analysis should be performed promptly in these cases. Cultured lymphocytes are yet the standard preparation at present. However, new non-isotopic hybridization techniques are becoming available which allow analysis of interphase cells and these may become more widely used as clinical experience with them is gained. Prognosis can usually be better defined once the chromosome analysis is complete. The information acquired may also be used to provide risk estimates for chromosomal abnormalities in future pregnancies of the parents of the affected infant and for other relatives. Empathetic counseling of the parents and family must be provided once the diagnosis is known. It must take into account the knowledge the chromosome analysis provides, be respectful of the parent's need for support, and be accurate as to prognosis of the condition diagnosed. When DS has been diagnosed care must be taken to emphasize the positive aspects of the prognosis. When a chromosomal abnormality with an extremely poor prognosis is identified, support for withdrawal of medical intervention must be sensitively provided. The diagnosis and care of an infant with a chromosomal abnormality will challenge all of the pediatrician's diagnostic, therapeutic, and communication skills [4].

The sequencing of HSA21 and the use of models of DS in mice have allowed us to relate genes and sets of genes to the neuropathogenesis of this syndrome and to better understand its phenotype. Research in PD and screening aims to find methods to identify fetuses with DS and reduce or eliminate the need for amniocentesis. Other areas of active research and clinical interest include the association of DS with celiac disease (CD) and Alzheimer's disease (AD) and improved median age of death. Medical management of the syndrome requires an organised approach of assessment, monitoring, prevention, and vigilance. Improvements in quality of life of individuals with DS have resulted from improvements in medical care, identification and treatment of psychiatric disorders (such as depression, disruptive behaviour disorders, and autism), and early educational interventions with support in typical educational settings. Approaches and outcomes differ throughout the world [5].

Epidemiology and Pathogenesis

The prevalence of chromosomal abnormalities in clinically recognized early pregnancy loss is greater than 50%. Fetuses with aneuploidy account for 6-11% of all still births and neonatal deaths. Chromosome abnormalities which are compatible with life but cause considerable morbidity occur in 0.65% of newborns and structural chromosomal rearrangements that will eventually affect reproduction occur in 0.2% of newborns. Consequently, although it is not possible to identify all aneuploidies antenatally, screening and diagnostic programs to detect the most common autosomal trisomies in liveborn infants, including DS, are well established [6].

DS is the most commonly identified genetic form of MR and the leading cause of specific birth defects and medical conditions. Traditional epidemiological studies to determine the prevalence, cause, and clinical significance of the syndrome have been conducted over the last 100 years. DS has been estimated to occur in approximately 1 in 732 infants in the United States of America (USA), although there is some evidence that variability in prevalence of estimates exist among racial/ethnic groups. Progress has been made in characterizing the specific types of chromosome errors that lead to DS and in identifying associated factors that increase the risk of chromosome 21 malsegregation, i.e., advanced maternal age and recombination. Studies to examine the variability of the presence of specific DS-associated birth defects and medical conditions provide evidence for genetic and environmental modifiers [7].

Much attention has been focused on the influence of the decline in mean maternal age on the incidence of DS. Decline in incidence and unchanged incidences have been reported. For mothers over 35 years old, a rise in incidence has been found in recent years in some societies. Environmental factors or seasonal fluctation might cause this trend. Data from antenatal diagnosis show a 30% higher incidence of DS for age groups over 35 than population studies do. Late abortions of trisomic fetuses, a high perinatal mortality, and a small rise in incidence for higher maternal ages in recent years may account for this fact. With the growing tendency toward younger maternal age at childbirth, paternal factors also have to be considered. Between 10% and 30% paternal failures have been found by non-disjunction studies applying chromosomal variants. The rate of paternal failures may reflect environmental influences and young maternal age distribution. The mortality rate in DS is still high in early childhood, especially perinatally and in the first year of life. After the age of 1 year mortality is reduced considerably and more and more cases will survive early childhood and live to rather old ages [8].

Trisomy, occurring in at least 4% of pregnancies, is the most common chromosome abnormality in humans. The majority of trisomies are associated with single additional chromosome. The presence of an additional sex chromosome is often associated with physical, behavioral, and intellectual impairment. The presence of an additional autosome is even more serious, being associated with severe mental and physical retardation and frequently with death in infancy. The incidence of trisomy varies widely among different chromosomes. This variation appears to reflect a real difference in the frequency of the primary event leading to trisomy as well as in differential selection. Studies of parental origin have shown a first maternal meiotic division error to be the most frequent source of the additional chromosome, regardless of the chromosome involved or the maternal age. Although the magnitude of risk varies among chromosomes, increased maternal age is an important risk factor in trisomy. The incidence of trisomy 21 increases from 0.05% of livebirths at maternal age 20 years to over 3% of all livebirths at age 45 years. (Tab. I, Figure 1-2) The effect of maternal age is most pronounced in double trisomies. It has been hypothesized that the relationship between increasing maternal age and trisomy is due to a gradient in the fetal ovary that affects chiasma frequency. While the basis for the maternal age effect remains unknown, it is almost certainly due to factors acting at or before conception. Epidemiologic studies suggest that maternal irradiation exposure may also lead to trisomy; however, the effective dosage level and the relationship to maternal age remain unknown. No effect of oral contraceptives, spermicides, or fertility drugs on the incidence of trisomy has been documented to date. Understanding of the mechanisms by which trisomies are produced represents a major challenge for human cytogenetics [9].

In fact, the maternal age effect remains an enigma. Rationale has been presented for a compromised microcirculation hypothesis which explains the cause of non-disjunction and why its occurrence changes with maternal age from menarche to menopause. It takes into account two facts:

1) 95% of DS children receive their extra chromosome from their mother and in 80% or more of these the non-disjunction occurred in the first meiotic division which is completed in the ovary;
2) the ovarian follicle containing the primary oocyte has no internal circulation.

Table I. Trisomy 21 cases/1000 births in relation to mother's age

Mother's age (years)	Number of cases/1000 births	%
20-24	0.5	0.05
25-29	0.8	0.08
30-34	1.5	0.15
35-39	2.6	0.26
40-44	14.3	1.43
45 and more	34.2	3.42

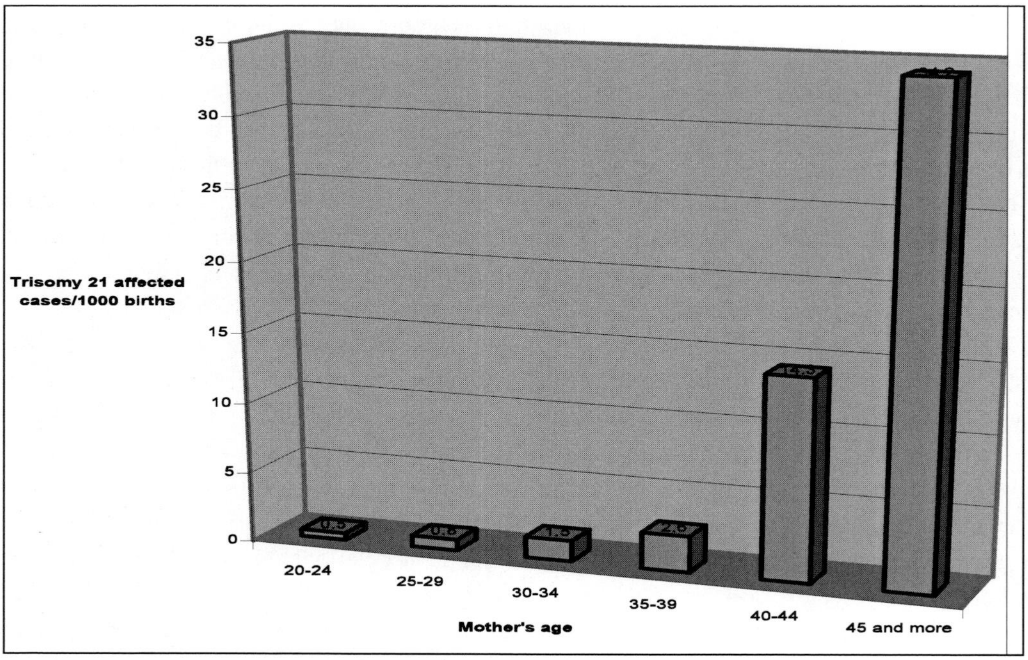

Figure 1. Trisomy 21 cases/1000 births in relation to mother's age.

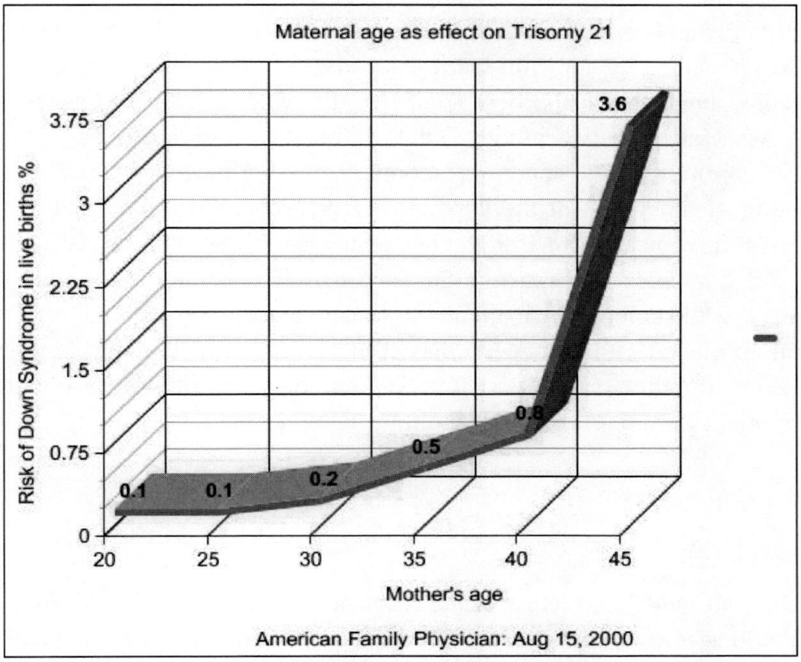

Figure 2. Trisomy 21 cases/100 births in relation to mother's age [10].

The hypothesis proposes that aneuploid oocytes arise from a concatenation of events. It begins with hormonal imbalance that causes a less-than-optimal microvasculature to develop around the maturing and mature follicles. The resulting decrease in the size of the perifollicular capillary bed reduces the volume of blood flow through the area, leading to an oxygen deficit and a concomitant increase inside the follicle of carbon dioxide (CO_2) and anaerobic products, such as lactic acid. This in turn causes a decrease in the intracellular pH of the oocyte which diminishes the size of the spindle with consequent displacement and non-disjunction of a chromosome. The compromised microcirculation hypothesis explains the occurrence of aneuploidy in primary and secondary oocytes, sperm precursor cells, tumor, and embryonic cells. It also explains why women of all reproductive ages may have a DS child [11].

Thus, a prevalent hypothesis concerning the cause of the rise in aneuploid conceptions with maternal age is that the changes that accompany normal ovarian aging increase the rate of meiotic errors in the oocyte. Biological aging of the ovary is accompanied by a decline in both the total oocyte pool and the number of antral follicles maturing per cycle, as well as changes in the levels of circulating reproductive hormones. The biological aging hypothesis predicts that aneuploidy rates should be higher in women with a prematurely reduced oocyte pool and that women with trisomic conceptions should show signs of earlier ovarian aging than women of the same chronological age without trisomic conceptions. Comprehensive studies of aneuploidy in groups of women with known causes of premature ovarian failure (POF) remain to be done, though anecdotal evidence does suggest increased rates of pregnancy loss and aneuploidy. Smoking, which is a well-documented cause of earlier ovarian aging, is not associated with an increase in aneuploid conceptions. Evidence from women with unilateral ovariectomies is inconsistent. Support for the biological aging hypothesis was provided by showing that menopause occurs about a year earlier in women with a trisomic spontaneous abortion compared to women with chromosomally normal conceptions. Associations between high follicle-stimulating hormone (FSH) and pregnancies with DS and chromosomally abnormal spontaneous abortions have also been reported. However, the most direct test of the hypothesis which compared antral follicle counts and hormonal levels in women with trisomic pregnancies and those with chromosomally normal pregnancies failed to find a difference in the expected direction. A prospective study of FSH levels in women with subfertility also failed to find an association with the rate of pregnancy loss. The bulk of evidence thus suggests that, if the processes of biological aging are indeed related to aneuploidy, they probably involve factors other than those measured by oocyte or antral follicle pool size and reproductive hormone levels [12].

Genetics

The analysis of the fine structure of the chromatids permits the identification of different regions on the long arm of chromosome 21. The preponderant role of the distal third of the long arm in the syndrome of trisomy 21 is now well established. Thus, trisomy of only band 21q22 results in a state identical to that caused by complete trisomy 21. If the trisomy involves only a part of band 21q22, the intensity of the symptoms is diminished, but the appearance of the patient is still reminiscent of DS. Monosomy for band 21q22 results in a pathologic condition in which the morphological anomalies are the inverse of those observed in trisomic patients. This syndrome, as a “contre-type” to trisomy 21, is lethal. Trisomy of the proximal long arm region of chromosome 21 (21q21 leads to 21q22) is not associated with malformations but is accompanied by MR. Monosomy of the same region results in a pathologic condition which does not have features of the contre-type of trisomy 21 (Figure 3a-3b) [13].

A major question in human genetics concerns the relationship between the extra chromosome material in DS and its effects. It is suggested that a generalized disruption of evolved genetic balance in cells of affected individuals leads to decreased developmental and physiological buffering against genetic and environmental forces. Examples of consequences in DS of this model of disruption of homeostasis are:

1) increased variance for metric traits;
2) amplified instability of developmental pathways;
3) reduced precision of physiological homeostatic controls;
4) generalized increased morbidity.

Evolution has selected for interacting systems. When this evolved balance is disrupted, as in autosomal aneuploidy, the organism is generally disrupted. The model emphasizes the role of environment in producing much of the DS phenotype. Traits less buffered than others in the general population are the ones most disturbed in DS and account for much of the DS phenotype [14].

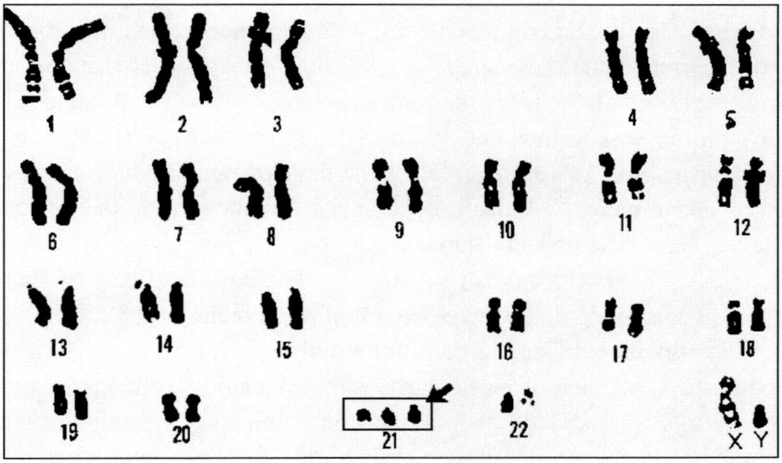

Figure 3a. Trisomy 21 karyotype.

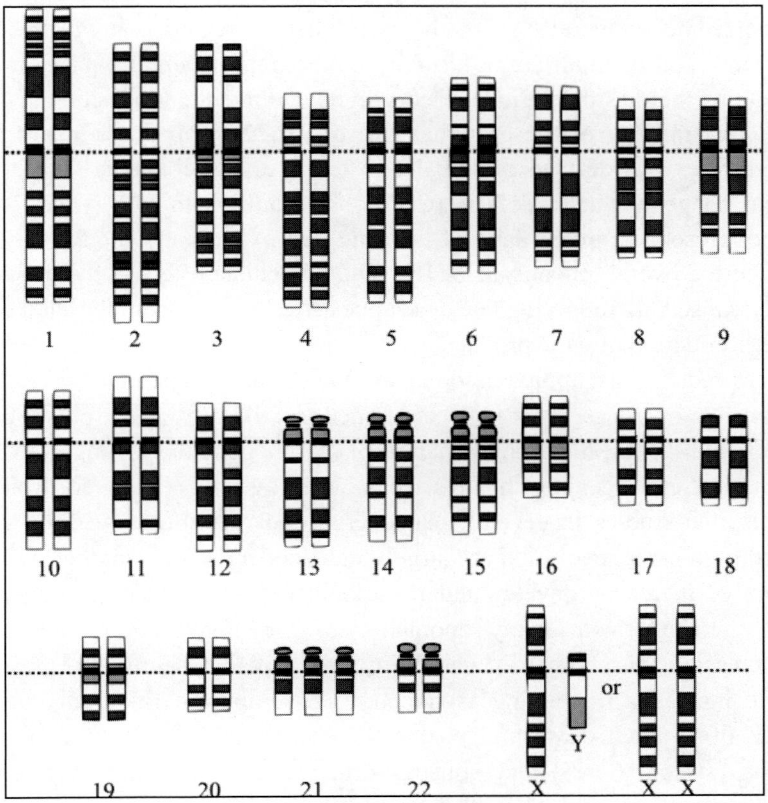

Figure 3b. Trisomy 21 karyotype.

Several hypotheses have been proposed to explain the mechanisms by which aneuploidy (especially trisomy) disrupts development. These mechanisms include specific gene dosage effects, generalized disruption of genetic homeostasis, and the influence of the parental origin of the duplicated chromosome. The availability of specific chromosomal rearrangements in mice, coupled with selective breeding schemes, permits generation of aneuploidy of specific chromosomes or chromosomal segments on controlled genetic backgrounds, thus enabling the systematic study of the causes and consequences of defined aneuploidy. Genetic homology between mouse chromosome 16 and HSA21 has led investigators to suggest that analogous mechanisms will be responsible for the developmental abnormalities produced in these respective aneuploidies. Analysis of trisomy 16 mice from the organismal to the subcellular level has revealed a number of phenotypic characteristics (particularly neurobiologic ones) shared with human trisomy 21. The dosage effects of shared genes (or their products) may contribute to the development of these features [15].

Review of the clinical cytogenetic literature provides compelling evidence for a specific relationship between imbalance of particular chromosomes or chromosomal regions and the appearance of defined patterns of phenotypic abnormalities. In many instances, detailed phenotypic mapping has made it possible to assign portions of a phenotype to relatively small chromosome segments, which are sometimes referred to as "critical regions" (CR). However, since these regions are usually defined by a subset of the phenotypic manifestations of an aneuploidy syndrome – generally those anomalies that are regarded as most characteristic or readily observable – it is important not to fall into the trap of thinking that it is imbalance of only these regions that has deleterious effects on development and function. Thus, in DS the presence of an extra copy of the proximal part of 21q22.3 appears to result in the typical physical phenotype – as defined principally in terms of the characteristic facial and hand anomalies and congenital heart defects (CHD) – in addition to MR. Therefore, it remains likely that loci present on many parts of the long arm of chromosome 21 play a role in the development of the overall phenotype of DS. The immediate effect at the molecular level of an aneuploidy-caused alteration in gene dose appears to be a non-compensated commensurate change in the production of gene products [16].

However, a reductionist approach to explain the DS phenotype in a "linear" manner from the DNA sequence of the segment will be doomed to failure from the outset because of the open, complex, non-linear, hierarchical nature of morphogenetic systems. Neo-Darwinism is under strong attack; most genetic changes accumulated over time may very well be of neutral effect, and detailed studies in several related groups of vertebrate species has shown that molecular and organismal evolution are largely independent of one another. DS impresses us as a paradigm of increased developmental variability due to a deceleration of the rate of development (neoteny) with many anomalies of incomplete morphogenesis (vestigia), atavisms, increased morphometric variability with many decreased means, increased variances, and increased fluctuating asymmetry. These abnormalities, together with highly increased risk of prenatal death and postnatal morbidity, impaired growth, and abnormal central nervous system (CNS) and gonadal structure and function characteristic of most aneuploidy syndromes, suggest to us that the pathogenesis of DS is best viewed in terms of the mechanisms of speciation. Transgenic experiment involving sequential or overlapping pieces of "the consensus segment" on distal 21q22.1-22.3 may help decide to what extent the DS phenotype can be resolved into the additive effect of several pleiotropic oligogenes with epistatic interaction or the indirect secondary "mass" effect of a specific segment of 21q with epistatic interaction involving multiple loci on 21q and other chromosomes [17].

As we told before, there are several evidences that DS is a gene dosage disease. This means that overproduction of certain proteins, encoded by normal genes on the extra chromosome, distorts the delicate balance of some biochemical pathways which are important for proper development and function of the organs affected in DS. It has been shown that only the distal segment of the long arm of chromosome 21 is involved in the pathogenesis of DS. Great efforts to define this "DS specific" segment have been made with the aim to find the "DS responsible" genes. It is suggested that as few as 10-20 genes might be responsible for the DS phenotype. Although several genes have been mapped on chromosome 21, not one single feature of DS has been proved to be an effect of any single gene [18].

Parental age is the most important etiological factor in trisomy formation in humans. Cytogenetic studies on germ cells imply that:

1) 2-4% sperms are aneuploid and 8.6% oocytes from in vitro fertilization (IVF) are hyperploid;
2) a paternal age effect may exist;
3) oocytes of aged women contain precociously separated chromatids in metaphase II.

Trisomy data suggest that most aneuploidy is generated during meiosis I of oogenesis and is maternal age-dependent. Trisomy of individual chromosomes may remain low, linearly rise, or exponentially increase with advanced maternal age. Maternal age related trisomies involve achiasmatic and normochiasmate chromosomes and chromosomes with disturbed recombination and distally located chiasmata. One model relates to altered cell cycle and protein phosphorylation in oocytes of aged mammals and accounts for most of the observed data in humans and in experimental studies. Aneuploidy may thus involve a predetermined component but is possibly also influenced by extrinsic factors reducing oocyte quality or depleting the oocyte pool precociously [19].

Since the early 1970s numerous attempts have been made to learn whether specific segments of chromosome 21, when triplicated, are responsible for the clinical condition DS. Studies were reported in which positive or negative clinical diagnoses of DS were made in the presence of partial trisomy of one or another segment of the chromosome. The distal half of the long arm of 21 (21q22) possesses most of the gene transcribing sites of the chromosome. It was this region that was thought to contain loci essential to production of the clinical syndrome. Subsequent studies identified subregions of this band as "minimal" or "critical" sites necessary and sufficient to produce the clinical condition. A major problem with these assignments was that different investigators defined "different critical/minimal regions". In 1994 evidence was presented in which regions of most of the long arm of chromosome 21 were said to contribute to the DS phenotype. Soon after, a report described a child with DS and partial tetrasomy of the short arm and proximal long arm of 21, segments clearly distinct from the previously identified critical areas. Thus, the clinical diagnosis of DS can be made in the presence of partial aneuploidy of nearly all segments of chromosome 21. It must be concluded that no evidence exists that individual loci on 21 are singularly responsible for specific phenotypic abnormalities in DS. Without exception, each of the clinical findings associated with DS is a multifactorial trait. The analysis of each trait in DS should thus be similar to analyses of the same traits in the general population with a focus on the way aneuploidy affects expression of multifactorial characteristics [20].

Two hypotheses exist to explain the DS phenotype. The "gene dosage effect" hypothesis states that the phenotype is a direct result of the cumulative effect of the imbalance of the individual genes located on the triplicated chromosome or chromosome region. In a nut shell the phenotype results directly from the overexpression of specific chromosome 21 genes.The "amplified developmental instability" hypothesis contends that most manifestations of DS may be interpreted as the results of a non-specific disturbance of chromosome balance, resulting in a disruption of homeostasis. This hypothesis was proposed in an attempt to explain the similarities between the phenotypes of different aneuploid states and the observation that all of the phenotypic traits in DS are also seen in the general population but at lower frequency, with less severity and usually only present as a single trait [21].

Recently genetic mapping studies of trisomy 21 families have led to the identification of the first molecular correlate of human non-disjunction; i.e., altered levels and positioning of meiotic recombinational events. Specifically, increases in 0 exchange events or in distal-only or pericentromeric exchanges are significantly increased in trisomy 21-generating meioses. These observations have led to the idea that chromosome 21 non-disjunction requires "two hits": first, the establishment in prophase I of a "vulnerable" bivalent and second, abnormal processing of the bivalent at metaphase I or II [22].

In recent years mutations in mitochondrial DNA (mtDNA) have been associated with a growing number of disorders, including those associated with spontaneous deletions of mtDNA (deltamtDNAs). Intriguingly, these pathogenic deltamtDNAs, which are present at extremely high levels in certain patients, are also present at extremely low levels (detectable only by polymerase chain reaction [PCR]) in normal individuals. The proportion of such deltamtDNAs in normal muscle is a function of age; the shape of this curve is exponential, with the accelerating part of the curve beginning at approximately 30-40 years. As well as muscle and brain, a similar time-dependent accumulation of deltamtDNAs also occurs in normal oocytes. Since deltamtDNAs are functionally inactive, an accumulation of such aberrant genomes could eventually compromise ATP-dependent energy utilization in these cells. Furthermore, these deficiencies would also affect the function of the somatic follicular cells that surround, and secrete important paracrine factors to, the oocyte. If there is indeed an age-associated relationship between deltamtDNAs and oocyte age, perhaps errors in meiosis (which is almost certainly an energy, and ATP, dependent process) are related to mutations in mtDNA (primarily deletions but perhaps point mutations as well) in oocytes and/or the surrounding somatic cells, which result in deficiencies in both mitochondrial function in general and oxidative energy metabolism in particular. This hypothesis would explain many of the non-Mendelian features associated with maternal age-related trisomies, e.g. DS [23].

The entire DNA sequence for human chromosome 21 is now complete and it is predicted to contain only about 225 genes, which is approximately three-fold fewer than the number initially predicted almost 20 years ago. Although many of the phenotypic traits show large individual variation, neuromotor dysfunction and cognitive and language impairment are observed in virtually all individuals. Currently there are no efficacious biomedical treatments for these CNS-associated impairments. To develop novel therapeutic strategies the effects of gene dosage imbalance need to be understood within the framework of those critical biological events that regulate brain organization and function [24].

Clinics

While certain external anomalies are specific and almost constant features in DS, internal anomalies seem to be more variable in terms of frequency and severity. They may affect any organ system and are more often of minor clinical significance. However, severe malformations may occur. When they affect the cardiovascular system, postnatal survival is impaired, which is responsible for a distinctly higher incidence of cardiac and other malformations in younger children or neonates with DS. Fetuses with trisomy 21 at midterm pregnancy show even more frequent manifestation of developmental disorders suggesting an increased spontaneous abortion rate in the second half of pregnancy. The analysis of malformations and minor anomalies in DS compared to those of other chromosomal aberrations shows no absolute specificity but a tendency for certain developmental disturbances. These are characterized not so much by the organ system involved but much more by the time in which the disturbance of a developmental process becomes evident, thus influencing type and localization of an anomaly [25].

In past decades most individuals with DS were usually not afforded adequate medical care. Many children with DS were institutionalized and they were often deprived of all but the most elementary medical services. Fortunately there have been major improvements in the health care provision during the past 40 years. Professionals who are providing services to persons with DS need to be aware of those clinical conditions that are more often observed in this population. Certain congenital anomalies (congenital cataracts, anomalies of the gastrointestinal [GI] tract, and CHD) often require immediate attention, as some of them may be life threatening. During the subsequent childhood years a number of clinical conditions and disorders such as infectious diseases, increased nutritional intake, periodontitis, seizure disorders, sleep apnea, visual impairment, audiologic deficits, thyroid dysfunction, and skeletal problems usually occur at a higher prevalence. During adolescence specific aspects of maturation and certain health issues (skin infections, thyroid disorders, increased weight gain, and others) as well as mental health concerns need to be taken into consideration. Similar concerns may also be observed during adulthood which in addition is often marked by accelerated aging and the threat of AD in some persons with DS. Special attention needs to be paid to these disorders and conditions during the lifetime of a person with DS. Appropriate medical care should be provided to and no form of treatment should be withheld from a person with DS that would be given unhesitatingly to an individual without this chromosome disorder [26].

The family physician's holistic approach to patients forms the basis of good health care for adults with DS. Patients with DS are likely to have a variety of illnesses including diabetes, depression, and obsessive-compulsive disorder. In addition to routine health screening, patients with DS should be screened for signs and symptoms of spinal cord compression and dementia. Patients with DS may have an unusual presentation of an ordinary illness or condition and behavior changes or a loss of function may be the only indication of medical illnesses. Plans for long-term living arrangements, estate planning, and custody arrangements should be discussed with the parents or guardians. Because of improvements in health care and better education and because more people with this condition are being raised at home, most adults with DS can expect to function well enough to live in a group home and hold a meaningful job [27].

As the child with DS enters the second decade of life some of the original medical issues such as cardiac, vision, and hearing problems, continue to concern parents. Dermatologic and pediatric problems may become particularly bothersome. Although the child may be doing well, monitoring for thyroid and CD continues to be needed. Continued vigilance is needed for arthritis, diabetes, leukemia, neck subluxation, and seizures. Prevention and treatment of dental and obesity problems are important. Psychiatric and behavioral problems may compromise the adolescent's opportunities. Sexuality and the associated issues of abuse, pregnancy, and menstrual hygiene must be addressed [28].

Oncology

Solid tumors are poorly understood in DS. Cancers are in excess in this condition because of the 20-fold excess of leukemias, whereas malignant solid tumors seem to be globally underrepresented as compared with those in the general population. However, among these tumors some are in excess: lymphomas, gonadal and extragonadal germ cell tumors, and possibly retinoblastomas and pancreatic and bone tumors. Neoplasms in excess are seen earlier, sometimes in fetal life (leukemias and testicular germ cell tumors) or neonatally (leukemias and lymphoma) and affect mainly male subjects. There seems to exist an excess of rare karyotypes. Other tumors are underrepresented, particularly neuroblastomas and nephroblastomas, in young children, and perhaps common epithelial tumors in adults. These observations suggest that DS has a particular tumor profile with some tissues more affected by malignant diseases (hematopoietic tissue and germ cells) and others that seem to be protected (central and peripheral nervous system, renal tissue, and epithelial tissues). The mechanism is mainly genetic but differences in exposure to exogenous agents compared with the general population must be kept in mind. These findings are of interest for the management of these patients and early detection of cancers. Better knowledge of this tumor profile could help us to understand the mechanisms of carcinogenesis and should be compared to the current knowledge of genes on chromosome 21 [29].

According to the currently prevailing perception sporadic cancer arises as a result of somatic mutations in a cell that lead to its uncontrolled proliferation. It is generally accepted that somatic mutations occur randomly and that they are generally either "spontaneous" or due to various external agents (physical or chemical carcinogens). Constitutional genetic conditions, which modify cancer risk, may become instrumental in opening new concepts in carcinogenesis. Evidence gathered from DS individuals has challenged the above perceived explanation since somatic mutations in these patients markedly differ from those arisen in the general population and do not seem to occur at random. There is no global increase or decrease of somatic mutations in all genes in DS. Instead, specific mutations have been detected on particular loci depending on the tissue type and the age of the DS person. In the context of constitutional trisomy 21 where cancer have a very particular and striking distribution, biochemical, physiological, and architectural imbalances in specific tissues may be responsible for a vulnerable state leading to carcinogenesis. Conversely, in tissues of DS patients which seem resistant to cancer the proliferative and maturation state of the cells would lead to a refractory state of neoplastic transformation. Experimentally, the proliferation of tumor cells in extracellular matrix produced by trisomic 21 fibroblasts appears to be inhibited when compared to that of those placed on an extracellular matrix produced by euploid fibroblasts. These observations challenge the current somatic mutation theory of carcinogenesis and strongly suggest instead a critical role of cells and tissues in the microenvironment where carcinogenesis occurs [30].

Hematology and Immunology

Hematologic abnormalities are common in individuals with DS. Increased erythrocyte mean corpuscular volume (MCV) is frequently found among DS infants and remains elevated throughout life in 2/3 of patients, making interpretation of red cell indices for diagnosis of nutritional anemias or bone marrow failure disorders more challenging. Transient leukemoid disorders (TMD) associated with pancytopenia, hepatosplenomegaly, and circulating immature white blood cells (WBCs), is found almost exclusively in DS infants with an incidence of approximately 10%. In most cases TMD regresses spontaneously within the first 3 months of life, but in some children it can be life threatening or even fatal. Despite the high rate of spontaneous regression, TMD can be a preleukemic disorder in 20-30% of children with DS. The types of malignancy, response to therapy, and clinical outcome in children with DS are also unique. There is an increased risk of leukemia with an equal incidence of lymphoid (LL) and myeloid leukaemia (ML). Acute megakaryoblastic leukemia (AMKL) subtype is the most common form of AML in this setting, and is uncommon in children without DS. Somatic mutations of the gene encoding the hematopoetic growth factor (HGF) GATA1 have been shown to be specific for TMD and AMKL in children with DS. Myelodysplastic syndrome can precede AML. Children with DS and leukemia are more sensitive to some chemotherapeutic agents such as methotrexate (MTX) than other children which requires careful monitoring for toxicity. Although the risk for leukemia is higher in individuals with DS, these patients have a lower risk of developing solid tumors with the exception of germ cell tumors and perhaps retinoblastoma and lymphoma [31].

Over the past decade a series of clinical reports have described the experience of DS children treated for AML. Whereas prior to the first reports in the early 1980s it was felt that DS children with AML had poor outcomes, these clinical trials concluded that DS had a better outcome than non-DS children with AML. With these recent reports it is clear that DS children have a better outcome utilizing less intensive chemotherapy regimens. They also tolerate the more intensive regimens less well than the non-DS children. Regimens of varying intensity have all had similar outcomes. In general the remission rates are approximately 90% with event-free survival (EFS) approximating 70-80%. Most recently the clinical trials have been large enough to explore prognostic factors specifically in the DS children. This has identified that the younger DS children fair significantly better than the older children. AML in DS is unique. The significantly better outcomes for DS children likely represents a combination of the unique AML seen in DS children and the heightened sensitivity to cytosine arabinoside (araC) that DS-AML cells have. Future trials should focus on age-stratified approaches that exploit the greater sensitivity of DS-AML to araC [32].

Subjects with DS have a high mortality due to infections and a high risk of developing malignancies. These observations, together with the demonstration of a frequent occurrence of hepatitis B antigen (HBsAg) carrier state and of autoantibodies, have prompted investigations of the immune function in DS. Thymic morphological and functional abnormalities have been demonstrated. Peripheral blood mononuclear cells of DS subjects have been shown to include a high number of T-lymphocytes with low avidity for sheep erythrocytes and a very high percentage of cells with a natural killer (NK) phenotype. However, NK activity is low in DS. Production of some important cytokines such as interleukin-2 (IL-2) is depressed, thus contributing to T-cell derangement. Abnormalities of the B-cell compartment were also demonstrated with a tendency towards high immunoglobulin G (IgG) and low IgM serum levels. Controversial results have been obtained with regard to antigen-specific antibody response. Also phagocytes of DS subjects display some characteristic functional impairments with low chemotactic ability and reduced production of oxygen radicals. Despite the clearly established and rather detailed evidence of immune derangements, therapeutic trials have been anecdotal and resulted in marginal effects. Hepatitis B virus (HBV) vaccination is highly advisable in DS because of the high risk of becoming chronic HBV carriers once infected [33].

Therefore, DS may be considered as a model of precocious, abnormal ageing of the thymus-dependent system in man. In DS children less than 6 years of age the levels of serum Ig do not differ from healthy controls, but after that age considerable hyper-IgG and -IgA are found. Furthermore, high levels of IgG1 and IgG3 have been found, whereas a progressive decline of IgG2 and IgG4 with age has been observed. The frequency of HBV carriers even in the youngest age group is much higher among DS children. It has been reported that an IgG response is detectable in 75% of controls after HBsAg vaccination as compared to the 16.6% of DS patients. The presence of autoantibodies against human thyroglobulin shows a positive association with HBsAg carriers, but only in the oldest DS subjects. Natural antibodies against intestinal antigens are low, while in the presence of cow's milk abnormally high titres against casein and beta-lactoglobulin were present. High levels of IgG antibodies against gliadin have been observed. In spite of a normal percentage of CD3- and CD2-positive lymphocytes, a high proportion of cells express low-avidity receptors for sheep erythrocytes. Although the proportion of CD4+ T-lymphocyte helper-cells is normal, a marked imbalance in the CD4+ subpopulations has been documented. The percentage of suppressor-cytotoxic CD8+ lymphocytes is markedly increased. The responses to phytohemagglutinin and concanavalin A are within the normal range in the first decade of life and decline progressively thereafter. A recent study reported defective proliferative response to allo-mixed lymphocyte culture with decreased expression of the membrane CD25, low secretion of IL-2 in the supernatant, and depressed allo-specific cytotoxic activity [34].

Neurology

The brain of a child with DS develops differently from a normal one, attaining a form reduced in size and altered in configuration. Directly related to MR are neuronal modifications manifest as alterations of cortical lamination, reduced dendritic ramifications, and diminished synaptic formation. However, selected cholinergic marker enzymes such as choline acetyl transferase and acetyl cholinesterase have shown no alterations in young children with DS. The pace of the neuronal transformations is related to stage of maturation. With early growth and development the normal dendritic tree continuously expands. In DS at 4 months of age the neurons show a relatively expanded dendritic tree, but during the first year the dendrites stop growing and become atrophic relative to control neurons. Accompanying these neuronal irregularities are subtle alterations of other cell types: astrocyte, oligodendrogliocyte, microglia, and endothelial cell. In early infancy one of the astrocytic markers, GFAP, is not altered but there is greater expression of S-100 protein in the temporal lobe in DS. Oligodendrogliocyte dysfunction is reflected in delayed myelination in pathways of frontal and temporal lobes. Microglia appear more prominent in DS. A minority of children with DS have vascular dysplasias and focal calcification of basal ganglia. In young children expression of beta-amyloid in DS is no different than in normal children but disappears after age two, only to reappear in adults. As some of these studies suggest, the identification of genes on chromosome 21 and the determination of the gene product allow the production of specific antibodies and, through immunohistochemical techniques, the identification of the expression of these proteins in both normal development and DS. Specifically, the localization and appearance in development of proteins such as the beta-subunit of S-100, beta-amyloid (A4 protein), superoxide dismutase (SOD), and OK-2 are providing the means for better understanding the morphogenesis of the cellular and eventually molecular basis for MR in DS [35].

DS brain is characterized by a reduced cerebellar volume and number of granular cells, defective cortical lamination and reduced cortical neurons, malformed dendritic trees and spines, and abnormal synapses. These neurological alterations, also found in trisomic mouse models, result from gene-dosage effects of HSA21 on the expression of critical developmental genes. HSA21 sequencing, mouse ortholog gene identification, and DS mouse model generation lead to determine HSA21 gene functions and the effects of protein-dosage alterations in neurodevelopmental and metabolic pathways in DS individuals. Trisomic brain transcriptome of DS patients and trisomic mouse models identified some molecular changes determined by gene-overdosage and associated dysregulation of some disomic gene expression in DS brains. These transcriptional variations cause developmental alterations in neural patterning and signal transduction pathways that may lead to defective neuronal circuits responsible for the pathogenesis of MR in DS. Recently, the first altered molecular pathway responsible of some DS phenotypes, including neurological and cognitive disorders has been identified. In this pathway two critical HSA21 genes (DYRK1A and DSCR1) act synergistically to control the phosphorylation levels of NFATc and NFATc-regulated gene expression. Interestingly, the NFATc mice show neurological dysfunctions similar to those seen in DS patients and trisomic mouse models. Treatment of DS mouse models with

GABA(A) antagonists allows post-drug rescue of cognitive defects, indicating a hopeful direction in clinical therapies for MR in children with DS [36].

Dermatology

Owing to advances in medical care and changes in attitude, the median age of death in this population has increased to 49 years and the life expectancy of a 1-year-old person with DS today is more than 60 years and is likely to improve. With the increase in the number of individuals with DS in the population and an increased life span, dermatologists are more likely to encounter the wide spectrum of dermatological disorders that occurs in these patients. Furthermore, new reports of possible associations are frequent in the literature. DS is associated with rare dermatological disorders and increased frequency of some common dermatoses [37].

The cutaneous manifestations of DS are numerous, yet they seldom receive appropriate attention. DS is associated with an increased incidence of numerous dermatological conditions, some of which may be related to an immunological deficiency. Along with the importance of understanding the physical and psychosocial aspects of DS, an appreciation of the dermatological manifestations of this condition is integral to comprehensive medical care [38].

Ophthalmology

The isolated occurrence of any one of the most of the protean systemic and ocular features of DS is not specific to the disorder. The associated occurrence of several of these features, however, has distinguished affected individuals as having a distinct entity for nearly 150 years. Associated ocular disorders can significantly affect the quality of life of individuals with DS. As more children with DS live into adulthood, the ophthalmologist will play an increasing role in allowing them to lead productive and meaningful lives [39].

Otolaryngology

Otolaryngologic or ear, nose, and throat (ENT) problems are common in children with DS. This includes problems with chronic ear infections and chronic middle ear effusions with associated hearing loss, airway obstruction, and sleep apnea, as well as problems with chronic rhinitis and sinusitis. As the care of children with DS has become more consistent and proactive, outcomes from the treatment of these ENT manifestations have improved. Aggressive interventions, both medical and surgical, have led to a decreased incidence of hearing loss, good control of the chronic rhinitis, and a better awareness of the incidence of sleep apnea and sleep-disordered breathing in individuals with DS. In addition, many of these ENT problems require surgical interventions and there are special anesthesia considerations that need to be addressed in children with DS. These include subglottic stenosis, post-operative airway obstruction, and cervical spine concerns [40].

In fact, the DS patient has clear anatomic differences in the head and neck region when compared with the general population. These anomalies include a flat occiput, oblique palpebral fissures, epicanthal folds, speckled irides, a protruding tongue, prominent malformed ears, and a flat nasal bridge. Congenital otologic anomalies and acquired conditions such as otitis media are also more frequently observed in the DS population. The DS patient is predisposed to obstructive sleep apnea and the diagnosis of sleep apnea in DS patients is more likely to be delayed. A child with DS who has a narrowed nasopharynx, large tongue, and a subglottis which is smaller than normal must be given special consideration at the time of intubation. Such a patient requires an endotracheal tube two sizes smaller than the standard size appropriate for the patient's age. The child should also be suspected of having and be evaluated for obstructive sleep apnea, to ensure that appropriate precautions are taken in the perioperative period. Finally, any DS patient undergoing preoperative evaluation for a general anesthetic should have a careful assessment of the cervical spine to avoid dislocation or spinal cord injury. Hearing loss may be suspected in any congenital syndrome. In DS there is a clearly increased incidence of congenital temporal bone anomalies, external auditory canal stenosis, and otitis media. All DS patients should undergo hearing assessment in the neonatal period with follow-up as appropriate. Aggressive treatment of conductive hearing loss and early amplification may be necessary to maximize speech and language development [41].

Pneumology

Involvement of the lungs by a characteristic form of subpleural cystic disease is well described in the pathology literature. The imaging characteristics of changes caused by this disease have not been described in detail in the radiology literature, possibly because they are not well appreciated on plain chest radiographs [42].

Cardiology

The frequency of CHD in children with DS is high and ranges between 40% and 50% of cases. It was evident for many years that patients with trisomy 21 present certain CHD (atrioventricular canal, ventricular septal defect, tetralogy of Fallot) and seem to be "protected" from others (situs inversus and situs ambiguus, ventricular inversion, transposition of the great arteries). Recent observations also suggest that left-sided obstructive lesions and the muscular ventricular septal defect are very rare. The role of a suspected "increased adhesiveness of trisomy 21 cells" and of the anomalies of neural crest needs to be investigated. The interaction between studies of clinicians and basic research will improve the knowledge of these genetically determined heart defects [43].

If there is significant concern about a current pregnancy, a fetal echocardiogram can provide important information. The presence of a cardiac defect in and of itself constitutes a major birth defect and should stimulate the search for other problems. When other anomalies are found and an identifiable syndrome is present, then care of the infant is dictated by the heart defect along with other features of the syndrome. Of note, when a syndrome that frequently has a heart defect in its spectrum of anomalies is identified it is quite reasonable to perform a thorough cardiovascular evaluation to determine whether a cardiac defect is present. All children with DS should have a thorough cardiac evaluation early in life, including a cardiac ultrasound. Knowledge about the genetics and etiology of cardiac defects is changing yearly. It is expected that more information will be available for physicians to pass on to the families of children born with CHD [44].

Orthopedics

Orthopedic manifestations occur frequently. Approximately 20% of all patients with DS experience orthopedic problems; most are related to hypotonia, joint hypermobility, and ligamentous laxity. Atlanto-occipital and atlanto-axial hypermobility, as well as bony anomalies of the cervical spine, can produce atlanto-occipital and cervical instability. Methods of screening for this instability, particularly with regard to participation in sports, are a subject of controversy. Scoliosis, hip instability, slipped capital femoral epiphysis, patellar instability, and foot deformities are other musculoskeletal conditions found in patients with DS that can be challenging for the orthopedic surgeon to treat [45].

Upper cervical spine instability has the most potential for morbidity and, consequently, requires close monitoring. Other conditions such as scoliosis, hip instability, patellar instability and foot problems can cause disability if left untreated. In some of these conditions early diagnosis can prevent severe disability. Surgical intervention in children with DS has a high risk of complications, particularly infection and wound healing problems. Careful anesthetic airway management is needed because of the associated risk of cervical spine instability [46].

Odontology

DS craniofacial features include midfacial hypoplasia with a resultant flattened face, ocular hypotelorism, and mandibular prognathism. The universal characteristic of the DS face is the upward slanting of the palpebral fissures and epicanthic folds (Figure 4). Dental features include tooth size reduction, hypodontia, reduced root lengths, changes in tooth shape, and excessive tooth wear [47].

Cross-sectional as well as longitudinal studies indicate that the prevalence of periodontal disease in persons with DS under the age of 30 years is extremely high. It is even noted in the deciduous dentition. The progression of the disease is rapid, especially in the younger age groups. Severe periodontal breakdown with horizontal bone loss is often present in the lower anteriors. The large amount of plaque and calculus alone cannot explain the severity of periodontal disease in DS persons.

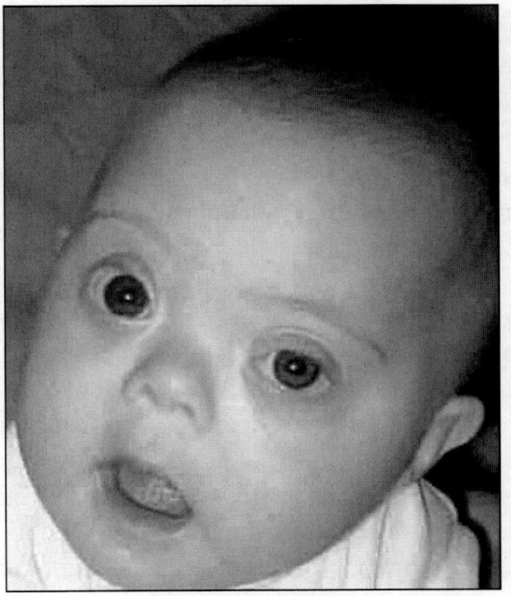

Figure 4. Typical facial trisomy 21 features (HealthNews-Stat).

Abnormal capillary morphology, disorders in connective tissue and anatomical aspects of teeth are some of those considered to be of influence. Alteration in immunological response may also play a role in the progression of the disease process. Disorders in the polymorphonuclear leucocyte function and monocyte function have been reported in persons with DS. T-cell functioning declines after the first 10 years of life. T-cell lymphocyte counts are low and an immature subset of T-lymphocytes is present. This latter effect occurs especially in institutions where the immunological system is under stress. The altered immune response, together with higher calculus scores, may explain the difference in severity of periodontal disease between institutionalized DS children and those living at home [48].

Gastroenterology

DS is recognized as one of the most common predisposing conditions for a group of serious GI anomalies. Up to 77% of DS children have associated GI abnormalities, which may be structural or functional in nature. Functional disturbances may in turn affect the outcome of corrective surgical procedures, prompting to caution. Tracheo-esophageal fistula, duodenal obstruction with or without pyloric stenosis, annular pancreas, imperforate anus, and Hirschsprung's disease (HSCR) are the most prevalent lesions. Understanding of the morphogenetic mechanisms responsible for this range of abnormalities is far from clear, as none of the lesions is specific to the trisomic state and the underlying defects (i.e., failure of foregut canalization, failure of neural crest cell migration into the myenteric and submucosal plexuses or malformation of the anterior abdominal wall, etc.) are encountered in unaffected infants. Segregation analysis of inheritance patterns points to multi-factorial traits and random genetic action provide appropriate models (to a certain extent) for describing the observations. Furthermore, intestinal anomalies can be found in many other genetic disorders with recent evidence suggesting the presence of GI developmental regulatory genes on chromosome 13q. A possible common pathway to the observed anomalies might be enhanced epithelial adhesiveness, as demonstrated in vitro experiments with fibroblasts. Molecular genetic techniques applied to the smallest human autosome could provide the needed insight into the ultimate mechanisms determining morphogenesis. The development of a murine model is a promising tool for the successful approach to these extraordinarily complex questions [49].

It is becoming clear that the processes affecting the enteric nervous system (ENS) in DS not only affect the micro-anatomy but also nerve function and there is some histological evidence of ENS variations in both human and DS animal models. This suggests that developmental disorders of the ENS are probably fundamental to the functional GI disturbances encountered in patients with DS. The anomalous brain development, function, and resulting intellectual impairment associated with DS appears to result from the genetic imbalance created by the trisomy of chromosome 21. The possible links between the brain, GI, and ENS involvement are not as yet entirely clear. Neurotropic factors affecting brain development during embryogenesis are probably interlinked with ENS development, but the precise mechanism of how this occurs has yet to be established. Functional motor disturbances of the esophagus and colon are not uncommon and may be congenital or acquired in nature. The most prominent of these include esophageal dysmotility syndromes (e.g., achalasia, gastroesophageal reflux, dysphagia) as well as a higher incidence of chronic constipation and HSCR (2-15%) occurring in association with DS. Chromosome 21 itself is thought to be the site of a modifier gene for HSCR. Recently identified candidate genetic mechanisms provide unique insights into the genetic background of the neurological and cognitive disorders associated with DS. Although the role of the triplicated chromosome 21 and genetic dosage remain important, the additional role of other chromosome 21 genes in the etiology of ENS developmental anomalies remains undetermined and requires ongoing research [50].

Nephrology and Urology

Renal and urological anomalies in DS have received little attention compared with the nephrourological findings described in other chromosomal abnormalities. Renal hypoplasia, hydroureteronephrosis, ureterovesical and ureteropelvic junction obstruction, and glomerular microcysts have been associated with DS. Children with DS may have an increased risk for developing posterior urethral valves and obstructive uropathy. Furthermore, they may also develop chronic renal failure secondary to posterior urethral valves. Therefore, infants with DS should be screened with ultrasonography for renal and urological abnormalities early in life and, if abnormal, a contrast voiding cystourethrogram should be performed to rule out posterior urethral valves or other bladder or urethral abnormalities [51].

Decreased creatinine clearance has also been noted. Developmental anomalies such as megaureter and vesicoureteral reflux have been reported. Dysfunctional voiding and urinary retention have been found in these patients. Hypospadias has also been seen. The testicular abnormalities most frequently reported are cryptorchidism, testicular cancer, and infertility. Improved understanding and identification of the various urological anomalies associated with DS will aid in the care of these patients. In addition, an awareness of perioperative issues will further facilitate a smooth clinical course [52].

Anesthesiology

In the course of various studies on pain transmission in Down patients the reduced tolerance of pain and the incapacity to give a qualitative and quantitative description emerged in a powerful way. All of these aspects cause difficulty in evaluating pain. This is linked to several learning difficulties. However, it cannot be excluded that in these anomalies of pain perception both the anatomical and the neurotransmitter alteration, typical of this syndrome, may hold a certain importance. This fact may have important clinical repercussions that could affect the choice of therapeutic and rehabilitative schemes for treatment of pathologies in which pain is the dominant symptom, such as postoperative pain. It could influence research on analgesics that are more suitable for these patients, the evaluation of the depth of analgesia during surgical operation, and ultimately absence of obvious pain manifestations [53].

During preoperative evaluation for anesthesia in the Down patient it is important to focus attention on the functional conditions of him and systems that frequently show anomalies. One of the challenges of evaluating pre-operative conditions and potential risks in the Down patient is the lack of a gold-standard evaluation score; cervical spine abnormalities, reduced dimensions and malformations of the airways, neurological changes, respiratory and cardiac disease, as well as endocrinological and metabolic alterations [54].

Screening and Prenatal Diagnosis

In the last decade numerous markers and strategies for DS screening have been developed. Algorithms that combine ultrasound and serum markers in the first and second trimesters have been evaluated (Tab. II). Furthermore, the practice of using age cut-offs to determine whether women should be offered screening or invasive diagnostic testing has been challenged [55].

Invasive Prenatal Diagnosis

PD of fetal chromosomal abnormalities is the most common indication for invasive prenatal testing [56].

In some cases a Mendelian disorder may be identified by obtaining a thorough prenatal genetic history. In virtually all cases of prenatally detected fetal malformations chromosome analysis is indicated. Amniocentesis is the most common means of fetal chromosome analysis but usually takes at least 2 weeks for results.

Table II. First and second trimester trisomy 21 screenings

Screening	Weeks gestation	Detectio n rate	False positive rate	Description
Triple test	15–20	75%	8.5%	This test measures the maternal serum alpha-feto protein (AFP, a fetal liver protein), unconjugated estriol (uE3, a pregnancy hormone), and human chorionic gonadotropin (hCG, a pregnancy hormone).
Quadruple test	15–20	79%	7.5%	This test measures the maternal serum AFP, uE3, hCG, and high inhibin-alpha (INHA).
AFP/free beta-hCG screening	13–22	80%	2.8%	This test measures the AFP, produced by the fetus, and free beta-hCG, produced by the placenta.
Nuchal translucency (NT)/free beta-hCG/pregnancy-associated plasma protein-A (PAPP-A) screening	10–13.5	91%	5%	Uses ultrasound to measure NT in addition to the free beta-hCG and PAPP-A. National Institute of Health (NIH) has confirmed that this first trimester test is more accurate than second trimester screening methods.

In cases where the gestation is approaching the legal limit for elective termination rapid karyotyping by percutaneous umbilical cord sampling (UCS) should be considered and referral to a center familiar with this procedure is suggested. Chromosome analysis from fetal blood takes approximately 3 days to accomplish.

Alternatively, rapid karyotyping by transabdominal chorionic villus sampling (CVS) may also be accomplished. If a chromosomal abnormality is identified genetic counseling should be arranged to discuss prognosis, cause, recurrence risks, and to help the parents through this difficult time. If applicable the option of pregnancy termination should be offered. Not all parents faced with a chromosomally abnormal fetus will wish to terminate their pregnancy and others may be too late in gestation to consider this option. In these cases discussions with other families raising similarly affected children, social workers, clergy, psychiatrists, and geneticists may be helpful to the parents. Late pregnancy cytogenetic PD may be beneficial both to the parents in helping prepare them psychologically and emotionally for an adverse outcome and in guiding obstetric management [57].

Amniocentesis will undoubtedly continue to hold an important place in PD and has great importance in diagnosing neural tube defects (NTD) and DS through widespread maternal serum alpha-fetoprotein (AFP) screening. Patients now have a choice in prenatal diagnostic procedures for most genetic disorders. Many are already choosing CVS despite the questions that remain regarding risks and diagnostic accuracy. Risk figures for miscarriages due to the procedure and for intrauterine infection are especially needed. The issues of maternal contamination in laboratory analyses and chromosomal mosaicism that may not be present in the fetus are also of prime importance. Collaborative efforts continue to answer these and other questions so that in the future patients will be better able to make informed decisions regarding PD [58].

Maternal Serum Screening

In the absence of prenatal screening (PS) and diagnosis prevalence at birth in the USA would currently exceed 1:600. The purpose of PS is to identify those women at increased risk for an affected pregnancy and to maximize the options available to these women. Second trimester serum screening involves combining the maternal age-specific risk for an affected pregnancy with the risks associated with the concentrations of maternal serum AFP, unconjugated estriol (uE3), and human chorionic gonadotrophin (hCG) (triple testing). A forth analyte, inhibin-alpha (INHA), is increasingly being utilized (quadruple testing). Optimal second trimester screening requires the integration of a number of clinical variables, the most important of which is an accurate assessment of gestational age. In addition to DS the triple and quadruple tests preferentially identify fetal trisomy 18, Turner syndrome (TS), triploidy, trisomy 16 mosaicism, fetal death, Smith-Lemli-Opitz syndrome, and steroid sulfatase deficiency. Some programs modify the DS risks generated through maternal serum screening (MSS) tests with fetal biometric data obtained by ultrasound. Other second trimester tests have shown promise, including the analysis of maternal urine and fetal cells in the maternal circulation, but none are in routine clinical use. The second trimester triple and quadruple tests provide benchmarks for evaluating new screening protocols. The combination of fetal biometry, new test development, as well as clarification of the role of co-factors that affect the concentrations of analytes in existing tests should lead to greater efficacy in screening for DS [59].

In 1968 the first antenatal diagnosis of DS was made and screening on the basis of selecting women of advanced maternal age for amniocentesis was gradually introduced into medical practice. In 1983 it was shown that low maternal serum AFP was associated with DS. Later, raised maternal serum hCG and low uE3 were found to be markers of DS. In 1988 the three biochemical markers were used together with maternal age as a method of screening and this has been widely adopted. Methods of screening need to be fully evaluated before being introduced into routine clinical practice. This included choosing markers for which there is sufficient scientific evidence of efficacy, quantifying performance in terms of detection and false positive rates, and establishing methods of monitoring performance. Screening needs to be provided as an integrated service, coordinating and managing the separate aspects of the screening process. A large number of serum markers have been found to be associated with DS between 15 and 22 weeks of pregnancy. The principal markers are AFP, hCG or its individual subunits (free alpha- and free beta-hCG), uE3, and INHA. Screening performance varies according to the choice of markers used and whether ultrasound is used to estimate gestational age. When an ultrasound scan is used to estimate gestational age the detection rate for a 5% false positive rate is estimated to be 59% using the double test (AFP and hCG), 69% using the triple test (AFP, hCG, uE3), and 76% using the quadruple test (AFP, hCG, uE3, INHA), all in combination with maternal age. Other factors that can usefully be taken into account in screening are maternal weight, the presence of insulin-dependent diabetes mellitus (IDDM), multiple pregnancy, ethnic origin, previous DS pregnancy, and whether the test is the first one in a pregnancy or a repeated one. Factors such as parity and smoking are associated with one or more of the serum markers, but the effect is too small to justify adjusting for these factors in interpreting a screening test. Urinary beta-core fragment (beta CF) of hCG has been investigated in a number of studies and shown to be raised in pregnancies with DS. This area is currently the subject of active research and the use of urine in future screening programmes may be a practical possibility. Other urinary markers such as total E3 and free beta-hCG may also be of value. Fetal cells can be identified in the maternal circulation and techniques such as fluorescence in situ hybridization (FISH) can be used to identify aneuploidies including DS and trisomy 18. This approach may, in the future, be of value in screening or diagnosis. Currently, the techniques available do not have the performance, simplicity, or economy needed to replace existing methods. Demonstration projects are valuable in determining the feasibility of screening and in refining the practical application of screening. They are of less value in determining the performance of different screening methods. There are a number of ultrasound markers of DS at 15-22 weeks, including nuchal fold thickness, cardiac abnormalities, duodenal atresia, femur length (FL), humerus length (HL), pyelectasis, and hyperechogenic bowel [60].

Various other serum markers of DS have been reported, but at present they do not have a place in routine antenatal screening for DS. The role of amniotic fluid acetylcholinesterase measurement, alone and in combination with amniotic fluid AFP measurement, in the antenatal diagnosis of open NTD has recently been clarified. The best policy is to perform an amniotic fluid AFP measurement as the primary test and an acetylcholinesterase determination for those women who have an amniotic fluid AFP measurement of two times the normal median or greater. The acetylcholinesterase can be measured either by the standard method (gel electrophoresis) or by a new quantitative monoclonal antibody method [61].

In the past two decades the second trimester of pregnancy has been the most common time for PD of fetal anomalies and chromosomal aneuploidies. More recently, screening for and diagnosis of chromosomal abnormalities are increasingly being performed in the first trimester. With improvements and technological advances in ultrasound it is now possible to identify many fetal structural anomalies at 11 to 13 weeks' gestation. At 10 to 11 weeks' gestation biochemical markers in serum pregnancy-associated plasma protein-A (PAPP-A), free beta-hCG, AFP, and uE3 combined with sonographic measurement of an enlarged thickness of the subcutaneous fluid-filled space at the back of the neck of the developing fetus (referred to as "nuchal translucency" [NT]) (Figure 5) and the presence/absence of the nasal bone can achieve a DS detection rate of 97.5% at a false-positive rate of 5%. Structural anomalies of the CNS, and the cardiac, renal, and GI tracts can now be diagnosed by either transabdominal (TA) or transvaginal (TV) scanning, achieving detection of up to 80% of CNS anomalies by 13 weeks' gestation. In future the emphasis in PD will likely be in the first trimester [62].

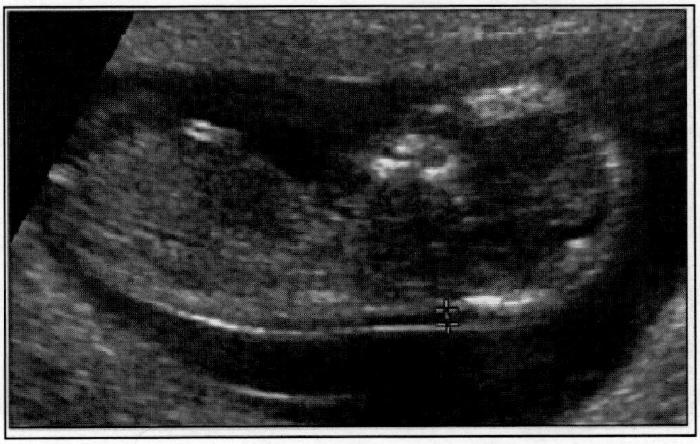

Figure 5. Nuchal translucency detected with first trimester fetal ultrasonography (Ontario Multiple Marker Screening [MMS] Program).

First trimester screening for chromosomal abnormalities offers potential advantages over second trimester screening. Studies in the 1990s demonstrated an association between chromosomal abnormalities and the ultrasonographic finding of abnormally increased NT between 10 and 14 weeks of gestation. First trimester screening using NT, free beta-hCG, and PAPP-A has comparable detection rates and positive screening rates for DS as second trimester screening using 4 serum markers (AFP, beta-hCG, uE3, and INHA). Although first trimester screening for DS and trisomy 18 is an option, it should be offered only if certain criteria can be met [63].

The acceptability of PS and diagnosis of DS is dependent in part on the gestational age at which the testing is offered. First trimester screening could be advantageous if it has sufficient efficacy and can be effectively delivered. Two first trimester maternal serum markers (MSM), PAPP-A and free beta-hCG, are useful for identifying women at increased risk for fetal DS. In addition, measurement of NT has been demonstrated to be an indicator for these high-risk pregnancies. When these three parameters are combined estimates for DS efficacy exceed those currently attainable in the second trimester. Women who are screen-positive in the first trimester can elect to receive cytogenetic testing of a CVS. The first trimester tests could also, theoretically, be combined with the second trimester MSS tests (integrated screening) to obtain even higher levels of efficacy. There are, however, several practical limitations to first trimester and integrated screening. These include scheduling of testing within relatively narrow gestational age intervals, availability of appropriately trained ultrasonographers for NT measurement, risks associated with CVS, and costs. There is also increasing evidence that an enlarged NT measurement is indicative of a high risk for spontaneous abortion and for fetal abnormalities that are not detectable by cytogenetic analysis. Women whose fetuses show enlarged NT, therefore, need first trimester counseling regarding their DS risks and the possibility of other adverse pregnancy outcomes. Follow-up ultrasound and fetal echocardiography in the second trimester are also indicated. First trimester screening appears to be a highly effective method to screen for DS. Women with screen-positive results based on NT measurement appear to be at increased risk for diverse fetal abnormalities. The finding of a normal fetal karyotype may not, therefore, carry a high level of reassurance for a normal baby [64].

Maternal Urine Screening

Most Down's screening protocols have concentrated on the analysis of oncofetal antigen levels present in serum. Urine has largely been ignored, but mass screening based on a urine text has several logistical advantages. Beta CF is a major immunoreactive degradation product of hCG and in particular its beta-subunit. Elevated maternal serum hCG is the single most effective biochemical marker of DS and levels are more than doubled. Measurement of elevated free beta-subunit has been shown to be a superior discriminator than measurement of intact or total hCG. This was shown by an increase in comparative serum levels from 2.04 to 2.41 multiple of the median (MoM). The median MoM value of beta CF for Down's cases in studies has varied between 4.38 and 6.28. The proportion of true Down's cases having a beta CF value greater than the 95th centile of the controls varied from 61% to 93%. This is far superior to any single serum marker. If other complimentary urinary markers can be found urinary screening could replace serum screening not only because of the logistical advantages but also of the increased sensitivity [65].

Ultrasound screening

DS incidence rises with maternal age, thus prompting the current practice of offering genetic amniocentesis to women 35 years of age or older. However, even if every pregnant woman of advanced maternal age ($\geq$ 35 years) were to undergo karyotyping, only 20% of fetuses with DS would be detected. Until approximately 10 years ago karyotyping of the fetuses of older women was practically the only antenatal method of identifying any fetus with trisomy 21. In 1984 it was first reported the use of a low level of serum AFP as a screening tool for identifying affected fetuses in younger women. Combining the criteria based on both maternal age and serum AFP resulted in identifying 40% of fetuses with DS, as well as 6.8% of unaffected fetuses. Still at least 60% of fetuses with DS remained undetected with these screening techniques. It was logical to expect that sonographic imaging of the second trimester fetus itself would result in the optimal detection of the anatomical features of DS. To this end many researchers have attempted to identify sonographic findings that would serve to detect fetuses likely to have DS [66].

So antenatal DS screening begins with maternal age-specific risks. It also may incorporate the MSS and antenatal ultrasound. These complementary tests improve the efficacy of maternal age in DS screening. Ultrasound enhances antenatal DS screening by:

1) precise dating of a pregnancy for the interpretation of serum screen results;
2) detecting major structural anomalies that occur in approximately 20% of all second trimester DS fetuses;

3) detecting minor markers, such as nuchal fold thickness, pyelectasis, echogenic bowel, short long bones, sandal gap, and hypoplasia of the mid-phalanx of the fifth digit, which are more commonly seen in second trimester fetuses with DS;
4) acting in combination with serum screening in the first trimester using fetal NT as the marker.

Ultrasound, therefore, enhances the efficacy of either age or age and the serum screening for the antenatal detection of DS [67].

The first sonographic sign of DS, the thickened nuchal fold, was first described in 1985. Since that time multiple sonographically-identified markers have been described as associated with DS. The so-called "genetic sonogram", involving a detailed search for sonographic signs of aneuploidy, can be used to both identify fetuses at high risk for aneuploidy and, when normal, can be used to decrease the risk for aneuploidy for a pregnancy when no sonographic markers are identified. Combining the genetic sonogram with MSS has been the best method of assessing aneuploidy risk for women who desired such an assessment in the second trimester. Trisomy 18, trisomy 13, and triploidy are typically associated with sonographically identified abnormalities and have a high prenatal detection rate. The use of these sonographic signs in low-risk women requires further investigation, however patients at increased risk for aneuploidy due to advanced maternal age or abnormal serum screening can benefit from a genetic sonogram screening for sonographic signs of aneuploidy to adjust their baseline risk of an affected fetus [68].

The genetic sonogram is therefore an ultrasound examination done on second trimester fetuses that not only evaluates the fetus for structural malformations but also searches for the sonographic markers of fetal DS. The main markers that comprise the genetic sonogram include the nuchal fold, short femur and humerus, pyelectasis, hyperechogenic bowel, echogenic intracardiac focus, and any major abnormality. The absence of any marker on a second trimester scan conveys a 60-80% reduction in prior risk of DS based on advanced maternal age or serum screening risk. The presence of sonographic markers, either singly or in combination, will raise the baseline risk of DS using likelihood ratios calculated for each individual marker. Using this approach approximately 75% of fetuses with DS can be identified by modifying the patient's baseline risk according to the results of the ultrasound. The second trimester scan will likely continue to play an important role in the future in the detection of aneuploidy [69].

The usefulness of ultrasonography in detecting fetuses with DS in the second trimester has been the subject of considerable debate during the past years. Conflicting reports have led to increasing confusion about the subject in the medical community and among the public. A review of the existing literature indicates that structural malformations that are chiefly cardiac are present in half of DS fetuses but are not consistently found during routine second trimester ultrasonography. Although excess posterior nuchal skin-fold thickness is frequently present in infants with DS, it is also not consistently identified during second trimester ultrasonographic examinations. Studies evaluating the efficacy of screening programs that are based on FL shortening associated with DS have revealed markedly discrepant intercenter results. Although variations in methods may account for some of the observed variability, the magnitude of femoral shortening in DS suggests that this measurement may be only marginally useful. Antenatal ultrasonography allows for the detection of only those fetuses with DS who have multiple characteristic phenotypic features or anomalies. Moreover, second trimester ultrasonography did not appear to be either sensitive or specific enough to be used as a unique DS screening modality; however, it has been a useful adjunct to maternal age and serum biochemical markers in the assignment of risk for DS [70].

The utility of ultrasound screening for DS should therefore be judged by whether the pertinent markers are reliably obtained and by whether they efficiently discriminate between fetuses with DS and euploid fetuses. Furthermore, the markers must be reliable at a gestational age early enough to be clinically useful. Screening for characteristic congenital malformations will result in a low detection rate of DS and many of these cases will be identified only after 24 weeks of gestation. The subtlety of many of the ultrasound findings of DS in the second trimester requires significant technical expertise if ultrasonographic screening is to be used. Investigation thus far has centered on identifying patients at increased risk of DS and no data are available on how much a normal ultrasound might decrease the risk associated with advanced maternal age or abnormal biochemical screening. The ultimate value of ultrasound may be to help further define the risk assigned by age and biochemical screening, to provide each patient with an aggregate risk. The decision on whether or not to offer an amniocentesis could then be based on the findings of these various examinations, with the goal to improve the accuracy of age or biochemical screening alone [71].

Ultrasound evidence for aneuploidy may be found in almost every organ of the fetus and can be used to modify the risk of aneuploidy. The diagnosis of these minor anomalies on second trimester ultrasonography will increase the risk of an abnormal karyotype whereas the absence of these findings may reduce this danger. The most specific and most ominous isolated markers for fetal aneuploidy are nuchal findings (edema or cysts), indicating the need to obtain a fetal karyotype in all cases irrespective of maternal age or results of biochemical serum screening. Hyperechogenic fetal bowel is apparently also a strong indicator of fetal aneuploidy. Other isolated sonographic markers may increase the risk of an abnormal karyotype three- to ninefold. Most sonographic markers for aneuploidy specify an increased risk for DS but choroid plexus cysts are apparently more specific for trisomy 18 [72].

In the presence of normal ultrasonographic results the negative prediction can be combined with maternal age-related or biochemical prediction of trisomy 21 to help in the informed consent process in counseling women about the benefits and harms of genetic amniocentesis. Genetic amniocentesis should be considered in women of any age when second trimester ultrasonography reveals the presence of one or more of the following: fetal structural malformations, short femur (determined by biparietal diameter [BPD]-to-FL ratio), combination of short femur and humerus, abnormal ($\geq$ 6 mm) nuchal fold thickening, echogenic bowel, or short ear length [73].

Second trimester sonographic findings of fetal trisomy may then include structural abnormalities or sonographic markers of fetal aneuploidy. Unlike structural anomalies, sonographic markers of fetal aneuploidy are insignificant by themselves with regard to outcome, are non-specific – most frequently seen in normal fetuses, and are often transient. The sensitivity of sonography for detection of fetal trisomic conditions varies with the type of chromosome abnormality, gestational age at the time of sonography, reasons for referral, criteria for positive sonographic findings, and the quality of the sonography. As an estimate,

1 or more sonographic findings can be identified in approximately 90% of fetuses with trisomy 13, 80% of fetuses with trisomy 18, and 50% to 70% of fetuses with trisomy 21. The presence or absence of sonographic markers can substantially modify the risk of fetal DS and is the basis of the genetic sonogram. Because maternal biochemical and sonographic markers are largely independent, combined risk estimates will result in even higher detection rates than either alone [74].

However, non-specific markers are more commonly observed than structural abnormalities, which are detected in less than 20% of cases in a non-selected population. Also, the actual sensitivity of a genetic sonogram will depend on various factors including the markers sought, gestational age, reasons for referral, and of course the quality of the ultrasound. Appropriate use of a genetic sonogram can help to modify the risk of fetal DS by decreasing the risk when the ultrasound is normal or increasing the risk when specific ultrasound markers are detected. The postultrasound risk can be estimated by applying specific likelihood ratios, reflecting the strength of individual markers with the a priori risk based on maternal age alone or combined with biochemical markers when known [75].

In fact, not every aspect of sonographic examination reveals karyotypic abnormalities. Ultrasound examination of a fetus with trisomy 21 generally reveals normal amniotic fluid, normal placentation, and normal fetal growth. In addition, other chromosomal abnormalities have many of the same sonographic findings as DS and many findings have a large overlap with phenotypically normal fetuses. The importance of second trimester ultrasound screening for DS has remained great because of its ease of use and relative effectiveness. Trained sonographers can adjust the relative risk for trisomy 21 and alter the need for genetic amniocentesis. It is important that parents understand the limitations of a screening test and the risks and benefits of possible subsequent confirmatory testing. If a major structural abnormality is identified on ultrasound karyotype determination should be considered. The predictive value of all the markers depends on the population studied and can be modified by a host of biochemical markers and historical factors. If fetal karyotype analysis could be performed without sampling through the uterus, PD could be offered to all pregnant women and screening would be unnecessary. Despite its limitations, ultrasound will have an important role in PD at least until isolating and testing fetal cells from maternal blood or other sources becomes practical and widely available [76].

Among high-risk mothers (advanced maternal age, abnormal triple screen, or both), while many undoubtedly will choose to have invasive testing as a first option, others will instead use the information derived from genetic sonography to obtain an adjusted risk for DS to guide their decision about genetic amniocentesis. Accordingly, it is imperative that these patients have accurate and detailed counseling regarding their degree of risk reduction when the genetic sonogram is normal. Genetic sonography is a patient-driven service and the information obtained at the time of ultrasound is an important component of the patient's decision of whether or not to proceed with invasive testing [77].

Genetic sonography identifies between 60% and 93% of fetuses with trisomy 21. One of the reasons for the variation in sensitivity is because of the under-detection of CHD. Although CHD are present in 56% of second trimester fetuses and 44% of newborns with trisomy 21, most studies evaluating second trimester fetuses at risk for trisomy 21 detect less than 10% of heart malformations. The cardiovascular examination consists of three levels. In the level I examination only non-cardiac markers are evaluated for a detection rate of 60% and false-positive rate of 5.9%. The level II examination incorporates the four-chamber view with non-cardiac markers. If the examiner can identify atrial and/or ventricular chamber disproportion, then the sensitivity is increased to 75% with a false-positive rate of 6.4%. The level III examination utilizes grayscale and color Doppler ultrasound to evaluate the fetal heart. If the examiner can identify ventricular septal defects, atrioventricular septal defects, pericardial effusion, tricuspid regurgitation, and chamber disproportion, then the sensitivity of genetic sonography increases to 91% with a false-positive rate of 14% [78].

During the last decade fetal ultrasound screening has led to frequent situations characterised by clinical uncertainty due to the disclosure of soft markers in the unborn child. Soft markers are minor anatomical variations indicating a somewhat increased likelihood that the fetus has a chromosomal aberration, most frequently trisomy 21. An analysis of the literature makes evident that many ultrasound examiners have counseled individual pregnant women on the basis of insufficient data. Moral dilemmas have thus emerged as a direct result of advancing medical technology and healthy fetal lives prove to have been lost due to invasive diagnostic testing aimed at resolving clinical uncertainty. Ultrasound examiners have warned against a policy of disclosing all findings of soft markers to expectant parents, but no exploration of experiential aspects linked to the disclosure of fetal soft markers has yet been published in the medical literature. The emotional reactions of mothers are important to consider given their potential impact on the biological development of the fetus [79].

The value of all non-invasive prenatal tests must therefore be viewed with the perspective of the consequences of invasive testing. Regarding second trimester non-invasive testing, biochemical screening is more accurate in establishing risk than maternal age alone. One or more major ultrasound abnormalities, NT, or a shortened humerus should raise concern for DS regardless of the patient's a priori risk based on age or biochemical markers. Isolated minor ultrasound markers should not be used in calculating risk in low-risk patients regarding DS unless the biochemical profile already places the patient at risk or in a borderline risk zone. If the ultrasound finding is hyperechogenic bowel, problems other than aneuploidy may be the cause, including cystic fibrosis (CF), infection, or hemorrhage, and these problems must be considered if hyperechogenic bowel is an isolated finding. Improved risk adjustment seems to be applicable to a priori high-risk patients with completely normal sonograms. Genetic sonograms with specific risk adjustment schemata may be used to adjust a priori risk (either maternal age or biochemical screening results) at centers in which this has proven to be accurate, but whether this is statistically sound remains to be determined. The goal of second trimester ultrasound screening is to identify at-risk fetuses better and offer invasive testing to a more selected group of patients. As the value of first trimester screening becomes more evident and practical and if the risk of CVS becomes an acceptable norm, the patient population that reaches the second trimester of pregnancy will be selected. Therefore, second trimester screening and invasive testing may be needed only in a minority of cases and the practice standards of prenatal testing and sonography (including minor ultrasound markers) will change entirely [80].

Over the past 10 years the use of ultrasound in aneuploidy risk estimation has allowed patients to obtain more personalized risk assessment and has allowed many women a reasonable alternative to invasive testing. The addition of soft markers to the sonographic screening for aneuploidy has been extremely beneficial, especially when considered in combination with other ultrasound findings. The best estimate of risk seems to be achieved through the combined use of ultrasound, MSS, and maternal age. The literature supports the use of soft markers only when applied to the high-risk population, where the prevalence of aneuploidy is increased. If this information is applied to the low-risk populations, especially in isolation, the lower prevalence of aneuploidy makes the positive predictive value too low to be of any value in counseling patients. As with many screening tests, it occasionally misses the diagnosis and every patient needs to understand this potential shortcoming. It is a personal decision regarding their willingness to accept the risk of a missed diagnosis versus the risk of fetal loss from an invasive procedure. Although it is far from perfect, in the right hands and with appropriate counseling ultrasound is an excellent tool. This is such an important decision for women and their families and it is worth the time it takes to explain the benefits and limitations of this test [81].

The genetic sonogram, in fact, can be considered a composite algorithm combining multiple individual markers to increase DS risk prediction. Transformation of sonographic information into a standard mathematical format represented an early challenge that has now been surmounted. Using increasingly sophisticated mathematical techniques individual patient risk can be estimated. High diagnostic accuracy comparable to standard mid-trimester serum algorithms has been reported. Most recently a few studies have reported the ability to combine serum and biochemical markers to achieve diagnostic accuracy comparable to first trimester screening. Even fewer studies have reported combinations of ultrasound and maternal urine markers (MUM). While it is clear that consistently high sensitivity and specificity for DS can be achieved, almost all the studies are based on high-risk groups. Studies in low-risk populations have suffered from lack of standardization. The relevance of genetic sonogram in a low-risk population thus remains to be proven. The most significant challenge, however, remains the development of uniform and reproducible sonographic and measurement standards. This is likely to be the most important factor in optimizing the accuracy of the mid-trimester genetic sonogram [82].

Screening for fetal aneuploidy is now possible during the first trimester using sonographic and biochemical markers. Although early studies showed wide variation in detection of fetal DS when using NT, more recent studies showed sensitivities of approximately 70% to 80% for a 5% false-positive rate. Maternal serum biochemical screening can be used as a test for aneuploidy during the first trimester. The two MSM that appear to be most useful in the late first trimester are the free beta subunit of hCG and PAPP-A. Together with maternal age, these markers yield a detection rate for trisomy 21 of approximately 60% for a 5% false-positive rate. Because sonographic and biochemical markers appear to be largely independent, their combined risk results in improved detection rates compared with either method alone. As a result the combination of NT, biochemical markers, and maternal age has achieved a detection rate of approximately 85% for a 5% false-positive level for detection of trisomy 21. A newly proposed "integrated" approach using a panel of first and second trimester markers suggests that further improvement in the screening performance is possible [83].

NT sonography, therefore, is the most powerful single prenatal marker for DS. In fact, as seen above, its detection rate is 75% at a 5% false-positive rate. The combination of NT and maternal serum-free beta-hCG and PAPP-A can identify 85% to 90% of fetuses with DS for a false-positive rate of 5%. This method can also identify more than 90% of fetuses with trisomies 18 and 13, TS, and triploidy for a screen-positive rate of 1% [84].

Increased NT can also identify a high proportion of other chromosomal abnormalities and is associated with major defects of the heart and great arteries and a wide range of skeletal dysplasias and genetic syndromes. In monochorionic twins discordancy for increased NT is an early marker of twin-to-twin transfusion syndrome (TTTS) [85].

In addition to increased NT important sonographic markers for chromosomal abnormalities include fetal growth restriction, tachycardia, abnormal flow in the ductus venosus, megacystis, exomphalos, and single umbilical artery. Most pregnant women prefer screening in the first rather than in the second trimester. As with all aspects of good clinical practice those care givers who perform first trimester screening should be trained appropriately and their results should be subjected to external quality assurance [86].

Already in 1866 John Langdon Down noted that common features of patients with trisomy 21 are a skin being too large for the body and a flat face with a small nose. The additional soft markers in the first trimester are fetal nasal bone, Doppler velocity waveform in the ductus venosus, and tricuspid regurgitation and these markers can be used to further increase the detection rate of trisomy 21. In addition increased NT thickness can also identify other chromosomal defects (mainly trisomy 13 and 18 and monosomy X) and major congenital malformations (mainly cardiac defects) and genetic syndromes [87].

Thus, anatomic examination of the fetus in the first trimester has been emphasized because it allows for early diagnosis of many conditions. The prevalence of absent nasal bone, a marker for trisomy 21, in euploid fetuses depends on ethnicity. Nasal bone hypoplasia is another marker for DS. Studies on genetic screening in the first trimester have involved various serum analytes, adjustments in timing and calculations, use in multiple gestations, and the association of extreme measurements with adverse outcomes. A first trimester integrated screening approach, which incorporates NT, nasal bone, crown-rump length (CRL), PAPP-A, and free beta-hCG, has the potential to maximize detection rates of DS and trisomy 18 and minimizes the screen-positive rate. The value of combining first and second trimester results in sequential, contingent, or integrated screening protocols has been assessed. Isolated mild ventriculomegaly (10-12 mm) may prove to be a normal variant and the role of soft ultrasound markers in genetic counseling continues to be debated. Anomaly or high-risk status detection in the second trimester has been enhanced by the use of Doppler, 3D/4D ultrasound, and magnetic resonance imaging (MRI). Imaging techniques have been critical in the development of screening methods for DS or trisomy 18 and for euploid fetuses at high risk for adverse outcomes [88].

The debate over the application of NT measurement in DS screening is still unresolved in some clinicians' minds. Although different authors report a range of sensitivities for DS, none question the validity of the association between increased NT and fetal aneuploidy. The published literature reveals a lack of congruence over a standard, reproducible method for measuring NT. Only with the adoption of uniform methodology and the establishment of international standards for NT measurement is the true potential of this test likely to be realized. The increasing use of first trimester ultrasound has focused attention on the value of this investigation in confirming fetal viability, estimation of gestational age, and screening for congenital abnormality [89].

Multiple and Assisted Reproduction Techniques Pregnancies

First or second trimester screening in twin pregnancies is feasible and still efficacious by using either a combination of ultrasound and maternal serum biochemistry in the first trimester or maternal serum biochemistry in the second trimester. Special care, however, should be emphasized in what concerns biochemical screening since it is much less sensitive in multiples. These "pseudo-risks" have been challenged for their scientific and clinical validity, however. Until more data are available from larger studies on the distribution of markers in concordant or discordant twins, NT estimated for each fetus should be the predominant factor by which women who present with increased risk should be counseled regarding invasive testing. In dizygotic pregnancies pregnancy-specific risk should be calculated by summing the individual risk estimates for each fetus. In monozygotic twins the risk should be calculated based on the geometric mean of both NT measurements, not forgetting that the false-positive rate of NT screening is expectantly higher than in singletons [90].

Assisted reproduction techniques (ART) have increased both the number of pregnancies in women beyond the age of 35 and the incidence of multiple pregnancies. Specific problems were encountered when methods of screening for DS are applied for twin pregnancies. Overall, more women with twin pregnancies (mainly those who conceived via ART) are found to be false positive for DS. This is because mid-trimester MSS is associated with a higher false-positive rate secondary to changes in the feto-placental endocrinologic metabolism reflected mainly in high hCG levels in the ART pregnancies. First trimester NT measurement in twin pregnancies is not affected by the problems encountered in serum screening. This sonographic screening approach enables a fetus-specific identification of those fetuses at high risk of DS and is associated with a lower false-positive rate than mid-trimester serum screening. DS screening in ART twins presents several challenges in determining the most appropriate screening test modality. Whether there is any significant benefit of adding first trimester biochemistry or nasal bone scanning in screening ART-conceived twins awaits further investigation [91].

Personal Experience with Nuchal Translucency Assessment

We conducted a study to assess the detection of fetal structural defects with an ultrasound scan at 11-14 weeks of gestation performed on fetuses of women with singleton pregnancies undergoing first trimester fetal karyotyping by amniocentesis or CVS because of advanced maternal age, parental anxiety, or family history of a chromosomal abnormality in the absence of balanced parental translocation. In the 4-year period from January 1998 to December 2001 we submitted 3,157 pregnant women to a routine ultrasound examination at 11-14 weeks. The patients were then submitted to an ultrasound scan in the second or third trimester of pregnancy. The same type of ultrasound machine and standardized approach were used in all patients. The measurement of fetal NT was performed by mid-sagittal section. Fetal NT thickness was measured twice by each examiner on a regular-sized image and subsequently on the same still image magnified. An isolated increased NT thickness (> 95th percentile thickness of the normal range for CRL between 38 and 84 mm) was not considered an abnormality. These patients, however, were submitted to an early echocardiographic evaluation. Fetal structural abnormalities were classified as major or minor and of early or late onset. The study protocol included first-trimester combined NT and MSM (free beta-hCG and PAPP-A) testing. Karyotyping was advised when:

1) NT was ≥ 3 mm;
2) the MSM-related risk was ≥ 1 in 250 at term.

Karyotyping was delayed until after a maternal blood sample had been taken. NT and MSM were expressed as MoM and risks were calculated and tailored to the study population. A combined risk for NT and MSM was estimated retrospectively. The second trimester triple serum screening included AFP, intact hCG, and uE3. After excluding aneuploidies, miscarriages, anatomical anomalies, and cases with incomplete follow-up, the serum samples of normal cases were assessed and correlated. To determine if the risk for fetal trisomies during the first trimester of pregnancy can be derived by combining data from maternal serum PAPP-A and fetal NT thickness, likelihood ratios for trisomies 21, 18, and 13 in relation to PAPP-A, in MoM for CRL, were derived from the overlapping Gaussian frequency distribution curves for normal and abnormal pregnancies. Moreover, we compared the potential value of maternal serum total hCG and free beta-hCG in predicting the risk for fetal trisomies during the first trimester of pregnancy and to examine whether data on maternal hCG and fetal NT thickness can be combined to derive risks. Clinical examination of the neonates was performed by a pediatrician. Long-term follow-up was completed through a questionnaire filled in by parents and pediatricians.

A detection rate of 4.3% (135 cases) of abnormalities was found and 22.6% of these (30 cases) were diagnosed with the ultrasound scan at 11-14 weeks, including 7 cardiac defects associated with increased NT. The antenatal ultrasound detection rate was 73.5% and 33.2% were diagnosed in the first trimester assessment. A rate of 76.8% of the major defects were diagnosed by the prenatal scan and 35.8% by the scan at 11-14 weeks. Fetal structural defects with the ultrasonography at 11-14 weeks were diagnosed in about 24.3% of the cases, therefore, a second trimester abnormality is important in routine antenatal care to increase the prenatal assessment of fetal anomalies. The incidence of trisomies 21, 18, or 13 was significantly associated with both maternal age ($r = 0.92$) and fetal NT thickness ($r = 0.70$). The sensitivity, specificity, and relative risk (RR) for all aneuploidies were 25%, 91%, and 5.77, respectively, and no difference was found between trisomy 21 and other types of aneuploidy. The sensitivity, specificity, and RR were significantly higher at 11 weeks than at 14 weeks. The likelihood of aneuploidy increased with increasing thickness of the NT. Where the karyotype was found to be normal there was complete resolution of this ultrasound appearance by the second trimester. Spontaneous abortion, intrauterine, and neonatal death occurred in 2.9%, 1.6%, and 1.0%, respectively. The incidence of immature delivery was 1.6% and of premature delivery 6.5%. The only adverse pregnancy outcome recorded that was associated with increased NT was spontaneous abortion. The likelihood ratio for the occurrence of a spontaneous abortion was 3.6 for measurements between 3.0 and 3.9 mm and 7.3 for measurements ≥ 4 mm. NT measurement increased by about 12% per week. Expressing the result as a MoM-NT for a given CRL allowed for this increase with gestational age and yielded a distribution of values that was approximately Gaussian. About 91% of values lay between 0.5 and 2.0 MoM. The variance and therefore the false-positive rate of NT were significantly reduced by recording several measurements and using the average: for example, the false-positive rate reduced from 7.8% to 4.5% if the average of six measurements were used instead of one (a potential 40% reduction in the false-positive rate if the test were used in screening). Inter-observer repeatability of regular-sized image measurements showed a significant difference ($p < 0.01$) but the mean difference (+/- standard deviation – SD) of 0.05 (0.13) mm was negligible. Similarly, inter-observer repeatability of the magnified-image measurements yielded a significant difference ($p < 0.02$) but again with a small mean difference of 0.08 (0.21) mm. NT increases with gestational but not maternal age. Reproducibility is poor: by repeating measurements with a different operator, the same operator using a different still image, or the same operator using the same still image, 13.8%, 12.5%, or 11.9% of NT measurements, respectively, change their classification as normal or abnormal.

The findings of this study demonstrate the feasibility of introducing scanning at 11-14 weeks' gestation and the measurement of fetal NT thickness in routine maternity units. This study also demonstrates that first trimester NT measurement is an effective method of screening for fetal chromosomal abnormality [92].

Non-Invasive Prenatal Diagnosis

Although the first finding that fetal cells can enter the maternal circulation was made more than a century ago, it is still unclear if this finding will be translated into a clinically useful diagnostic tool in the foreseeable future. However, significant progress has been made via the analysis of cell-free fetal DNA in maternal plasma/serum and clinical services are now already being offered for the determination of fetal Rhesus D (Rh[D]) status and sex. Currently, however, this technology is really only suited for the analysis of fetal genetic loci completely absent from the maternal genome. The detection of more subtle fetal genetic traits such as point mutations involved in Mendelian disorders (thalassemia, CF) is considerably more complex. Preliminary reports indicate that the detection of fetal aneuploidies might be possible using epigenetically modified genes, e.g. maspin on chromosome 18. Additionally, an exiting recent development is that it might be feasible to detect DS via the quantitative assessment of placentally derived cell-free mRNA of chromosome-21-specific genes such as PLAC4 [93].

The data accumulated thus far indicate that fetal nucleated red blood cells (NRBCs) are the target cell type of choice in maternal blood for most investigators although some groups continue to work with the trophoblast. Reports of persistent circulation of hematopoietic stem cells, lymphoid/myeloid progenitors, and lymphocytes mandate that removal of these cell types must occur before clinical diagnosis of the current pregnancy can be made. In selected cases accurate detection of fetal aneuploidy has been made from fetal cells in maternal blood. At present detection of uniquely fetal, paternally inherited gene polymorphisms or mutations such as the Rh(D) antigen is possible only because the mother lacks these genes; hence, maternal cell contamination does not hinder diagnosis. Currently the presence of large numbers of maternal cells in enriched samples precludes single-gene diagnosis for conditions in which the mother carries a mutant gene because her cells are preferentially amplified and difficult to distinguish from those of the fetus. It is likely, however, that as techniques of individual fetal cell isolation are perfected maternal cell contamination will no longer be an issue and the entire fetal genome will become available for diagnosis and therapy. Pediatricians need to be aware of the progress of research in this field because fetal cell isolation from maternal blood not only could change PD but would change the amount of genetic information that arrives with a newborn infant at birth [94].

The diagnostic use of circulating fetal DNA in maternal plasma is currently limited to genes which are present in the fetus but not in the mother. From a clinical perspective the most advanced application is for non-invasive detection of fetal Rh(D) genotype. The results of studies performed by four different groups showed that PD of fetal Rh(D) status by molecular analysis of maternal plasma or serum is routinely possible beginning in the second trimester. Non-invasive fetal genotyping should be useful for the treatment of sensitized Rh(D)-negative women whose partners are heterozygous for the Rh(D) gene because no further diagnostic or therapeutic procedures are necessary if the fetus is Rh(D) negative. Future clinical applications of fetal DNA may be in its use as a screening test for DS, preeclampsia, or preterm labor. However, these applications currently rely on the detection of Y chromosomal sequences and consequently are limited presently to male fetuses. The recent discovery of high concentrations of fetal DNA in maternal plasma represents a promising non-invasive approach to PD. Compared with the analysis of the cellular fraction of maternal blood the analysis of fetal DNA extracted from maternal plasma has the advantage of being rapid, robust, and easy to perform. The fetal DNA detected is limited to the current pregnancy. However, universal fetal gene sequences must be identified that allow analysis of genetic material from both male and female fetuses. Study of fetal DNA in maternal plasma can improve our understanding of feto-maternal biology and physiology. The long-term effects of maternal exposure to relatively high amounts of foreign DNA are unknown but represent an exciting area for future inquiry [95].

Both intact fetal cells as well as cell-free fetal DNA are present in the maternal circulation and can be recovered for non-invasive prenatal genetic diagnosis. Although methods for enrichment and isolation of rare intact fetal cells have been challenging, diagnosis of fetal chromosomal aneuploidy including trisomy 21 in first and second trimester pregnancies has been achieved with a 50-75% detection rate. Similarly, cell-free fetal DNA can be reliably recovered from maternal plasma and assessed by quantitative PCR to detect fetal trisomy 21 and paternally derived single gene mutations. Real-time PCR assays are robust in detecting low-level fetal DNA concentrations with sensitivity of approximately 95-100% and specificity near 100%. Comparing intact fetal cell versus cell-free fetal DNA methods for non-invasive PS for fetal chromosomal aneuploidy reveals that the latter is at least four times more sensitive. These preliminary results do not support a relationship between frequency of intact fetal cells and concentration of cell-free fetal DNA. The above results imply that the concentration of fetal DNA in maternal plasma may not be dependent on circulating intact fetal cells but rather be a product of growth and cellular turnover during embryonic or fetal development [96,97].

Circulating fetal DNA levels are elevated in pregnancies complicated by fetal trisomies 13 and 21, but not 18. Measurement of fetal DNA levels improves the performance of the current standard maternal serum screen by increasing the detection of DS cases by 5% with no increase in the false-positive rate. Fetal DNA levels are elevated in women who have developed clinical symptoms of preeclampsia but they are also elevated by the early second trimester in women who will eventually develop preeclampsia. Fetal DNA and mRNA gamma globin measurement may have clinical utility as markers for feto-maternal hemorrhage in the late first trimester. Cell-free fetal DNA levels are quite high in the amniotic fluid, permitting fetal genomic isolation and analysis using comparative genomic hybridization techniques. Fetal DNA crosses the blood-brain barrier and is detectable in maternal cerebrospinal fluid in a subset of pregnant women. The biological implications of this are currently unknown. Review of the literature suggests that the placenta is the predominant source of the circulating fetal nucleic acids. However, detection of gamma globin mRNA sequences in the plasma of pregnant women suggests that fetal blood cells also contribute to the pool of nucleic acids. Widespread incorporation of fetal nucleic acid measurement into routine prenatal care depends on the identification of a readily accessible gender-independent fetal marker [98].

Non-invasive PD offers the opportunity to eliminate completely the risky procedures of amniocentesis and CVS. The development of non-invasive PD tests has largely centred around the isolation and analysis of fetal cells in the maternal circulation and the analysis of free fetal DNA in maternal plasma. Both of these techniques offer difficult technical challenges and at the current moment in time the use of free fetal DNA is the simplest and most effective method of defining paternally inherited fetal genes for diagnosis. Post-genomics technologies that explore the proteins (proteomics) and transcripts (transcriptomics) released by the placenta into the maternal circulation offer new opportunities to identify genes and their protein products that are key diagnostic markers of disease (in particular DS) and might replace the current screening markers in use for prediction of risk of DS. In the ideal situation these markers are sufficiently diagnostic not to require invasive sampling of fetal genetic material. Post-genomics techniques might also offer better opportunities for defining fetal cell-specific markers that might enhance their isolation from maternal blood samples [99].

Quality Assessment and Cost-Effective Analysis of Prenatal Screening

PS for trisomy 21 uses a risk estimate as the screening variable. Modifying the age-associated risk by measuring biochemical markers or fetal measurements requires more sophisticated mathematical techniques than calculating the observed estimates of the likelihood ratio. Frequently the screening performance is reported on the same data used to generate the model. This can lead to an overestimate of the performance likely to be achievable in practice. In order to determine whether a proposed model for screening is better (or worse) than an established model the two should be directly compared on a reasonably sized dataset of cases and controls that was not used to derive either of the models. At best only marginal gains in screening performance can be expected using new or refined models for assigning DS risk [100].

Epidemiologic monitoring is a process which uses data generated from the screened population as a quality control measure. Most commonly laboratories monitor the percentage of women with screen positive test results, i.e., with test results falling at or above a specified MoM for open NTD screening or with a risk at or above a specified risk cut-off for DS screening. These percentages are sensitive to inaccurate and imprecise assays, inappropriate reference data, and long term assay drift. In fetal DS screening it is necessary to simultaneously monitor two or more assays, which is accomplished by monitoring the median MoM for each assay (which should be 1.0 within statistical limits) calculated using patient MoM values. Monitoring the median MoM can identify inappropriate adjustment factors for variables which affect the MoM such as maternal weight. Epidemiologic monitoring is a useful tool for identifying problems which are not readily apparent using traditional quality control measures [101].

Statistical modeling is used to predict screening detection and false-positive rates for policies using different marker combinations and screening modalities. Parameters are derived wherever possible from meta-analyses. Screening with four serum markers yields a similar detection rate in the first trimester as it does in the second and both have a similar detection rate to that of ultrasound NT screening. Ultrasound anomaly screening has a low detection rate. The integration of the different screening modalities can yield very high detection rates. Some methods of integration are preferable to others. The concurrent use of first trimester serum markers and ultrasound NT is the most practical. The combination of three modalities with non-disclosure of the intermediate results is more efficient but the gain in detection is too small to warrant the wait for up to 4 weeks for results. The sequential use of modalities with intermediate disclosure is more practical but will generate higher false-positive rates [102].

With increasing concerns regarding rapidly expanding health care costs, cost-effectiveness analysis (CEA) provides a methodology to assess whether marginal gains from new technology are worth the increased costs. In the arena of PD particular methodological and ethical concerns include whether the effects of such testing on individuals other than the patient are included, how termination of pregnancy is included in the models, redundancy of screening and diagnostic methods, and how screening may reassure or cause anxiety in patients depending on their results. The existing literature has demonstrated cost-effectiveness of screening and diagnosis of NTD, DS, and CF in the general population. Screening for genetic disorders which have a higher prevalence among particular groups has also been shown to be cost effective, including diseases such as hemoglobinopathies and Tay-Sachs disease. Understanding the methodology and salient issues of CEA is critical for researchers, editors, and clinicians to accurately interpret results of the growing body of cost-effectiveness studies in PD [103].

Counseling

Based on the ethical principles of respect for autonomy, beneficence, and justice, routinely offering first trimester risk assessment in centers qualified to provide it is ethically obligatory and routinely withholding the results of first trimester risk assessment is ethically unjustified. As risk for trisomy 21 occurs along a continuum, no pregnant woman is without risk; thus, offering diagnostic testing to all women is ethically justified. Informed consent and personal choice regarding diagnostic testing and termination of pregnancy shape patients' decisions to undergo first trimester risk assessment for trisomy 21. Appropriate counseling is required to allow for individual choice regarding timing of disclosure [104].

Despite methodological difficulties recent publications strongly suggest that genetic counseling is successful in educating counselees about diagnostic and risk information. In general investigators suggest that there is room for improvement and the factors leading to imperfect recall of information need to be elucidated. Process studies suggest that the educational priorities of counselors and counselees may not always be consistent. The contribution of these inconsistencies to outcome measures needs further study. Also it appears that differing counseling approaches may be equally effective in achieving educational goals. Studies on the reproductive outcome of genetic counseling show no strong impact of counseling; there appears to be a net increase of desire for more children following counseling. Precounseling reproductive intentions rather than counseling were found to be a major factor in determining postcounseling outcome. Process studies suggest that although many counselees say that they were influenced by genetic counseling it is uncertain what they mean, since for many counselees reproductive decisions seem to have been made prior to counseling [105].

Choice in prenatal care has moved on from a paternalistic approach to increased patient autonomy and informed decision-making. Knowledge scores can be improved and decisional conflict reduced by group counseling, individual sessions, and by use of leaflets. None of the interventions leads to a raise in anxiety scores or influence uptake rates. Using medical words rather than lay terms significantly alter risk perception. Information can increase the level of knowledge and reduce decisional conflict without raising anxiety scores. A clarification of the women's expectations seems paramount to obtain a perception of good information and informed consent. The information provided about DS and screening tests does not empower an informed consent based on relevant knowledge [106].

After being informed of the risks and advantages of serum screening a patient may elect to be screened. Counseling must emphasize that serum screening for these disorders is voluntary and patients must be aware that further evaluation, if their results are classified as positive, may include amniocentesis. Physicians should have access to genetic services and reliable laboratories to assist them in the management of MSS and genetic procedures. Special attention must be given to the older gravida to help her make an appropriate personal decision regarding screening and genetic testing. Patients receiving positive results from a definitive test (karyotype or, possibly, ultrasonography) should have access to adequate counseling including the availability of support groups and pediatric surgeons [107].

Although the pediatrician's initial contact with the child is usually during infancy, occasionally the pregnant woman who has been given the PD of DS will be referred for counseling [108].

The role of the pediatrician as genetic counselor is ideal because pediatricians have medical knowledge and experience with genetic disorders. Moreover, pediatricians can provide comprehensive care in a medical home to patients with genetic disorders. However, changes in the curriculum of the pediatric resident are necessary to address the future challenges of effectively communicating genetic information to patients. Pediatricians and residents lack essential knowledge of genetics and communication skills for effective counseling of patients. Successful communication of genetic information involves a number of important skills and considerations. It is likely that these skills and considerations are universally required for the communication of most complex specialized medical information. In the past communication skills have not been considered a priority. Today these skills have become a demanding professional and even legal obligation. However, the challenges involved in communicating complex medical information cannot be successfully addressed with universal, one-size-fits-all recommendations. Residency training programs require changes to adequately prepare future pediatricians for the growing challenge of communicating genetic information. Four important skills should be considered in the training of residents to improve the communication of complex information to patients. These skills are:

1) discriminating;
2) understanding;
3) simplifying;
4) explaining information [109].

Prevention

DS patients are known to be of short stature, prone to infections, autoimmune disease, hypothyroidism, leukemia, heart defects, and later AD. They tend to have older mothers like AD patients. The latter tend to have sibs with either DS or lymphoma/leukemia. Evidence, looking at DS patients, suggests that multiple food allergies, gluten-gliadin sensitivity, or intolerance are causing a CD-like picture with a malabsorption state for essential vitamins, minerals, and severe autoimmune disease. It is hoped that missed gluten-gliadin sensitivity or intolerance with or without CD will be considered as a cause of abnormal oogenesis and spermatogenesis resulting in trisomy 21 and other aneuploidies. The mechanism most likely is low B1 interfering with sufficient release of cAMP for normal meiosis. Alternatively exorphins and peptides from foods may suppress prostaglandin E1 (PGE1) synthesis or food sensitivities may alter toxic metal absorption mechanisms which are thought to play a role in the development of AD. Adequate vitamin/mineral supplementation, especially B1, prior to conception and in the first trimester is recommended for mothers at risk for DS, especially older mothers and a gluten free diet for those with CD or gluten-gliadin sensitivity/intolerance. Hopefully this will prevent conception of a DS child or prevent heart defects/stigmata if one is conceived. DS children should be investigated for the above and commence a food allergy free diet with relevant supplements to meet their needs as early as maximum development [110].

Folate is an important vitamin that contributes to cell division and growth and is therefore of particular importance during infancy and pregnancy. Folate deficiency has been associated with slowed growth, anemia, weight loss, digestive disorders, and some behavioural issues. Adequate folate intake around the time of conception and early pregnancy can reduce the risk of certain problems including NTD. It has been suggested that certain versions (polymorphisms) of some genes can increase the risk of conceiving a baby with DS. If this is the case, then people with DS may be more likely to carry these forms of these genes and to experience associated problems in folate metabolism. Studies to date have found conflicting results suggesting that these gene variants may be part of a more complex picture [111].

Treatment

DS has a variable physical expression but CHD, transient myelodysplasia of the newborn, and duodenal atresia are highly specific for this chromosomal disorder. Routine health maintenance is important because infants and children with DS are more likely to have otitis media, thyroid disease, congenital cataracts, leukemoid reactions, dental problems, and feeding difficulties. Since infants with this syndrome are prone to respiratory infections, immunization recommendations should be followed closely. Motor, language, social, and adaptive skills should be assessed at each office visit. The psychosocial aspects of care should be discussed with the parents of an infant with DS. If necessary the parents should be referred to family support and specialty resources. Institutionalization of infants with DS is now unlikely. With newer surgical techniques, early therapy to minimize developmental delay, and proper health supervision the functional prognosis for infants with DS is considerably improved [112].

A comprehensive systematic review provides no positive evidence that any combination of drugs, vitamins, and minerals enhance either cognitive function or psychomotor development in people with DS. However, because of the small number of subjects involved and the overall unsatisfactory quality of the trials an effect cannot be excluded at this point. At present there is no justification for the use of such regimes outside the context of large well designed trials. Parents of children with DS should be actively discouraged from giving these “miracle drugs” to their children [113].

In their role as committed advocates parents of children with DS have always sought alternative therapies mainly to enhance cognitive function but also to improve their appearance. Nutritional supplements have been the most frequent type of complementary and alternative therapy used. Cell therapy, plastic surgery, hormonal therapy, and a host of other therapies such as massage therapy have been used. There is a lack of well-designed scientific studies on the use of alternative therapies in individuals with DS. Antioxidants hold theoretical promise for treatment of the cognitive, immune, malignancy, and premature aging problems associated with DS. Medications for treatment of AD may also result in benefit for the population of individuals with DS [114].

Trisomy 21 is a common condition encountered by the pediatric surgeon. The surgical anomalies associated with DS now have treatment options that were previously considered futile. An effective surgical team approach to these children involves knowledge of the unique pathophysiology of trisomy 21 and an appreciation for the desires of the family and the needs of the child. Surgical techniques benefit children with DS equally as typical children. Pessimism regarding the outcome of surgical treatment of colorectal anomalies is fading with evidence of nearly equivalent outcomes. Several autoimmune disorders impact children with DS. Idiosyncratic susceptibility to infections and malignancy is noted. Unique anesthetic complications and aerodigestive tract disorders have been identified. Many anomalies have surgical options that enhance the quality of life. There is optimism in the surgical treatment of children with DS. Improved operations, better anesthetic management, and recognition of problems specific to the child with trisomy 21 make it safer and ethical to offer surgical solutions. Societal acceptance and mainstream participation are on the rise. The astute, compassionate pediatric surgeon does much to enhance the quality of life of these children and of the families who love them [115].

The number of people over the age of 60 years with lifelong developmental delays is predicted to double by 2030. DS is the most frequent chromosomal cause of developmental delays. As the life expectancy of people with DS increases, changes in body function and structure secondary to aging have the potential to lead to activity limitations and participation restrictions for this population. As individuals with DS age, a shift in emphasis from disability prevention to the prevention of conditions that lead to activity and participation limitations must occur. Exercise programs appear to have potential to positively affect the overall health of adults with DS thereby increasing the quality of life and years of healthy life for these individuals [116].

Although physical fitness has been suggested to improve physical and psychosocial health for a variety of population profiles, there is insufficient evidence to support improvement in physical or psychosocial outcomes of aerobic exercise in adults with DS. Although evidence exists which supports improvements in physiological and psychological aspects from strategies using mixed physical activity programmes, well-conducted research which examines long-term physical outcomes, adverse effects, psychosocial outcomes, and costs are required before informed practice decisions can be made [117].

Conclusion

DS remains one of the most common causes of MR. Although knowledge of pathogenesis remains incomplete, recent molecular biologic techniques have identified regions of the 21st chromosome critical for expression of the DS phenotype and animal models have helped elucidate the origins of the neurochemical and neuropathologic abnormalities. There also has been an improved understanding of the spectrum of medical complications of this disorder and the need for anticipatory management, including the search for atlanto-axial subluxation and hypothyroidism. With its increased risk of AD, DS is proving to be a useful model for studying aging. Accompanying greater knowledge has been improved functional outcome. Better medical care has made individuals with DS healthier, remaining at home through childhood has increased their cognitive function, and availability of increased numbers of group homes and supported employment opportunities has permitted the young adult with DS to live a more independent and full life. In this climate the role of the pediatrician in early intervention and anticipatory guidance cannot be overemphasized [118].

In the era of human functional genomics the chromosome 21 has represented a prototype for pioneering global biotechnologies. Its relatively low gene content enabled studying DS at the chromosomal scale for which the last years have seen intense research activity aiming at genotype-phenotype correlations. The global gene-dose dependent upregulation of gene expression seen in the context of trisomy and preliminary functional annotation of chromosome 21 genes points towards candidate genes and molecular pathways potentially associated with the cognitive defects observed in DS [119].

DS has been recognized as a clinical entity for about 150 years but it is only recently that there has been hope for the possibility to understand its pathogenesis and to use this information to devise approaches for the prevention and treatment of its numerous features. The earlier pessimism was due to several reasons including:

1) the nature of the genetic defect that leads to the syndrome;
2) the multiplicity of systems involved;
3) the high degree of variability of the phenotype.

However, science has now caught up with the problem and recent developments, especially in genetics, genomics, developmental biology, and neuroscience suggest that these potential impediments might not be as arduous as once appeared. As a result basic research on DS is now rapidly accelerating and there is hope that the findings will be translatable into benefit for people with DS [120].

Improved social and educational opportunities and access to informed healthcare are helping today's generations of people with DS to achieve more and live longer. This progress is bringing new challenges. Scientific research is steadily improving our understanding of the condition. Future improvements in the lives of people with DS will require multidisciplinary efforts and more applied or translational research with practical outcomes [121].

The discovery of cell-free fetal DNA and RNA in the maternal circulation has driven developments in non-invasive PD for the past decade. Detection of paternally derived alleles in cell-free fetal DNA is becoming well established. Now much interest is focusing on non-invasive PD of fetal chromosomal abnormalities such as trisomy 21 which is a considerable challenge because this demands accurate quantitative measurements of the amounts of specific cell-free fetal DNA or cell-free fetal RNA sequences in maternal blood samples.

Emerging strategies for distinguishing and quantifying the fetal nucleic acids in the maternal circulation promise continued development of the field and pose a number of unanswered questions [122].

Interest in cytogenetics may be traced to the development of the chromosomal theory of inheritance that emerged from efforts to provide the basis for Darwin's theory "On the origin of species by means of natural selection". Despite their fundamental place in biology chromosomes and genetics had little impact on medical practice until the 1960s. The discovery that a chromosomal defect caused DS was the spark responsible for the emergence of medical genetics as a clinical discipline. PD of trisomies, biochemical disorders, and NTD became possible and hence the proliferation of genetic counseling clinics. MSS for NTD and DS followed taking the new discipline into social medicine. Safe amniocentesis needed ultrasound and ultrasound soon found other applications in obstetrics including scanning for fetal malformations. Progress in medical genetics demanded a gene map and cytogeneticists initiated the mapping workshops that led to the human genome project and the complete sequence of the human genome. As a result conventional karyotyping has been augmented by molecular cytogenetics and molecular karyotyping has been achieved by microarrays. Genetic diagnosis at the level of the DNA sequence is with us at last. It has been a remarkable journey from disease phenotype to karyotype to genotype and it has taken < 50 years. Our mission now is to ensure that the recent advances such as prenatal screening, microarrays, and non-invasive PD are available to our patients. History shows that it is by increased use that costs are reduced and better methods discovered. Chromosome research has been behind the major advances in our field and it will continue to be the key to future progress, not least in our appreciation of chromosomal variation and its importance as a mechanism in Darwinian evolution [123].

References

[1] Roubertoux, PL; Kerdelhué, B. Trisomy 21: from chromosomes to mental retardation. *Behav Genet,* 2006 36, 346-354.

[2] Finley, WH; Finley, SC. The diagnosis of genetic disorders before birth. *South Med J,* 1976 69, 1486-1492.

[3] Epstein, CJ. Developmental genetics. *Experientia,* 1986 42, 1117-1128.

[4] Seashore, MR. Chromosomal abnormalities in the newborn period. *Semin Perinatol,* 1993 17, 312-317.

[5] Roizen, NJ; Patterson, D. Down's syndrome. *Lancet,* 2003 361, 1281-1289.

[6] American College of Obstetricians and Gynecologists Committee on Practice Bulletins – Obstetrics. ACOG Practice Bulletin. Clinical Management Guidelines for Obstetrician-Gynecologists. Prenatal diagnosis of fetal chromosomal abnormalities. *Obstet Gynecol,* 2001 97 suppl, 1-12.

[7] Sherman, SL; Allen, EG; Bean, LH; Freeman, SB. Epidemiology of Down syndrome. *Ment Retard Dev Disabil Res Rev,* 2007 13, 221-227.

[8] Mikkelsen, M. Epidemiology of trisomy 21: population, peri- and antenatal data. *Hum Genet Suppl,* 1981 2, 211-226.

[9] Hassold, TJ; Jacobs, PA. Trisomy in man. *Annu Rev Genet,* 1984 18, 69-97.

[10] Newberger, DS. Down syndrome: prenatal risk assessment and diagnosis. *Am Fam Physician,* 2000 62, 825-832.

[11] Gaulden, ME. Maternal age effect: the enigma of Down syndrome and other trisomic conditions. *Mutat Res,* 1992 296, 69-88.

[12] Warburton, D. Biological aging and the etiology of aneuploidy. *Cytogenet Genome Res,* 2005 111, 266-272.

[13] Rethoré, MO. Structural variation of chromosome 21 and symptoms of Down's syndrome. *Hum Genet Suppl,* 1981 2, 173-182.

[14] Shapiro, BL. Down syndrome – A disruption of homeostasis. *Am J Med Genet,* 1983 14, 241-269.

[15] Gearhart, JD; Oster-Granite, ML; Reeves, RH; Coyle, JT. Developmental consequences of autosomal aneuploidy in mammals. *Dev Genet,* 1987 8, 249-265.

[16] Epstein, CJ. The consequences of chromosome imbalance. *Am J Med Genet Suppl,* 1990 7, 31-37.

[17] Opitz, JM; Gilbert-Barness, EF. Reflections on the pathogenesis of Down syndrome. *Am J Med Genet Suppl,* 1990 7, 38-51.

[18] Annerén, G; Edman, B. Down syndrome – A gene dosage disease caused by trisomy of genes within a small segment of the long arm of chromosome 21, exemplified by the study of effects from the superoxide-dismutase type 1 (SOD-1) gene. *APMIS Suppl,* 1993 40, 71-79.

[19] Eichenlaub-Ritter, U. Parental age-related aneuploidy in human germ cells and offspring: a story of past and present. *Environ Mol Mutagen,* 1996 28, 211-236.

[20] Shapiro, BL. The Down syndrome critical region. *J Neural Transm Suppl,* 1999 57, 41-60.

[21] Pritchard, MA; Kola, I. The "gene dosage effect" hypothesis versus the "amplified developmental instability" hypothesis in Down syndrome. *J Neural Transm Suppl,* 1999 57, 293-303.

[22] Hassold, T; Sherman, S. Down syndrome: genetic recombination and the origin of the extra chromosome 21. *Clin Genet,* 2000 57, 95-100.

[23] Schon, EA; Kim, SH; Ferreira, JC; Magalhães, P; Grace, M; Warburton, D; Gross, SJ. Chromosomal non-disjunction in human oocytes: is there a mitochondrial connection? *Hum Reprod,* 2000 15, 160-72.

[24] Capone, GT. Down syndrome: advances in molecular biology and the neurosciences. *J Dev Behav Pediatr,* 2001 22, 40-59.

[25] Rehder, H. Pathology of trisomy 21 – With particular reference to persistent common atrioventricular canal of the heart. *Hum Genet Suppl,* 1981 2, 57-73.

[26] Pueschel, SM. Clinical aspects of Down syndrome from infancy to adulthood. *Am J Med Genet Suppl,* 1990 7, 52-56.

[27] Smith, DS. Health care management of adults with Down syndrome. *Am Fam Physician,* 2001 64, 1031-1038.

[28] Roizen, NJ. Medical care and monitoring for the adolescent with Down syndrome. *Adolesc Med,* 2002 13, 345-358.

[29] Satgé, D; Sommelet, D; Geneix, A; Nishi, M; Malet, P; Vekemans, M. A tumor profile in Down syndrome. *Am J Med Genet,* 1998 78, 207-216.

[30] Satgé, D; Bénard J. Carcinogenesis in Down syndrome: what can be learned from trisomy 21? *Semin Cancer Biol,* 2008 18, 365-371.

[31] Dixon, N; Kishnani, PS; Zimmerman, S. Clinical manifestations of hematologic and oncologic disorders in patients with Down syndrome. *Am J Med Genet C Semin Med Genet,* 2006 142C, 149-157.
[32] Gamis, AS. Acute myeloid leukemia and Down syndrome evolution of modern therapy – State of the art review. *Pediatr Blood Cancer,* 2005 44, 13-20.
[33] Ugazio, AG; Maccario, R; Notarangelo, LD; Burgio, GR. Immunology of Down syndrome: a review. *Am J Med Genet Suppl,* 1990 7, 204-212.
[34] Nespoli, L; Burgio, GR; Ugazio, AG; Maccario, R. Immunological features of Down's syndrome: a review. *J Intellect Disabil Res,* 1993 37, 543-551.
[35] Becker, L; Mito, T; Takashima, S; Onodera, K. Growth and development of the brain in Down syndrome. *Prog Clin Biol Res,* 1991 373, 133-152.
[36] Rachidi, M; Lopes, C. Mental retardation and associated neurological dysfunctions in Down syndrome: a consequence of dysregulation in critical chromosome 21 genes and associated molecular pathways. *Eur J Paediatr Neurol,* 2008 12, 168-182.
[37] Madan, V; Williams, J; Lear, JT. Dermatological manifestations of Down's syndrome. *Clin Exp Dermatol,* 2006 31, 623-629.
[38] Barankin, B; Guenther, L. Dermatological manifestations of Down's syndrome. *J Cutan Med Surg,* 2001 5, 289-293.
[39] Catalano, RA. Down syndrome. *Surv Ophthalmol,* 1990 34, 385-398.
[40] Shott, SR. Down syndrome: common otolaryngologic manifestations. *Am J Med Genet C Semin Med Genet,* 2006 142C, 131-140.
[41] Kanamori, G; Witter, M; Brown, J; Williams-Smith, L. Otolaryngologic manifestations of Down syndrome. *Otolaryngol Clin North Am,* 2000 33, 1285-1292.
[42] Gyves-Ray, K; Kirchner, S; Stein, S; Heller, R; Hernanz-Schulman, M. Cystic lung disease in Down syndrome. *Pediatr Radiol,* 1994 24, 137-138.
[43] Marino, B. Congenital heart disease in patients with Down's syndrome: anatomic and genetic aspects. *Biomed Pharmacother,* 1993 47, 197-200.
[44] Ardinger, RH Jr. Genetic counseling in congenital heart disease. *Pediatr Ann,* 1997 26, 99-104.
[45] Caird, MS; Wills, BP; Dormans, JP. Down syndrome in children: the role of the orthopaedic surgeon. *J Am Acad Orthop Surg,* 2006 14, 610-619.
[46] Mik, G; Gholve, PA; Scher, DM; Widmann, RF; Green, DW. Down syndrome: orthopedic issues. *Curr Opin Pediatr,* 2008 20, 30-36.
[47] Kieser, J; Townsend, G; Quick, A. The Down syndrome patient in dental practice, part I: Pathogenesis and general and dental features. *N Z Dent J,* 2003 99, 5-9.
[48] Reuland-Bosma, W; van Dijk, J. Periodontal disease in Down's syndrome: a review. *J Clin Periodontol,* 1986 13, 64-73.
[49] Levy, J. The gastrointestinal tract in Down syndrome. *Prog Clin Biol Res,* 1991 373, 245-256.
[50] Moore, SW. Down syndrome and the enteric nervous system. *Pediatr Surg Int,* 2008 24, 873-883.
[51] Kupferman, JC; Stewart, CL; Kaskel, FJ; Fine, RN. Posterior urethral valves in patients with Down syndrome. *Pediatr Nephrol,* 1996 10, 143-146.
[52] Mercer, ES; Broecker, B; Smith, EA; Kirsch, AJ; Scherz, HC; A Massad, C. Urological manifestations of Down syndrome. *J Urol,* 2004 171, 1250-1253.
[53] Mafrica, F; Schifilliti, D; Fodale, V. Pain in Down's syndrome. *ScientificWorldJournal,* 2006 6, 140-147.

[54] Santamaria, LB; Di Paola, C; Mafrica, F; Fodale, V. Preanesthetic evaluation and assessment of children with Down's syndrome. *ScientificWorldJournal,* 2007 7, 242-251.
[55] ACOG Committee on Practice Bulletins. ACOG Practice Bulletin No. 77: screening for fetal chromosomal abnormalities. *Obstet Gynecol,* 2007 109, 217-227.
[56] American College of Obstetricians and Gynecologists. ACOG Practice Bulletin No. 88, December 2007. Invasive prenatal testing for aneuploidy. *Obstet Gynecol,* 2007 110, 1459-1467.
[57] Donnenfeld, AE; Mennuti, MT. Sonographic findings in fetuses with common chromosome abnormalities. *Clin Obstet Gynecol,* 1988 31, 80-96.
[58] Blakemore, KJ. Prenatal diagnosis by chorionic villus sampling. *Obstet Gynecol Clin North Am,* 1988 15, 179-213.
[59] Benn, PA. Advances in prenatal screening for Down syndrome: I. general principles and second trimester testing. *Clin Chim Acta,* 2002 323, 1-16.
[60] Wald, NJ; Kennard, A; Hackshaw, A; McGuire, A. Antenatal screening for Down's syndrome. *J Med Screen,* 1997 4, 181-246.
[61] Wald, NJ; Kennard, A. Prenatal biochemical screening for Down's syndrome and neural tube defects. *Curr Opin Obstet Gynecol,* 1992 4, 302-307.
[62] Ndumbe, FM; Navti, O; Chilaka, VN; Konje, JC. Prenatal diagnosis in the first trimester of pregnancy. *Obstet Gynecol Surv,* 2008 63, 317-328.
[63] ACOG Committee Opinion #296: first-trimester screening for fetal aneuploidy. *Obstet Gynecol,* 2004 104, 215-217.
[64] Benn, PA. Advances in prenatal screening for Down syndrome: II first trimester testing, integrated testing, and future directions. *Clin Chim Acta,* 2002 324, 1-11.
[65] Iles, RK. Urinary analysis for Down's syndrome: is the measurement of urinary beta-core the future of biochemical screening for Down's syndrome. *Early Hum Dev,* 1996 47 Suppl, S41-S45.
[66] Benacerraf, BR. The second-trimester fetus with Down syndrome: detection using sonographic features. *Ultrasound Obstet Gynecol,* 1996 7, 147-155.
[67] Egan, JF. The role of ultrasound in screening for fetal Down syndrome. *Curr Womens Health Rep,* 2002 2, 52-58.
[68] Shipp, TD; Benacerraf, BR. Second trimester ultrasound screening for chromosomal abnormalities. *Prenat Diagn,* 2002 22, 296-307.
[69] Benacerraf, BR. The role of the second trimester genetic sonogram in screening for fetal Down syndrome. *Semin Perinatol,* 2005 29, 386-394.
[70] Lockwood, CJ; Lynch, L; Berkowitz, RL. Ultrasonographic screening for the Down syndrome fetus. *Am J Obstet Gynecol,* 1991 165, 349-352.
[71] Norton, ME. Biochemical and ultrasound screening for chromosomal abnormalities. *Semin Perinatol,* 1994 18, 256-265.
[72] Drugan, A; Johnson, MP; Evans, MI. Ultrasound screening for fetal chromosome anomalies. *Am J Med Genet,* 2000 90, 98-107.
[73] Vintzileos, AM; Egan, JF. Adjusting the risk for trisomy 21 on the basis of second-trimester ultrasonography. *Am J Obstet Gynecol,* 1995 172, 837-844.
[74] Nyberg, DA; Souter, VL. Sonographic markers of fetal trisomies: second trimester. *J Ultrasound Med,* 2001 20, 655-674.
[75] Nyberg, DA; Souter, VL. Use of genetic sonography for adjusting the risk for fetal Down syndrome. *Semin Perinatol,* 2003 27, 130-144.

[76] Graupe, MH; Naylor, CS; Greene, NH; Carlson, DE; Platt, L. Trisomy 21. Second-trimester ultrasound. *Clin Perinatol,* 2001 28, 303-319.
[77] Yeo, L; Vintzileos, AM. The use of genetic sonography to reduce the need for amniocentesis in women at high-risk for Down syndrome. *Semin Perinatol,* 2003 27, 152-159.
[78] DeVore, GR. The role of fetal echocardiography in genetic sonography. *Semin Perinatol,* 2003 27, 160-172.
[79] Getz, L; Kirkengen, AL. Ultrasound screening in pregnancy: advancing technology, soft markers for fetal chromosomal aberrations, and unacknowledged ethical dilemmas. *Soc Sci Med,* 2003 56, 2045-2057.
[80] Budorick, NE; O'Boyle, MK. Prenatal diagnosis for detection of aneuploidy: the options. *Radiol Clin North Am,* 2003 41, 695-708.
[81] Stewart, TL. Screening for aneuploidy: the genetic sonogram. *Obstet Gynecol Clin North Am,* 2004 31, 21-33.
[82] Bahado-Singh, RO; Oz, UA; Mendilcioglu, I; Mahoney, MJ. The mid-trimester genetic sonogram. *Semin Perinatol,* 2005 29, 209-214.
[83] Souter, VL; Nyberg, DA. Sonographic screening for fetal aneuploidy: first trimester. *J Ultrasound Med,* 2001 20, 775-790.
[84] Said, S; Malone, FD. The use of nuchal translucency in contemporary obstetric practice. *Clin Obstet Gynecol,* 2008 51, 37-47.
[85] Nicolaides, KH; Heath, V; Cicero, S. Increased fetal nuchal translucency at 11-14 weeks. *Prenat Diagn,* 2002 22, 308-315.
[86] Nicolaides, KH. Nuchal translucency and other first-trimester sonographic markers of chromosomal abnormalities. *Am J Obstet Gynecol,* 2004 191, 45-67.
[87] Witters, I; Fryns, JR. Fetal nuchal translucency thickness. *Genet Couns,* 2007 18, 1-7.
[88] Filkins, K; Koos, BJ. Ultrasound and fetal diagnosis. *Curr Opin Obstet Gynecol,* 2005 17, 185-195.
[89] Hyett, J; Thilaganathan, B. First trimester screening for fetal abnormalities. *Curr Opin Obstet Gynecol,* 1999 11, 563-569.
[90] Matias, A; Montenegro, N; Blickstein, I. Down syndrome screening in multiple pregnancies. *Obstet Gynecol Clin North Am,* 2005 32, 81-96.
[91] Maymon, R; Neeman, O; Shulman, A; Rosen, H; Herman A. Current concepts of Down syndrome screening tests in assisted reproduction twin pregnancies: another double trouble. *Prenat Diagn,* 2005 25, 746-750.
[92] Borruto, F; Comparetto, C; Acanfora, L; Bertini, G; Rubaltelli, FF. Role of ultrasound evaluation of nuchal translucency in prenatal diagnosis. *Clin Exp Obstet Gynecol,* 2002 29, 235-241.
[93] Hahn, S; Zhong, XY; Holzgreve, W. Recent progress in non-invasive prenatal diagnosis. *Semin Fetal Neonatal Med,* 2008 13, 57-62.
[94] Bianchi, DW. Prenatal diagnosis by analysis of fetal cells in maternal blood. *J Pediatr,* 1995 127, 847-856.
[95] Pertl, B; Bianchi, DW. Fetal DNA in maternal plasma: emerging clinical applications. *Obstet Gynecol,* 2001 98, 483-490.
[96] Bischoff, FZ; Sinacori, MK; Dang, DD; Marquez-Do, D; Horne, C; Lewis, DE; Simpson, JL. Cell-free fetal DNA and intact fetal cells in maternal blood circulation: implications for first and second trimester non-invasive prenatal diagnosis. *Hum Reprod Update,* 2002 8, 493-500.

[97] Fan, HC; Quake, SR. Detection of aneuploidy with digital polymerase chain reaction. *Anal Chem,* 2007 79, 7576-7579.
[98] Wataganara, T; Bianchi, DW. Fetal cell-free nucleic acids in the maternal circulation: new clinical applications. *Ann N Y Acad Sci,* 2004 1022, 90-99.
[99] Avent, ND; Plummer, ZE; Madgett, TE; Maddocks, DG; Soothill, PW. Post-genomics studies and their application to non-invasive prenatal diagnosis. *Semin Fetal Neonatal Med,* 2008 13, 91-98.
[100] Palomaki, GE. Down's syndrome epidemiology and risk estimation. *Early Hum Dev,* 1996 47 Suppl, S19-S26.
[101] Knight, GJ. Quality assessment of a prenatal screening program. *Early Hum Dev,* 1996 47 Suppl, S49-S53.
[102] Cuckle, H. Integrating antenatal Down's syndrome screening. *Curr Opin Obstet Gynecol,* 2001 13, 175-181.
[103] Caughey, AB. Cost-effectiveness analysis of prenatal diagnosis: methodological issues and concerns. *Gynecol Obstet Invest,* 2005 60, 11-18.
[104] Sharma, G; McCullough, LB; Chervenak, FA. Ethical considerations of early (first vs. second trimester) risk assessment disclosure for trisomy 21 and patient choice in screening versus diagnostic testing. *Am J Med Genet C Semin Med Genet,* 2007 145C, 99-104.
[105] Kessler, S. Psychological aspects of genetic counseling: VI. A critical review of the literature dealing with education and reproduction. *Am J Med Genet,* 1989 34, 340-353.
[106] Dahl, K; Kesmodel, U; Hvidman, L; Olesen, F. Informed consent: providing information about prenatal examinations. *Acta Obstet Gynecol Scand,* 2006 85, 1420-1425.
[107] ACOG educational bulletin. Maternal serum screening. Number 228, September 1996 (replaces no. 154, April 1991). Committee on Educational Bulletins of the American College of Obstetricians and Gynecologists. *Int J Gynaecol Obstet,* 1996 55, 299-308.
[108] American Academy of Pediatrics. Committee on Genetics. American Academy of Pediatrics: Health supervision for children with Down syndrome. *Pediatrics,* 2001 107, 442-449.
[109] Rosas-Blum, E; Shirsat, P; Leiner, M. Communicating genetic information: a difficult challenge for future pediatricians. *BMC Med Educ,* 2007 7, 17.
[110] Reading, CM. Down's syndrome: nutritional intervention. *Nutr Health,* 1984 3, 91-111.
[111] Patterson, D. Folate metabolism and the risk of Down syndrome. *Downs Syndr Res Pract,* 2008 12, 93-97.
[112] Saenz, RB. Primary care of infants and young children with Down syndrome. *Am Fam Physician,* 1999 59, 381-390.
[113] Salman, M. Systematic review of the effect of therapeutic dietary supplements and drugs on cognitive function in subjects with Down syndrome. *Eur J Paediatr Neurol,* 2002 6, 213-219.
[114] Roizen, NJ. Complementary and alternative therapies for Down syndrome. *Ment Retard Dev Disabil Res Rev,* 2005 11, 149-155.
[115] Allshouse, MJ. Trisomy 21 and the pediatric surgeon. *Curr Opin Pediatr,* 2006 18, 298-304.
[116] Barnhart, RC; Connolly, B. Aging and Down syndrome: implications for physical therapy. *Phys Ther,* 2007 87, 1399-1406.

[117] Andriolo, RB; El Dib, RP; Ramos, LR. Aerobic exercise training programmes for improving physical and psychosocial health in adults with Down syndrome. *Cochrane Database Syst Rev,* 2005 3, CD005176.
[118] Hayes, A; Batshaw, ML. Down syndrome. *Pediatr Clin North Am,* 1993 40, 523-535.
[119] Kahlem, P. Gene-dosage effect on chromosome 21 transcriptome in trisomy 21: implication in Down syndrome cognitive disorders. *Behav Genet,* 2006 36, 416-428.
[120] Antonarakis, SE; Epstein, CJ. The challenge of Down syndrome. *Trends Mol Med,* 2006 12, 473-479.
[121] Buckley, F. New and old directions. *Downs Syndr Res Pract,* 2007 12, 1-4.
[122] Puszyk, WM; Crea, F; Old, RW. Noninvasive prenatal diagnosis of aneuploidy using cell-free nucleic acids in maternal blood: promises and unanswered questions. *Prenat Diagn,* 2008 28, 1-6.
[123] Ferguson-Smith, MA. Cytogenetics and the evolution of medical genetics. Genet Med, 2008 10, 553-559.

In: Handbook of Down Syndrome Research
Editors: Dominicus Jelinek and Gijs Dvorak
ISBN 978-1-60741- 690-6

Chapter 2

Gene Expression Regulation in Down Syndrome: Dosage Imbalance Effects at Transcriptome and Proteome Levels

Mohammed Rachidi*[*1,2] *and Carmela Lopes [1,2,3]
[1]Molecular Genetics of Human Diseases (GMMH), BP 130228, F-98717 Punaauia, Tahiti, French Polynesia
[2]Laboratory of Genetic dysregulation models: Trisomy 21 and Hyperhomocysteinemia, EA 3508, University Paris 7-Denis Diderot, Paris, France
[3]University of French Polynesia, Dept of Sciences, Tahiti, French Polynesia

Abstract

Trisomy of human chromosome 21 (HSA21) is the most frequent genetic cause of mental retardation and other phenotypic abnormalities, including developmental defects, hematological and solid tissue malignancies, heart and cranio-facial abnormalities, cognitive impairment and Alzheimer's disease, collectively known as Down syndrome. The expression of these characteristic features is due to the dosage imbalance of HSA21 genes.

DNA sequencing of HSA21 and gene annotation improve identification of the gene products. These sequencing data and the development of molecular analysis tools allow large-scale application of gene expression analysis. Genotype/phenotype correlation, transcriptome, proteome and functional genomics studies have shown genetic program perturbation by gene-dosage effects caused by trisomy of HSA21. The elevated gene expression, that is especially critical in Down syndrome, is a product of genetic effects on different cells, structures, and functions throughout development, many of which may have cascading effects to produce clinically observed phenotypic end points in a given individual with trisomy 21. The developmental regulated expression of trisomic genes and their downstream effects, direct and indirect, on the expression of other genes is

[*] Corresponding author: Mohammed RACHIDI, Molecular Genetics of Human Diseases (GMMH), BP 130228, F-98717 Punaauia, Tahiti, French Polynesia. Email: mrachidi2@yahoo.fr.

linked to phenotypic consequences, not only in fully differentiated cells, but also at all stages where euploid and trisomic developmental processes diverge.

The important contribution of the molecular biology of understanding the molecular mechanisms underlying Down syndrome becomes of the most interest in the molecular medicine and provides potential directions for clinical therapeutics.

1. Developmental Effects of Trisomy 21 and Down Syndrome

Down syndrome is a collection of features that are caused by trisomy for human chromosome 21 (HSA21) affecting 1 in 700 live births (LeJeune et al., 1959). The incidence of most clinical phenotypes seen in Down syndrome is variable and the severity of a given feature is highly variable. This clinical presentation is complex that occurs to some degree in every individual, includes hypotonia, characteristic facial dysmorphology, skeletal traits, dermatoglyphic features, cardiac, intestinal, immunological and endocrinological defects, neurological alterations and mental retardation (Roizen and Patterson, 2003). In addition to this complex phenotype, trisomy 21 is also a risk factor for a number of diseases. The incidence of congenital heart disease (Ferencz et al., 1989), the atherosclerosis (Murdoch et al., 1977; Yla-Herttuala et al., 1989), the leukaemia and the Hirschsprung disease are significantly elevated in individuals with trisomy 21, and metabolic diseases are also observed including a higher frequency of diabetes and obesity (Puffenberger et al, 1994; Epstein, 1995; Cohen, 1999).

Among these features, only two are constantly observed: mental retardation (Jackson et al., 1976; Epstein CJ 1993) and the neuropathological modifications (in persons with Down syndrome over 35 years of age) identical to those observed in the brains of patients with Alzheimer's disease (Wisniewski et al., 1985; Berg et al., 1993).

Compared to others trisomies resulting in prenatal loss, such as trisomy 13 (1/7000) or trisomy 18 (1/3500), the high frequency of postnatal survival for trisomy 21 (1/700) is thought to be principally a function of the small number of genes on HSA21, the smallest and least gene-dense of the autosomes.

The HSA21 complete sequence (Hattori et al., 2000; International Human Genome Sequencing Consortium, 2004), the gene annotation improvement, the development of molecular analysis tools, and the identification of the gene products allow whole genome approaches of gene expression studies. Transcriptome studies are performed by quantitative RT-PCR (qRT-PCR), microarrays and Serial Analysis of Gene Expression (SAGE), to investigate gene expression variation in trisomic tissues compared to the euploid ones using human tissues and cell lines (FitzPatrick et al., 2002; Mao et al., 2003; Giannone et al., 2004; Malago et al., 2005; Mao et al., 2005; Deutsch et al., 2005; Li et al., 2006; Prandini et al., 2007; Ait Yahya-Graison et al., 2007; Chou et al., 2008). Transcriptome studies of the brain, the cerebellum or neuronal cell lines are particularly abundant, considering their major interest in the understanding of the molecular mechanisms involved in mental retardation pathogenesis in Down syndrome (Chrast et al., 2000a; Mao et al., 2003; Saran et al., 2003;

Amano et al., 2004; Wang et al., 2004; Kahlem et al., 2004; Lyle et al., 2004; Mao et al., 2005; Dauphinot et al., 2005; Potier et al., 2006; Sultan et al., 2007).

While elevated expression of mRNA transcript levels of these HSA21 genes is primarily responsible of the characteristic phenotypic overabundance, it is likely that multiple genetic mechanisms underlie the numerous ways in which development and function diverge in individuals with trisomy 21 compared to euploid individuals.

Defining the etiology of genetic mechanisms in Down syndrome requires knowledge of the trisomic genes, their expression patterns in time and space, their developmental regulated expression and their downstream effects, direct and indirect, on the expression of other genes. This information must be linked to a precise description of phenotypic consequences, not only in fully differentiated cells, but also at all stages where euploid and trisomic developmental processes diverge.

Our current progress in gene expression studies presented herein, including gene expression, transcriptome and proteome studies in human and mouse models of Down syndrome, represent a central challenge of genetic research to define and correlate the direct genotype-phenotype effects of trisomic gene expression on development and function. We explain also the impact of elevated gene expression that is especially critical in Down syndrome, which is a product of genetic effects on different cells, structures, and functions throughout development, many of which may have cascading effects to produce clinically observed phenotypic end points in a given individual with trisomy 21.

Studies of variation of gene expression and its genomic regulation/control, and functional studies of these genes and other conserved DNA elements are two fundamental research priorities. An important effort could be also concentrated on the microRNAs of the human chromosome 21 to elucidate their biological role in Down syndrome, because it has been demonstrated recently that microRNAs show an increasing importance in the gene expression control and have been shown to play a fundamental role in diverse biological and pathological processes, including cell proliferation, differentiation, apoptosis, carcinogenesis, and cardiovascular disease (Bushati and Cohen, 2007; Wang et al., 2007).

Considering the hypothesis that trisomic 21 gene dosage overexpression of HSA21-derived miRNAs results in the decreased expression of specific target proteins and contributes, in part, to features of the neuronal and cardiac Down syndrome phenotype; HSA21-derived microRNAs may provide novel therapeutic targets in the treatment of individuals with Down syndrome (Kuhn et al., 2008).

2. Gene Dosage Imbalance in Down Syndrome: Transcriptomic and Proteomic Effects

Down syndrome results of an extra-copy of chromosome 21 in all cells of the afflicted individuals (LeJeune et al., 1959). The most commonly accepted hypothesis for the molecular origins of Down syndrome is that the extra-copy of HSA21 genes contributes to Down syndrome phenotypes (Antonarakis, 1998). This pathology results neither from a gene deletion, point mutation, chimerism, transposable element insertion, or triple repeat expansion, but rather from the overdosage of genes on chromosome 21 and that could be responsible for the complex phenotype in Down syndrome patients.

A central question of genetic research in Down syndrome is to define the specific phenotypes, which results from complex genetic effects on different tissues and functions during development. Other fundamental question is to identify the genes involved in Down syndrome phenotypes and to determine their individual role in these specific phenotypes.

2.1. Primary and Secondary Gene Effects

The 1.5-fold increase in the dosage of genes on the trisomic chromosome 21 may determine a primary effect on gene expression consisting in a 1.5 fold increase of expression level. Nevertheless, genes on the trisomic chromosome 21 coding transcription factors, scaffold proteins and other proteins that can directly or indirectly influence gene expression, could produce a secondary genome-wide transcriptional downstream misregulation. This secondary effect of the chromosomal imbalance, which may consist in gene overexpression different than 1.5-fold, and also in down-regulation, is complex and highly variable in the different cells and during lifespan. Moreover, the secondary effect can concern genes located on both chromosome 21 and the other chromosomes (Epstein, 1986; 1988; FitzPatrick, 2005).

On chromosome 21, gene expression may also be regulated by dosage compensation or other mechanisms such that only a subset of those genes is expressed at the expected 1.5 fold. The indirect effects on genes located on other chromosomes are widely used in antenatal screening programs for trisomy 21, which detect abnormal levels of fetal proteins in maternal serum. Although, the genes encoding alpha-fetoprotein and chorionic gonadotrophin map to 4q11–13 and 19q13, respectively, the level of alpha-fetoprotein is reduced (Newby et al., 1997), while human chorionic gonadotrophin is increased (Aitken et al., 1993), in trisomy 21. In addition, the effects of three copies of a gene may be even more complex at the protein level, as additional regulatory points are introduced, such as post-translational modifications that can alter the function or stability of the protein.

The global effect of the gene over-dosage can produce complex effects by direct and indirect mechanisms to produce a specific and morbid effect on development and on adult functions. However, to explain the highly variable phenotypes in trisomic adults directly with the presence of three copies of individual genes appears to be simplistic. The initial genetic insult determines a trisomy-induced alteration of the phenotype in one cell can cause concomitant changes in gene expression in downstream cells. The changes in secondarily affected cells are undoubtedly a result of aneuploidy, but could represent a perfectly normal response, in terms of gene expression, to the signals received from the first, directly affected cell.

The variability of the Down syndrome phenotypes may be determined directly from the overexpression of human chromosome 21 gene products or indirectly from the interaction of these human chromosome 21 gene products with the whole genome, transcriptome and proteome.

2.2. Transcriptomic Effects in Down Syndrome

The overdosage of HSA21 genes determines gene expression variation that can be responsible for the complex Down syndrome phenotype. The expression studies in normal and trisomic tissues contribute to understanding the role of the HSA21 genes and the contribution of their dosage alterations in Down syndrome pathogenesis, allowing the identification of HSA21 genes potentially involved in a given Down syndrome phenotype. In this way, a gene expressed in developing and/or adult brain, particularly when its transcription is restricted to key brain regions involved in cognitive functions may be a good candidate gene for mental retardation in Down syndrome.

The complete HSA21sequence (Hattori et al., 2000; International Human Genome Sequencing Consortium, 2004), gene annotation improvement, the development of molecular analysis tools, and the identification of gene products, allow whole genome approaches to the molecular biology of chromosome 21 genes, in combination with comparison studies of the variation in their genotype, expression, and function in the normal population and in Down syndrome individuals, with well-characterized phenotypic traits.

Transcriptome studies are performed by quantitative RT-PCR (qRT-PCR), microarrays and Serial Analysis of Gene Expression (SAGE), to study gene expression variation in trisomic tissues compared to the euploid ones using human tissues and cell lines (FitzPatrick et al., 2002; Mao et al., 2003; Giannone et al., 2004; Malago et al., 2005; Mao et al., 2005; Deutsch et al., 2005; Li et al., 2006; Prandini et al., 2007; Ait Yahya-Graison et al., 2007; Chou et al., 2008), or mouse trisomic model tissues (Chrast et al., 2000a; Saran et al., 2003; Amano et al., 2004; Kahlem et al., 2004; Lyle et al. 2004; Wang et al., 2004; Dauphinot et al., 2005; Potier et al., 2006; Sultan et al., 2007). Interestingly, transcriptome studies of the brain, the cerebellum or neuronal cell lines are particularly abundant, considering their major interest in the understanding of the molecular mechanisms involved in mental retardation pathogenesis in Down syndrome (Chrast et al., 2000a; Mao et al., 2003; Saran et al., 2003; Amano et al., 2004; Wang et al., 2004; Kahlem et al., 2004; Lyle et al., 2004; Mao et al., 2005; Dauphinot et al., 2005; Potier et al., 2006; Sultan et al., 2007).

These works demonstrated that transcript levels are elevated about 1.5-fold for the majority of trisomic genes in human trisomic tissues and across a broad range of tissues of trisomic mouse models (Epstein, 1986; FitzPatrick et al., 2002; Mao et al., 2003; Kahlem et al., 2004; Lyle et al., 2004; Amano et al., 2004; Wang et al., 2004; Dauphinot et al., 2005; Mao et al., 2005; Potier et al., 2006; Prandini et al., 2007; Sultan et al., 2007; Ait Yahya-Graison et al. 2007). These results indicate that the triplicated genes are overexpressed in a dosage-dependent manner, supporting the hypothesis that a global HSA21 dosage imbalance causes the heterogeneous phenotypes of Down syndrome (Shapiro, 1983; 1997). Moreover, the overexpression of a limited number of genes on HSA21 could also be responsible for the Down syndrome phenotypic features (Korenberg et al., 1990).

There is not always a direct correlation between genomic imbalance and not all genes are overexpressed ~1.5-fold compared to euploid (Saran et al., 2003; Lyle et al., 2004; Kahlem et al., 2004; Dauphinot et al., 2005; Potier et al., 2006; Ait Yahya-Graison et al. 2007), and a decreased expression is also found for some genes, such as Ets2 (Greber-Platzer et al., 1999; Engidawork and Lubec, 2003; Wang et al., 2004), HMGN1 (Engidawork and Lubec, 2003), and CCT8 (Engidawork and Lubec, 2003), DSCR3 (Engidawork and Lubec, 2003), GRIK1 (Saran et al., 2003), and SOD1 (Engidawork and Lubec, 2003; Wang et al., 2004). For these dysregulated genes, the initial overexpression of genes from the aneuploid chromosome was modified by subtle compensatory mechanisms to the gene-dosage effect that may, in turn, result in the extensive variability of the phenotype that characterizes Down syndrome (Lyle et al., 2004; Kahlem et al., 2004; Dauphinot et al., 2005).

In human and Down syndrome mouse models, some euploid genes showed also a differential expression (over or under-expression) (Chrast et al. 2000; Bahn et al. 2002; FitzPatrick et al., 2002; Mao et al. 2003; Saran et al. 2003; Mao et al., 2005; Dauphinot et al., 2005; Potier et al., 2006). These findings support a model of a subtle primary upregulation of genes on the trisomic chromosome resulting in a more generalized secondary transcriptional misregulation (FitzPatrick et al., 2002). Evaluation of difference of gene expression in two independent experiments suggests that the global perturbation includes a significant stochastic component. In this way, the dosage imbalance of 124 genes in Ts65Dn mouse model of Down syndrome alters the expression of thousands of genes to create a variable trisomic transcriptome (Saran et al., 2003).

Nevertheless, expression studies have been found that the expression variation for a given gene can change in the different tissues, including brain, (Rachidi et al., 2000; 2005a; 2006; Saran et al., 2003; Lyle et al., 2004; Kahlem et al., 2004; Dauphinot et al., 2005; Mao et al., 2005; Sultan et al., 2007) and during developmental stages (Rachidi et al., 2000; 2005a; 2006; Dauphinot et al., 2005; Potier et al., 2006; Sultan et al., 2007), suggesting tissue- and cell-specific changes of gene expression in trisomy 21 during fetal development of human and mouse models of Down syndrome.

Quantitative differences in gene expression have been proposed to explain variation in natural populations, participating to the evolution and contributing to phenotypic diversity (King and Wilson, 1975). Several studies indicate that variation in gene expression levels within and among populations is abundant, with significant inter-individual variation (Oleksiak et al., 2002; Brem et al., 2002; Schadt et al., 2003; Cheung et al., 2003) and most of the differentially expressed genes had significant heritability (Brem et al., 2002; Yvert et al., 2003; Monks et al., 2004; Morley et al., 2004; Storey et al., 2007; Spielman et al., 2007). This inter-individual gene expression variation has also been found for HSA21 genes in Down syndrome (FitzPatrick et al., 2002; Deutsch et al., 2005; Stranger et al., 2005; Sultan et al., 2007; Prandini et al., 2007; Ait Yahya-Graison et al. 2007) and significant eQTLs have been identified. In particular, a cis-eQTL was identified for CCT8 corresponding to a single nucleotide polymorphism (SNP) located within cis-regulatory region of CCT8 (Deutsch et al., 2005). These findings support the model in which the variability of phenotypic manifestations of trisomy 21 is a threshold effect of expression of HSA21 genes that show variable levels of expression in the population (Antonarakis et al., 2004). Based on this variation in gene expression observed among normal individuals, it has been predicted that for many HSA21 genes there is a considerable overlap in total expression levels between normal and trisomy 21 individuals due to allelic variation (Deutsch et al., 2005; Sultan et al., 2007; Prandini et al., 2007; Ait Yahya-Graison et al. 2007).

The expression variations can explain the differences in the penetrance and variability of the Down syndrome phenotypes. The overexpressed genes, showing low levels of expression variation, would be predicted to lead to the more penetrant phenotypes. In contrast, genes with high variation in expression would contribute to incompletely penetrant/variable Down syndrome -related phenotypes (Deutsch et al., 2005; Prandini et al., 2007; Sultan et al., 2007; Ait Yahya-Graison et al. 2007). Moreover, the existence of expression variations suggest caution in the analyses of the gene expression changes, particularly for low variation ratios (less than 2 fold), because of overlapping of gene expression variation in Down syndrome and normal individuals in this variation interval (Deutsch et al., 2005; Sultan et al., 2007; Prandini et al., 2007; Ait Yahya-Graison et al. 2007).

A recent study of inter-individual gene expression variations between HSA21 genes in trisomic and normal cell lines showed a global gene dosage-dependent expression of chromosome 21 genes whether the RNAs are pooled. In contrast, when inter-individual gene expression variations were analyzed, most of the HSA21 genes results compensated for the gene-dosage effect (Ait Yahya-Graison et al., 2007). This suggests that overexpressed genes are likely to be involved in Down syndrome phenotypes, in contrast to the compensated genes. Interestingly, it has been found a group of euploid genes showing greater expression variance in human trisomy 21 tissues than in euploid tissues, and that the number of euploid genes with elevated variance was significantly higher in Down syndrome tissues than in the euploid tissues (Chou et al., 2008) suggesting that the gene imbalance determined a more generalized instability in the transcriptional regulation.

Recently, new aspects of gene expression acquire more importance in Down syndrome studies with the discovery of new transcripts, the microRNAs (miRNAs) that play a role in gene expression regulation. The miRNAs are small, non-protein coding RNAs that link specific mRNA targets and leads to translational repression or mRNA cleavage (Bartel, 2004; Bushati and Cohen, 2007; Wang et al., 2007). These miRNAs have been shown to play a fundamental role in diverse biological and pathological processes, including cell proliferation, differentiation, apoptosis, carcinogenesis, and cardiovascular disease (Bushati and Cohen, 2007; Wang et al., 2007), and it has been demonstrated that each miRNA can potentially regulate a large number of protein-coding genes, and many miRNAs can act in combination to regulate the same target genes (Bushati and Cohen, 2007; Wang et al., 2007).

Recent bioinformatic studies demonstrate that HSA21 harbors five miRNA genes: miR-99a, let-7c, miR-125b-2, miR-155, and miR-802 (Kuhn et al., 2008). Interestingly, HSA21 miRNA expression analyses demonstrate that they are overexpressed in fetal brain and heart specimens from individuals with Down syndrome when compared with controls (Sethupathy et al., 2007; Kuhn et al., 2008). Some miRNAs, located on other chromosome than HSA21, have been found overexpressed or under-expressed in hippocampus specimens from individuals with Down syndrome when compared to controls (Kuhn et al., 2008). The overexpression of the five HSA21 miRNAs in Down syndrome individuals may result in the aberrant expression of a large number of proteins in a variety of tissues. The inhibition or knock-down of these miRNAs should normalize the expression level of all miRNA/mRNA targets back to non-trisomic 21 levels, suggesting that HSA21 miRNAs may provide new therapeutic targets in the treatment of individuals with Down syndrome.

2.3. Proteomic Effects in Down Syndrome

The molecular effects of the 1.5 gene overdosage may be even more complex at the protein level, as additional regulatory points are introduced, such as post-transcriptional, translational and post-translational regulations and post-translational modifications. Modification in the levels of proteins involved in multicomplex protein formation, in protein-protein interactions and in metabolic and regulatory networks can determine alterations in these interactions because of the loss of the correct ratio among the proteins and, finally, can alter the function or stability of the proteins. The determination of protein levels changes, that not always correspond to the quantity of the corresponding mRNAs, in Down syndrome cells, is also necessary to understand the real genotype/phenotype correlation operating in Down syndrome pathogenesis.

In initial studies, some level changes in individual or small number of proteins were identified. Among the proteins encoded on HSA21, COL6A1, was decreased in Down syndrome tissues compared to the normal tissues (Engidawork et al., 2001a), while HMG14 (Epstein, 2001), S100B (Griffin et al., 1998), carbonyl reductase (Balcz et al., 2001), and synaptojanin (Arai et al., 2002) were increased in Down syndrome tissues compared to the normal tissues. Some proteins encoded on other chromosomes than HSA21 also show level changes: EF1A1 and EF2 (Freidl et al., 2001), ATP-sensitive potassium channels (Kim and Lubec, 2001), synaptosomal associated protein 25 subunits, drebrin, nucleoside diphosphate kinase B, Rab GDP-dissociation inhibitor beta subunit, histidine triad nucleotide-binding protein (Weitzdoerfer et al., 2001), and stathmin (Cheon et al., 2001) were decreased in Down syndrome tissues compared to the normal tissues, while alcohol dehydrogenase (Balcz et al., 2001) and nicotinic acetylcholine receptor beta 2 subunits were found increased in Down syndrome tissues compared to the normal tissues (Engidawork et al., 2001b).

The analysis of expression levels of 31 proteins encoded on HSA21 (Cheon et al., 2003a; 2003b; 2003c; 2003d; Ferrando-Miguel et al. 2004) showed that only three proteins have different expression levels in Down syndrome compared to controls: Hematopoietic adapter containing Src homology 3 domain and sterile α motifs (HACS1) was decreased in Down syndrome, compared to controls (Cheon et al., 2003b); Synaptojanin-1 was increased in Down syndrome, compared to controls (Cheon et al., 2003c); and DSCR5 (PIG-P), a component of glycosylphosphatidylinositol-N-acetylglucosaminyltransferase (GPI-GnT), was overexpressed about 2-fold in Down syndrome, compared to controls (Ferrando-Miguel et al. 2004).

Other proteomic approaches, using 2D-gel electrophoresis, identified 11 proteins, among the 49 proteins analyzed, that are deregulated in cerebral cortex of fetal Down syndrome, none of which encoded on HSA21 (Engidawork et al., 2003). Using the same approach, Kadota and co-workers (2004) have used an *in vitro* neuronal differentiation system of mouse ES cells containing a single human chromosome 21 (TT2F/hChr21) (Shinohara et al., 2001), using TT2F parental ES cells as a control. This allows the identification of only 18 proteins with significantly altered levels, including SOD1 and CCT8, which are encoded on HSA21 (Kadota et al., 2004). Among the other 16 proteins, they found matrix and structural proteins, heat shock/stress proteins, protein or translational regulators, nuclear transcriptional factors, and enzymes for energy and macromolecular metabolism (Kadota et al., 2004). Between these 16 proteins encoded on other human chromosomes, the authors identified seven proteins that were over-expressed: Protein subunits Atp6v1a1 and Atp6v1b2 of the vacuolar ATPase proton pump, which mediate acidification of intracellular organelles for energy production and convention, actin- (T-plastin and Vil2), filament- (Krt2– 8) and phospholipid- (Anxa4) related cytoskeleton proteins. In constrast, nine proteins were under-expressed significantly in TT2F/hChr21 cells compared with TT2F cells: AI850305, Eef1D and UchL1, involved in protein catabolism or translation regulation, heat shock proteins Hsp84–1, Hsp70 and Hsp86–1, microtubule- (Mapre2) and calmodulin- (Cnn3) related architectural proteins were under-expressed. Moreover, splicing regulatory elements, HnrnpF and HnrnpC, displayed contradictory expression patterns of over-expression and underexpression respectively (Kadota et al., 2004). Comparison between mRNA and protein level change in TT2F/hChr21 cells compared with TT2F cells, different features were identified. The expression of *Anxa4*, *Atp6v1a1*, *Atp6v1b2*, *Krt2–8*, *Vil2* (overexpressed), and of *HnrnpC*, *Mapre2*, *UchL1*, *AI850305* (under-expressed) showed consistent mRNA transcription and protein translation. In contrast, *Cnn3*, *Eef1D*, *Hsp70*, *Hsp84*, *Hsp86*, *HnrnpF* and *T-plastin* showed disagreement, suggesting the existence of post-transcriptional regulation or translational modification (Kadota et al., 2004).

In an other proteomic study, using a mouse model for Down syndrome carrying the 141G6 YAC and polytransgenic for HSA21 genes DSCR3, 5, 6, 9, and TTC3, it has been identified 45 proteins showing altered expression levels, among the 422 polypeptides, which were the products of 239 different genes, in mouse transgenic hippocampus compared to control (Shin et al., 2006). These abnormal protein expressions may lead to impairment of cognitive functions. Interestingly, the CaMKII protein was decreased in the 141G6 mouse hippocampus (Shin et al., 2006), and it is known that alteration of the CaMKII-pathway lead a downstream alteration of the CREB pathway associated with impairment of fear memory (Bourtchuladze et al., 1994). 141G6 mice showed a lower performance in fear conditioning against sound as acoustic conditional stimulus (Chabert et al., 2004) that could be explained by these abnormal protein levels of CaMKII (Shin et al., 2006).

The protein alterations exist as polymorphisms among wild-type mice of different inbred strains, and these polymorphic variations complicate the interpretation of the variation of protein level changes and their correlation to a given disease. Recently, Mao and co-workers (2007) conceived a simplified approach to analyze the effect of gene-dosage imbalance on proteome in a controlled environment by using mouse embryonic stem (ES) cells. Investigation of four cell lines contained one single overexpressed gene (App, Snca, Dyrk1a, and Dopey2) and two cell lines with duplication or deletion, respectively, of a HSA21 segment containing 14 genes, identified globally 255 proteins showing expression variation in the six cell lines. The results demonstrated that: i) the same numbers (70-110) of proteins showed expression alterations in each line, with dosage imbalance in only one or 14 genes; ii) the dosage alteration of a single gene led to quantitative changes in a large number of proteins; iii) many proteins showed changed expression levels in several cell lines (38 proteins have alteration in at least 3 lines); iv) 114 proteins were altered only in one cell line (Mao et al., 2007). These data suggest that the protein level changes may also be explained in part by a global response of the cellular proteome to the gene dosage defect, restoring the balance in the cellular proteome, on the hypothesis that quantitative changes of the proteome by gene dosage effects can be compensated by a rearrangement restoring a new balance. Thus, the cellular proteins were defined as balancer proteins, with altered quantity in several lines, and cell line-specific proteins, when altered only in one cell line. These balancers proteins would function as buffers in the proteome homeostasis without a direct functional correlation with the transgene(s) and among them, in contrast to the cell line-specific proteins, likely including proteins participating to common functional networks of the transgene(s) (Mao et al., 2007). The balancers have more non-synonymous SNPs in coding regions than cell line-specific proteins, indicating that these balancers may have more tolerance towards quantitative changes, whereas cell line-specific proteins need more precise correlation between expression level and function (Mao et al., 2007).

3. Chromosome 21 Candidate Genes for Mental Retardation in Down Syndrome

Down syndrome is considered as a complex trait where the ultimate phenotypes could represent the epistatic and synergistic effects of overdosage of many genes localized in HSA21. Moreover, the genetic evidence between mouse and human supports the essential use of the mouse models to study the disruption of the developmental process and the genetic pathways caused by trisomy 21. The elevated gene expression, due to trisomy, is very comparable between mice and humans and show similar complexity and comparable genetic effect. The highly parallel outcomes that result when the same evolutionarily conserved genetic programs are perturbed by gene dosage imbalance in mouse models of Down syndrome and Down syndrome individuals validate the studies that focus on dissecting comparable phenotypes, particularly neurological alterations and mental retardation.

The principal interest of the genetic dissection is the identification of the gene(s) responsible of each phenotypic trait in Down syndrome. Several HSA21 genes have been identified as candidates for Down syndrome neurological phenotypes, particularly neurological alterations and mental retardation. These candidate genes show a strong expression in the key brain regions, altered in the brain of Down syndrome patients, which play crucial roles in cognitive functions. These genes are overexpressed in the brain of Down syndrome patients and/or in Down syndrome mouse models, and for most of these genes, mouse models overexpressing them have impaired behaviours and cognitive defects, similar to those observed in Down syndrome indivuduals.

ETS2 encodes a transcription factor ETS2 (Watson et al., 1985), it is expressed in neurons and is crucial for the normal formation of the neuromuscular junction (de Kerchove D'Exaerde et al., 2002). Moreover, ETS2 is overexpressed in trisomic tissues (Saran et al., 2003; Lyle et al., 2004; Dauphinot et al., 2005). Transgenic mice overexpressing ETS2 develop neurocranial and cervical skeletal abnormalities (Sumarsono et al., 1996), similarly to trisomy 16 mice and Down syndrome patients. The overexpression of ETS2 induces neuronal apoptosis, suggesting that overexpression of ETS2 may contribute to the increased rate of apoptosis of neurons in Down syndrome (Wolvetang et al., 2003).

APP gene encodes the beta-amyloid precursor protein, a protein involved in senile plaque formation in Down syndrome and Alzheimer's disease (Kang et al., 1987). In Down syndrome individuals and Ts65Dn mouse models, APP is expressed at more than the expected 1.5-fold (Epstein, 2001; Hunter et al., 2003; Lyle et al., 2004; Kahlem et al. 2004). Hippocampal neurons lacking APP show significantly enhanced amplitudes of evoked AMPA- and NMDA-receptor-mediated excitatory postsynaptic currents (EPSCs), and increased size of the readily releasable synaptic vesicle pool, indicating that lack of APP increases the number of functional synapses (Priller et al., 2006), suggesting a role of APP in the neurophysiology of Alzheimer's disease and Down syndrome. Transgenic mice over-expressing APP in the neocortex and hippocampus showed dystrophic neuritis associated with congopholic plaques (Sturchler-Pierrat et al., 1997) and learning defects (Lamb et al., 1993; Janus, 2004), mimicking features of Down syndrome and Alzheimer's disease like pathology.

SOD1 gene encodes the Cu-Zn superoxide dismutase, a key enzyme in the metabolism of oxygen-derived free radicals. Transcriptome and proteome studies show that both mRNA and protein levels are increased in human and mouse trisomic tissues (Epstein et al., 1987; Saran et al., 2003; Lyle et al., 2004; Kadota et al., 2004; Mao et al., 2005). The motor unit numbers are reduced in mice lacking SOD1 suggesting that axonal sprouting are functionally impaired in the absence of SOD1 (Shefner et al., 1999). The overexpression of Sod1 in transgenic mice leads to an impairment in LTP (Gahtan et al., 1998) and defects in distal motor neuron terminals, indicating that this gene affect principally motor neurons (Avraham et al., 1991; Gurney et al., 1994). These transgenic mice showed decreased cell number in several brain areas and decreased LTP in the pyramidal neuron CA1 (Zang et al., 2004; Harris-Cerruti et al., 2004). Transgenic mice over-expressing human SOD1 show a reduction in proteasome activities in the cortex and an associated increase in the content of oxidized SOD1 protein (Le Pecheur et al., 2005) and show impairment in the ability to adjust their posture in response to a moving surface and mild deficits in sensori-motor responsiveness (Lalonde et al., 2004; 2005) suggesting a central role of SOD1 in the development of motor neurons and axons.

GIRK2 or KCNJ6 encodes the G-protein coupled inward rectifying potassium channel subunit 2 (Lesage et al., 1994; Ohira et al., 1997). This is a member of the ATP-sensitive potassium channels involved in increase of the intracellular ATP concentration, linking cellular metabolism to the electrical excitability of the plasma membrane. Girk2 mutation in mouse causes the weaver phenotype, a drastically reduced cerebellum due to the reduction of granular cell neurons (Patil et al., 1995). Girk2 homozygous mice show a higher level of locomotion, suggesting hyperactivity and reduced anxiety in Girk2 null mice (Harashima et al., 2006a). GIRK2 is highly expressed in the cerebellar granule cells, suggesting a role of Girk2 in granule cell differentiation (Goldowitz and Smeyne, 1995). GIRK2 is overexpressed in trisomic tissues (Saran et al., 2003; Lyle et al., 2004; Khalem et al., 2004) and in the brain of Down syndrome mouse model Ts65Dn (Harashima et al., 2006b). This over-expression determines an increase of GIRK channel density in Ts65Dn neurons and a 2-fold increase of $GABA_B$-mediated GIRK current (Best et al., 2006). GIRK2 overexpression seems to alter the GIRK1/GIRK2 ratio, which likely affects the balance between excitatory and inhibitory neuronal transmission in Ts65Dn and thus overexpression of GIRK2 could contribute to Down syndrome neurophysiological phenotypes (Best et al., 2006; Harashima et al., 2006a; 2006b).

S100B is a calcium-binding protein synthesized and released by astrocytes. It is an important extracellular neurotrophic agent during normal fetal brain development, with effects on neuroblasts and glia, involving the neuronal cytoskeleton (Morii et al. 1991; Azmitia et al., 1992). S100B RNA and protein are overexpressed in Down syndrome brain and Alzheimer disease (Griffin et al., 1998; Epstein, 2001). S100b null mice have enhanced LTP in the hippocampal CA1 region and also enhanced spatial memory (Nishiyama et al., 2002). Transgenic mice overexpressing S100B show alterations in astrocyte morphology and axonal sprouting (Reeves et al., 1994; Bell et al., 2003; Shapiro and Whitaker-Azmitia, 2004) and decreased spatial learning and memory (Gerlai and Roder, 1996; Whitaker-Azmitia et al., 1997; Winocur et al., 2001; Bell et al., 2003). Transgenic mice overexpressing mouse S100β or human S100B show changes in cytoskeletal markers, such as the dendritic spine marker, drebrin, leading to an increased density of dendrites within the hippocampus (Shapiro and Whitaker-Azmitia, 2004) and appearing decreased in Down syndrome and Alzheimer's disease brain regions (Shin and Lubec, 2002; Kojima and Shirao, 2007). These findings indicate that over-expression of S100B contribute to glial-neuronal interactions and dendritic abnormalities in Down syndrome and suggest this gene as a glial modulator of neuronal synaptic plasticity and of information processing in the brain.

SIM2 encodes a transcription factor/helix-loop-helix protein (Crews et al., 1988; Dahmane et al., 1995), it is expressed in the neuroepithelium of D1 and D2 neuromeric regions of embryonic brain of mammals (Dahmane et al., 1995; Ema et al., 1996; Fan et al., 1996; Rachidi et al., 2005a), and in discrete human brain regions, including cortical layers, hippocampus and cerebellum (Rachidi et al., 2005a). Sim2 is overexpressed about 1.5 fold in the brain of Ts1Cje mouse fetuses (Vialard et al., 2000) and in trisomic tissues (Lyle et al., 2004). Transgenic mice overexpressing Sim2 show reduced sensitivity to pain and mild impairment of learning (Ema et al., 1999; Chrast et al., 2000b), similar to some phenotypes observed in trisomic mouse models for Down syndrome, Ts65Dn and Ts1Cje (Coussons-Read and Crnic, 1996; Sago et al., 1998; Martinez-Cue et al., 1999), and in Down syndrome individuals (Hennequin et al., 2000). Functional studies indicated that SIM2 protein control the Shh expression in the brain (Epstein et al., 2000) involved in cell growth and differentiation in the brain, and that SIM2 can inhibit cell cycle by inhibition of cyclin E expression (Meng et al., 2006) suggesting a key role of SIM2 in neulogical alterations seen in Down syndrome.

DOPEY2, a member of the Dopey family containing leucine zipper-like domains involved in protein-protein interactions (Rachidi et al., 2005b), is highly expressed in differentiating zones of embryonic human and mouse brains (Lopes et al., 2003; Rachidi et al., 2006), suggesting a role of DOPEY2 in cell differentiation and developmental patterning. This role is also supported by the high homology of DOPEY2 with the *C. elegans Pad-1*, required for embryonic patterning during gastrulation (Guipponi et al., 2000), the yeast *Dop1* and *DopA*, required for normal growth patterning, cell differentiation and organogenesis in Fungi (Dujon, 1996; Pascon and Miller, 2000). DOPEY2 expression becomes restricted to cerebellum, cortex and medial temporal-lobe system during human fetal development and in mouse adult brain (Lopes et al., 2003; Rachidi et al., 2006). Interestingly, the medial temporal-lobe system, including the hippocampal formation and perirhinal cortex, works as control centres of the memory (Milner et al., 1998; Krasuski, 2002), and present neuronal alterations in Down syndrome brain (Golden and Hyman, 1994; Raz et al., 1995). DOPEY2 is overexpressed in Down syndrome lymphoblasts 1.5-2 fold compared to normal lymphoblasts (Lopes et al., 2003) and in trisomic tissues (Lyle et al., 2004). Transgenic mice carrying the human YAC 230E8 (Smith et al., 1995), over-expressing DOPEY2 (Lopes et al., 2003; Rachidi et al., 2005b), show increased cortical cell density (Smith et al., 1997; Rachidi et al., 2005b) and a new cerebellar phenotype characterized by elongation of the antero-posterior axis, increased length of rostral folia of the vermis and abnormal culmen and declivus lobules (Rachidi et al., 2007). These phenotypes could explain the learning and memory deficits of these mouse models (Smith et al., 1997; Rachidi et al., 2005b; Rachidi et al., 2007), suggesting a role of the DOPEY2 gene in neuropathological defects and mental retardation in Down syndrome.

TPRD or TTC3 encodes a protein containing 2-3 units of a 34-amino acid repeat similar to the tetratricopeptide (TPR) motif that are involved in protein-protein interactions (Das et al. 1998; Groves and Barford, 1999), in the different splicing forms (Dahmane et al., 1998). During mouse and human brain development, TPRD shows higher expression in differentiating areas than in proliferating ones, suggesting a role of TPRD in neuronal cell differentiation (Lopes et al., 1999; Rachidi et al., 2000). Interestingly, it has been demonstrated that TPRD/TTC3 protein interacts to Citron kinase (CIT-K) and Citron N (CIT-N), two effectors of the RhoA small GTPase involved in neuronal proliferation and differentiation and that TPRD/TTC3 overexpression strongly inhibits neurite extension, while its knockdown stimulates the neurite extension (Berto et al., 2007). In agreement to previous results (Lopes et al., 1999; Rachidi et al., 2000), these dose-dependent effects are Rho-dependent, suggesting an important role of the TPRD-RhoA-CIT-K in neuronal differentiation (Berto et al., 2007). Transgenic mice YAC-141G6 containing entire TPRD gene (Smith et al., 1997) showed lower performances in fear conditioning against sound as acoustic conditional stimulus (Chabert et al., 2004). In addition, the 141G6 mice showed aberrant protein expression that may potentially lead to impairment of cognitive functions. Interestingly, these mice showed decreased CaMKII protein in hippocampus (Shin et al., 2006) taking into consideration that alteration of CaMKII-pathway lead to a downstream alteration of the CREB pathway associated with impairment of fear memory (Bourtchuladze et al., 1994; Shin et al., 2006).

DSCAM, an axon guidance molecule (Yamakawa et al., 1998; Schmucker et al., 2000), expressed in the developing spinal cord and cortex, may be involved in determination of the spinal cord dorsal–ventral axis and neuronal fates of the cortex (Barlow et al., 2002). In Down syndrome brains, DSCAM protein level is increased in the Purkinje cells at all ages, and in the cortical neurons during adulthood. In demented Down syndrome patients, DSCAM protein appeared in the core and periphery of senile plaques. This expression pattern suggests that DSCAM may play a role as an adhesion molecule regulating myelination (Saito et al., 2000). DSCAM *Drosophila melanogaster* homolog, dDscam, has been involved in neuronal wiring specificity (Chen et al., 2006; Hattori et al., 2007). DSCAM is expressed on spinal commissural axons, binds netrin-1, and is required for commissural axons to grow towards and across the midline. The overexpression of DSCAM, by causing enhanced netrin-DSCAM interactions, could contribute to the axonal wiring defects seen in Down syndrome (Ly et al., 2008).

Synaptojanin 1 (SYNJ1) is a polyphosphoinositide phosphatase that dephosphorylates the phosphatidylinositol-4,5-bisphosphate, that regulates membrane transduction and membrane trafficking in the endocytic pathway at synapses. Synaptojanin is highly expressed in the brain and located at nerve terminals, and it is associated with synaptic vesicles and coated endocytic intermediates (McPherson et al., 1994; Haffner et al., 1997). The rapid degradation of phosphatidylinositol by synaptojanin 1 is of critical importance for efficient synaptic vesicle regeneration and for the recovery of normal presynaptic function after an exocytic burst. In the absence of synaptojanin 1, sustained activity leads to a kinetic delay in synaptic vesicle reformation and to an increased, transient backup of synaptic membrane (Kim et al., 2002). These findings provide direct evidence for the hypothesis that synaptojanin 1 plays a key physiologic role in the transition from early endocytic compartments to newly reformed synaptic vesicles and suggest a critical role of phosphoinositide in synaptic physiology (Kim et al., 2002). The phosphoinositide metabolism is altered in the brain of Ts65Dn mice and in transgenic mice overexpressing Synj1. The Synj1 transgenic mice exhibit deficits in learning performances, suggesting that phosphoinositide dyshomeostasis caused by gene dosage imbalance for Synj1 may contribute to brain dysfunction and cognitive disabilities in Down syndrome (Voronov et al., 2008).

Intersectin 1 (ITSN1) is a SH3-containing domain protein, commonly found in signal transduction and cytoskeletal proteins (Pawson, 1995) and which interact with proline-rich domain-containing proteins involved in clathrin-mediated synaptic vesicle endocytosis (McPherson, 1999). ITSN1 encodes two isoforms: the long form is neuronal-specific and the short form is expressed in glial cells (Hussain et al., 1999; Ma et al., 2003). ITSN1 seems to function as a scaffolding protein, providing a link between the components of endocytosis and actin cytoskeleton and has a role in signal transduction (Roos and Kelly, 1998; Yamabhai et al., 1998; Hussain et al., 1999; Martina et al., 2001; Jenna et al., 2002). ITSN1 over-expression blocks clathrin-mediated endocytosis (Sengar et al., 1999), and also blocks epidermal growth factor (EGF) mediated MAPK activation by inhibiting Ras activation directly, most probably by preventing the Ras/mSos interaction, suggesting a role for ITSN1 in Ras activation (Tong et al., 2000). Itsn1 null mice show reduced number of exocytosis in chromaffin cells, slowing of endocytosis in neurons, increased endosome size in neurons and reduced NGF levels and decreased levels of Choline Acetyl Transferase (ChAT) positive cells in the septal region of the brain (Yu et al., 2008). Interestingly, the presence of enlarged endosomes in the neurons of Down syndrome is an early sign of Alzheimer's disease, suggesting that ITSN1 could contribute to the disturbance in endocytosis in early Alzhaimer's disease pathogenesis in Down syndrome (Yu et al., 2008).

DYRK1A encodes a serine-threonine kinase (Kentrup et al., 1996) expressed in cortex, hippocampus and cerebellum (Guimera et al., 1996; Rahmani et al., 1998; Guimera et al., 1999) and overexpressed in mouse trisomic model Ts65Dn (Guimera et al., 1999) and in Down syndrome fetal brain and other trisomic tissues (Saran et al., 2003; Lyle et al., 2004). The heterozygote mice *Dyrk1A*$^{+/-}$ show a decreased size in several brain regions (Fotaki et al., 2002) and show smaller size of the pyramidal cell somata, shorter dendritic length, lower spine number, and altered spine distribution (Benavides-Piccione et al., 2005). The reduction in brain size and behavioural defects observed in *Dyrk1A*$^{+/-}$ mice suggests that this kinase is involved in dendritic alterations and in monosomy 21 associated mental retardation

(Benavides-Piccione et al. 2005). Transgenic mouse models overexpressing DYRK1A showed neurodevelopmental defects and motor dysfunction (Altafaj et al., 2001; Fotaki et al., 2002), an increased brain and neuronal sizes (Smith et al., 1997; Branchi et al., 2004; Rachidi et al., 2007), and exhibit spatial learning and memory defects (Smith et al., 1997; Altafaj et al., 2001; Ahn et al., 2006), indicating that the correct dosage of DYRK1A gene is crucial for brain hippocampal and prefrontal cortex functions, particularly concerning a cognitive dysfunction of the reference memory. Dyrk1A proteins are also localized in the neuron dendrites, where it is co-localized with Dynamin (DYN1), a GTPase putative substrate of DYRK1A, involved in synaptic vesicle recycling, membrane trafficking and neurite outgrowth (Chen-Hwang et al., 2002; Hammerle et al., 2003), and regulate their development (Hammerle et al., 2003). Dyrk1A proteins also modulate the activity of the c-AMP response element-binding protein (CREB), which participates in signal transduction pathways involved in synaptic plasticity and neuronal differentiation (Hammerle et al., 2003). Recently, it has been demonstrated that DYRK1A influence the NFATc pathways through its kinase activity (Arron et al., 2006; Gwack et al., 2006).

Down syndrome Critical Region 1 gene (DSCR1) or Regulator of the Calcineurin 1 protein (RCAN1) directly modulates the activity of the protein phosphatase calcineurin. The calcipressin 1, the protein encoded by DSCR1, interacts with calcineurin A (Fuentes et al., 2000) to inhibit calcineurin activity (Rothermel et al., 2000). DSCR1 is over-expressed in brain of Down syndrome fetuses (Fuentes et al., 2000), in brains of Down syndrome patients with Alzheimer's disease (Ermak et al., 2001), and in brain of Down syndrome mouse models (Amano et al., 2004; *Lyle et al., 2004; Dauphinot et al., 2005)*. The over-expression of DSCR1 in rat primary neurones causes formation of aggresome-like inclusion bodies similar to those observed in Down syndrome and Alzheimer's disease brains, as well as reducing the expression of the synaptic vesicle protein, synaptophysin, in neural processes (Ma et al., 2004). Loss-of-function and over-expression of *Drosophila* orthologue DSCR1, both display severe learning defects in several basic learning assays, indicating that DSCR1 may affect regulatory pathways of synaptic transmission (Chang et al., 2003). DSCR1 knock-out mice displayed neurological phenotype and show faster overall movements and a significant impairment in working memory (Sanna et al., 2006). DSCR1 knock-out mice also exhibit deficits in spatial learning and memory, reduced associative cued memory, and impaired late-phase long-term potentiation (L-LTP), phenotypes similar to those of transgenic mice with increased calcineurin activity, demonstrating that DSCR1 play a central role in long-term potentiation, memory and synaptic plasticity (Hoeffer et al., 2007).

Recently, five miRNA genes harbored on HSA21 including miR-99a, let-7c, miR-125b-2, miR-155, and miR-802 have been identified (Kuhn et al., 2008). The five HSA21-derived miRNAs are overexpressed in Down syndrome tissues when compared with normal tissues (Sethupathy et al., 2007; Kuhn et al., 2008). Moreover, other miRNAs, localized on other chromosomes, have also been identified showing expression alteration (over- or down-expression) in Down syndrome tissues when compared with normal tissues (Kuhn et al., 2008). These findings suggest that trisomic 21 gene dosage overexpression of HSA21-derived miRNAs results in the decreased expression of specific target proteins and contribute to features of the neuronal and cardiac Down syndrome phenotype.

4. Dosage Balance in Gene Regulation and Genetic Pathways Involved in Developmental Functions in Down Syndrome

Trisomy of human chromosome 21 (HSA21) is the most frequent genetic cause of mental retardation, which is the invariable hallmark disorder of Down syndrome and the most invalidating pathological aspect, contributing to about 30% of all moderate-to-severe cases of mental retardation (Lejeune, 1990; Stoll et al., 1990; Pulsifer, 1996). This major neurological disorder of Down syndrome is mainly a consequence of functional and developmental brain alterations in neurogenesis, neuronal differentiation, myelination, dendritogenesis and synaptogenesis.

In the brain, the presence of the chromosomal imbalance determines misexpression and interaction of genes/proteins that play crucial roles in neuromorphogenesis and neurogenic cascades. The developmental genetic error caused by trisomy 21 during neural patterning and signal transduction pathways may lead to defective functioning neuronal circuitry and could be responsible for the pathogenesis of mental retardation in Down syndrome, as we proposed recently in a genetic and molecular mechanism (Rachidi and Lopes, 2007).

It is imperative to elucidate the molecular pathways involving the HSA21 gene functions, and which of these genes are perturbed in trisomy 21 and are relevant to neurological and cognitive disorders in Down syndrome. An altered genetic pathway involved in some Down syndrome phenotypes has been identified in which two HSA21 dosage-sensitive genes are involved, DYRK1A and DSCR1. It has been demonstrated that DYRK1A and DSCR1 regulate NFAT activity and their overexpression dysregulates the NFATc pathways (Arron et al., 2006). The NFATc signaling pathways are activated by the entry of calcium into the cell and results in activation of calcineurin, the catalytic subunit of the Ca^{2+}/calmodulin-dependent protein phosphatase PP2B. In the cytoplasm, the activated calcineurin remove phosphate groups from NFATc factors and the dephosphorylated NFATc proteins enter the nucleus and activate their target genes. DSCR1 encodes an inhibitor of calcineurin (Fuentes et al., 2000; Rothermel et al., 2000) and decreases NFATc dephosphorylation in the cytoplasm. Once in the nucleus, NFATc may be phospharylated by DYRK1A serine-threonine protein kinase and the phosphorylated forms of NFATc return into the cytoplasm, decreasing gene transcription activity.

In transgenic mice overexpressing Dyrk1A or DSCR1 alone, or both Dyrk1A and DSCR1, NFATc is mostly phosphorylated and found in the cytoplasm, suggesting that overexpression of Dyrk1A and DSCR1 reduces NFATc transcriptional activity by increase of the phosphorylated forms of NFATc proteins, which leads to their cytoplasmic localization. Interestingly, the mice lacking NFATc2 and NFATc4, such as transgenic mice overexpressing DYRK1A and/or DSCR1, have similar phenotypes to those seen in trisomic mouse models, Ts65Dn and Ts1Cje, and Down syndrome patients, including neuronal and behavioral phenotypes (Arron et al., 2006).

Interestingly, DYRK1A and DSCR1 are known to be involved in synaptic development, maturation and plasticity. In the nuclei, DYRK1A is localised to the nuclear speckles that represent the splicing compartment (Alvarez et al., 2003), and several splicing factors and proteins involved in splicing regulation are DYRK1A substrates (de Graaf et al., 2004) indicating that DYRKIA is involved in splicing control. Overexpression of DYRK1A in Down syndrome may dysregulate the splicing control and may determine several developmental and functional alterations, particularly in the brain and thus participate to neurological and cognitive alterations seen in Down syndrome patients.

DSCR1 inhibites calcineurin and, indirectly, affects its substrates, which include dynamin and SYNJ1 (Cousin et al., 2001), and is a critical point of connection between the calcineurin and the MAPK pathway (Rothermel et al., 2003), which is involved in regulation of synaptic plasticity and memory (Sweatt, 2001; Sweatt and Weeber, 2003; Thomas and Huganir, 2004). Dysregulation of MAPK affects long term potentiation (LTP) and spatial learning, which correspond to some defects observed in children with Down syndrome (Pennington et al., 2003) and in Ts65Dn mice (Hyde et al., 2001; Stasko and Costa, 2004; Kleschevnikov et al., 2004).

In addition, dysregulation of calcineurin activity is associated with cognitive and behavioral deficits, including spatial learning (Mansuy, 2003; Lee and Ahnn, 2004) that are related to Down syndrome. Inhibition of calcineurin reduces the level of synaptic vesicle recycling as well as the total vesicle pool size in synaptic terminals (Kumashiro et al., 2005), indicating a potential role for endogenous calcineurin inhibitors in regulating synaptic transmission. The over-expression of DSCR1, as observed in Down syndrome and Alzheimer's disease, may affect at least two calcineurin-dependent pathways by blocking calcineurin activity. In a first pathway, the elevated levels of DSCR1 may disrupt endocytosis and vesicle recycling due to the inhibition of calcineurin-dependent dephosphin dephosphorylation. In a second pathway, the over dosage of DSCR1 contributes to the hyperphosphorylation of Tau by reducing calcineurin phosphatase activity, leading to Alzheimer's disease (Ermak et al., 2001). DSCR1 knock-out mice showed increased enzymatic activity of both calcineurin and decreased phosphorylation of calcineurin substrates, consistent with an elevation in calcineurin activity in the hippocampus, demonstrating a essential role for DSCR1 in learning-memory and in mental retardation in Down syndrome (Hoeffer et al., 2007).

5. Conclusion and Perspectives

Great efforts on gene expression, transcriptome, proteome and functional genomics studies, in human, trisomic and transgenic mouse models have shown similar genotype/phenotype correlations and parallel outcomes suggesting that the same evolutionarily conserved genetic programs are perturbed by gene-dosage effects. The expression variations caused by this gene-dosage imbalance may firstly induce brain developmental variations at cellular level, as primary phenotypes, and finaly induce neurological alterations and cognitive deficits as secondary phenotypes.

The identification of trisomic candidates genes overexpressed in the brain, including microRNAs, and their function, their developmental regulated expression and their downstream effects, their interaction with other proteins, and their involvement in regulatory and metabolic pathways help us to best understand the developmental origin of the mental retardation in Down syndrome. This lead to the identification of potential targets in the altered molecular pathways involved in mental retardation pathogenesis, such as Calcineurin, NFATs and MAPK pathways, that may be potentially corrected, in the perspective of new therapeutic approaches. The efforts are focused particularly in pathways involved in learning and memory processes in mouse models of Down syndrome towards identification of targets for therapeutics that will correct the mental retardation features in Down syndrome individuals.

Hopefully, a novel biomedical era for prevention, intervention and therapy of mental retardation in Down syndrome begins.

Acknowledgments

We are grateful to J.M. Delabar (University Paris 7) for his continuous support. We thank our colleagues of the Department of Molecular Biology-Jacques Monod at the Pateur Insitute (Paris) for their advices and support. We also thank L. Peltzer (University of French Polynesia) and C. Tetaria (Hospital Centre of French Polynesia) for their continuous support.

References

Ahn, K. J., Jeong, H. K., Choi, H. S., Ryoo, S. R., Kim, Y. J., et al. (2006) DYRK1A BAC transgenic mice show altered synaptic plasticity with learning and memory defects. *Neurobiol. Dis., 22,* 463-472.

Aït Yahya-Graison, E., Aubert, J., Dauphinot, L., Rivals, I., Prieur, M., et al. (2007) Classification of human chromosome 21 gene-expression variations in Down syndrome: impact on disease phenotypes. *Am. J. Hum. Genet., 81,* 475-491.

Aitken, D. A., McCaw, G., Crossley, J. A., Berry, E., Connor, J. M., Spencer, K. and Macri, J.N. (1993) First-trimester biochemical screening for fetal chromosome abnormalities and neural tube defects. *Prenat. Diagn., 13,* 681–689.

Altafaj, X., Dierssen, M., Baamonde, C., Marti, E., Visa, J., Guimera, J., Oset, M., Gonzalez, J. R., Florez, J., Fillat, C. and Estivill, X. (2001) Neurodevelopmental delay, motor abnormalities and cognitive deficits in transgenic mice overexpressing Dyrk1A (minibrain), a murine model of Down's syndrome. *Hum. Mol. Genet., 10,* 1915–1923.

Alvarez, M., Estivill, X. and de la Luna, S. (2003) DYRK1A accumulates in splicing speckles through a novel targeting signal and induces speckle disassembly. *J. Cell Sci., 116,* 3099-3107.

Amano, K., Sago, H., Uchikawa, C., Suzuki, T., Kotliarova, S. E., Nukina, N., Epstein, C. J. and Yamakawa, K. (2004) Dosage-dependent over-expression of genes in the trisomic region of Ts1Cje mouse model for Down syndrome. *Hum. Mol. Genet., 13,* 1333-1340.

Antonarakis, S. E. (1998) 10 years of genomics, chromosome 21, and Down syndrome, *Genomics 51,* 1–16.

Antonarakis, S. E., Lyle, R., Dermitzakis, E. T., Reymond, A. and Deutsch, S. (2004) Chromosome 21 and Down syndrome: from genomics to pathophysiology. *Nat. Rev. Genet., 5,* 725-738.

Arai, Y., Ijuin, T., Takenawa, T., Becker, L. E. and Takashima, S. (2002) Excessive expression of synaptojanin in brains with Down syndrome. *Brain Dev., 24,* 67–72.

Arron, J. R., Winslow, M. M., Polleri, A., Chang, C. P., Wu, H., Gao, X., Neilson, J. R., Chen, L., Heit, J. J., Kim, S. K., Yamasaki, N., Miyakawa, T., Francke, U., Graef, I. A. and Crabtree, G. R. (2006) NFAT dysregulation by increased dosage of DSCR1 and DYRK1A on chromosome 21. *Nature, 441,* 595-600.

Avraham, K. B., Sugarman, H., Rotshenker, S. and Groner, Y. (1991) Down's syndrome: morphological remodelling and increased complexity in the neuromuscular junction of transgenic CuZn-superoxide dismutase mice. *J. Neurocytol., 20,* 208-215.

Azmitia, E. C., Griffin, W. S. T., Marshak, D. R., Van Eldik, L. J. and Whitaker-Azmitia, P. M. (1992) S100b and serotonin: a possible astrocytic-neuronal link to neuropathology of Alzheimer's disease. *Prog. Brain Res., 92,* 459–473.

Balcz, B., Kirchner, L., Cairns, N., Fountoulakis, M. and Lubec G. (2001) Increased brain protein levels of carbonyl reductase and alcohol dehydrogenase in Down syndrome and Alzheimer's disease. *J. Neural. Transm., 61,* 193–201.

Barlow, G. M., Micales, B., Chen, X. N., Lyons, G. E. and Korenberg, J. R. (2002) Mammalian DSCAMs: roles in the development of the spinal cord, cortex, and cerebellum? *Biochem. Biophys. Res. Commun., 293,* 881-891.

Bartel, D. P. (2004) MicroRNAs: genomics, biogenesis, mechanism, and function. *Cell, 116,* 281–297.

Bell, K., Shokrian, D., Potenzieri, C. and Whitaker-Azmitia, P. M. (2003) Harm avoidance, anxiety, and response to novelty in the adolescent S-100beta transgenic mouse: role of serotonin and relevance to Down syndrome. *Neuropsychopharmacology, 28,* 1810-1816.

Benavides-Piccione, R., Dierssen, M., Ballesteros-Yaöez, I., Martinez de Lagran, M., Arbones, M. L., et al. (2005) Alterations in the phenotype of neocortical pyramidal cells in the Dyrk1A$^{+/-}$ mouse. *Neurobiol. Dis., 20,* 115-122.

Berg, J. M., Karlinsky, H. and Holland, A. J. (1993) Alzheimer's disease, Down syndrome and their relationship. New York (NY), Oxford University Press.

Berto, G., Camera, P., Fusco, C., Imarisio, S., Ambrogio, C., et al. (2007) The Down syndrome critical region protein TTC3 inhibits neuronal differentiation via RhoA and Citron kinase. *J. Cell Sci., 120,* 1859-1867.

Best, T. K., Siarey, R. J. and Galdzicki, Z. (2006) Ts65Dn, a mouse model of Down syndrome, exhibits increased GABAB induced potassium current. J. Neurophysiol. In press.

Bourtchuladze, R., Frenguelli, B., Blendy, J., Cioffi, D., Schutz, G., et al. (1994) Deficient long-term memory in mice with a targeted mutation of the cAMP-responsive element-binding protein. *Cell, 79,* 59-68.

Branchi, I., Bichler, Z., Minghetti, L., Delabar, J. M., Malchiodi-Albedi, F., Gonzalez, M. C., Chettouh, Z., Nicolini, A., Chabert, C., Smith, D. J., Rubin, E. M., Migliore-Samour, D. and Alleva, E. (2004) Transgenic mouse in vivo library of human Down syndorme Critical Region 1: association between *DYRK1A* overexpession, brain development abnormalities, and cell cycle protein alteration. *J. Neuropathol. Exp. Neurol., 63,* 429-440.

Brem, R. B., Yvert, G., Clinton, R. and Kruglyak, L. (2002) Genetic dissection of transcriptional regulation in budding yeast. *Science, 296,* 752–755.

Bushati, N. and Cohen, S. M. (2007) microRNA functions. *Ann. Rev. Cell. Develop. Biol., 3,* 175–205.

Chabert, C., Jamon, M., Cherfouh, A., Duquenne, V., Smith, D. J., et al. (2004) Functional Analysis of Genes Implicated in Down Syndrome: 1. Cognitive Abilities in Mice Transpolygenic for Down Syndrome Chromosomal Region-1 (DCR-1). *Behav. Genet., 34,* 559-569.

Chang, K. T., Shi, Y. J. and Min, K. T. (2003) The Drosophila homolog of Down's syndrome critical region 1 gene regulates learning: implications for mental retardation. *Proc. Natl. Acad. Sci., 100,* 15794–15799.

Chen, H., Chrast, R., Rossier, C., Morris, M. A., Lalioti, M. D. and Antonarakis, S. E. (1996) Cloning of 559 potential exons of genes of human chromosome 21 by exon trapping. *Genome Res., 6,* 747-760.

Chen-Hwang, M. C., Chen, H. R., Elzinga, M. and Hwang, Y. W. (2002) Dynamin is a minibrain kinase/dual specificity Yak1-related kinase 1A substrate. *J. Biol. Chem., 277,* 17597-17604.

Cheon, M. S., Fountoulakis, M., Dierssen, M., Ferreres, J. C. and Lubec, G. (2001) Expression profiles of proteins in fetal brain with Down syndrome. *J. Neural. Transm. Suppl., 61,* 311–319.

Cheon, M. S., Kim, S. H., Yaspo, M. L., Blasi, F., Aoki, Y., et al. (2003a) Protein levels of genes encoded on chromosome 21 in fetal Down syndrome brain: challenging the gene dosage effect hypothesis (Part I). *Amino Acids, 24,* 111–117.

Cheon, M. S., Bajo, M., Kim, S. H., Claudio, J. O., Stewart, A. K., et al. (2003b) Protein levels of genes encoded on chromosome 21 in fetal Down syndrome brain: challenging the gene dosage effect hypothesis (Part II). *Amino Acids, 24,* 119–125.

Cheon, M. S., Kim, S. H., Ovod, V., Kopitar Jerala, N., Morgan, J. I., et al. (2003c) Protein levels of genes encoded on chromosome 21 in fetal Down syndrome brain: challenging the gene dosage effect hypothesis (Part III). *Amino Acids, 24,* 127–134.

Cheon, M. S., Shim, K. S., Kim, S. H., Hara, A. and Lubec, G. (2003d) Protein levels of genes encoded on chromosome 21 in fetal Down syndrome brain: challenging the gene dosage effect hypothesis (Part IV). *Amino Acids, 25,* 41–47.

Cheung, V. G., Conlin, L. K., Weber, T. M., Arcaro, M., Jen, K. Y., et al. (2003) Natural variation in human gene expression assessed in lymphoblastoid cells. *Nature Genet., 33,* 422–425.

Chou, C. Y., Liu, L. Y., Chen, C. Y., Tsai, C. H., Hwa, H. L., et al. (2008) Gene expression variation increase in trisomy 21 tissues. *Mamm. Genome, 19,* 398-405.

Chrast, R., Scott, H. S., Papasavvas, M. P., Rossier, C., Antonarakis, E. S., Barras, C., Davisson, M. T., Schmidt, C., Estivill, X., Dierssen, M., Pritchard, M. and Antonarakis, S. E. (2000a) The mouse brain transcriptome by SAGE: differences in gene expression between P30 brains of the partial trisomy 16 mouse model of Down syndrome (Ts65Dn) and normals. *Genome Res., 10,* 2006-2021.

Chrast, R., Scott, H. S., Madani, R., Huber, L., Wolfer, D. P., Prinz, M., Aguzzi, A., Lipp, H. P. and Antonarakis, S. E. (2000b) Mice trisomic for a bacterial artificial chromosome with the single-minded 2 gene (Sim2) show phenotypes similar to some of those present in the partial trisomy 16 mouse models of Down syndrome. *Hum. Mol. Genet., 9,* 1853-1864.

Cohen, W. I. (1999) Health care guidelines for individuals with Down syndrome: 1999 revision. *Down Syndrome Quarterly, 4,* 1-16.

Cousin, M. A., Tan, T. C. and Robinson, P. J. (2001) Protein phosphorylation is required for endocytosis in nerve terminals: potential role for the dephosphins dynamin I and synaptojanin, but not AP180 or amphiphysin. *J. Neurochem;, 76,* 105–116.

Coussons-Read, M. E. and Crnic, L. S. (1996) Behavioral assessment of the Ts65Dn mouse, a model for Down syndrome: altered behavior in the elevated plus maze and open field. *Behav. Genet., 26,* 7-13.

Crews, S. T., Thomas, J. B. and Goodman, C. S. (1988) The Drosophila singleminded gene encodes a nuclear protein with sequence similarity to the per gene product, *Cell, 52,* 143–151.

Dahmane, N., Charron, G., Lopes, C., Yaspo, M. L., Maunoury, C., Decorte, L., Sinet, P. M., Bloch, B. and Delabar, J. M. (1995) Down syndrome critical region contains a gene homologous to Drosophila sim expressed during rat and human central nervous system development, *Proc. Natl. Acad. Sci. USA*, *92,* 9191–9195.

Dahmane, N., Ait Ghezala, G. A., Gosset, P., Chamoun, Z., Dufresne-Zacharia, M. C., Lopes, C., Rabatel, N., Gassanova-Maugenre, S., Chettouh, Z., Abramowski, V., Fayet, E., Yaspo, M. L., Korn, B., Blouin, J. L., Lehrach, H., Poutska, A., Antonarakis, S. E., Sinet, P. M., Creau, N. and Delabar, J. M. (1998) Transcriptional map of the 2.5-Mb CBR–ERG region of chromosome 21 involved in Down syndrome. *Genomics, 48,* 12–23.

Das, A. K., Cohen, P. W. and Barford, D. (1998) The structure of the tetratricopeptide repeats of protein phosphatase 5: implications for TPR-mediated protein-protein interactions. *EMBO J., 17,* 1192-1199.

Dauphinot, L., Lyle, R., Rivals, I., Dang, M. T., Moldrich, R. X., Golfier, G., Ettwiller, L., Toyama, K., Rossier, J., Personnaz, L., et al. (2005) The cerebellar transcriptome during postnatal development of the Ts1Cje mouse, a segmental trisomy model for Down syndrome. *Hum. Mol. Genet., 14,* 373-384.

Deutsch, S., Lyle, R., Dermitzakis, E. T., Attar, H., Subrahmanyan, L., et al. (2005) Gene expression variation and expression quantitative trait mapping of human chromosome 21 genes. *Hum. Mol. Genet., 14,* 3741-3749.

Dujon, B. (1996) The yeast genome project: what did we learn? *Trends Genet., 12,* 263-270.

Ema, M., Suzuki, M., Morita, M., Hirose, K., Sogawa, K., Matsuda, Y., Gotoh, O., Saijoh, Y., Fujii, H., Hamada, H. and Fujii-Kuriyama, Y. (1996) cDNA cloning of a murine homologue of Drosophila single-minded, its mRNA expression in mouse development, and chromosome localization. *Biochem. Biophys. Res. Commun., 218,* 588-594.

Ema, M., Ikegami, S., Hosoya, T., Mimura, J., Ohtani, H., Nakao, K., Inokuchi, K., Katsuki, M. and Fujii-Kuriyama, Y. (1999) Mild impairment of learning and memory in mice overexpressing the mSim2 gene located on chromosome 16: an animal model of Down's syndrome, *Hum. Mol. Genet., 8,* 1409-1415.

Engidawork, E., Balic, N., Fountoulakis, M., Dierssen, M., Graber-Platzer, S. and Lubec, G. (2001a) b-Amyloid precursor protein, ETS-2 and collagen alpha 1 (VI) chain precursor, encoded on chromosome 21, are not overexpressed in fetal Down syndrome: further evidence against gene dosage effect. *J. Neural Transm. Suppl., 61,* 335–346.

Engidawork, E., Gulesserian, T., Balic, N., Cairns, N. and Lubec, G. (2001b) Changes in nicotinic acetylcholine receptor subunits expression in brain of patients with Down syndrome and Alzheimer's disease. *J. Neural. Transm., 61,* 211–222.

Engidawork, E., Gulesserian, T., Fountoulakis, M. and Lubec, G. (2003) Aberrant protein expression in cerebral cortex of fetus with Down syndrome. *Neuroscience, 122,* 145-154.

Engidawork, E. and Lubec, G. (2003) Molecular changes in fetal Down syndrome brain. *J. Neurochem., 84,* 895–904.

Epstein, C. J. (1986) *The Consequences of Chromosome Imbalance: Principles, Mechanisms, and Models,* New York, Cambridge University Press.

Epstein, C. J. (1988) Mechanisms of the effects of aneuploidy in mammals. *Annu. Rev. Genet., 22,* 51-75.

Epstein, C. J. (1993) The phenotypic mapping of Down syndrome and other aneuploid conditions. In C. J. Epstein (Ed.), *Progress in Clinical and Biological Research. Proceedings of a National Down Syndrome Society Conference. 1993 Jan 14-15; New York, USA.* (pp. 1-26) New York, Wiley-Liss.

Epstein, C. J. (1995) Down syndrome (trisomy 21). In C. R. Scriver, A. L., Beaudet, W. S., Sly, and D. Valle (Eds.), *The Metabolic and Molecular Bases of Inherited Disease* (pp.749–794) New York, McGraw-Hill.

Epstein, J. (2001) Down syndrome. In C. R. Scriver, A. L. Beaudet, W. S. Sly., and D. Valle (Eds.), *The Metabolic and Molecular Bases of Inherited Disease* (7th edn., Vol. I, pp. 1223–1256) New York, McGraw-Hill, Inc.

Epstein, C. J., Avraham, K. B., Lovett, M., Smith, S., Elroy-Stein, O., Rotman, G., Bry, C. and Groner, Y. (1987) Transgenic mice with increased Cu/Zn-superoxide dismutase activity: animal model of dosage effects in Down syndrome. *Proc. Natl. Acad. Sci., 84,* 8044-8048.

Epstein, D. J., Matinu, L., Michaud, J. L., Losos, K. M., Fan, C. M., et al. (2000) Members of the bHLH-PAS family regulate Shh transcription in forebrain regions of the mouse CNS. *Development, 127,* 1701-1709.

Ermak, G., Morgan, T. E. and Davies, K. J. (2001) Chronic overexpression of the calcineurin inhibitory gene DSCR1 (Adapt78) is associated with Alzheimer's disease. *J. Biol. Chem., 276,* 38787-38794.

Fan, C. M., Kuwana, E., Bulfone, A., Fletcher, C. F., Copeland, N. G., Jenkins, N. A., Crews, S., Martinez, S., Puelles, L., Rubenstein, J. L. and Tessier-Lavigne, M. (1996) Expression patterns of two murine homologs of Drosophila single-minded suggest possible roles in embryonic patterning and in the pathogenesis of Down syndrome. *Mol. Cell. Neurosci., 7,* 1-16.

Ferencz, C., Neill, C. A., Boughman, J. A., Rubin, J. D., Brenner, J. I. and Perry, L. W. (1989) Congenital cardiovascular malformations associated with chromosome abnormalities: An epidemiologic study. *J. Pediatr., 114,* 79-86.

Ferrando-Miguel, R., Cheon, M. S. and Lubec, G. (2004) Protein levels of genes encoded on chromosome 21 in fetal Down syndrome brain (Part V); overexpression of phosphatidyl-inositol-glycan class P protein (DSCR5). *Amino Acids., 26,* 255-261.

FitzPatrick, D. R. (2005) Transcriptional consequences of autosomal trisomy: primary gene dosage with complex downstream effects. *Trends Genet., 21,* 249-253.

FitzPatrick, D. R., Ramsay, J., McGill, N. I., Shade, M., Carothers, A.D. and Hastie, N. D. (2002) Transcriptome analysis of human autosomal trisomy. *Hum. Mol. Genet., 11,* 3249-3256.

Fotaki, V., Dierssen, M., Alcantara, S., Martinez, S., Marti, E., et al. (2002) Dyrk1A haploinsufficiency affects viability and causes developmental delay and abnormal brain morphology in mice. *Mol. Cell. Biol., 22,* 6636-6647.

Freidl, M., Gulesserian, T., Lubec, G., Fountoulakis, M. and Lubec, B. (2001) Deterioration of the transcriptional, splicing and elongation machinery in brain of fetal Down syndrome. *J. Neural. Transm. Suppl., 61,* 47–57.

Fuentes, J. J., Genesca, L., Kingsbury, T. J., Cunningham, K. W., Perez-Riba, M., Estivill, X. and de la Luna, S. (2000) DSCR1, overexpressed in Down syndrome, is an inhibitor of calcineurin-mediated signaling pathways. *Hum. Mol. Genet., 9,* 1681–1690.

Gahtan, E., Auerbach, J. M., Groner, Y. and Segal, M. (1998) Reversible impairment of long-term potentiation in transgenic Cu/Zn-SOD mice. *Eur. J. Neurosci., 10,* 538-544.

Gerlai, R. and Roder, J. (1996) Spatial and nonspatial learning in mice: effects of S100 beta overexpression and age. Neurobiol. *Learn. Mem., 66,* 143-154.

Giannone, S., Strippoli, P., Vitale, L., Casadei, R., Canaider, S., et al. (2004) Gene expression profile analysis in human T lymphocytes from patients with Down syndrome. *Ann. Hum. Genet., 68,* 546-554.

Golden, J. A. and Hyman, B. T. (1994) Development of the superior temporal neocortex is anomalous in trisomy 21. J. Neuropathol. *Exp. Neurol., 53,* 513–552.

Goldowitz, D. and Smeyne, R. J. (1995) Tune into the weaver channel. *Nat. Genet., 11,* 107-109.

de Graaf, K., Hekerman, P., Spelten, O., Herrman, A., Packman, L. C., et al. (2004) Characterization of cyclin L2, a novel cyclin with an arginine/serine-rich domain: phosphorylation by DYRK1A and colocalization with splicing factors. *J. Biol. Chem. 279,* 4612–4624.

Greber-Platzer, S., Schatzmann-Turhani, D., Cairns, N., Balcz, B. and Lubec, G. (1999) Expression of the transcription factor ETS2 in brain of patients with Down syndrome-evidence against the overexpression-gene dosage hypothesis. *J. Neural. Transm., 57(Suppl),* 269–281.

Griffin, W. S. T., Sheng, J. G., McKenzie, L. E., Royston, M. C., Gentleman, S. M., Brumback, R. A., Cork, L. C., Del Bigio, M. R., Roberts, G. W. and Mrak, R. E. (1998) Life-long over-expression of S100b in Down's syndrome: implications for Alzheimer's pathogenesis. *Neurobiol. Aging, 19,* 401–405.

Groves, M. R. and Barford, D. (1999) Topological characteristics of helical repeat proteins. *Curr. Opin. Struct. Biol., 9,* 383-389.

Guimera, J., Casas, C., Pucharcos, C. Solans, A., Domenech, A., Planas, A. M., Ashley, J., Lovett, M., Estivill, X. and Pritchard, M. A. (1996) A human homologue of Drosophila minibrain (MNB) is expressed in the neuronal regions affected in Down syndrome and maps to the critical region. *Hum. Mol. Genet., 5,* 1305–1310.

Guimera, J., Casas, C., Estivill, X. and Pritchard, M. (1999) Human minibrain homologue (MNBH/DYRK1): characterization, alternative splicing, differential tissue expression, and overexpression in Down syndrome, Genomics, 57, 407–418.

Guipponi, M., Brunschwig, K., Chamoun, Z., Scott, H. S., Shibuya, K., Kudoh, J., Delezoide, A. L., El Samadi, S., Chettouh, Z., Rossier, C., Shimizu, N., Mueller, F., Delabar, J. M. and Antonarakis, S. E. (2000) *C21orf5*, a novel human chromosome 21 gene, has a *Caenorhabditis elegans* ortholog (*pad-1*) required for embryonic patterning. *Genomics, 68,* 30–40.

Gurney, M. E., Pu, H., Chiu, A. Y., Dal Canto, M. C., Polchow, C. Y., Alexander, D. D., Caliendo, J., Hentati, A., Kwon, Y. W., Deng, H. X. et al. (1994) Motor neuron degeneration in mice that express a human Cu,Zn superoxide dismutase mutation. *Science, 264,* 1772-1775.

Gwack, Y., Sharma, S., Nardone, J., Tanasa, B., Iuga, A., et al. (2006) A genome-wide *Drosophila* RNAi screen identifes DYRK-family kinases as regulators of NFAT. *Nature, 441,* 646-650.

Haffner, C., Takei, K., Chen, H., Ringstad, N., Hudson, A., et al. (1997) Synaptojanin 1: localization on coated endocytic intermediates in nerve terminals and interaction of its 170 kDa isoform with Eps15. *FEBS Lett., 419,* 175–180.

Hammerle, B., Carnicero, A., Elizalde, C., Ceron, J., Martinez, S. and Tejedor, F. J. (2003) Expression patterns and subcellular localization of the Down syndrome candidate protein MNB/DYRK1A suggest a role in late neuronal differentiation. *Eur. J. Neurosci., 17,* 2277-2286.

Harashima, C., Jacobowitz, D. M., Stoffel, M., Chakrabarti, L., Haydar, T. F., et al. (2006a) Elevated expression of the G-protein-activated inwardly rectifying potassium channel 2 (GIRK2) in cerebellar unipolar brush cells of a Down syndrome mouse model. *Cell. Mol. Neurobiol., 26,* 719-734.

Harashima, C., Jacobowitz, D. M., Witta, J., Borke, R. C., Best, T. K., Siarev, R. J. and Galdzicki, Z. (2006b) Abnormal expression of the G-protein-activated inwardly rectifying potassium channel 2 (GIRK2) in hippocampus, frontal cortex, and substantia nigra of Ts65Dn mouse: a model of Down syndrome. *J. Comp. Neurol., 494,* 815-833.

Harris-Cerruti, C., Kamsler, A., Kaplan, B., Lamb, B., Segal, M., Groner, Y. (2004) Functional and morphological alterations in compound transgenic mice overexpressing Cu/Zn superoxide dismutase and amyloid precursor protein. *Eur. J. Neurosci., 19,* 1174-90. (Erratum in: *Eur. J. Neurosci., 19,* 2913).

Hattori, D., Demir, E., Kim, H. W., Viragh, E., Zipursky, S. L., et al. (2007) Dscam diversity is essential for neuronal wiring and self-recognition. *Nature, 449,* 223-227.

Hattori, M., Fujiyama, A., Taylor, T. D., Watanabe, H., Yada, T., Park, H. S., Toyoda, A., Ishii, K., Totoki, Y., Choi, D. K., Groner, Y., Soeda, E., Ohki, M., Takagi, T., Sakaki, Y., Taudien, S., Blechschmidt, K., Polley, A., Menzel, U., Delabar, J., Kumpf, K., Lehmann, R., Patterson, D., Reichwald, K., Rump, A., Schillhabel, M., Schudy, A., Zimmermann, W., Rosenthal, A., Kudoh, J., Schibuya, K., Kawasaki, K., Asakawa, S., Shintani, A., Sasaki, T., Nagamine, K., Mitsuyama, S., Antonarakis, S. E., Minoshima, S., Shimizu, N., Nordsiek, G., Hornischer, K., Brant, P., Scharfe, M., Schon, O., Desario, A., Reichelt, J., Kauer, G., Blocker, H., Ramser, J., Beck, A., Klages, S., Hennig, S., Riesselmann, L.,

Dagand, E., Haaf, T., Wehrmeyer, S., Borzym, K., Gardiner, K., Nizetic, D., Francis, F., Lehrach, H., Reinhardt, R., Yaspo, M. L. Chromosome 21 mapping and sequencing consortium. (2000) The DNA sequence of human chromosome 21. *Nature*, *405,* 311–319.

Hennequin, M., Morin, C. and Feine, J. S. (2000) Pain expression and stimulus localisation in individuals with Down's syndrome. *Lancet, 356,* 1882-1887. (Erratum in: *Lancet , 357,* 890.

Hoeffer, C. A., Dey, A., Sachan, N., Wong, H., Patterson, R. J., et al. (2007) The Down syndrome critical region protein RCAN1 regulates long-term potentiation and memory via inhibition of phosphatase signaling. *J. Neurosci., 27,* 13161-13172.

Hunter, C. L., Isacson, O., Nelson, M., Bimonte-Nelson, H., Seo, H., Lin, L., Ford, K., Kindy, M. S. and Granholm, A. C. (2003) Regional alterations in amyloid precursor protein and nerve growth factor across age in a mouse model of Down's syndrome. *Neurosci, Res., 45*, 437-445.

Hussain, N. K., Yamabhai, M., Ramjaun, A. R., Guy, A. M., Baranes, D., et al. (1999) Splice variants of intersectin are components of the endocytic machinery in neurons and nonneuronal cells. *J. Biol. Chem., 274,* 15671-15677.

Hyde, L. A., Frisone, D. F. and Crnic, L. S. (2001) Ts65Dn mice, a model for Down syndrome, have deficits in context discrimination learning suggesting impaired hippocampal function. Behav. Brain Res., 118, 53–60.

International Human Genome Sequencing Consortium (2004) Finishing the euchromatic sequence of the human genome. *Nature, 431,* 931-945.

Jackson, J. F., North, E. R. 3rd. and Thomas, J. G. (1976) Clinical diagnosis of Down syndrome. *Clin. Genet., 9,* 483-487.

Janus, C. (2004) Search strategies used by *APP* transgenic mice during navigation in the Morris water maze. *Learn. Mem., 11,* 337-346.

Jenna, S., Hussain, N. K., Danek, E. I., Triki, I., Wasiak, S., et al. (2002) The activity of the GTPase-activating protein CdGAP is regulated by the endocytic protein intersectin. *J. Biol. Chem., 277,* 6366-6373.

Kadota, M., Nishigaki, R., Wang, C. C., Toda, T., Shirayoshi, Y., Inoue, Gojobori, T., Ikeo, K., Rogers, M. S. and Oshimura, M. (2004) Proteomic signatures and aberrations of mouse embryonic stem cells containing a single human chromosome 21 in neuronal differentiation: an *in vitro* model of Down syndrome. *Neuroscience, 129,* 325–335.

Kahlem, P., Sultan, M., Herwig, R., Steinfath, M., Balzereit, D., Eppens, B., Saran, N. G., Pletcher, M. T., South, S. T., Stetten, G. et al. (2004) Transcript level alterations reflect gene dosage effects across multiple tissues in a mouse model of downsyndrome. *Genome Res., 14,* 1258-1267.

Kang, J., Lemaire, H. G., Unterbeck, A., Salbaum, J. M., Masters, C. L., et al. (1987) The precursor of Alzheimer's disease amyloid A4 protein resembles a cell-surface receptor. *Nature,* 325, 733-736.

Kentrup, H., Becker, W., Heukelbach, J., Wilmes, A., Schurmann, A., Huppertz, C., Kainulainen, H. and Joost, H. G. (1996) Dyrk, a dual specificity protein kinase with unique structural features whose activity is dependent on tyrosine residues between subdomains VII and VIII. *J. Biol. Chem., 271,* 3488-3495.

de Kerchove D'Exaerde, A., Cartaud, J., Ravel-Chapuis, A., Seroz, T., Pasteau, F., et al. (2002) Expression of mutant Ets protein at the neuromuscular synapse causes alterations in morphology and gene expression. *EMBO Reports, 3,* 1075-1081.

Kim, S. H. and Lubec, G. (2001) Decreased alpha-endosulfine, an endogenous regulator of ATP-sensitive potassium channels, in brains from adult Down syndrome patients. *J. Neural. Transm. Suppl., 61,* 1-9.

Kim, W. T., Chang, S., Daniell, L., Cremona, O., Di Paolo, G., et al. (2002) Delayed reentry of recycling vesicles into the fusion-competent synaptic vesicle pool in synaptojanin 1 knockout mice. *Proc. Natl. Acad. Sci., 99,* 17143-17148.

King, M. C. and Wilson, A. C. (1975) Evolution at two levels in humans and chimpanzees. *Science, 188,* 107–116.

Kleschevnikov, A. M., Belichenko, P. V., Villar, A. J., Epstein, C. J., Malenka, R. C. and, Mobley, W. C. (2004) Hippocampal long-term potentiation suppressed by increased inhibition in the Ts65Dn mouse, a genetic model of Down syndrome. *J. Neurosci., 24,* 8153-8160.

Kojima, N. and Shirao, T. (2007) Synaptic dysfunction and disruption of postsynaptic drebrin-actin complex: A study of neurological disorders accompanied by cognitive deficits. *Neurosci. Res., 58,* 1-5.

Korenberg, J. R., Kawashima, H., Pulst, S. M., Ikeuchi, T., Ogasawara, N., Yamamoto, K., Schonberg, S. A., West, R., Allen, L., Magenis, E. et al. (1990) Molecular definition of a region of chromosome 21 that causes features of the Down syndrome phenotype, *Am. J. Hum. Genet., 47,* 236–246.

Krasuski, J. S., Alexander, G. E., Horwitz, B., Rapoport, S. I. and Schapiro, M. B. (2002) Relation of medial temporal lobe volumes to age and memory function in nondemented adults with Down's syndrome: implications for the prodromal phase of Alzheimer's disease. *Am. J. Psychiatry, 159,* 74-81.

Kuhn, D. E., Nuovo, G. J., Martin, M. M., Malana, G. E., Pleister, A. P., et al. (2008) Human chromosome 21-derived miRNAs are overexpressed in Down syndrome brains and hearts. *Biochem. Biophys. Res. Commun., 370,* 473-477.

Kumashiro, S., Lu, Y. F., Tomizawa, K., Matsushita, M., Wei, F. Y., et al. (2005) Regulation of synaptic vesicle recycling by calcineurin in different vesicle pools. *Neurosci. Res., 51,* 435-443.

Lalonde, R., Dumont, M., Paly, E., London, J. and Strazielle, C. (2004) Characterization of hemizygous SOD1/wild-type transgenic mice with the SHIRPA primary screen and tests of sensorimotor function and anxiety. *Brain Res. Bull., 64,* 251-258.

Lalonde, R., Le Pecheur, M., Strazielle, C. and London, J. (2005) Exploratory activity and motor coordination in wild-type SOD1/SOD1 transgenic mice. *Brain Res. Bull., 66,* 155-162.

Lamb, B. T., Sisodia, S. S., Lawler, A. M., Slunt, H. H., Kitt, C. A., Kearns, W. G., Pearson, P. L., Price, D. L. and Gearhart, J. D. (1993) Introduction and expression of the 400 kilobase amyloid precursor protein gene in transgenic mice. *Nat. Genet., 5,* 22-30.

Le Pecheur, M., Bourdon, E., Paly, E., Farout, L., Friguet, B., London, J. (2005) Oxidized SOD1 alters proteasome activities in vitro and in the cortex of SOD1 overexpressing mice. *FEBS Lett., 579,* 3613-3618.

Lee, J; I. and Ahnn, J. (2004) Calcineurin in animal behavior. *Mol. Cells, 17,* 390–396.

Lejeune, J. (1990) Pathogenesis of mental deficiency in trisomy 21. *Am. J. Med. Genet. Suppl., 7,* 20-30.

Lejeune, J., Gautier, M., and Turpin, R. (1959) Etude des chromosomes somatiques de neufs enfants Mongoliens, *C. R. Acad. Sci. Paris*, *248,* 1721-1722.

Lesage, F., Duprat, F., Fink, M., Guillemare, E., Coppola, T., Lazdunski, M. and Hugnot, J. P. (1994) Cloning provides evidence for a family of inward rectifier and G-protein coupled K+ channels in the brain. *FEBS Lett., 353,* 37-42.

Li, C. M., Guo, M., Salas, M., Schupt, N., Silvermann, W., et al. (2006) Cell type-specific over-expression of chromosome 21 genes in fibroblasts and fetal hearts with trisomy 21. *BMC Med. Genet., 7,* 24.

Lopes, C., Chettouh, Z., Delabar, J. M., and Rachidi, M. (2003) The differentially expressed *C21orf5* gene in the medial temporal-lobe system could play a role in mental retardation in Down syndrome and transgenic mice, *Biochem. Biophys. Res. Commun*., *305,* 915-924.

Lopes, C., Rachidi, M., Gassanova, S., Sinet, P. M. and Delabar, J. M. (1999) Developmentally regulated expression of mtprd, the murine ortholog of tprd, a gene from the Down syndrome chromosomal region 1. *Mech. Dev., 84,* 189-193.

Ly, A., Nikolaev, A., Suresh, G., Zheng, Y., Tessier-Lavigne, M., et al. (2008) DSCAM is a netrin receptor that collaborates with DCC in mediating turning responses to netrin-1. *Cell, 133,* 1241-1254.

Lyle, R., Gehrig, C., Neergaard-Henrichsen, C., Deutsch, S. and Antonarakis, S. E. (2004) Gene expression from the aneuploid chromosome in a trisomy mouse model of down syndrome. *Genome Res., 14,* 1268-1274.

Ma, H., Xiong, H., Liu, T., Zhang, L., Godzik, A., et al. (2004) Aggregate formation and synaptic abnormality induced by DSCR1. *J. Neurochem., 88,* 1485-1496.

Ma, Y. J., Okamoto, M., Gu, F., Obata, K., Matsuyama, T., et al. (2003) Neuronal distribution of EHSH1/intersectin: molecular linker between clathrin-mediated endocytosis and signalling pathways. *J. Neurosci. Res., 71,* 468-477.

Malago, W. Jr., Sommer, C. A., Del Cistia Andrade, C., Soares-Costa, A., Abrao Possik, P., et al. (2005) Gene expression profile of human Down syndrome leukocytes. *Croat. Med. J., 46,* 647-656.

Mansuy, I. M. (2003) Calcineurin in memory and bidirectional plasticity. *Biochem. Biophys. Res. Commun., 311,* 1195–1208.

Mao, L., Zabel, C., Herrmann, M., Nolden, T., Mertes, F., et al. (2007) Proteomic shifts in embryonic stem cells with gene dose modifications suggest the presence of balancer proteins in protein regulatory networks. *PLoS ONE, 2,* e1218.

Mao, R., Zielke, C. L., Zielke, H. R. and Pevsner, J. (2003) Global up-regulation of chromosome 21 gene expression in the developing Down syndrome brain. *Genomics, 81,* 457-467.

Mao, R., Wang, X., Spitznagel Jr, E. L., Frelin, L. P., Ting, J. C., Ding, H., Kim, J-W., Ruczinski, I., Downey T. J. and Pevsner, J. (2005) Primary and secondary transcriptional effects in the developing human Down syndrome brain and heart. *Genome Biology, 6,* R107.

Martina, J. A., Bonangelino, C. J., Aguilar, R. C. and Bonifacino, J. S. (2001) Stonin 2: an adaptor-like protein that interacts with components of the endocytic machinery. J. Cell. Biol., (153) 1111-1120.

Martinez-Cue, C., Baamonde, C., Lumbreras, M. A., Vallina, I. F., Dierssen, M. and Florez, J. (1999) A murine model for Down syndrome shows reduced responsiveness to pain. *Neuroreport, 10,* 1119–1122.

McPherson, PS. (1999) Regulatory role of SH3 domain-mediated protein-protein interactions in synaptic vesicle endocytosis. *Cell Signal, 11,* 229-238.

McPherson, P. S., Takei, K., Schmid, S. L. and De Camilli, P. (1994) p145, a major Grb2-binding protein in brain, is co-localized with dynamin in nerve terminals where it undergoes activity-dependent dephosphorylation. *J. Biol. Chem., 269,* 30132–30139.

Meng, X., Shi, J., Peng, B., Zou, X. and Zhang, C. (2006) Effect of mouse Sim2 gene on the cell cycle of PC12 cells. *Cell Biol. Int., 30,* 349-353.

Milner, B., Squire, L. R. and Kandel, E. R. (1998) Cognitive neuroscience and the study of memory, *Neuron, 20,* 445–468.

Monks, S. A., Leonardson, A., Zhu, H., Cundiff, P., Pietrusiak, P., et al. (2004) Genetic inheritance of gene expression in human cell lines. *Am. J. Hum. Genet., 75,* 1094-1105

Morii, K., Tanaka, R., Takahashi, Y., Minoshima, S., Fukuyama, R., et al. (1991) Structure and chromosome assignment of human S100 alpha and beta subunit genes. *Biochem. Biophys. Res. Commun., 175,* 185-191.

Morley, M., Molony, C. M., Weber, T. M., Devlin, J. L., Ewens, K. G., et al. (2004) Genetic analysis of genome-wide variation in human gene expression. *Nature, 430,* 743-747.

Murdoch, J. C., Rodger, J. C., Rao, S. S., Fletcher, C. D. and Dunnigan, M.G. (1977) Down's syndrome: An atheroma-free model. *Br. Med. J., 2,* 226-228.

Newby, D., Aitken, D. A., Crossley, J. A., Howatson, A. G., Macri, J. N. and Connor, J. M. (1997) Biochemical markers of trisomy 21 and the pathophysiology of Down's syndrome pregnancies. *Prenat. Diagn., 17,* 941–951.

Nishiyama et al., 2002).

Ohira, M., Seki, N., Nagase, T., Suzuki, E., Nomura, N., Ohara, O., Hattori, M., Sakaki, Y., Eki, T., Murakami, Y., Saito, T., Ichikawa, H. and Ohki, M. (1997) Gene identification in 1.6-Mb region of the Down syndrome region on chromosome 21. *Genome Res., 7,* 47-58.

Oleksiak, M. F., Churchill, G. A. and Crawford, D. L. (2002) Variation in gene expression within and among natural populations. *Nature Genet., 32,* 261–266.

Pascon, R. C. and Miller, B. L. (2000) Morphogenesis in Aspergillus nidulans requires Dopey (DopA), a member of a novel family of leucine zipper-like proteins conserved from yeast to humans. *Mol. Microbiol., 36,* 1250-1264.

Patil, N., Cox, D. R., Bhat, D., Faham, M., Myers, R. M. and Peterson, A. S. (1995) A potassium channel mutation in weaver mice implicates membrane excitability in granule cell differentiation. *Nat. Genet., 11,* 126-129.

Pawson, T. (1995) Protein modules and signalling networks. Nature, 373, 573-580.

Pennington, P. F., Moon, J., Edgin, J., Stedron, J. and Nadel, L. (2003) The neuropsychology of Down syndrome: evidence for hippocampal dysfunction. *Child Dev., 74,* 75-93.

Potier, M. C., Rivals, I., Mercier, G., Ettwiller, L., Moldrich, R. X., Laffaire, J., Personnaz, L., Rossier, J. and Dauphinot, L. (2006) Transcriptional disruptions in Down syndrome: a case study in the Ts1Cje mouse cerebellum during post-natal development. *J. Neurochem., 97 Suppl. 1,* 104-109.

Prandini, P., Deutsch, S., Lyle, R., Gagnebin, M., Delucinge Vivier, C., et al. (2007) Natural gene-expression variation in Down syndrome modulates the outcome of gene-dosage imbalance. *Am. J. Hum. Genet., 81,* 252-263.

Priller, C., Bauer, T., Mitteregger, G., Krebs, B., Kretzschmar, H. A., et al. (2006) Synapse Formation and Function Is Modulated by the Amyloid Precursor Protein. *J. Neurosci., 26,* 7212-7221.

Puffenberger, E. G., Kauffman, E. R., Bolk, S., Matise, T. C., Washington, S. S., Angrist, M., Weissenbach, J., Garver, K. L., Mascari, M. and Ladda, R. (1994) Identity-by-descent and association mapping of a recessive gene for Hirschsprung disease on human chromosome 13q22, *Hum. Mol. Genet., 3,* 1217–1225.

Pulsifer, M B. (1996) The neuropsychology of mental retardation. *J. Int. Neuropsychol. Soc., 2,* 159-176.

Rachidi, M. and Lopes, C. (2007) Mental retardation in Down syndrome: from gene dosage imbalance to molecular and cellular mechanisms. *Neurosci. Res., 59,* 349-369.

Rachidi, M., Lopes, C., Vayssettes, C., Smith, D. J., Rubin, E. M., et al. (2007) New cerebellar phenotypes in YAC transgenic mouse *in vivo* library of human Down syndrome critical region-1. *Biochem. Biophys. Res. Commun., 364,* 488-494.

Rachidi, M., Lopes, C., Delezoide, A. L. and Delabar, J. M. (2006) C21orf5, a human candidate gene for brain abnormalities and mental retardation in Down syndrome. *Cytogenet. Genome Res., 112,* 16-22. (Erratum in: *Cytogenet. Genome Res., 112,* 226.)

Rachidi, M., Lopes, C., Charron, G., Delezoide, A. L., Paly, E., Bloch, B. and Delabar, J. M. (2005a) Spatial and temporal localization during embryonic and fetal human development of the transcription factor SIM2 in brain regions altered in Down syndrome. *Int. J. Dev. Neurosci., 23,* 475-484.

Rachidi, M., Lopes, C., Costantine, M. and Delabar, J. M. (2005b) C21orf5, a new member of dopey family involved in morphogenesis, could participate in neurological alterations and mental retardation in down syndrome. *DNA Res., 12,* 203-210.

Rachidi, M., Lopes, C., Gassanova, S., Sinet, P. M., Vekemans, M., Attie, T., Delezoide, A. L. and Delabar, J. M. (2000) Regional and cellular specificity of the expression of TPRD, the tetratricopeptide Down syndrome gene, during human embryonic development. *Mech. Dev., 93*, 189–193.

Rahmani, Z., Lopes, C., Rachidi, M. and Delabar, J. M. (1998) Expression of the mnb (dyrk) protein in adult and embryonic mouse tissues. *Biochem. Biophys. Res. Commun., 253,* 514–518.

Raz, N., Torres, I. J., Briggs, S. D., Spencer, W. D., Thornton, A. E., Loken, W. J., Gunning, F. M., McQuain, J. D., Driesen, N. R. and Acker, J.D. (1995) Selective neuroanatomic abnormalities in Down_s syndrome and their cognitive correlates: evidence from MRI morphometry. *Neurology, 45,* 356–366.

Reeves, R. H., Yao, J., Crowley, M. R., Buck, S., Zhang, X., Yarowsky, P., Gearhart, J. D. and Hilt, D. C. (1994) Astrocytosis and axonal proliferation in the hippocampus of S100b transgenic mice. *Proc. Natl. Acad. Sci. USA., 91,* 5359-5363.

Roizen, N. J. and Patterson, D. (2003) Down's syndrome. *Lancet, 361,* 1281-1289.

Roos, J. and Kelly, R. B. (1998) Dap160, a neural-specific Eps15 homology and multiple SH3 domain-containing protein that interacts with Drosophila dynamin. *J. Biol. Chem., 273,* 19108-19119.

Rothermel, B. A., Vega, R. B. and Williams, R. S. (2003) The role of modulatory calcineurin-interacting proteins in calcineurin signaling. *Trends Cardiovasc. Med., 13,* 15–21.

Rothermel, B., Vega, R. B., Yang, J., Wu, H., Bassel-Duby, R., et al. (2000) A protein encoded within the Down syndrome critical region is enriched in striated muscles and inhibits calcineurin signaling. *J. Biol. Chem., 275,* 8719-8725.

Sago, H., Carlson, E. J., Smith, D. J., Kilbridge, J., Rubin, E. M., Mobley, W. C., Epstein, C. J. and Huang, T. T. (1998) Ts1Cje, a partial trisomy 16 mouse model for Down syndrome, exhibits learning and behavioural abnormalities. *Proc. Natl. Acad. Sci. USA., 95,* 6256-6261.

Saito, Y., Oka, A., Mizuguchi, M., Motonaga, K., Mori, Y., et al. (2000) The developmental and aging changes of Down's syndrome cell adhesion molecule expression in normal and Down's syndrome brains. *Acta Neuropathol., 100,* 654-664.

Sanna, B., Brandt, E. B., Kaiser, R. A., Pfluger, P., Witt, S. A., et al. (2006) Modulatory calcineurin-interacting proteins 1 and 2 function as calcineurin facilitators *in vivo*. *Proc. Natl. Acad. Sci., 103,* 7327-7332.

Saran, N. G., Pletcher, M. T., Natale, J. E., Cheng, Y. and Reeves, R. H. (2003) Global disruption of the cerebellar transcriptome in a Down syndrome mouse model. *Hum. Mol. Genet., 12,* 2013-2019.

Schadt, E. E., Monks, S. A., Drake, T. A., Lusis, A. J., Che, N., et al. (2003) Genetics of gene expression surveyed in maize, mouse and man. *Nature, 422,* 297–302.

Schmucker, D., Clemens, J. C., Shu, H., Worby, C. A., Xiao, J., et al. (2000) Drosophila Dscam is an axon guidance receptor exhibiting extraordinary molecular diversity. *Cell, 101,* 671-684.

Sengar, A. S., Wang, W., Bishay, J., Cohen, S. and Egan, S. E. (1999) The EH and SH3 domain Ese proteins regulate endocytosis by linking to dynamin and Eps15. *EMBO J., 18,* 1159-1171.

Sethupathy, P., Borel, C., Gagnebin, M., Grant, G. R., Deutsch, S., et al. (2007) Human microRNA-155 on chromosome 21 differentially interacts with its polymorphic target in the AGTR1 3' untranslated region: a mechanism for functional single-nucleotide polymorphisms related to phenotypes. *Am. J. Hum. Genet., 81,* 405-413.

Shapiro, B. (1983) Down syndrome – A disruption of homeostasis. *Amer. J. Medical Genet., 14,* 241-269.

Shapiro, B. L. (1997) Down syndrome critical regions? *Hum. Genet., 99,* 421-423.

Shapiro, L. A. and Whitaker-Azmitia, P. M. (2004) Expression levels of cytoskeletal proteins indicate pathological aging of S100B transgenic mice: an immunohistochemical study of MAP-2, drebrin and GAP-43. *Brain Res., 1019,* 39-46.

Shefner, J. M., Reaume, A. G., Flood, D. G., Scott, R. W., Kowall, N. W., et al. (1999) Mice lacking cytosolic copper/zinc superoxide dismutase display a distinctive motor axonopathy. *Neurology, 53,* 1239-1246.

Shin, J. H., Gulesserian, T., Verger, E., Delabar, J. M. and Lubec, G. (2006) Protein dysregulation in mouse hippocampus polytransgenic for chromosome 21 structures in the Down syndrome critical region. *J. Proteome Res., 5,* 44-53.

Shin, K. S. and Lubec, G. (2002) Drebrin, a dendritic spine protein, is manifold decreased in brains of patients with Alzheimer's disease and Down syndrome. *Neurosci. Lett., 324,* 209-212.

Shinohara, T., Tomizuka, K., Miyabara, S., Takehara, S., Kazuki, Y., Inoue, J., Katoh, M., Nakane, H., Iino, A., Ohguma, A., Ikegami, S., Inokuchi, K., Ishida, I., Reeves, R. H. and Oshimura, M. (2001) Mice containing a human chromosome 21 model behavioral impairment and cardiac anomalies of Down's syndrome. *Hum. Mol. Genet., 10,* 1163–1175.

Smith, D. J., Zhu, Y., Zhang, J., Cheng, J. F. and Rubin, E. M. (1995) Construction of a panel of transgenic mice containing a contiguous 2-Mb set of YAC/P1 clones from human chromosome 21q22.2. *Genomics, 27,* 425-434.

Smith, D. J., Stevens, M. E., Sudanagunta, S. P., Bronson, R. T., Makhinson, M., Watabe, A. M., O'Dell, T. J., Fung, J., Weier, H. U., Cheng, J. F. and Rubin, E. M. (1997) Functional screening of 2Mb of human chromosome 21q22.2 in transgenic mice implicates minibrain in learning defects associated with Down syndrome. *Nature Genet., 16,* 28–36.

Spielman, R. S., Bastone, L. A., Burdick, J. T., Morley, M., Ewens, W. J., et al. (2007) Common genetic variants account for differences in gene expression among ethnic groups. *Nature Genet., 39,* 226–231.

Stasko, M. R. and Costa, A. C. (2004). Experimental parameters affecting the Morris water maze performance of a mouse model of Down syndrome. *Behav. Brain Res., 154,* 1–17.

Stoll, C., Alembik Y., Dott, B. and Roth, M. P. (1990) Epidemiology of Don syndrome in 118,265 consecutive births. *Am. J. Med. Genet., 7(Suppl.),* 79-83.

Storey, J. D., Madeoy, J., Strout, J. L., Wurfel, M., Ronald, J., et al. (2007) Gene-expression variation within and among human populations. *Am. J. Hum. Genet., 80,* 502–509.

Stranger, B. E., Forrest, M. S., Clark, A. G., Minichiello, M. J., Deutsch, S., et al. (2005) Genome-wide associations of gene expression variation in humans. *PLoS Genet., 1,* e78.

Sturchler-Pierrat, C., Abramowski, D., Duke, M., Wiederhold, K. H., Mistl, C., Rothacher, S., Ledermann, B., Burki, K., Frey, P., Paganetti, P. A., Waridel, C., Calhoun, M. E., Jucker, M., Probst, A., Staufenbiel, M. and Sommer, B. (1997) Two amyloid precursor protein transgenic mouse models with Alzheimer disease-like pathology. *Proc. Natl. Acad. Sci. USA., 94,* 13287-13292.

Sultan, M., Piccini, I., Balzereit, D., Herwig, R., Saran, N. G., et al. (2007) Gene expression variation in Down's syndrome mice allows prioritization of candidate genes. *Genome Biol., 8,* R91.

Sumarsono, S. H., Wilson, T. J., Tymms, M. J., Venter, D. J., Corrick, C. M., Kola, R., Lahoud, M. H., Papas, T. S., Seth, A. and Kola, I. (1996) Down's syndrome-like skeletal abnormalities in Ets2 transgenic mice. *Nature, 379,* 534-537.

Sweatt, J. D. (2001) The neuronal MAP kinase cascade: a biochemical signal integration system subserving synaptic plasticity and memory. *J. Neurochem., 76,* 1–10.

Sweatt, J. D. and Weeber, E. J. (2003) Genetics of childhood disorders: LII. Learning and memory, part 5: human cognitive disorders and the ras/ERK/CREB pathway. *J. Am. Acad. Child Adolesc. Psychiatry, 42,* 873–876.

Thomas, G. M. and Huganir, R. L. (2004) MAPK cascade signalling and synaptic plasticity. *Nature Rev. Neurosci., 5,* 173–183.

Tong, X. K., Hussain, N. K., de Heuvel, E., Kurakin, A., Abi- Jaoude, E., et al. (2000) The endocytic protein intersectin is a major binding partner for the Ras exchange factor mSos1 in rat brain. *EMBO J., 19,* 1263-1271.

Vialard, F., Toyama, K., Vernoux, S., Carlson, E. J., Epstein, C. J., Sinet, P. M. and Rahmani, Z. (2000) Over-expression of mSim2 gene in the zona limitans of the diencephalon of segmental trisomy 16 Ts1Cje fetuses, a mouse model for trisomy 21: a novel whole-mount RNA hybridization assay. *Dev. Brain Res., 121,* 73–78.

Voronov, S. V., Frere, S. G., Giovedi, S., Pollina, E. A., Borel, C., et al. (2008) Synaptojanin 1-linked phosphoinositide dyshomeostasis and cognitive deficits in mouse models of Down's syndrome. *Proc. Natl. Acad. Sci., 105,* 9415-9420.

Wang, C. C., Kadota, M., Nishigaki, R., Kazuki, Y., Shirayoshi, Y., Rogers, M. S., Gojobori, T., Ikeo, K. and Oshimura, M. (2004) Molecular hierarchy in neurons differentiated from mouse ES cells containing a single human chromosome 21. *Biochem. Biophys. Res. Commun., 314,* 335–350.

Wang, Y., Stricker, H. M., Gou, D. and Liu, L. (2007) MicroRNA: past and present. *Frontiers Biosci., 12,* 2316–2329.

Watson, D. K., McWilliams-Smith, M. J., Nunn, M. F., Duesberg, P. H., O'Brien, S; J., et al. (1985) The ets sequence from the transforming gene of avian erythroblastosis virus, E26, has unique domains on human chromosomes 11 and 21: both loci are transcriptionally active. *Proc. Natl. Acad. Sci.,* 82, 7294-7298.

Weitzdoerfer, R., Fountoulakis, M., Dierssen, M. and Lubec, G. (2001) Aberrant expression of dihydropyrimidinase-related proteins-2-3, and -4 in fetal Down syndrome brain. *J. Neural. Transm., Suppl. 61,* 95–107.

Whitaker-Azmitia, P. M., Wingate, M., Borella, A., Gerlai, R., Roder, J. and Azmitia, E. C. (1997) Transgenic mice overexpressing the neurotrophic factor S-100 beta show neuronal cytoskeletal and behavioral signs of altered aging processes: implications for Alzheimer's disease and Down's syndrome. *Brain Res., 776,* 51–60.

Winocur, G., Roder, J. and Lobaugh, N. (2001). Learning and memory in S100-beta transgenic mice: an analysis of impaired and preserved function. *Neurobiol. Learn. Mem., 75,* 230–243.

Wisniewski, K. E., Wisniewski, H. M. and Wen, G. Y. (1985) Occurrence of neuropathological changes and dementia of Alzheimer's disease in Down's syndrome. *Ann. Neurol., 17,* 278-282.

Wolvetang, E. J., Bradfield, O. M., Hatzistavrou, T., Crack, P. J., Busciglio, J., et al. (2003) Overexpression of the chromosome 21 transcription factor Ets2 induces neuronal apoptosis. *Neurobiol. Dis., 14,* 349-356.

Yamabhai, M., Hoffman, N. G. , Hardison, N. L., McPherson, P. S., Castagnoli, L., et al. (1998) Intersectin, a novel adaptor protein with two Eps15 homology and five Src homology 3 domains. *J. Biol. Chem., 273,* 31401-31407.

Yamakawa, K., Huot, Y. K., Haendelt, M. A., Hubert, R., Chen, X. N., et al. (1998) DSCAM: a novel member of the immunoglobulin superfamily maps in a Down syndrome region and is involved in the development of the nervous system. *Hum. Mol. Genet., 7,* 227-237.

Yla-Herttuala, S., Luoma, J., Nikkari, T. and Kivimaki, T. (1989) Down's syndrome and atherosclerosis. Atherosclerosis, 76, 269-272.

Yu, Y., Chu, P. Y., Bowser, D. N., Keating, D. J. and Dubach, D. (2008) Mice deficient for the chromosome 21 ortholog Itsn1 exhibit vesicle trafficking abnormalities. *Hum. Mol. Genet., 17,* 3281-3290.

Yvert, G., Brem, R. B., Whittle, J., Akey, J. M., Foss, E., et al. (2003) Trans-acting regulatory variation in Saccharomyces cerevisiae and the role of transcription factors. *Nature Genet., 35,* 57–64.

Zang da, W., Yang, Q., Wang, H. X., Egan, G., Lopes, E. C. and Cheema, S. S. (2004). Magnetic resonance imaging reveals neuronal degeneration in the brainstem of the superoxide dismutase 1 transgenic mouse model of amyotrophic lateral sclerosis. *Eur. J. Neurosci., 20,* 1745–1751.

In: Handbook of Down Syndrome Research
Editors: Dominicus Jelinek and Gijs Dvorak

ISBN 978-1-60741- 690-6

Chapter 3

Total (Birth + Fetal) Prevalence, Possible Causes and Prevention of Down Syndrome in Hungary

***Andrew E. Czeizel**[*1] **and Julia Métneki**[2]*
[1]Foundation for the Community Control of Hereditary Diseases, Budapest, Hungary, and
[2]Hungarian Congenital Anomalies Registry and Surveillance,
National Centre for Healthcare Audit and Inspection, Budapest, Hungary

Abstract

The recent significant increase of cases with Down syndrome in Hungary (1.1/1000 total births between 1973 and 1988, 1.57/1000 between 1989 and 1999 and 1.71/1000 between 2000 and 2006) is explained mainly by the higher proportion of prenatally diagnosed cases. Less important segment of this increase is a somewhat higher proportion of mothers with advanced maternal age and the more complete ascertainment due to the extra effort to reveal all cases in the study.

The data of the Hungarian Surveillance of Germinal Mutations based on the Hungarian Congenital Abnormality Registry did not show significant increase in the two forms (pure trisomy 21 as indicator of genom mutations and Robertsonian translocation due to chromosomal mutations) of Down syndrome after the fall-out deposition from Chernobyl in Hungary. In addition the rate of sentinel anomalies (new mutations of autosomal dominant disorders) and unclassified multiple congenital abnormalities (as the most sensitive indicator of environmental hazards) did also not indicate any increase in germinal mutations in Hungary after 1986.

The Hungarian Congenital Abnormality Registry detected a very obvious spatial cluster of Down syndrome and other congenital abnormalities in a small Hungarian village, 1989 and 1990. The number of inhabitants in this village was 456 and they had 15 livebirths in 1989 and 1990, and out of these 15 babies, 11 (73.3%) were affected with congenital abnormalities, 4 were affected with Down syndrome. The case-control

[*] Address of corresponding author: Dr. Czeizel, Endre/Andrew, 1026. Törökvész lejtő 32, Budapest, Hungary. Tel/Fax: 36 1 3944 712, e-mail: czeizel@interware.hu.

field study identified trichlorfon used in the fishfarms of the village, as an environmental agent that can induce Down syndrome in very large doses. This observation was confirmed in animal investigations. Thus our finding is an important argument for the necessity and importance of population-based registries of congenital abnormalities.

We studied the association between the use of nutritional supplements during the first gestational month and the origin of Down syndrome, and we found a significant protective effect of large doses (about 6 mg/day) of folic acid and iron (150-300 mg/day of ferrous sulfate) for the occurrence of cases with Down syndrome. In general, folic acid and iron were used together, therefore it was difficult to separate these effects due to the limited number of cases and controls. However, the main message of our study is that a pharmacological dose of folic acid and iron supplement appears to have a primary preventive effect for Down syndrome.

Introduction

Down syndrome (DS) (trisomy 21) may be the result of germinal aneuploidy or a chromosomal mutation. The additional chromosome 21 arises most commonly as a result of non-disjunction in maternal meiosis I [1]. Robertsonian translocations account for approximately 3% of all cases [2], and about two-thirds of these cases had parents with normal karyotype, i.e. DS is a consequence of a new chromosomal mutation. About 2% of DS cases are caused by mosaicism due to an error of mitosis after conception [2]. Thus, about 98% of DS cases are the result of a *de novo* event, familial cases are rare.

The aim of this review paper is to present the trend in occurrence of DS in Hungary, in addition to summarize the results of our previous studies regarding the detection of possible causes and primary prevention of DS.

Total (Birth + Fetal) Prevalences of Cases with Down Syndrome

The population-based large data set of the Hungarian Congenital Abnormality Registry (HCAR) provides data continuously for the evaluation of occurrence of different structural birth defects, i.e. congenital abnormalities (CAs), and among them, DS [3]. These recorded total (birth + fetal) prevalences of different CAs are appropriate for the detection of significant changes in time and spatial occurrences (the so-called clusters) of different CAs. However, this type of registries is not appropriate for the determination the so-called true occurrence: prevalence or incidence of CA due to the prenatal selection and underreporting (i.e. underascertainment) of different CA-entities.

There are two types of occurrence in the evaluation of diseases including CAs. Incidence is the rate at which a new event (i.e. fresh disorder of index patients or cases) occurs in the study population during a certain period. Prevalence is the rate of all index patients or cases with a defined disorder, e.g. CA in the study population at a given point of time or during a given period. The concept of incidence cannot be applied to most CAs because many malformed fetuses are selected out before birth mainly in the early period of pregnancy (e.g.

such as miscarriage). Thus we used the term prevalence at birth (or birth prevalence) at the evaluation of occurrence of index patients/cases with different CAs in the past based on all live- and stillbirths in the demoninator of this rate. However, recently we have been able to evaluate the prenatally diagnosed malformed fetuses in the second and third trimester of pregnancies as well, thus it was necessary to introduce a new term: informative offspring and we estimate the total (birth + fetal) prevalence of different CAs

In the 1990s an increase was found in the reported total prevalence rate of cases with DS. Thus we decided to check whether there was a real increase in the total prevalence of DS or it was the consequence of a more complete ascertainment, therefore we attempted to achieve a complete data set of cases with DS in an *ad hoc* study [4].

Material and Methods

A registry of malformed cases was established in Hungary in 1962, but HCAR has been launched officially in the Department of Human Genetics and Teratology, National Institute of Public Health in 1970 [3]. Notification of CAs is mandatory for physicians and most are reported by obstetricians (in Hungary practically all deliveries occur in inpatient obstetric clinics), and by paediatricians (who are working in the neonatal units of inpatient obstetric clinics and various general and special inpatient and outpatient paediatric clinics), and by 13 prenatal diagnostic centres (since 1984). An autopsy was obligatory for all infant deaths and usual in stillborn fetuses during the study period. Pathologists were asked to send a copy of autopsy report to the HCAR in stillborn fetuses and dead infants were affected with CA. In addition to the name and address of cases, the notified data included the date of pregnancy outcome: livebirth, stillbirth and elective termination of pregnancy, sex of infant or fetus, singleton-multiple birth, birth weight-gestational age, maternal age, region of parents' residence. The recorded *total* (birth + fetal) prevalence of malformed cases, diagnosed from the second trimester of pregnancy through the age of one year was calculated for 1000 *informative offspring* (liveborn infants, stillborn fetuses and electively terminated malformed fetuses). However, the number of electively terminated fetuses was not known during the whole study period therefore the denominator includes only total (live and still) births. Isolated and multiple CAs have been differentiated, thus the unit of the HCAR is the affected subject and a case with two or more CAs is considered as a multi-malformed person [5].

Cases with DS have been classified as a specified multiple CA entity. In the first level of registration, the clinical diagnosis was accepted because in general DS is recognizable on the basis of clinical symptoms [6]. However, a chromosomal diagnosis is recommended in these cases because karyotyping offers the confirmation of clinical diagnosis and the knowledge of DS types help us to have a more accurate recurrence risk estimation for the next pregnancy. Thus, the second level of registration includes the karyotyped cases.

Three extra efforts have been made to supplement the data set of the HCAR in 2000.

1 *The Hungarian Case-Control Surveillance of Congenital Abnormalities* [7] was created in 1980. Cases with isolated and multiple CAs (including DS) who were reported in the first three months after birth or pregnancy termination were included

into this Surveillance. A post-paid questionnaire and explanatory letter were mailed immediately after the selection of cases to their parents. The questionnaire provides an opportunity (i) to ask mothers to check the accuracy of data previously reported by medical doctors to the HCAR as these are mentioned on each questionnaire, (ii) to complete or revise the previous diagnosis of CA on the basis of recent medical examinations, (iii) to complement our data set concerning paternal age, parental occupation and employment status, birth and pregnancy order, marital status, outcomes of previous pregnancies, family history, (iv) to obtain the name and address of cases' paediatricians and (v) to provide a written informed consent for further registration of personal data and for invitation in possible studies. The data of recorded cases with DS were checked and supplemented by this source.

2 All *cytogenetic laboratories* were visited in Hungary, their records were reviewed and the available data set of the HCAR was checked and corrected if necessary, in addition the so-called new cases were added to the data set of the study. We supposed that all cases with DS had cytogenetic examination, except early lethal cases. Unfortunately, the maternal age was not recorded in the records of cytogenetic laboratories and we had no right to contact the parents of these cases.

3 All *prenatal diagnostic centres* were visited, their records were reviewed and the available data set of the HCAR was checked and revised, in addition new cases were also included to the data set of the study.

The demographic data of the Hungarian pregnant population at large (e.g., maternal age distribution) were obtained by the series of Demographic Yearbooks [8].

On the other hand after 2000 we decided to complete continuosly the number of cases with DS in the HCAR, therefore we followed the method of previously mentioned *ad hoc* study in each year. These data are published first here.

For the statistical analysis in general the chi-square and z test was used.

Results

Table 1 shows Hungarian basic data of cases with DS yearly between 1970 and 2006 based on two different approaches.

The recorded number of cases with DS was 3,312 in the HCAR between 1970 and 1999. Our extra efforts have resulted in 1,714 new cases; therefore the revised number of cases with DS was 5,026. Thus, the completeness of cases with DS in the HCAR was 65.9% during the first study period. The point is that the recorded rate of DS, i.e., 0.77 per 1000 increased to 1.21 per 1000 due to the study.

The second period of our data covers cases with DS between 2000 and 2006. The recorded number of cases with DS was 1,061 in the HCAR, our extra efforts have resulted in 104 new cases; therefore the revised number of cases with DS was 1,165. Thus, the completeness of recorded cases with DS was 91.1% in the HCAR during the second study period, much higher than in the first period. This good finding may be connected with the continuous control of reporting. The recorded rate of cases with DS, i.e., 1.56 per 1000 increased to 1.71 per 1000 due to our extra effort.

Table 1. Annual number and rate (per 1000 total births) of cases with Down syndrome (DS), in addition distribution of pregnancy outcomes of informative offspring with DS between 1970 and 2006. (The number of prenatally diagnosed fetuses with DS, but without termination is shown in bracket and they are included in the group of livebirths)

Year	Total births	HCAR		New cases		Revised dataset		Livebirth		Stillbirth		Prenatal diagnosis	
	No.	No.	Rate	No.	%	No.	Rate	No.	%	No.	%	No.	%
1970	153,339	93	0.61	27	22.5	120	0.78	120	100.0	-	-	-	-
1971	152,159	111	0.73	29	20.7	140	0.92	140	100.0	-	-	-	-
1972	154,668	115	0.74	32	21.8	147	0.95	147	100.0	-	-	-	-
1973	157,623	138	0.88	28	16.9	166	1.05	165	99.4	1	0.6	-	-
1974	187,957	174	0.93	26	13.0	200	1.06	198	99.0	2	1.0	-	-
1975	195,847	167	0.85	37	18.1	204	1.04	198	97.1	6	2.9	-	-
1976	186,916	167	0.89	32	16.1	199	1.06	195	98.0	4	2.0	-	-
1977	179,152	164	0.92	48	22.6	212	1.18	211	99.5	1	0.5	-	-
1978	169,524	154	0.91	50	24.5	204	1.25	202	100.0	-	-	2	0.1
1979	161,677	129	0.80	56	30.3	185	1.14	185	100.0	-	-	-	-
1980	149,829	141	0.94	51	26.6	192	1.28	188	97.9	3	1.6	1	0.5
1981	144,062	122	0.79	35	22.3	157	1.09	154	98.1	3	1.9	-	-
1982	134,579	124	0.86	39	23.9	163	1.21	163	100.0	-	-	-	-
1983	128,160	88	0.69	42	32.3	130	1.01	129	99.2	1	0.8	-	-
1984	126,158	80	0.63	32	28.6	112	0.89	108	96.4	1	0.6	3	2.7
1985	131,008	113	0.86	56	33.1	169	1.29	161	95.3	1	-	7	4.1
1986	129,032	88	0.68	45	33.8	133	1.03	128	96.2	-	-	5(1)	3.8
1987	126,722	108	0.85	62	36.5	170	1.34	161	94.7	-	0.6	9	5.3
1988	125,060	105	0.84	52	33.1	157	1.26	148	94.3	1	-	8	5.1
1989	123,957	115	0.92	73	38.8	188	1.52	169	89.9	-	0.5	19(3)	10.1
1990	126,378	116	0.92	72	38.3	188	1.49	170	90.4	1	-	17(2)	9.0
1991	127,782	132	1.03	69	34.3	201	1.57	168	83.6	-	-	33(1)	16.4
1992	122,233	90	0.74	126	58.3	216	1.77	171	79.2	-	-	45(2)	20.8
1993	117,458	68	0.58	109	61.6	177	1.51	123	69.5	-		54	30.5
1994	116,006	76	0.66	94	55.3	170	1.46	124	72.9	1	0.6	45(1)	26.5
1995	112,447	72	0.64	103	58.9	175	1.56	132	75.4	-	-	43(1)	24.6
1996	105,669	67	0.63	75	52.8	142	1.34	107	75.4	1	0.7	34	23.9
1997	100,830	61	0.60	72	54.1	133	1.32	79	59.4	-		54(2)	40.6
1998	97,857	56	0.57	62	52.5	118	1.21	76	64.4	1	0.8	41	34.8
1999	95,116	78	0.82	80	50.6	158	1.66	88	55.7	-	-	70(2)	44.3
2000	97,597	145	1.49	3	2.0	148	1.52	78	52.7	-	-	70	47.3
2001	97,047	145	1.49	17	10.5	162	1.67	85	52.1	1	0.6	76	46.6
2002	96,804	161	1,66	18	10.0	179	1.85	95	53.1	3	1.7	81	45.3
2003	94,647	135	1.43	23	14.6	158	1.67	98	62.0	-	-	60	38.0

Table 1. (Continued)

Year	Total births	HCAR		New cases		Revised dataset		Livebirth		Stillbirth		Prenatal diagnosis	
	No.	No.	Rate	No.	%	No.	Rate	No.	%	No.	%	No.	%
2004	95,137	152	1.60	13	7.9	165	1.73	79	47.9	-	-	86	52.1
2005	97,496	152	1.56	30	16.5	182	1.87	91	50.0	1	0.5	90	49.5
2006	99,871	171	1.71	0	0.0	171	1.71	72	42.1	3	1.8	96	56.1
Total	4,915,404	4,373	0.89	1,818	29.4	6,191	1.26	5,106	82.5	36	0.6	1,049	16.9

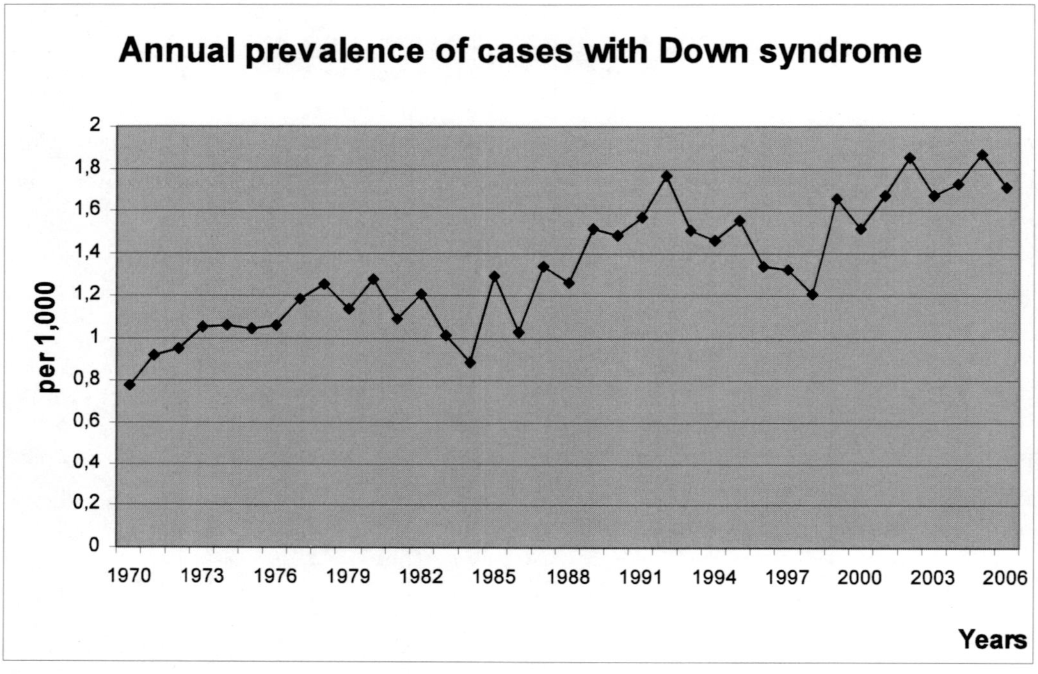

Figure 1. The annual revised rate of cases with DS reflects four periods in Hungary between 1970 and 2006.

The first period covers the first three years (1970-1972), particularly 1970, with the rate of DS less than 1.0 per 1000. Obviously these years had an underascertainment as seen by the high number of new cases in the revised dataset. The second period may represent the previous Hungarian birth prevalence of DS between 1.0-1.3 per 1000. These years cover the period between 1973 and 1988 (except for 1984) with the usual random fluctuation around 1.1 per 1000. The third period contains years between 1989 and 1999, the mean rate of cases with DS was 1.57 per 1000. This higher figure of cases with DS cannot be explained by chance because it indicates a significant increase ($z= -2.18$; $p=0.03$). The maximum rate of cases with DS was found in 1992 when its birth prevalence was 1.77 per 1000; however, the rates of years between 1996 and 1998 reflected the birth prevalences of the second period. Finally the fourth period between 2000 and 2006 confirmed the recent higher rate of cases with DS because its mean birth prevalence was 1.71 per 1000 and new maxmum values were seen in 2002 (1.85/1000) and 2005 (1.87/1000).

Of 5,026 cases, 2,720 were male and 2,306 female, thus the proportion of males was 54.1% in *ad hoc* study between 1970 and 1999. There was no secular change in the distribution of sex during the study period. Of 5,026 informative offspring, 57 (1.1%) were twins. Six twin pairs (i.e. 12 twins) were concordant for DS, while 45 discordant.

Table 1 also summarized three pregnancy outcomes of informative offspring with DS; however, it is worth differentiating two periods, i.e. 1970-1999 and 2000-2006. First we show the data of the first period. The stillbirth rate was 0.6% within informative offspring. In Hungary fetal chromosomal examination was introduced in the late 1970s, but a higher proportion of prenatal diagnosis in women over 35, but mainly over 40 years old was performed after 1988. The number of prenatally diagnosed and terminated fetuses was 490. However, an obvious increase was seen in their proportion, about one-third (32.3%) of cases with DS were diagnosed prenatally after 1992. Of 505 fetuses with the prenatal diagnosis of DS, 15 (3.0%) were not terminated, thus they are among live-born babies. The distribution of pregnancy outcomes shows a very different pattern in the second period. The proportion of stillbirths was the same, but there was a drastic change in the ratio of livebirths and elective termination of pregnancies, the previous 89.7% and 9.7%, i.e. 9.3:1.0 changed to 59.8% and 55.9%, i.e. 1.1:1.0. The explanation is the much more frequently used integrated maternal screening based on serum markers (AFP, estriol, beta component of hCG, inhibin, PAPP) and two untrasound signs in younger mothers.

Of 4,508 live-born cases with DS, 924 died (20.5%) between 1970 and 1999. However, there was a drastic decrease in the infant mortality of DS during the study period, while it was 23.7% in 1970-1972 and 4.1% in 1993-1999.

Of 5,026 cases, 3,390 (67.4%) had a cytogenetic diagnosis in our *ad hoc* study based on the year 1970 and 1999. While the proportion of cytogenetically confirmed cases was under 40% in the first 5 years, all years had a percentage figure of >73% between 1983 and 1999. Thus, there was a significant increase in the proportion of cytogenetically confirmed diagnoses achieving a maximum level of 91.8% in 1999. Of 3,390 cases with cytogenetically diagnosed DS, 3,085 had full trisomy 21 (91.0%), while 156 (4.6%) had a Robertsonian translocation and 149 (4.4%) had mosaicism. Among translocations, the percentage figure of males (60.9%) was somewhat higher than that of karyotyped cases with full trisomy 21 (55.1%), but the difference was not significant ($\chi2_1=1.94$, p=0.16).

Unfortunately, of 5,026 cases with DS between 1970 and 1999, only 3,420 (68.0%) had known maternal age. The proportion with unknown maternal age decreased significantly during the study period. This figure was less than 10% between 1984 and 1999. There was an obvious decrease in the mean maternal age of prenatally diagnosed cases; it was 40.5, 38.6 and 36.6 years during the years of 1985-1989, 1990-1994 and 1995-1999, respectively.

The maternal age distribution of cases with DS according to the three cytogenetic types is shown in Table 2. There is an exponential increase in the rate of cases with DS parallel with maternal age-groups particularly in cases with full trisomy 21 (Figure 2). However, a similar but much slighter trend is also seen in cases with mosaicism and in cases without karyotype. A higher rate of cases with DS can be found over 40 years in cases with translocation but based on only 7 cases.

The number and rate of informative offspring with DS according to maternal age in this Hungarian data set were compared with the data of eight surveys combined by Cuckle et al

[9] (Figure 2). However, the maternal age was known only in 3,420 informative offsping with DS (i.e., 68.3% of the data set), but we may suppose a similar specific rate of maternal age distribution in the rest 31.7%. The maternal age distribution of total births showed a slight change in the Hungarian pregnant population during the study period, because there was a decreasing trend in the age groups of 19 or less and 20-24 while an increase in 25-29 and more advanced groups except ≥45 years. The time trend in the rate of DS depending on maternal age also showed an increasing trend in each maternal age group according to the 5 years of the study period particularly in the age groups of 30-35 and ≥40 years.

Discussion

Our previous epidemiological study [10] estimated that the total birth prevalence of case with DS was 1.17 per 1000 in Budapest during the 1970s. The proportion of underascertainment and misdiagnosis in the recorded cases with DS in the HCAR was 25% and 5%, respectively.

The total birth prevalence rate estimate of DS in Budapest was in agreement with the findings of other countries as in North-Eastern France, 1979-1987: 1.17 [11], in South Australia, 1960-1989: 1.19 [12], in the USA, 1970-1989: 1.17-1.22 [13] and in Scotland, 1978-1992: 1.24 [14]. However, these prevalence rates are affected by the maternal age distribution of the population, extent of elective termination of affected pregnancies, completeness of ascertainment and accuracy of diagnosis. Thus we can compare only prevalence rates adjusted for the effects of maternal age [15, 16] and for elective termination [17].

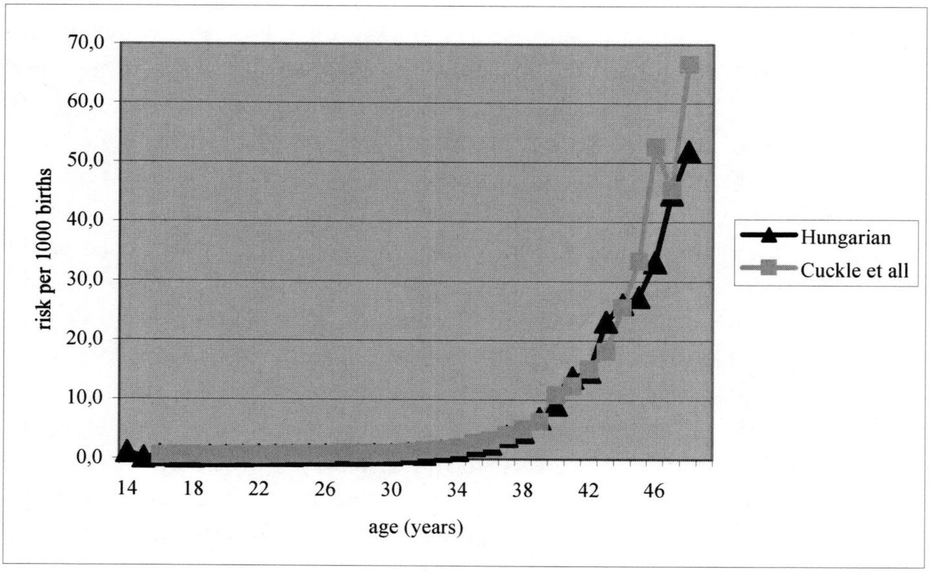

Figure 2. Maternal age specific DS rate per 1,000 and risk of DS by maternal age in the Hungarian study and in the eight studied combined by Cuckle et al [9].

Table 2. Distribution of maternal age groups in the Hungarian population (total births) and in different cytogenetic types of cases with DS, in addition their rate per 1000 during the study period (1970-1999). Exceptional cases are shown in footnote

Maternal Age Group (yr)	Total birth		Full trisomy 21			Robertsonian translocation			Mosaicism			Cases without karyotype			Total		
	No.	%	No.	%	Rate	No.	%	Rate	No.	%	Rate	No.	%	Rate	No.	%	Rate
-19	561,224	13.6	134	5.3	0.24	13	10.5	0.02	7	6.7	0.01	51	7.5	0.09	205	6.0	0.37
20-24	1,637,382	39.6	521	20.8	0.32	36	29.0	0.02	20§	19.2	0.01	160	23.8	0.10	737	21.6	0.45
25-29	1,196,860	28.9	547	21.7	0.46	38o	30.6	0.03	19§§	18.3	0.02	157	23.1	0.13	761	22.3	0.64
30-34	523,928	12.6	358x	14.2	0.68	22	17.8	0.04	16	15.4	0.03	103	15.1	0.20	499	14.6	0.95
35-39	180,498	4.4	502	20.0	2.78	8	6.5	0.04	26	25.0	0.14	102	15.0	0.57	638	18.6	3.53
40-44	37,441	0.9	406xx	16.2	10.84	6	4.8	0.16	15	14.4	0.40	91	13.4	2.43	518	15.1	13.84
45-	1,872	0.0	46	1.8	24.57	1	0.8	0.53	1	1.0	0.53	14	2.1	7.48	62	1.8	33.12
Total	4,139,205	100.0	2,514	84.5	0.61	124	79.5	0.03	104	69.8	0.03	678	41.4	0.16	3,420	68.0	0.83
Unknown	-	-	571	18.5	0.14	32	20.5	0.01	45	30.2	0.01	958	58.6	0.23	1606	32.0	0.39
Together	4,139,205	100.0	3085	100.0	0.75	156	100.0	0.04	149	100.0	0.04	1636	100.0	0.40	5026	100.0	1.21

x48,XXY,+21

xx48,XY,+18,+21

o46,XX/46,XX,t(21,13)

§46,X,+21/47,XX,+21

§§47,XX,+21/48,XXX,+21

Our recent studies were appropriate to estimate the proportion of underascertainment in the HCAR in Hungary during the last 37 years because a nationwide *ad hoc* field study was organized to reveal unreported cases to the HCAR in all cytogenetic labs and prenatal diagnostic centres. The proportion of newly ascertained cases was 34.1% thus the completeness of cases with DS (65.9%) in the HCAR was lower between 1970 and 1999 than in our previous Budapest study. There are two main reasons of underascertainment. Most physicians waited to have a final diagnosis of DS due to cytogenetic examination and later there was a lower notification activity due to this delay. In addition, prenatal diagnostic centres had a low notification rate despite mandatory obligation to report.

An important effect of our *ad hoc* epidemiological study as strong control of reporting of cases with DS was a significant change in the ascertainment rate of DS; this proportion was only 8.9% between 2000 and 2006. On the other hand there was a drastic increase in the proportion of prenatally diagnosed and terminated cases with DS.

Unfortunately, several cases with trisomy 21 were not karyotyped in the 1970s, however, the time trend showed a significant increase in the proportion of cytogenetically confirmed cases with DS. Recently this proportion was nearly 95% and most cases without karyotype had early neonatal deaths. The observed proportion of Robertsonian translocations (4.6%) and mosaicism (4.4%) between 1970 and 1999 was somewhat higher in this study than expected (about 3% and 2%) on the basis of international findings [1].

The slight male excess among cases with DS corresponds to international experiences [18-20]. However, among mosaic 46/47+21 cases, a female predominance was found [21, 22] which was not confirmed in our data set. We found a slightly higher proportion of males among cases with DS due to translocation.

The proportion of stillborn fetuses with DS was somewhat lower (0.6%) than the general stillbirth rate (about 1%) in Hungary during the study period and this finding may indicate an underascertainment of DS in stillbirths. Recently the proportion of prenatally diagnosed and terminated fetuses with DS has increased significantly. Of 505 cases, 15 fetuses were allowed to proceed to term after the diagnosis of DS in our *ad hoc* study; this 3.0% figure is lower than in other countries [23]

There was a 5.8 fold decrease in the proportion of infant mortality among cases with DS in the study period. The figure of infant mortality in the Hungarian population at large decreased from 3.4% to 1.1% between 1970 and 1999. A substantial improvement in the infant mortality of cases with DS was found in many countries [24]. In the USA, the median age of death of cases with DS increased from 25 years in 1983 to 49 years in 1977 [25].

We were able to confirm the well-known higher risk for DS parallel with maternal age and it was similar to the international observations (Figure 2). However, the comparison of the Hungarian and international trends shows that there was a lower Hungarian rate of DS in younger maternal age groups. An explanation for this discrepancy may be a higher proportion of unknown maternal age in these age groups because cytogenetic labs and prenatal diagnostic centres paid a higher attention for advanced maternal age.

Recently the question has been raised frequently whether the "incidence" of Down syndrome is increasing [26]. Our Hungarian data indicated a significant increase in the total rate of DS between 1989 and 2006. The statistical evaluation of this increase was against the random fluctuation. Our recent Hungarian figures are agreement with four recent estimates in other regions: 1.58 for West Berlin during 1980-1988 [27], 1.72 for selected states within USA during 1990-1993 [28, 29], 1.66 for Strasbourg region of France during 1979-1996 [30] and 1.71-2.49 for the Basque Country, Spain, 1990-1997 [31].

Four explanations are worth discussing regarding the increase rate of cases with DS in Hungary.

First, there was a significant increase in the proportion of prenatally diagnosed fetuses with DS. About 35% of conceptions affected with DS are selected during pregnancy as miscarriage [32]. At present amniocentesis (about 16-18th week of gestation) but mainly chorion villous sampling, i.e. CVS (about 13th week of gestation) may precede the time of certain part of miscarriages therefore now these previously undiagnosed cases are also ascertained. This possible explanation is confirmed by the increase in the proportion of prenatally diagnosed cases, recently about half of cases with DS have been ascertained from this source of cases in Hungary. Routine antenatal diagnosis (amniocentesis and CVS) for all women over the age of 35 for detecting trisomy 21 has been used for nearly two decades. The reduction of livebirth prevalence of DS was estimated as 20.6% during 1979-1980, 26.1% for 1980-1982, 27.8% for 1983-1985 and 31.9% for 1985-1989 with 66.9% of Danish pregnant women aged ≥35 years utilizing prenatal diagnosis during 1989 [33, 34]. This change in diagnostic method is the main explanation for the increasing trend of DS in other countries as well because the increase in early prenatal diagnoses of trisomy 21 in fetuses leading to terminations of pregnancy that would previously have aborted spontaneously [35-37].

Second, the possible effect of a change in maternal age was evaluated. In the 1960s an appropriate 33% decrease in the birth prevalence of DS was found due to the significant decrease of mean maternal age and the drastic decline in the proportion of women over 35 but particularly over 40 (<1%) [38]. Recently a relative increase was observed in babies born to mothers over 35 and mainly over 40. However, this redistribution of maternal age groups can explain only a minor segment of the recently found increase in the Hungarian rate of DS. In other countries some rise in recorded prevalences was also due to the demographic trend toward starting families later in life [39, 40]. After the adjustment for the number of terminations and the fetal losses that would have occurred naturally, the maternal age-specific risks of DS remained similar to those before the availability of prenatal diagnosis [41].

Third, a more complete ascertainment cannot be excluded due to the intensive field study.

Fourth, we cannot exclude possible new environmental causes of DS, e.g. drastic environmental pollution due to pesticides [42].

In conclusion, the recent significant increase of cases with DS in Hungary is explained mainly by the higher proportion of prenatally diagnosed cases. Less important segment of this increase is a somewhat higher proportion of mothers with advanced maternal age and the more complete ascertainment due to the extra effort to reveal all cases in the study.

II. Aetiological Studies in Down Syndrome

The true knowledge is the knowledge of causes, thus we have to do our best to understand better the aetiology, more exactly the causes of DS. The aim of our two previous studies was to confirm or to detect environmental cause of DS.

The Evaluation of Birth Prevalence of Cases with Down Syndrome after the Radiological Contamination Due to Chernobyl Nuclear Plant Accident in Hungary

At 1.23.43 a.m. on April 26, 1986 a massive explosion ripped open reactor No. 4 at the Soviet Union's nuclear power plant facility at Chernobyl. It was the largest reported accidental release of radioactive material in the world. An unusual pattern of north-westerly winds pushed the radioactive cloud towards the Baltic Sea. Later, changing wheather conditions altered its drift and the heaviest radionuclide deposition shifted to the south. Thus, a higher rate of radiation was measured in the surrounding countries of the Soviet Union including Hungary depending on the distance and prevailing meterological conditions [43].

In Hungary, the pathways likely to give the most significant exposure were external irradiation of the whole body from deposited materials, and internal radiation from the inhalation of the material in the cloud and from the ingestion of contaminated foods. The maximum beta activity in the air after the Chernobyl accident was found between April 28 and May 15, although beta activity of the fall-out had some late peaks up to the end of June. Hungary had the 13th highest ^{137}Cs deposition (7.9×10^{14} Bq) and the 10th-11th highest national collective 50 year total body dose (1.3×10^{-4} persons-Gy) but the 7th individual 50 year external dose ($6.3\text{x}10\text{-}^{4}$ Gy) and individual total body ingestion dose (5.9×10^{-4} Gy) among European countries [44]. In 1986, the estimated an extra dose due to the Chernobyl accident was about 0.1 mSv in the Hungarian population at large, the maximum was about 0.4 mSv in some regions of the country (Figure 3). These figures are only a fraction of the usual annual background dose of about 2.0 mSv.

Some previous human studies suggested an association of DS with ionizing radiation [45, 46]. Thus we decided to check the possible germinal mutagenic effect of these extra doses of radiation in Hungary [47]. Thus we evaluated the data of the Hungarian Surveillance of Germinal Mutations (HSGM) [48, 49]. As far as we know the HSGM was the first population-based public health system for the measurement of new germinal mutations in the human population. The basic data of the HCAR were used for these purpose. (See the description of the HCAR in Chapter I.).

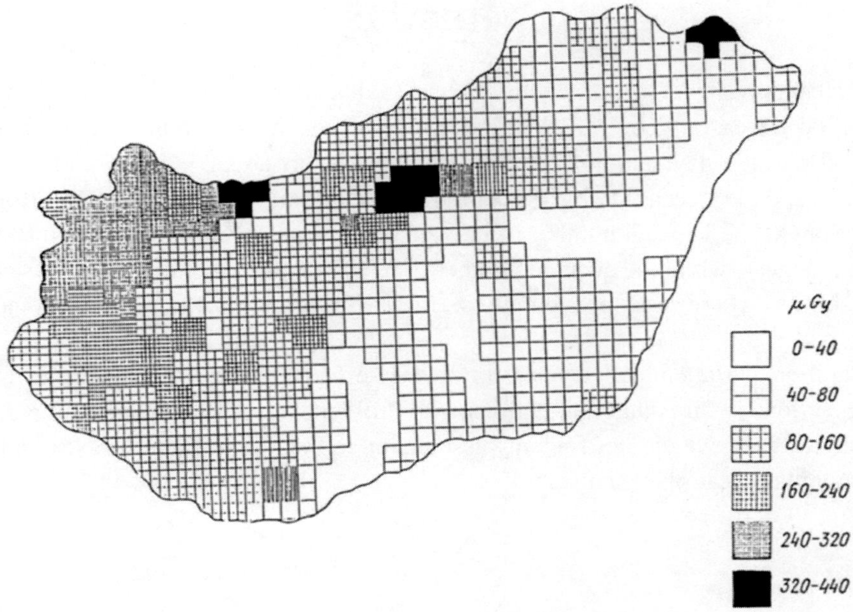

Figure 3. Territorial distribution of increased background radiation in Hungary after the Chernobyl accident. The highest radiocontaminations were caused by radiocontaminated transport vehicles. The increased general background radiation was most obvious in the western part of Hungary due to the direction of radioactice cloud, though North-East Hungary was nearest to Chernobyl.

The concept of the HSGM was that the evaluation of three indicator CA groups is appropriate for the estimation the rate of new germinal mutations in the Hungarian populations. These 3 indicators CA groups were as follows:

1. Sentinel anomalies are indicators of dominant gene mutations [50, 49]. Thus we selected 12 CAs with dominant inheritance and if these sentinel anomalies (e.g. achondroplasia or aniridia) occurred in a child without affected parents, this CA was considered as the first manifestation of new dominant germinal mutations.
2. DS may be the indicator partly and mainly of genom mutations (i.e. the error of meiosis I and II in gametogenesis) and partly chromosomal mutations (i.e. structural defects due to Robertsonian translocations) [51]. If these genom and chromosomal mutations did not occur in parents and DS was diagnosed in their children, it is the consequence of new germinal genom or chromosomal mutations.
3. Unclassified multiple CAs, i.e. children with 2 or more CAs without the identification of previously delineated CA-syndromes [5]. We have introduced a special protocol for the evaluation of multiple CAs including 2-11 component CAs [52] because evironmental mutagens in general cause CA-syndromes thus we have to expect a cluster of specified multiple CA-entities (i.e. new syndromes) after a drastic environmenal mutagenic effects.

The Chernonyl accident provided a sorrow opportunity to test the feasibility and efficacy of the HSGM. Here only the data of cases with DS are presented.

Results

The birth pervalence of cases with DS was evaluated between 1980 and 1989 (Figure 4). Rare familial DS cases were excluded from this analysis. We differentiated DS (pure trisomy 21) caused by non-disjunction in the gametogenesis, in about 90% of cases in maternal oogenesis, and DS caused by structural chromosomal mutations (i.e. Robertsonian translocations). The average number of new genom mutations was about 9 per 10,000 births yearly in Hungary, while the average number of new chromosomal mutations was about 3 per 100,000 births. There was no change in these figures after the Chernobyl accident in Hungary.

In addition we attempted to measure a dose-effect estimate based on the rate of new genom mutations in 20 Hungarian regions with different increased background radiation (see Figure 3), however, we did not find any association in the rate of DS with extra radiation due the Chernobyl nuclear plant accident.

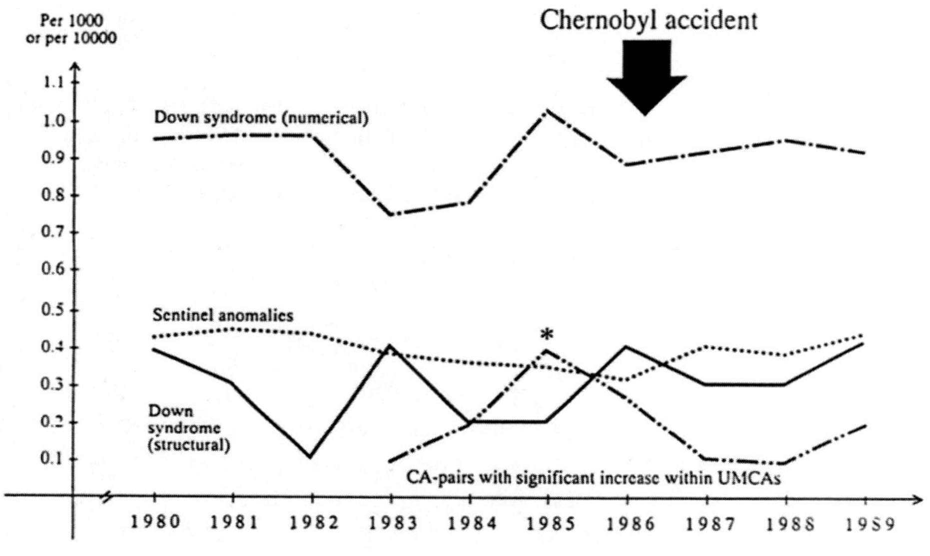

Figure 4. The annual rate of Down syndrome caused by numerical aberration: trisomy 21 (per 1000 total births) and Robertsonian translocation (per 10,000 total births), in addition of sentinel anomalies (per 1000 total births) and unclassified multiple CAs (UMCAs) (per 10,000 total births) in Hungary, between 1980 and 1989. (* shows significant increase)

(It is worth mentioning – as a good example for the chance events – that there was an obvious increase in DS due to new genom mutations and a significant increase in unidentified multiple CAs (UMCAs) in 1985, one year before the Chernobyl accident…)

In conclusion the HSGM seemed to be feasible but the HSGM was not able to detect any increase in the rate of DS due to new genom and chromosomal mutations. Thus our data suggested that there was no significant increase in the two forms of DS as a result of fall-out deposition from Chernobyl in Hungary. Similar negative findings were published in other countries [e.g. 53]. However, Sperling at al [27] reported a cluster of 10 cases with DS among the births in West Berlin 9 months after the radioactive contamination as resulting the Chernobyl accident. Our data did not support this debated observation. In addition the rate of sentinel anomalies and unclassified multiple CA did also not show any increase in the data set of the HSGM after 1986.

Thus it is necessary to differentiate the somatic and germinal mutations at the evaluation of environmental mutagens. While gene and chromosomal mutations are detectable in somatic cells after the effect of mutagens [54], it is not the case in children born to parents after the exposure of mutagens. Studies on the offspring of atomic bomb victims in Hiroshima and Nagasaki [55-57], children of cancer patients after radio- and/or chemotherapy [58] and the offspring of people who attempted suicide with extremely large doses of drugs and other chemicals [59, 60] did also not provide evidence for the effect of induced germinal mutations. The major explanation for these surprising findings is the very intensive germinal selection and early postconceptional (the so-called chemical pregnancies, i.e. positive pregnancy test without any clinical symptoms of pregnacy later) and early embryonic loss.

Environmental Trichlorfon and Cluster of Congenital Abnormalities in a Small Hungarian Village

A spatial cluster of CAs was detected in the population of the south-western Hungarian village of Rinyaszentiráky in 1990 by the HCAR. (The description of the HCAR was given in Chapter I.) The number of inhabitants in this village was 456 and they had 15 livebirths in 1989 and 1990, and out of these 15 babies, 11 (73.3%) were affected with CA. Hungarian epidemiological studies and the data of the HCAR suggested a birth prevalence of cases with CA about 4-6 %, i.e. only 1 in 15 livebirths [61]. Furthermore, of these 11 malformed babies, 4 were affected with DS. Thus we decided to explore this apparent cluster more thoroughly in a field study [62], because our first thought was the misdiagnosis of these cases with CA.

Materials and Methods

A team of expert (paediatrician, internist, medical geneticist, cytogeneticist, public health doctor) visited this village several times and all children born between 1980 amd 1991 were visited at home and thoroughly examined. Of 11 children affected with CA, 4 died, but we were able to get and evaluate their detailed autopsy report. The family tree of parents were drawn and the case history of the father, mother and all children were obtained through a personal interview using a structured questionnaire. Of course, we asked the parents of children about exposure to potential teratogens such as radiotherapy, diagnostic X-ray examination in abdominal-pelvic region, rubella and other infections, teratogenic drugs, etc.

Chromosomes of all malformed and healthy children born in 1989 and 1990 were examined in lymphocyte culture because we wanted to measure the possible chromosome breakages as the indicator of chromosome mutations. Prof. K. Sperling and his coworkers (Berlin) investigated dried blood samples of these cases from Guthrie card and of their parents and the origin of extra chromosomes 21 was analyzed by microsatellite and restriction fragment length polymorphism in their lymphocytes. Zygosity of twins was determined on the basis of placentation and genetic markers in blood or from Guthrie card.

In the next step we organized a case–control study, each case with CA had a control without CA born in Rinya in 1987-88 and three controls without CA born in the village nearest (5 km) to Rinyaszentkirály in 1989-90. All controls were examined and the necessary exposure data regarding the study pregnancy were obtained with the same structured questionnaire through interview from mothers at home visits.

After the preliminary findings of our field study we asked the authorities of the Hungarian Ministry of Welfare to order a detailed study of possible environmental exposures in air, water, and soil by the help of their institutions.

Results

After the recognition of this CA cluster in the data set of the HCAR, our first thought was the misdiagnosis of CAs. However, when we examined all children with CA and without CA in the village, all previous CA diagnoses were confirmed and new cases were not found. In addition it appeared that of these 15 live-born babies, 6 were twins, this 40% rate exceeded significatly the expected 2%.

Table 3. Children affected with CA and born in Rinyaszentkirály, 1989-1990

No.	Birth date	Sex	Birth weight (g)	Gestational age (wk)	CA	Comments
1.	06.01.89	M	1800	36	Ventricular septal defect + pulmonary atresia	Died (14.08.89), twin
2.	09.02.89	M	3540	40	Cong. ingunial hernia, left	His sib case 6
3.	09.12.89	F	2980	37	DS	
4.	30.12.89	M	2960	38	Stenosis of left bronchus (70%)	
5.	13.08.90	F	3300	40	Anal atresia	
6.	28.10.90	M	3300	38	Choanal atresia	Her sib case 2
7.	01.11.90	F	3300	38	Cleft lip, left	
8.	21.11.90	F	1790	33	DS (endocardial cushion defects)	Died (21.11.90)
9.	21.11.90	F	1980	33	DS (endocardial cushion defects)	Died (21.11.90)
10.	09.12.90	M	2600	26	DS	Died (09.12.90), twin
11.	09.12.90	M	2300	36	Robin sequence	Twin

Furthermore we examined all 61 children born in the village between 1980 and 1988, and 3 (4.9%) were affected with CA and twin birth did not occur.

Table 3 shows the most important data of children affected with CA. Case 1 had a healthy male twin-pair. Mother of case 9 was not in the village throughout pregnancy.

Chromosome examination confirmed the diagnosis of DS in all 4 children, their DS was caused by pure trisomy 21. In addition we wanted to measure the rate of chromosomal aberrations, mainly breakage as the indicator of somatic mutagenic effect. In the parents of cases with CA 1,600 cells were examined in peripheral lymphocyte cultures and 28 (1.7%) aberrant cells were found at the time of the study. This figure corresponded to the Hungarian population figure. However, this examinaiton was performed several months after the drastic environmental exposure.

Our second thought was connected with the important rule that most clusters are chance events. However, the propability of chance here is 1 in 380,000 births instead of the observed 11 CAs in 15 births. On the other hand, 8 different CAs were found in this cluster, but DS occurred in 4 cases. This birth prevalence of DS was 26.7 % and it is 223 times greater than that in the Hungarian population. The age of all mothers was less than 36. The critical period for DS caused by pure trisomy 21 was considered to be the day of conception or one day prior to conception, and all mothers lived in the village during this period. One pair with DS was monozygotic while two others were dizygotic. The final important argument for the causal association of this DS cluster with some environmental agent was that trisomy 21 in our evaluated cases was caused by the failure of the second maternal meiosis division. As it is well-known the characteristic maternal age dependent trisomy 21 is caused by the first maternal meiosis. Thus an association of this drastic DS cluster due to unusual origin of trisomy 21 with certain enironmental factor seemed to be obvious.

The other 7 children had different CAs, most of them multifactorial in origin and these CAs did not correspond with any known teratogenic CA syndrome. The critical period of these CAs was between March 18 and June 18, 1989 in 5 cases. All parents of cases were also examined and none had CA found in their children. Inbreeding was not characteritic for the people of this village, and there was no consanguinity between parents of children with CA.

The rate of fetal death (miscarriages and stillbirth) in the previous pregnancies of case mother and other women in the village did not exceed the expected rates in 1989-1990.

However, we did not find any difference in the well-known teratogenic exposures between case and control groups. Fortunately the discussion with the parents of cases helped us to find the possible cause. Of 11 case mothers, 9 had mentioned eating "contaminated" fish during early pregnancy. The rate of fish consumption was 33% (11/33) in controls, but in general not in early pregnancy.

Thus only one possibe cause of CAs was found and it was a drastic water pollution and according to our hypothesis this pollution attacked prepregnant and pregnant women through the eating of contaminated fish.

The area around Rinyaszentkirály has several ponds used for fish farming. This fish farm had a new director in 1987 and he introduced the so-called "chemical fast bathing" of fish. These fish were taken out of the water, and treated with 500 mg/L of Flibol® (40% of trichlorfon) for 5-10 minutes in barrels to eradicate parasites, and then returned to the pond.

These treatments were used several times between March and May in 1988-90. After treatment fish semed to be lifeless on the surface of the water for hours, even 1 or 2 days sometimes. Many dead fish were noted by both inhabitants and those supervising the cleaning operation. The inhabitants of the village were not told about this new technology, but fishing was prohibited during these periods. However, people were contnuous fish-eater, and they often taken out by hand fish from the surface of pond because fish were in a comatous state. Unfortunately these fish were stored in their refrigerators. Of 11 case mothers, 9 reported consumption of contaminated fish about the time of conception and during early pregnancy. Four DS occurred in this cluster, they were born from 3 women and these 3 women reported consumption of contaminated fish in the day of estimated conception. The critical period of these CAs in the fetuses was around Easter when fish is a traditional food locally.

Fish samples from this pond were examined at the Hungary's reference centre for food inspection on March 16, 1991. The content of trichlorfon averaged 0.15, 0.13, and 0.26 mg/kg in carp, amur, and European wels, respectively. These figures indicated a very high chemical pollution because trichlorfon disintegrates rapidly in biological organisms. According to the estimate of experts, the initial trichlorfon content of the fish could have been as high as 100 m/kg.

Discussion

The continuous analysis of the HCAR's data revealed an unusual cluster of CAs and particularly DS in a small Hungarian village in 1991. Pure chance was an unlikely explanation and the usual teratogens, familial inheritance and consanguinity have been excluded. Finally environmental pollution was suspected caused by the criminal use of trichlorfon in local fish-ponds.

Trichlorfon, an organophosphorous insecticide (2,2,2-trichloro-1-hydroxyethyl-phosphoric acid dimethyl ester, also known as chlorofos, metrifonate and trichlorphane; brand names include Flibol® and Dipterex^R) slowly releases dichlorvos which is estimated to be at least 100 times more potent an anticholinesterase agent than trichlorfon itself [63]. Trichlorfon is readily absorbed orally and is rapidly distributed to the tissues of the body. Peak blood concentrations are detected within 12 hours. In 1978 a joint FAO/WHO meeting on pesticide residue established an 'acceptable daily intake" as one not exceeding 0.01 mg/kg (i.e. 0.60 mg or so for an adult female) [64]. Estimated daily fish consumption was 250 g with an initial trichlorfon content of 25-100 mg in fish examned in the study thus it is very likely that the acceptable daily intake was significantly exceeded by pregnant women in Rinyaszentkirály.

The explanation of this CA cluster was the mistheory of the new director of the fishfarm. His idea was that fish were infected with parasites and these parasites avoided the increase of their body weight, Thus he hoped to have a larger body weight of fish (i.e. better economic profit) after the eradication of these parasites. However, Flibol® was labelled as a poison, nevertheless the director ordered to use this poison practically without dilution and did not measure the concentration of trichlorfon in the water and in the fish.

Thus the major finding of this sad field study was that the drastic cluster of DS (4 cases from 3 conceptions) was likely caused by trichlorfon. The adverse effect of trichlorfon on the gonads was demonstrated in animal investigations [63]. An inrease rate of chromosome aberrations was also observed in animals treated with trichlorfon [65-69]. Previously we were able to show a significant increase in numerical chromosome aberrations in lymphocytes in patients who attempted suicide with trichlorfon [70]. However, our study in Rinyaszentkirály indicated that trichlorfon is a more aggressive germinal than somatic mutagenic agent. We did not find a significantly higher rate of chromosomal aberrations in somatic cells several months after the poisoning while an extreme high rate of cases with DS occurred after the the exposure of germinal cells of their parents immediately after trichlorfon exposure. In addition for the 4 cases of DS, all with maternal exposure to trichlorfon during the critical period, the origin of non-disjunction was an error in maternal meiosis II. Typically non-disjunction occurs in maternal meiosis I, thus this unusual origin of trisomy 21 supports a drastic environmental exposure.

The other 7 CAs were heterogeneous both in their manifestation and in their origin. Trichlorfon can cross the placenta [71] and its teratogenic effect was shown in hamsters, mice and rats [72-75]. Different CAs have specific critical periods, thus teratogenic agents can induce CA only in gestation time specific period. Of 7 cases with different CA, 3 were born to mothers who consumed contaminated fish during the critical period of these CAs. In addition 2 other pregnant women mentioned the consumption of frozen storage fish in the critical period of CA in their children. Thus, a non-specific teratogenic role for trichlorfon cannot be ruled out in the origin of 5 CAs.

Higher rate of twins may also be connected with an environmental factor [76] and all twin pairs were conceived during the trichlorfon exposure period in Rinyaszentkirály.

In conclusion, the finger of suspicion is thus pointed at trichlorfon exposure as the explanation for the DS cases and, perhaps, some other CAs and the twins. As far as we know such a cluster of DS caused by an environmental factor has not been published.

Epilogue

There were three further important arguments due to the studies followed the publication of our paper in The Lancet in 1993 [62] for the above association.

1. This chemical treatment of fishfarm in Rinyaszentiráły was banned in March. 1991. All the 10 children born in 1991 and 1992 were healthy. In addition we checked again the births in Rinyaszentkirály until the end of 1996. Of 32 children, only one was affected with congenital inguinal hernia.
2. We had an extra effort to check the live-born babies of mothers who lived in the surrounding area of other fishfarms in Hungary, because trichlorfon was used in other fish-ponds as well. However, the head and workers of other fishfarms followed the international and Hungarian regulation of trichlorfon use, and these minimal doses did not associate with a higher risk for DS and other CA.

3. Last but not least a British [77, 78] and German [79-81] group tested the effect of trichlorfon in animal investigations and they were able to prove the aneugenic (i.e. non-disjunction causing) effect of large doses of trichlorfon. Yin et al [79] reported a higher risk for spindle aberrations and non-disjuction in mammalian oocytes after trichlorfon exposure. Sun et al [80] showed that trichlorfon induced spindle disturbances in V79 and aneuploidy in male mouse germ cells. These authors also demonstrated an obvious dose-dependent germinal mutagenic effect of trichlorfon. Finally Cukurcam et al [81] proved that trichlorfon predisposes to aneuploidy and interferes with spindle formation in *in vitro* maturing oocytes. Exposure 50 microgram/ml or more trichlorfon induced severe spindle aberrations at metaphase II and over one-third of the oocytes failed to align all chromosomes at the spindle equator (congression failure).

Thus our Hungarian study was able to detect an environmental agent which used in very large doses can induce DS. This observation was confirmed in animal investigations. Thus our finding is an important argument for the necessity and importance of population-based registries of CAs.

III. Prevention of Down Syndrome

The optimal prevention is the primary prevention that is avoiding the cause(s) of disorders, and among them, CAs. At present most fetuses affected with DS are diagnosed prenatally (see Chapter I) but after the recognition of this high risk for mental retardation and other defects, 97% of Hungarian pregnant women decided to terminate their pregnancy. Previously this approach was called as secondary prevention, i.e. prevention the birth of seriously malformed fetuses [82]. However, morally and scientifically it is not prevention, it is avoiding the birth of malformed fetuses, thus a special form of euthanasia, i.e. terathanasia. Major part of our societies accept and need it, but we have to know: it is not an optimal solution and we have to do our best to introduce primary preventive methods of DS.

The recent sequencing of chromosome 21 allows the identification of every gene on the chromosome 21 and at least 31 genes are involved in the pathogenesis of DS [83, 6]. Nevertheless, little is known about the etiology of DS. The strongest risk factor is older maternal age [84-86]. Numerous studies have already examined associations with different environmental factors such as ionizing radiation [45, 46], hepatitis [2], smoking [87], coffee drinking [88], contraceptive spermicids [2], etc. As we showed in Chapter II, certain chemicals, e.g., trichlorphon [62] can cause non-disjunction errors leading to trisomy 21.

Recently some studies have showed the importance of mitochondrial gene mutations in the origin of DS [89, 90] with an age-dependent increase. In addition, a possible link between DS and neural-tube defects has been published [91] indicating, among other factors, that mitochondrial dysfunction might cause ATP deficiency. On the other hand abnormal folate metabolism and mutations in the genes of methylenetetrahydrofolate-reductase (MTHFR) and methioninesynthase-reductase (MTRR) may also be a maternal risk factor for DS [92-94]. However, other studies have not confirmed this association [95, 96].

Maternal Use of Nutritional Supplements During the First Month of Pregnancy and Reduced Risk of Down Syndrome. A Case-Control Study

The objective of our study was to evaluate the possible association between antioxidant vitamins C and E, in addition folic acid use during the periconceptional period and the total prevalence of cases with DS [97]. Partly mitochondrial DNA (MtDNA) is sensitive to environmental factors, e.g. free radicals and their effects can be modified by vitamins C and E [98]. Partly we attempted to check the effect of high dose of folic acid for the occurrence of DS. Thus the prevalence of vitamin C and E, and folic acid use was compared in the pairs of cases with DS and their matched healthy controls without CA. In addition, the group of cases with DS was compared with the total population control group and all other CA groups as patient controls regarding the exposures of vitamin C, E and folic acid in the population-based large data set of the Hungarian Case-Control Surveillance of Congenital Abnormalities (HCCSCA) [7].

Materials and Methods

We identified fetuses-newborn infants as *cases* with DS and *patient controls* with all other CAs (except known Mendelian major gene and other chromosomal syndromes) from the previosuly shown population-based Hungarian Congenital Abnormality Registry (HCAR) between 1980 and 1996 [3]. The decription of the HCAR was given in Chapter I.

Cases with DS and patient controls with other CAs were selected from the HCAR for the HCCSCA who were reported in the three months after birth or after termination of pregnancy. This shorter time between the birth or pregnancy termination and data collection increases the accuracy of information on pregnancy history without undue loss of power since 77% of cases were reported during this time window to the HCAR.

We defined *population controls* as newborn infants without CAs matched to each case with CAs according to sex, week of birth in the year when the case was born and district of parent's residence. Population controls were selected from the National Birth Registry of the Central Statistical Office followed by 2 months after the notification of cases with CAs. In general each case with CAs had 2 population controls, but 3 newborn infants were selected for each case between 1986 and 1992. In this study we had a further matching procedure: one population control was matched for each case with DS on the basis of age ($\pm$3 years) of mothers and these pairs were evaluated separately.

We collected data on exposures from three sources [7]. First, we sent a post-paid structured questionnaire to the parents and we requested them to inform us, among others, on medicine (drug and pregnancy supplement) intakes during pregnancy, according to gestational months. We also supplied mothers with a list of medicines as a memory aid and mothers were asked to review them before they replied. The time difference between the end of pregnancy and questionnaire return was 3.8 $\pm$ 2.0 month for the cases with DS, 3.5 $\pm$ 1.2 months for patient controls and 5.2 $\pm$ 2.9 months for population controls. Second, mothers were requested to send us the *prenatal* care logbook and all other medical records concerning their child`s CA and diseases as well as maternal diseases and medicine intakes during the study pregnancy. In Hungary prenatal care obstetricians are obliged to record all pregnancy related medicines, complications, and maternal diseases in this logbook. Among respondents, prenatal care logbooks were available in 90.8% of cases with DS, 88.4% of patient controls and 93.8% of population controls. Third, regional district nurses visited and questioned all non-responding families of cases with DS and patient controls, but only 200 non-respondent families of population controls because the ethical committee considered this follow-up to be disturbing to the parents of all healthy infants [99]. Overall information were available for 95% of cases with DS (85% from reply, and 10% from visit), for 96% of patient controls (84% from reply, 12% from visit), for 83% of population controls (82.6% from reply and 0.4% from visit) without mothers with wrong or new unknown addresses.

For the comparison of case-control pairs we used conditional logistic regression model to estimate the adjusted OR and 95% CI for exposure of nutritional supplements. For the comparison between cases with DS and total population control or patient control groups we used unconditional logistic regression model to estimate the adjusted OR and 95% CI.

In Hungary, only one kind of folic acid tablet was available during the study period and it contained 3 mg. Tablets of vitamin C included 100 or 200 mg, while tablets of vitamin E contained 100 mg. The available iron supplements included 50 (10 mg elementary Fe^{2+}), 70 and 100 mg ferrous sulfate in one tablet. Multivitamins, more exactly the combination of micronutrients, containing folic acid (but low dose between 0.1-1.0 mg), vitamin C, E, other vitamins and minerals. Some women reported only vitamin use without the specification of product. Our validation study showed that about 90% of these women used vitamin C [99] because the "vitamin" in general is equal to vitamin C in Hungary. At the evaluation of nutritional supplements, those were evaluated which were used at least by one case-control pair during the *first* gestational month.

Five different aspects of nutritional supplements were considered: (i) source of information (medically recorded, maternal self-reported, both), (ii) the route of administration (always oral), (iii) dose, (iv) the onset according to gestational age and (v) duration of treatment during pregnancy. However, here we focused our analysis on the *first gestational month.* The gestational age was calculated from the first day of the last menstrual period, the first two weeks of gestation are therefore *before* conception, while the third and fourth weeks comprise the preimplantation and implantation processes of zygotes and blastocysts. Thus, this "periconceptional period" overlaps with the time of maternal non-disjunction in the oogenesis. Meiosis is the process of nuclear division which occurs during the final stage of gamete formation in two steps: the first meiotic division does not occur until ovulation, while the second meiotic division does not occur until fertilization.

Results

The number of cases with DS was 834, the pure trisomy 21 occurred in 781 cases (93.6%). Cases with DS caused by Robertsonian translocation and mosaicism were excluded from this analysis. The number of population controls was 38,151, 1.8 % of all Hungarian births during the study period. The number of patient controls with CA was 22,843.

Characteristics of 781 mothers, who had cases with DS caused by trisomy 21 showed the well-known advanced maternal age and concomittant higher birth order. Their matched controls had a somewhat lower mean maternal age (and birth order) on the contrary of matching criteria. The evaluation of maternal employment as an indicator of socio-economic status demonstrated a smaller proportion of higher (professional, managerial and skilled worker) and larger proportion of lower (semi- and unskilled workers, housewives and others) employment status in the mothers of cases with DS than in the mothers of their matched pairs and population controls, but there was no difference between cases with DS and patient controls. In Hungary most housewives belong to the lower socio-economic class.

The dose of folic acid was not reported in 51% of pregnant women. In our validation study (100) based on 600 pregnant women, 22.5%, 68.6% and 8.9% used 1 (3 mg), 2 (6 mg) and 3 (9 mg) tablets of folic acid per day, respectively, and these figures were in agreement with the reported data. The number and type of iron supplements were reported in 84% of pregnant women and their daily intake was between 150 and 300 mg of ferrous sulfate. The usual daily doses of vitamin C were 100-600 mg while in general daily 200 mg of vitamin E was used.

The proportion of medically recorded folic acid use was 29.4% and 32.7% during the first month of gestation, while these figures were 55.6% and 66.8% during the second-ninths months of gestation in the group of cases with DS and their matched control pairs, respectively. These figures were 73.5% and 75.5% in the first month, in addition 84.3% and 86.0% during the second and ninth month of gestation regarding iron use in the groups of cases with DS and their matched control pairs, respectively.

Among pregnancy supplements, only folic acid and iron showed a significantly lower prevalence during the first gestational month in cases with DS compared with their matched control pairs (Table 4). Similar difference was not seen at the comparison of II-IX months of gestation. At the comparison of groups with DS and population controls, the lowest use of folic acid and iron also was seen in group of DS, however, both in the first and II-IX months of gestation. At the comparison of groups with DS and patient controls, there was no difference in the use of pregnancy supplements either in the first month or in the II-IX months of pregnancy.

The prevalence of vitamin C and E was the lowest during the first month of pregnancy in the group of DS, but their use was rare. After the combination of vitamin C and "vitamins" in the first month, the prevalence of their use in cases with DS was lower than in their matched controls (7; 0.9%, vs 12; 1.5%), but the difference did not exceed the level of significance (OR with 95% CI: 0.6, 0.2-1.5). However, there was no difference in their use during II-IX months of gestation (99; 12.6%, vs 98; 12.5%). The prevalence of vitamin C + "vitamins" in the first month of gestation was 1.3% in the population control (OR with 95% CI: 0.7, 0.3-1.4) and 1.1% in the patient control (OR with 95% CI: 0.8, 0.4-1.6) groups. On the other hand, the use of micronutrients in the first month of pregnancy was not lower in the group of cases with DS.

Table 4. The occurrence of pregnancy supplement uses during the first (I) and second-ninth (II-IX) months of pregnancy in the study groups and the calculated adjusted OR with 95% CI for the total prevalence of Down syndrome (DS)

Pregnancy supplements	Cases with DS (N=781)				Matched controls (N=781)				Comparison between cases with DS and their matched control pairs				Population controls (N=38,151)				Comparison between cases with DS and population controls				Patient controls (N=22,843)				Comparison between cases with DS and patient controls			
	I.		II.-IX.		I.		II.-IX.		I.		II.-IX.		I.		II.-IX.		I.		II.-IX.		I.		II.-IX.		I.		II.-IX.	
	No.	%	No.	%	No.	%	No.	%	OR	95%CI	OR	95%CI	No.	%	No.	%	OR	95%CI	OR	95%CI	No.	%	No.	%	OR	95%CI	OR	95%CI
B1 (thiamin)	1	0.1	6	0.8	1	0.1	4	0.5	1.1	0.1-18.8	1.5	0.4-5.4	26	0.1	335	0.9	2.2	0.3-16.7	0.9	0.4-1.9	12	0.1	176	0.8	2.0	0.3-16.1	0.9	0.4-2.1
B6 (pyri-doxine)	14	1.8	55	7.0	22	2.8	59	7.6	0.8	0.4-1.5	1.0	0.7-1.4	715	1.9	3,370	8.8	1.1	0.6-1.8	0.9	0.7-1.1	288	1.3	1,725	7.6	1.5	0.9-2.7	1.0	0.8-1.3
B11 (folic acid)	16	2.1	349	44.7	42	5.4	364	46.6	0.4	0.2-0.7	0.9	0.7-1.1	1,526	4.0	19,239	50.4	0.5	0.3-0.9	0.8	0.7-0.9	684	3.0	10,591	46.4	0.7	0.4-1.2	0.9	0.8-1.1
B12 (cobalamin)	2	0.3	11	1.4	1	0.1	18	2.3	1.8	0.2-20.4	0.5	0.3-1.2	25	0.1	350	0.9	4.0	0.9-17.3	1.5	0.8-2.8	7	0.0	204	0.9	8.3	1.7-41.6	1.6	0.9-2.9
C (ascorbic acid)	3	0.4	35	4.5	5	0.6	34	4.4	0.6	0.1-2.6	1.0	0.6-1.7	226	0.6	1,431	3.8	0.6	0.2-2.0	1.3	0.9-1.8	105	0.5	792	3.5	0.8	0.2-2.4	1.3	0.9-1.9
D (cholecar-ciferol)	4	0.5	190	24.3	10	1.3	199	25.5	0.5	0.1-1.6	0.9	0.7-1.2	399	1.0	9,576	25.1	0.5	0.2-1.4	1.0	0.8-1.2	171	0.7	5,829	25.5	0.7	0.3-2.0	1.0	0.8-1.1
E (toco-pherol)	3	0.4	38	4.9	7	0.9	39	5.0	0.5	0.1-2.2	1.0	0.6-1.6	274	0.7	1,985	5.2	0.5	0.2-1.6	0.9	0.7-1.3	130	0.6	1,272	5.6	0.7	0.2-2.1	0.9	0.6-1.2
'Vitamins'	4	0.5	64	8.2	7	0.9	64	8.2	0.7	0.2-2.4	1.0	0.7-1.6	283	0.7	3,533	9.3	0.8	0.3-2.0	1.0	0.8-1.3	135	0.6	2,157	9.4	0.9	0.3-2.3	0.9	0.7-1.2
Micro-nutrients ("Multi-vitamins")	11	1.4	46	5.9	11	1.4	32	4.1	1.1	0.4-2.8	1.5	0.9-2.5	436	1.1	2,045	5.4	1.1	0.6-2.0	1.0	0.8-1.4	178	0.8	1,133	5.0	1.8	0.9-3.3	1.2	0.9-1.6
Calcium	1	0.1	56	7.2	1	0.1	66	8.5	1.2	0.1-20.8	0.9	0.6-1.3	184	0.5	3,402	8.9	0.3	0.0-1.9	0.8	0.6-1.1	73	0.3	1,745	7.6	0.4	0.1-2.8	0.9	0.7-1.2
Iron	19	2.4	464	59.4	45	5.8	477	61.1	0.5	0.3-0.8	1.0	0.8-1.2	1,869	4.9	24,882	65.2	0.5	0.3-0.8	0.8	0.7-0.9	869	3.8	13,859	60.7	0.7	0.4-1.0	1.0	0.8-1.1

In general folic acid and iron were used together, we attempted therefore to evaluate separately these two nutritional supplements, though there were only limited number of cases and controls with iron or folic acid alone during the first month of gestation (Table 5). Only iron alone showed a significant "protective" effect for DS. However, OR were much lower both in the group of folic acid alone and iron alone.

Table 5. A comparison of folic acid and iron use alone and together during the first month of pregnancy

Study groups	Folic acid + iron				Only folic acid				Only iron				Neither*		Total
	N	%	OR**	95% CI	N	%	OR**	95% CI	N	%	OR**	95% CI	N	%	N
Cases with DS	15	1.9	Referent		1	0.1	referent		4	0.5	Referent		813	97.5	834
Matched controls	40	4.6	0.4	0.2-0.7	6	0.8	0.3	0.1-1.8	9	1.2	0.5	0.2-1.7	779	93.4	834
Population controls	1,330	3.5	0.5	0.3-0.9	196	0.5	0.4	0.1-1.8	539	1.4	0.4	0.1-0.9	36,086	94.6	38,151
Patient controls	603	2.6	0.7	0.4-1.2	81	0.4	0.7	0.2-2.9	266	1.2	0.5	0.2-1.3	21,893	95.8	22,843

* we used the 'Neither' group as non-exposed group in all three comparisons
** adjusted for birth order, maternal age and employment status

Discussion

Our study provides risk estimates of different nutritional supplements taken during the periconceptional period on the odds of DS in the population-based data set of the HCCSCA. Only iron and folic acid showed significant protective effect for DS during the first month of pregnancy.

However, data on nutritional supplements in the first month of gestation were based mainly on maternal retrospective self-reported information because the usual time of first visit to the prenatal care is the 8th-10th week of gestation, i.e. after the periconceptional period. We found the maternal information is reliable in our validation study [99]. Nevertheless, the birth of an infant with CAs is a serious traumatic event for most mothers who therefore try to find a causal explanation, like medicine uses during pregnancy [101]. This does not occur after the birth of healthy newborn baby. Thus this recall bias may explain the somewhat higher proportion of nutritional supplement uses in case and patient control mothers due to the higher proportion of maternal self-reported information, but a *lower* consumption of folic acid and iron was reported by mothers of cases with DS in the study. However, it is possible that mothers of children with serious CAs such as DS will not only remember better the medicines they took during pregnancy, but the medicines including supplements that they did not take as well. In addition, it is possible to exclude recall bias by comparison of cases with DS and patient controls, in addition the use of nutritional supplements was evaluated only during the first month of gestation and we suppose an underreporting during the entire study pregnancy.

The results of our study demonstrated that the maternal use of folic acid and iron may have some preventive effect on the development of DS during the first month of gestation.

The time is an important argument because a similar association was not found after the first gestational month in case-control pairs of this data set. This protective effect was also found with the use of folic acid and iron *together,* thus it may be a combined effect or the iron effect might be explained by the concomitant use of folic acid. However, our analysis showed an independent protective effect of iron. We did not find any similar previous report in the international literature [102], however, Herbig and Stover [103] stated that "some reevaluation of the clinical literature regarding iron status to actual folate status is warranted".

Another important factor in the evaluation of the nutritional supplement is the dose. Multivitamins containing a relatively low dose (1 mg or less) of folic acid did not show protective effect for DS in the data set of the HCCSCA. Periconceptional multivitamin (including 0.8 mg of folic acid) supplementation in the two Hungarian intervention trials reduced the first occurrence of neural-tube defects [104, 105], and isolated CAs of cardiovascular system and urinary tract [106, 107], but not DS. Recent publications showed an association between polymorphism in genes involved in folate metabolism and maternal risk for DS. James et al [92] examined the 677C→T polymorphism of MTHFR gene and they found a higher frequency of both the C/T and T/T genotypes in the mothers of children with DS than in the control mothers. When the frequencies of mothers with at least one T allele were compared, the OR for mothers of children with DS was 2.6. This finding was confirmed by Hobbs et al [93] (OR with 95% CI: 1.9, 1.2-3.1) but not by O'Leary et al [94]. However, the homozygous mutation of MTRR 66A→G showed also 2.6 (1.3-5.0) increased risk in the study of Hobbs et al [93] and it was confirmed by O'Leary et al [94] who found a significantly higher frequency of the MTRR variant genotypes (AG, GG) (p=0.0028) in the mothers of children with DS compared to controls. Both studies showed the highest estimated risk in the combined present of both (MTHFR and MTRR) polymorphisms – it was 4.1 (1.9-8.6) in the study of Hobbs et al [93] and 3.0 (p=0.02) in the study of O'Leary et al [94].

Two Italian studies, however, were not able to confirm the association between MTHFR C6677T polymorphism and risk of DS [95, 96]. Bosco et al. [108] showed that elevated homocysteinemia and MTRR genetic polymorphism are two potent risk factors for DS in Sicily.

As we mentioned, two previous Hungarian intervention trials did not indicate a protective effect of periconceptional use of a multivitamin including 0.8 mg of folic acid for DS. This study shows a similar effect of multivitamins containing low dose of folic acid but some protective effect of high dose (in general 6 mg) of folic acid. Thus it is worth considering a dose dependent effect of folic acid. A similar finding was seen in isolated cleft lip ± palate and cleft palate only. While multivitamins including 0.8 mg of folic acid were not effective for the prevention of orofacial clefts [104, 105], a high dose (in general 6 mg or 10 mg) of folic acid was able to reduce the first occurrence [109] and recurrence [110] of cleft lip±palate, respectively. The US National Academy of Sciences [111] recommended to differentiate the physiological dose of folic acid (tolerable upper limit is 1 mg) for preventive purpose in healthy persons including pregnant women and the pharmacological dose of folic acid for the treatment of diseases (e.g. megaloblastic anemia) in patients after prescription and under medical control.

If the possible associations between some mitochondrial gene mutations, in addition nuclear gene mutations in folate metabolism and the incidence of DS are valid, the periconceptional use of the high dose of folic acid and/or iron, in addition to antioxidants may provide a chance for the primary prevention of DS.

In conclusion, we studied the association between the use of nutritional supplements during the first gestational month and the origin of DS, and a significant protective effect was seen with large doses (about 6 mg/day) of folic acid and iron (150-300 mg/day of ferrous sulfate) during the first gestational month for DS. In general, folic acid and iron were used together, therefore it was difficult to separate these effects due to the limited number of cases and controls. However, the main message of our study is that a pharmacological dose of folic acid and iron supplement appears to have a primary preventive effect for DS.

References

[1] Abruzzo MA, Hassold TJ. Etiology of nondisjunction in humans. *Envirum Mol Mutagen* 1999; 26: 38-47.

[2] Epstein,CJ. Morphogenesis of Down Syndrome. Wiley-Liss: New York. 1991.

[3] Czeizel AE. The first 25 years of the Hungarian Congenital Abnormality Registry. *Teratology* 1997; 55: 299-305.

[4] Métneki J, Czeizel AE. Incresing total prevalence rate of cases with Down syndrome in Hungary. *Eur J Epidemiol* 2005; 20: 525-535.

[5] Czeizel AE, Telegdi L, Tusnády G. Multiple Congenital Abnormalities. Akadémiai Kiadó. Budapest. 1988.

[6] Roizen NJ, Patterson D. Down's syndrome. *Lancet* 2003; 361: 1281-1289.

[7] Czeizel AE, Rockenbauer M, Siffel Cs, Varga E. Description and mission evaluation of the Hungarian Case-Control Surveillance of Congenital Abnormalities, 1980-1996. *Teratology* 2001; 63: 176-185.

[8] Demographic Yearbooks. 1970-2006. Központi Statisztikai Hivatal. (Hungarian Central Statistical Office) Budapest.

[9] Cuckle HS, Wald NJ, Thompson SG. Estimating a woman's risk of having a pregnancy associated with Down's syndrome using her age and serum alpha-fetoprotein level. *Br J Obstet Gynaecol* 1987; 94: 387-402.

[10] Czeizel AE. Some epidemiological characteristics of Down's syndrome in Hungary. *Acta Morph Hung* 1988; 36: 63-77.

[11] Stoll C, Alembik Y, Dott B, Roth M. Epidemiology of Down syndrome in 118,265 consecutive births. *Am J Med Genet* 1990; Suppl. 7: 79-83.

[12] Staples AJ, Sutherland GR, Haan EA, Clisby S. Epidemiology of Down syndrome in South Australia, 1960-89. *Am J Hum Genet* 1991; 49: 1014-1024.

[13] Krivchenia E, Huether CA, Edmonds LD, May D, Guckenberger S. Comparative epidemiology of Down syndrome in two United States population, 1970-1989. *Am J Epidemiol* 1993; 137: 828.

[14] Huether CA, Haraldson K, Ellis PM, Ramsay CN. Impact of prenatal diagnosed on revised livebirth prevalence estimates of Down syndrome in the Lothian Region of Scotland, 1978-1992. *Genet Epidemiol* 1996; 13: 367-375.

[15] Carothers AD, Boyd E, Lother G, Ellis PM, Couzin DA, Fead MJW, Robb A. Trends in prenatal diagnosis of Down syndrome and other autosomal trisomies in Scotland 1990 to 1994 with associated cytogenetic and epidemiological findings. *Genet Epidemiol* 1999; 16: 179-190.

[16] Morris JK, Mutton DE, Alberman E. Revised estimates of the maternal age specific live birth prevalence of Down's syndrome. *Physiol Res* 2000; 49: 227-231.

[17] Julian-Reynier C, Aurran Y, Dumaret A. Attitudes towards Down's syndrome: follow-up of a cohort of 280 cases. *J Med Genet* 1995; 32: 597-599.

[18] Ferguson-Smith MA. Abnormal sex ratios in the autosomal trisomy syndrome. *Lancet* 1962 ; 2: 357-358.

[19] Bernheim A, Chastang C, de Heaulme M, de Gronchy J. 1979. Exces de garcons dans la trisomie 21. *Ann Genet* 1979; 22: 122-124.

[20] Huether CA, Martin RLM, Stoppelman SM, O'Souza S, Bishop JK, Torfs CP, Lorey F, May KM, Hanna JS, Baird PA, Kelley JC. Sex ratio in fetuses and liveborn infants with autosomal aneuploidy. *Am J Med Genet* 1996; 63: 492-500.

[21] Mutton D, Alberman E, Hook EB. Cytogenetic and epidemiological findings in Down syndrome, England and Wales 1989 to 1993. *J Med Genet* 1996; 33: 387-394.

[22] Hook EB, Cross PK, Mutton DE. Female predominance (low sex ratio) in 47,+21 mozaics. *Am J Med Genet* 1999; 84: 316-319.

[23] Hook EB, Topol BB, Cross PK. The natural history of cytogenetically abnormal fetuses detected at midtrimester amniocentesis which are not terminated electively: new data and estimates of the excess and relative risk of late fetal death associated with 47,+21 and some other abnormal kariotypes. *Am J Hum Genet* 1989; 45: 855-861.

[24] Leonard B, Bower CK, Petterson B, Leonard H. Survival of infants born with Down' syndrome: 1980-96. *Paediatr Perinat Epid* 2000; 14: 163-171.

[25] Yang Q, Rasmussen SA, Friedman JM. Mortality associated with Down's syndrome in the USA from 1983 to 1997; a population-based study. *Lancet* 2002; 359: 1019-1025.

[26] Evans HJ, Lyon MF, Czeizel AE. Is the incidence of Down syndrome increasing? *Mut Res* 1986; 175: 263-266.

[27] Sperling K, Pelz J, Wegner RD, Schulake I, Struck E. Frequency of trisomy 21 in Germany before and after the Chernobyl accident. *Biomed Pharmacother* 1991; 45: 255-262.

[28] Bishop J, Huether CA. Revised estimates and projections of Down syndrome births in the United States, and the effects of prenatal diagnosis utilization, 1910-2002. *Prenat Diagn* 1987; 7: 261-271.

[29] CDC (Centers for Disease Control and Prevention). Down syndrome prevalence at birth - United States, 1983-1990. *MMWR* 1994; 43: 607-622.

[30] Stoll C, Alembik Y, Dott B. Study of Down syndrome in 238,942 consecutive births. *Ann Genet* 1998; 41: 44-51.

[31] Sixto G-M, Laiz S. Inreasing total prevalence of trisomy 21 in the Bask country, Spain. *Eur J Hum Genet* 1999; 7: 80. (Suppl 1)

[32] Hook EB, Mutton DE, Ide R, Alberman E, Bobrow M. The natural history of Down syndrome conceptuses diagnosed prenatally that are not electively terminated. *Am J Hum Genet* 1995; 57: 875-881.

[33] Mikkelsen M. The incidence of Down' syndrome and progress toward its reduction. *Philos Trans R Soc. London: Ser B.* 1988; 319: 315-324.

[34] Mikkelsen M. The impact of prenatal diagnosis on the incidence of Down syndrome in Denmark. *Birth Defects* 1992; 28: 44-51.

[35] Ramsay CN, Ellis PM, Zealley H. Down' syndrome in the Lothian region of Scotland - 1978 to 1989. *Biomed Pharmacother* 1991; 45: 267-272.

[36] Halliday J, Lumley J, Watson L. 1995. Comparison of women who do and do not have amniocentesis or chorionic villus sampling. *Lancet* 1995; 345: 704-709.

[37] Carothers AD, Hecht CA, Hook EB. International variation in reported livebirth prevalence rates of Down syndrome, adjusted for maternal age. *J Med Genet* 1999; 36: 386-393.

[38] Czeizel AE, Tusnády G. 1972. Some biological aspects of differential family planning. *Adv Biol Human Popul* 1972; 13: 193-203.

[39] Baird PA, Sadovnick AD. Maternal age-specific rates for Down syndrome: Changes over time. *Am J Med Genet* 1988; 29: 917-927.

[40] Carothers AD. Methods for maternal age-standardization of the incidence of congenital abnormalities. *Statistics Med* 1995; 14: 1797-1806.

[41] Snijders RJM, Noble P, Sebire N, Souka A, Nicolaides KH. UK multicenter project on the assessment of risk of trisomy 21 by maternal age and fetal nuchal-translucency thickness at 10-14 weeks of gestation. *Lancet* 1998; 351: 343-346.

[42] Czeizel AE. Human germinal mutagenic effects in relation to intentional and accidental exposure to toxic agents. *Environm Health Perspect* 1996; 104: 615-617.

[43] Anspaugh LR, Catlin RJ, Goldman M. Ths global impact of the Chernobyl reactor accient. *Nature* 1988; 242: 1513-1518.

[44] WHO (World Health Organization): Updated Background Information on the Nuclear Reactor Accident in Chernobyl, USSR June 12, 1986. WHO, Copenhagen, 1986.

[45] Verger P. Down syndrome and ionizing radiation. *Health Phys* 1997; 73: 882-893.

[46] Sankaranarayan K. Ionizing radiation and genetic risk. IV. Current methods, estimates of risk of Mendelian diseases, human data and lessons from biochemical and molecular studies of mutations. *Mutat Res* 1991; 258: 99-122.

[47] Czeizel AE, Elek Cs, Susánszky E. The evaluation of the germinal mutagenic impact of Chernobyl radiological contamination in Hungary. *Mutagenesis* 1991; 6: 285-288.

[48] Czeizel AE. Hungarian surveillance of germinal mutations. *Hum. Genet* 1989; 82: 359-366.

[49] Czeizel AE, Kis-Varga A. Mutation surveillance of sentinel anomalies. *Mutat Res* 1989; 212: 3-9.

[50] Mulvihill JJ, Czeizel AE. Perspectives in mutation epidemiology. 6. A 1983 view of sentinel phenotype. *Mutat Res* 1983; 123: 345-361.

[51] Hook EB, Gross PK. Survellance of human populations for germinal cytogenetic mutations. In. Sugimurs T., Kondo S, Takabe H (eds.) Environmental Mutagens and Carcinogens. Univesity of Tokyo Press - Alan R. Liss. New York, 1982.pp. 613-624.

[52] Kis-Varga A, Rudas T, Czeizel AE. A new aproach to germinal mutation surveillance: pair-wise evaluation of component elements in unidentified multipele congenital abnormalities. *Mutat Res* 1990; 238: 87-97.

[53] De Wals P, Bertrand F, De la Mata I, Lechat MF. Chromosomal anomaliees and Chernobyl. *Int J Epidemiol* 1988; 17: 230-231.

[54] Czeizel AE. Phenotypic and cytogenetic studies in self-poisoned patients. *Mutat Res* 1994; 313: 175-181.

[55] Neel JV, Schull WJ, Awa AA, Sotach C. The children of parents exposed to atomic bombs: estimates of the genetic doubling dose of radiation for humans. *Am J Hum Genet* 1990; 46: 1053-1072.

[56] Otake M, Schull WJ, Neel JV. Te effects of parental exposure to the atomic bombing of Hisroshima and Nagasaki on congenital malformations, stillbirths and early mortality among their children: a reanalysis. *Radiat Res* 1990; 122: 1-11.

[57] Yashimoto Y, Neel JV, Schull WJ, Kato H. Malignant tumors during the first two decades of life in the offspring of atomic bomb survivors. *Am J Med Genet* 1990; 46: 1041-1052.

[58] Mulvihill JJ. Sentinel and othert effects in offspring of cancer survivors. In: Mendelsohn ML, Albertini RJ (eds.) Mutation ans the Environment. Part C. Somatic and heritable Mutation, Adduction and Epidemiology. Wiley-Liss, New York, 1982. pp. 179-191.

[59] Czeizel AE, Szentesi I, Molnár G. Lack of effect of self-poisoning on subsequent reproductive outcome. *Mutat Res* 1984; 127: 175-182.

[60] Czeizel AE, Gidai J, Petik D, Timmermann G, Puho HE. Self-poisoning during pregnancy as a model for teratogenic risk estimation of drugs. *Toxicology and Industrial Health,* 2008; 24: 11-28.

[61] Czeizel AE, Intődy Zs, Modell B. What proportion of congenital abnormalities can be prevented? *Brit Med J* 1993; 306: 499-503.

[62] Czeizel AE, Elek Cs, Gundy S, Métneki J, Nemes E, Reis A, Sperling K, Timár L, Tusnády G, Virágh Z. Environmental trichlorphon and cluster of congenital abnormalities. *Lancet* 1993; 341: 539-542.

[63] IPCS (International Programme on Chemical Safety). Trichlorfon (Health Safety Guide. No. 66), WHO, Geneva, 1991.

[64] WHO (World Health Organization): Environmental Health Criteria 63: Organophosphorus insecticides: a general introduction, Geneva, 1986.

[65] Moutschen-Dahmen J, Moutschen-Dahmen M, Degraeve N. Metrifonate and dichlorvos: cytogenetic investigations. *Acta Pharmacol Toxicol (Copenh)* 1981; 49 (Suppl): 29-39

[66] Degraeve N, Chollet MC, Moutschen J. Evaluation of the mutagenic potential of four commercial mixtures of insecticides. *Food Chem Toxicol* 1984; 22: 683-687.

[67] Degraeve N, Chollet MC, Moutschen J. Cytoygenetic and genetic effects of subchronic treatment with organophosphorus insecticides. *Arch Toxicol* 1984; 56: 66-67.

[68] Degraeve N, Chollet MC, Moutschen J. Cytoygenetic effects induced by organophosphorus pesticides in mouse spermtocytes. *Toxicol Lett* 1984; 21: 315-319.

[69] Dzwonkowska A, Hubner H. Induction of chromosomal aberrations in the Syrian hamster by insecticides tested in vivo. *Arch Toxicol* 1986; 58: 152-156.

[70] Bao T van, Szabó I, Ruzsicska P, Czeizel AE. Chromosome aberrations in patients suffering acute organis phosphate insectice intoxication. *Humangenetik* 1994; 24: 33-57.

[71] Berge GN, Nafstad I. Distribution and placental transfer of trichlorfon in guinea pig. *Arch Toxicol* 1986; 59: 26-29.

[72] Martson LV. Teratological studies on chlorophos in golden hamsters and white mice. *Gigiena Sanitariya (USSR)* 1979; 7: 70-72.

[73] Staples RE, Goulding EH. Dipterex teratogenicity in the rat, hamster and mouse when given by gavage. *Environ Health Perspect* 1979; 30: 105-113.

[74] Courtney KD, Andrews JE, Springer J. Assessment of teratogenic potential of trichlorfon in mice and rats. *J Environm Sci Health* 1986; B21: 207-227.

[75] Nehéz M, Huszta E, Mazzeg E, Scheufler H, Schneider P, Fischer GW: Cytogenetic, genetic and embryotoxicity studies with dimethyl 2,2,2-trichlorfo-1-(2,2,2-tricholo-1-hydroxyethoxy)-ethylphosphonate,a hypothetical impurity in technical grade trichlorfon. *Ecotoxicol Envir Safety* 1987; 13: 216-224.

[76] Källen B. Congenital malformations in twins: A population study. *Acta Genet Med Gemellol* 1986; 35: 167-178.

[77] Parry JM, Al-Obaidly M, Al-Walhaib M, Kayani T, Nebeel J, Strefford EM, Parry EM. Spontaneous, induced aneuplidy, consideration which may influence shromosome mals egregation. *Mutat Res* 2002; 504: 119-129.

[78] Doherty AT, Ellard EM, Parry EM, Parry JM. A study of the aneugenic activity of trichorfon detected by centromere-specific probes in human lymphoblastoid cell lines. *Mutat Res* 1996; 372: 221-231.

[79] Yin FY, Cukurcam S, Betzendahl I, Adler I-D, Eichenlaub-Ritter U. Trichlorfon exposure, spindle aberrations and non-disjunction in mammalian oocytes. *Chromosome* 1998; 107: 514-522.

[80] Sun FY, Schmid TE, Schmid E, Baumgartner A, Adler I-D. Trichlorfon induces spindle disturbances in V79 cells and aneuploidy in male mouse germ cells. *Mutagenesis* 2000; 15: 17-24.

[81] Cukurcam S, Sun F, Betzendahl I, Adler I-D, Eichenlaub-Ritter U. Trichlorfon predisposes to aneuploidy and interfers with spindle formation in in vitro maturing mouse oocyte. *Mutat Res* 2004; 564: 165-178.

[82] Haddow JE. Antenatal screening for Down' syndrome: where are we and where next? *Lancet* 1998; 352: 336-337.

[83] Hattori M, Fujiyama A, Taylor TD et al. The DNA sequence of human chromosome 21. *Nature* 2000; 405: 311-319.

[84] Penrose LS. The relative effects of paternal and maternal age in mongolism. *J Genet* 1933; 27: 219-224.

[85] Yoon PW, Freeman SB, Sherman SL, Taft LF, Gu Y, Pettay D, Flansers DW, Khoury MJ, Hassold TJ. Advenced maternal age and the risk of Down syndrome characterized by the meiotic stage of the chromosomal error: A population-based study. *Am J Hum Genet* 1996; 58: 628-633.

[86] Hassold T, Sherman S. 2000. Down syndrome: genetic recombinaton and the origin of the extra chromosome 21. *Clin Genet* 2000; 57: 95-100.

[87] Källen B. Down's syndrome and maternal smoking in early pregnancy. *Genet Epidemiol* 1997; 14: 77-84.

[88] Kline J, Stein Z. Environmental causes of aneuploidy: Who so elusive. In: Dellarco VL, Voytek PE, Hollander A. Aneuploidy. Etiology and Mechanism. Plenum Press: New York. 1985. pp 149-164.

[89] Arbuzova S. Why it is necessary to study the role of the mitochondrial genome in trisomy 21 pathogenesis? *Downs Syndr Res Pract* 1998; 5: 26-29.

[90] Arbuzova S, Cuckle H, Mueller R, Sehmi I. Familial Down syndrome: evidence supporting cytoplasmic interitance. *Genet* 2001; 60: 456-462.

[91] Barkai G, Arbuzova S, Berkenstadt M, Heifetz S, Cuckle H. Frequency of Down's syndrome and neural-tube defects in the same family. *Lancet* 2003; 361: 1331-35.

[92] James SI, Pogribna J, Pogribny IP, Melnyk S, Hine RJ, Gibson JB. Abnormal folate metabolism and mutation in the methylenetetrahydrofolate-reductase gene may be maternal risk factors for Down syndrome. *Am J Clin Nutr* 1999; 70: 495-501.

[93] Hobbs CA, Sherman SL, Ping Y, Hopkins SE, Torfs CP, Hine J. Polymorphisms in genes involved in folate metabolism as maternal risk factors for Down syndrome. *Am J Hum Genet* 2000; 67: 623-630.

[94] O'Leary VB, Parle-McDermott A, Molloy AM. MTRR and MTHFR polymorphism: link to Down syndrome. *Am J Med Genet* 2002; 107: 151-155.

[95] Stuppia L, Gatta V, Gaspari AR, Antonucci I, Morizio E, Calabrese G. C677T mutation in the 5,10-MTHFR gene and risk of Down syndrome in Italy. *Eur J Hum Genet* 2002; 10: 388-390.

[96] Yanamandra K, Bochini JA, Jr., Thurmon TF. Absence of association of fetal MTHFR C677T polymorphism with prenatal Down syndrome pregnancy. *Eur J Hum Genet* 2003; 11: 5.

[97] Czeizel AE, Puho E. Maternal use of nutritional supplements during the first month of pregnancy and a reduced risk of Down's syndrome. A case-control study. *Nutrition* 2005; 21: 698-704.

[98] Bendich A, Butterworth CE (eds). Micronutrients in health and in disease prevention. Marcel Dekker Inc. New York, 1991.

[99] Czeizel AE, Petik D, Vargha P. Validation studies of drug exposures in pregnant women. *Pharmacoepid Drug Safety* 2003; 12: 409-416.

[100] Czeizel AE, Vargha P Periconceptional folic acid/multivitamin supplementation and twin pregnancy. *Am J Obstet Gynecol* 2004; 191: 790-794.

[101] Rockenbauer M, Olsen J, Czeizel AE, Pedersen L, Sorensen TH, EuroMAP Group. Recall bias in a case-control surveillance system on the use of medicine during pregnancy. *Epidemiology* 2001; 12: 461-466.

[102] Allen LH. Anemia and iron deficiency: Effect on pregnancy outcomes. *Am J Clin Nutr* 2000; 71: 12805-12845.

[103] Herbig AK, Stover PJ. Regulation of folate metabolism by iron. In: Massaro EJ, Rogers JM. eds). Folate and Human Development. Humana Press, Totowa, New Jersey, 2002. pp. 241-262.

[104] Czeizel AE, Dudás I. Prevention of the first occurrence of neural-tube defects by periconceptional vitamin supplementation. *N Engl J Med* 1992; 327: 1832-1835.

[105] Czeizel AE, Dobó M, Vargha P. Hungarian cohort-controlled trial of periconceptional multivitamin supplementation shows a reduction in certain congenital abnormalities. *Birth Defects Research Part A* 2004; 70: 853-861.

[106] Czeizel AE. Prevention of congenital abnormalities by periconceptional multivitamin supplementation. *Br Med J* 1993; 306: 1645-1648.

[107] Czeizel AE. Reduction of urinary tract and cardiovascular defects by periconceptional multivitamin supplementation. *Am J Med Genet* 1996; 62: 179-183.

[108] Bosco P, Gueant-Rodriguez RM, Anello G, Barone C, Namsur F, Caraci F. Methionine synthase (MTR) 2756 (A-G) polymorphism, double heterozygosity methionine synthase 2756 AG/methionine synthase reductase (MTRR) 66 AG, and elevated homocysteinemia are three risk factors having a child with Down syndrome. *Am J Med Genet* 2003; 121A: 219-224.

[109] Czeizel AE, Tímár L, Sárközi A. Dose-dependent effect of folic acid on the prevention of oral clefts. *Pediatrics* 1999; 104: e66.

[110] Tolarova M. Periconceptional supplementation with vitamins and folic acid to prevent recurrence of cleft lip. *Lancet* 1982; 2: 217.

[111] US National Academy of Sciences. Dietary Reference Intakes: Folate, Other B Vitamins and Choline. National Academy Press. Washington DC, 1998

In: Handbook of Down Syndrome Research
Editors: Dominicus Jelinek and Gijs Dvorak
ISBN 978-1-60741- 690-6

Chapter 4

Social Functioning In Down Syndrome: A Neuropsychological Perspective

Melanie A. Porter[1]
Clinical Neuropsychologist and Lecturer in Neuropsychology,
Psychology Department, Macquarie University, Sydney, Australia

Abstract

This chapter will commence with an overview of the literature on social functioning in Down syndrome (DS). The overview is structured according to Tager-Flusberg and Sullivan's (2000) model of social functioning, which differentiates social perceptual and social cognitive skills. Compared to the literature available for other developmental syndromes, there has been very little research exploring social abilities in DS, and studies have produced mixed findings. Following the overview, research limitations are discussed, then a research study is introduced which addresses some of the limitations and assesses social attribution in DS (N=17), Williams-Beuren syndrome (WBS, N=17), and in typically developing mental age matched controls (N=17, MAC) and chronological age matched controls (N=17, CAC). The research study compares individuals with DS, individuals with WBS, and MAC and CAC on the Social Attribution Task (SAT, Klin, 2000), which uses the Heider and Simmel (1944) silent cartoon animation in which geometric shapes enact a social plot. The SAT measures social abilities which are a fundamental basis of human social interaction (Klin, 2000). Findings indicated a comparable performance between DS, WBS, and MAC on all social cognitive indices from the SAT, but the DS group displayed reduced paralinguistic skills compared to MAC. All groups performed significantly below the level of CAC, except for their ability to attribute cognitive and affective mental states, which was comparable across the four groups. Findings are discussed in relation to Tager-Flusberg and Sullivan's model of social functioning and in relation to amygdala and frontal lobe brain impairments in DS.

[1] Phone: + 61 2 9850 6768, Fax: +61 2 9850 8062, E-mail: melanie.porter@psy.mq.edu.au.

Introduction

Down syndrome (DS), or trisomy 21, is a chromosomal disorder caused by the presence of an extra (third) copy of chromosome 21. DS is associated with impaired brain and cognitive development, physical impairments and a distinct facial appearance.

The cognitive difficulties associated with DS present a major challenge to those affected, and their families. Individuals with DS tend to have lower than average cognitive skills, with their intellectual abilities typically ranging from mild to moderate (within the bottom half to bottom two percent of the population). DS is one of the most common causes of intellectual disability, with a prevalence of around 1 per 800 births, although the statistics are heavily dependent on a number of factors, including the age of the mother (Nadel, 1999).

Despite their intellectual disabilities, individuals with DS are often portrayed as ‘friendly’, ‘affectionate’, ‘charming’, and ‘happy’ (Pitcairn and Wishart, 2000), leading to the attribution of a stereotyped sociable and outgoing personality. This stereotype also includes the belief that social development is relatively ‘protected’ in DS, despite their impaired cognitive development. Perhaps because of this stereotype, until recently there has been very little research exploring social abilities in DS. Recent empirical work is now emerging, however, and seems to challenge this notion of intact social functioning in DS.

These emerging empirical findings, which suggest impaired social understanding in DS, are perhaps not surprising given that: 1. Children and adults with intellectual impairments typically display deficits in social skills and problems in day-to-day social functioning (Kasari and Bauminger, 2000), although not all authors proclaim this (e.g. see Hobson, 1989); 2. Anecdotal reports from parents and teachers indicate that individuals with DS experience difficulties with day-to-day social interaction and with forming and maintaining friendships (Leonard, Msall, Bower, Tremont, and Leonard, 2002); and 3. Neurological studies highlight impairments in those regions of the brain which are thought to be heavily involved in social skill development, including the amygdala (e.g. see Marui, Iseki, Kosaka, Kato, Adachi, and Kenji, 1999; Raz, et al., 1995), and the frontal cortex (e.g. see Teipel, Alexander, Schapiro, Möller, Rapoport, and Hampel, 2004).

This chapter will provide an overview of research on social functioning in DS, focusing particularly on social perception and theory of mind (or the ability to attribute causal mental states in order to explain and/or predict one’s own and other people’s behavior, Premack and Woodruff, 1978), two dissociable aspects of social understanding according to Tager-Flusberg and Sullivan’s (2000) model. Research limitations are then discussed and a new study is introduced - an experimental study of social attribution in DS, comparing individuals with DS to typically developing mental age matched or chronological age matched controls, as well as a group of individuals with Williams-Beuren Syndrome (WBS, also known simply as ‘Williams syndrome’), a rare genetic disorder which, like DS, is associated with intellectual disability (also typically mild to moderate) and a stereotyped sociable and friendly personality (Bellugi, Mills, Jernigan, Hickok, and Galaburda, 1999). Unlike individuals with DS, some individuals with WBS display a relative strength in conversational language skills and in vocabulary (Bellugi, Lichtenberger, Jones, Lai, and St. George, 2000; Ypsilanti, Grouios, Alevriadou, and Tsapkini, 2005).

A Brief Overview of Neuropsychological and Neurological Functioning in DS[2]

The DS Cognitive Profile

In addition to their global intellectual disability, individuals with DS display a range of cognitive weaknesses, although compared to other developmental syndromes, such as WBS, their cognitive profile is more flat or more universally impaired. As Sigman (1999, p. 190) asserts, "the specific deficits of children with Down syndrome are less dramatic than are those of children with other developmental disorders, such as autism or Williams syndrome".

Research suggests a particular weakness in auditory processing within DS, in particular, a weakness in phonological short term memory (Jarrold, Baddley, and Hewes, 1999; Wang and Bellugi, 1994), as well as speech and language (Mervis, 1988; Wang, and Bellugi, 1994; also see Rondal, 1995 for a comprehensive review). In addition, Carlesimo, et al. (1997) and Nadel (1999) discuss learning and memory impairments in DS, suggesting this cognitive domain is also a relative weakness in DS compared to their global level of intellectual functioning. Rowe, Lavender, and Turk (2006) also suggest executive functioning deficits in DS compared to non-DS intellectually impaired participants, although future research is required before we can claim that executive functioning is a particular weakness in DS.

Neurological Impairments in DS

The above cognitive weaknesses are consistent with neurological findings within the syndrome. Although there are widespread brain abnormalities in DS, including an overall reduction in brain volume and disruption to myelination (e.g. see Nadel, 1999, and see Raz et al., 1995 for reviews); neuroimaging, electrophysiological and neuropathological studies indicate that the temporal regions of the brain are disproportionally affected, (Frangou, Aylward, Warren, Sharma, Barta, and Pearlson, 1997; Golden, and Hayman, 1994; Nadel, 1999; Risser, Lubec, Cairns, and Herra-Marshitz, 1997; Wang and Bellugi, 1994, see Raz, et al., 1995 for a review), including the superior temporal gyrus (Pinter, Eliez, Schmitt, Capone, and Reiss, 2001). Other regions that appear to be disproportionally affected in DS include the cerebellum (Raz, 1995; Weis, 1991), the frontal cortex (Conrad, Schmidt, Niccolos, Polak, Riniolo, and Burack, 2007; Nadel, 1999; Shapiro, Berman, Alexander, Weinberger, and Rapoport, 1999;Teipel at al., 2004), and the amygdala (Marui et al., 1999; Murphy, et al., 1992; Pearlson, et al., 1998).

These latter regions, particularly the frontal lobes and the amygdala, are specialized in processing social information (see Adolphs, 1999 for a review). The frontal lobes are particularly involved in monitoring, regulating and adapting social behavior, theory of mind, and use of mental state language (Castelli, Frith, Happè, and Frith, 2002). The amygdala

[2] A comprehensive review of neuropsychological and neurological functioning in DS is beyond the scope of this chapter; please see Nadel (1999); Sigman (1999); Raz et al., (1995); and Wang, (1996) for comprehensive reviews.

plays a particularly important role in emotion recognition (Adolphs, Tranel, Damasio, and Damasio, 1994) and in constantly monitoring and evaluating the environment for potential threat (Davis and Whalen, 2001). Given that these regions of the brain are impaired in DS, it is not surprising that functional impairments in many of these neuropsychological areas have also been reported in DS, including: inappropriate and over-friendly behaviors (Jones, 2000); poor emotion regulation (Jahromi, Gulsrud, Kasari, 2008); inappropriate use of affective linguistic devices (Bellugi, et al., 2000); and emotion recognition deficits (see below).

For example, research suggests low frustration tolerance in individuals with DS (Jahromi et al., 2008) and impaired behavioral inhibition (Karrer, Karrer, Bloom, Chaney, and Davis, 1998), and other research indicates that people with DS use significantly less affective prosody than individuals with WBS or mental age matched controls, and they refer to a character's affective state and use sound effects less often than their WBS counterparts (Bellugi, Korenberg, and Klima, 2001; Reilly et al., 1990; Reilly et al., 1995).

Recent neuroimaging research also implicates the amygdala and the frontal lobes in WBS (Galaburda and Bellugi, 2000; Gaser et al., 2006; Mobbs, et al., 2007; Meyer-Lindenberg et al., 2005; Porter, Coltheart, and Langdon, 2007), and individuals with WBS also display difficulties with social functioning, including social cognition and behavior and emotion regulation (see below, and see Bellugi, Adolphs, et al., 1999; Gosch, and Pankau, 1994; Porter, 2008; Tager-Flusberg and Sullivan, 2000).

A Model of Social Understanding Applied to DS

Tager-Flusberg and Sullivan (2000) make an important distinction between *perceptual* and *cognitive* components of social knowledge. *Social perception* is generally termed 'person perception', and includes skills like the capacity to distinguish between people and objects, and to make on-line rapid judgments about people's mental states (intentions, emotions, personality traits) from their facial, body and vocal expressions. In contrast, *social cognition* is said to involve a capacity to make more complex cognitive inferences about the content of mental states, it incorporates what has traditionally been referred to as 'theory of mind' or understanding the mind as a representational system (Premack and Woodruff, 1978). Theory of mind is a social domain which is characteristically impaired in autism, leading to the term 'Mindblindness' as a descriptive term for the social deficits observed in these individuals (e.g. see Baron-Cohen, Leslie, and Frith, 1985; Leslie and Frith, 1988).

Developmentally, according to Tager-Flusberg and Sullivan (2000), social perceptual abilities are said to emerge very early on, with newborns selectively orienting toward human faces and voices (Mehler and Dupoux, 1994), and by 4 to 12 months of age, responding differently to various facial expressions of emotion (Baron-Cohen, 1994; Serrano, Iglesias, and Loeches, 1995). In contrast, Tager-Flusberg and Sullivan propose that social cognitive skills develop from around the age of 3 years and continue to develop into middle childhood and beyond. Some theorists also argue that social cognitive (or theory of mind) skills build upon these more early social perceptual abilities (e.g. see Wellman and Woolley, 1990).

Tager-Flusberg and Sullivan (2000) assert that social perceptual skills rely less on general cognitive abilities or language, and are more closely connected to the affective system, whereas social cognitive skills are thought to interact closely with other non-social cognitive domains such as language and information processing capabilities (Tager-Flusberg and Sullivan, 2000). However, dissociations have been found between social cognition (theory of mind) and non-social cognitive capabilities such as intellect (e.g. see Castelli, et al., 2002) and language (Leslie and Frith, 1988; Perner, Frith, Leslie, and Leekham, 1989). For example, individuals with Asperger syndrome display intact intellectual functions, but impaired social cognition (Castelli, et al., 2002), and individuals with specific language impairment have been known to pass theory of mind tasks (Leslie and Frith, 1988).

Moreover, Tager-Flusberg and Sullivan (2000) propose that social perceptual and social cognitive abilities depend upon "distinct underlying neuro-cognitive mechanisms" (p. 63). The amygdala is said to be involved in social perception, while the prefrontal cortex is said to mediate social cognition. It is now known, however, that the limbic system (which includes the amygdala) and the frontal cortex are both heavily connected, and that each of these areas is likely to play a role in both social perception and social cognition (Adolphs, 1999; Siegel and Varley, 2002).

Similarly, most social tasks generally tap both social perception and social cognition. It would be difficult, for example, to find a social perceptual task that does not rely somewhat on social cognitive processes. Nevertheless, some tasks rely more heavily on one or the other component of social functioning. An overview of social perceptual and then social cognitive skills in DS is now provided, exploring the possibility of a dissociation between these skills within DS. Such a dissociation would provide support for Tager-Flusberg and Sullivan's (2000) proposal that social perception and social cognition are independent abilities (i.e. can be selectively impaired).

Social Perception and Social Cognition in DS: A Selective Impairment in Social Perception?

Social perceptual tasks most commonly administered to individuals with DS have included: (1.) general face processing (e.g. face perception and recognition of facial identity, Hippolyte, Barisnikov, and Van der Linden, 2008, and see Pitcairn and Wishart, 2000 for a review); (2.) emotion perception and emotion recognition, including matching facial, body, and vocal expressions of emotion, and labeling facial, body, and vocal expressions of emotion (see Kasari and Sigman, 1996 for a review; see also Kasari, Freeman, and Hughes, 2001; Porter, et al., 2007), (3.) orientation of attention toward social information (such as attention toward people versus objects, and face and eye gaze); and (4.) social and emotion expression (e.g. the production of facial expressions and nonverbal communication, Carvajal, and Iglesias, 2006; see also Wishart and Pitcairn, 2000). Social cognition or theory of mind has also been assessed in DS (Baron-Cohen, et al., 1985; Kasari and Sigman, 1996; Porter, 2008). While findings tend to be mixed in all of these social domains, overall, findings implicate impaired social perception and relatively spared social cognition (theory of mind) abilities in DS.

Social Perception in DS

1. Face Perception Difficulties in DS

In terms of face perception, Pitcairn and Wishart (2000) asked children with DS (aged 8 to 14 years), children with non-specific intellectual impairments (aged 8 to 14 years) and mental age matched controls (3 to 5 years of age) to match photographs of faces based on their identity. Pitcairn and Wishart found no significant difference in performance across the three groups and suggested intact face perception (or at least intact facial identity recognition) in individuals with DS.

In contrast, in a later study, Williams, Wishart, Pitcairn, and Willis (2005) found that their group of individuals with DS (aged 7 to 15 years) performed more poorly than a group of children with non-specific intellectual disability on the Benton Facial Recognition Test, a more complex face perception task which requires participants to recognize the same face under different lighting and orientation conditions (Benton, Hamsher, Varney, and Spreen, 1983).

Similarly, in their review, Bellugi, et al. (2000, p. 25) indicated "across a range of tasks involving faces, individuals with WMS [Williams syndrome] outperform those with DNS [Down syndrome]". They report DS and WBS individuals have been compared on a range of standardized face processing tasks including the Mooney Closure Test (Mooney, 1957), Benton Test of Facial Recognition (Benton, et al., 1983), and the Warrington Recognition Memory Test (Warrington, 1984), and that people with WBS always outperformed DS participants (Bellugi, Lichtenberger, Jones, Lai, and St. George, 2000).

Thus, research to date most strongly supports the notion of impaired face perception in individuals with DS. Their perceptual difficulties are, however, not specific to faces or to social stimuli, and more than likely relate to more general attention and spatial deficits, including a general bias in attention toward processing global information (Porter and Coltheart, 2006) and spatial-perceptual deficits (Bihrle, Bellugi, Delis, and Marks, 1989).

2. Emotion Recognition Difficulties in DS

Consistent with findings of impaired face perception, the majority of research indicates general impairments in emotion recognition abilities amongst children and adults with DS, with some studies suggesting a more specific difficulty in recognizing the emotions of fear (Kasari, et al., 2001; Pitcairn and Wishart, 2000), anger (Kasari et al., 2001), sadness (Porter, Coltheart, and Langdon, 2007) and surprise (Wishart and Pictairn, 2000; Hippolyte, Barisnikov, and Van der Linden, 2008). These emotion recognition deficits seem to extend beyond the facial modality, however, including not only the perception of affect in faces, but also in bodies and voices (Porter, 2008).

Kasari, Hughes, and Freeman (1994, as cited by Kasari and Sigman, 1996) did not find evidence to suggest emotion recognition deficits in DS in their early studies. Kasari and colleagues examined emotion recognition in four to six year old children with DS and included a typically developing chronological age matched control group and a typically developing mental age matched control group. They used three independent tasks to assess recognition of happy, sad, angry and scared expressions: (a.) verbally labelling facial expressions of puppets, (b.) choosing the correct puppet when the experimenter said an emotion, and (c.) stating the emotion of a puppet following a story (e.g. one puppet giving another an ice cream to depict happiness). Kasari et al. (1994, as cited by Kasari and Sigman, 1996) reported no group differences in the ability to verbalize, recognize, or identify emotions across the various tasks. Using these same tasks, however, Kasari, et al. (2001) found that while children with DS whose developmental age was around 3 years of age performed similarly to mental age matched typically developing controls, by the developmental age of around 4 years, the DS group was less accurate.

Also, using an emotion matching task to assess recognition of happiness, sadness, anger, fear, surprise and disgust, Williams, et al. (2005) found that their group of individuals with DS (aged 7 to 18 years) performed more poorly than children with non-specific intellectual disabilities and typically developing controls.

In a recent study, we compared emotion recognition abilities in DS and WBS. We administered the Diagnostic Analysis of NonVerbal Accuracy scale (or DANVA, Nowicki and Duke, 1994) to individuals with DS or WBS aged 5 to 44 years, and to mental age matched and chronological age matched typically developing controls (Porter, Coltheart, & Langdon, 2007). The DANVA is a standardized battery assessing emotion recognition across three modalities (faces, body postures and voices). The main effect for group was significant, and there was a significant emotion by group interaction. Overall, the WBS group performed similarly to mental age matched typically developing controls, and both of these groups significantly outperformed the DS group. In addition, the DS group displayed a particular difficulty in recognizing sadness compared to WBS and mental age matched control groups.

Thus, research to date suggests emotion recognition deficits in DS, with some suggestion of more specific difficulties pertaining to particular emotions, although the latter emotion-specific difficulties remain equivocal and require further research before any firm conclusions can be made.

3. Abnormal Social Attention in DS

Results also tend to indicate some anomalies in the way that individuals with DS attend to social information. For example, Kasari, Mundy, Yirmiya, and Sigman (1990) found that compared to typically developing controls, children with DS were significantly more attentive to the experimenter's face and less attentive to a toy that was out of reach; this phenomenon has also been noted by Pitcairn and colleagues (e.g. see Pitcairn and Wishart, 2000), and by Jones (1990), who found that infants with DS attend more often to the faces of caregivers and strangers than do typically developing infants. Similarly, other literature suggests that individuals with DS fixate for longer periods than typically developing controls during social interactions (Landry, and Chapieski, 1990).

This tendency to over-fixate on social stimuli is similar to observations of individuals with WBS, who also spend an unusual amount of time attending to people and to faces (Bellugi, Adolphs, Cassady and Chiles, 1999; Frigerio, Burt, Gagliardi, Cioffi, Martelli,

Perrett, and Borgatti, 2006; Porter, et al., 2007). Unlike individuals with DS, however, individuals with WBS seem to particularly fixate on the eye region of the face (Porter, Shaw, and Marsh, Submitted; Riby, and Hancock, 2008).

In addition to these anomalies in social attention amongst individuals with DS, there is also evidence to suggest that individuals with DS may experience abnormal social referencing when exposed to an ambiguous situation (Kasari, Freeman, Mundy, Sigman, 1995; Knieps, Walden, Tedra, and Baxter, 1994). Kasari et al. (1994) found that when a toy robot entered the room, individuals with DS showed less emotion than typically developing children and did not use social referencing to appraise the situation (that is, they did not take their mother's facial expression of either fear or joy into account). Similarly, Knieps, et al. (1994) found that infants with DS fail to monitor the emotional expressions displayed by their mother during a social referencing task. These social referencing difficulties are likely to relate, at least partially, to their inability to accurately recognize facial expressions of emotion, but may also indicate anomalies in the way in which DS individuals use their attention to gain information about the world.

In contrast to the above anomalies in social attention, Yirmiya, Pilowsky, Solomonica-Levi, and Shulman (1999) reported that in their study, individuals with DS spent a similar amount of time looking in the experimenter's eyes to that of typically developing controls, suggesting no abnormalities in DS; this was compared to poor eye gaze observed in their participants with autism.

4. Impaired Social and Emotional Expression in DS

There is very little research exploring emotional expression in DS, however, Carvajal and Iglesias (2006) provide evidence to suggest impairments in this area. For example, Carvajal and Iglesias (2006) explored how accurately adults could perceive facial and vocal emotions in infants with DS and found that the adults were less accurate in perceiving the emotion displayed by infants with DS than they were at perceiving the emotion displayed by typically developing controls. Berger and Cunningham (1983) also found that even adults familiar to the child with DS experienced difficulty perceiving facial expressions of emotion.

Similarly, Lacroix, Bernicot, and Reilly (2004) explored mental state expression in DS and WBS during mother-and-child interactions; they noted that children with DS produced less expressive mental states than children with WBS. Also, although not technically emotion expression, DS individuals have been shown to experience a weakness in nonverbal requesting skills (see Hines and Bennet, 1996; Mundy, Sigman, and Kasari, 1988).

In contrast to these impairments in social and emotional expression, other research indicates intact nonverbal social and emotional interaction in DS, at least in infancy (see Carvajal and Iglesias, 2002 for a review, and see Caselli, Vicari, Longobardi, Lami, Pizzoli, and Stella, 1998; Mundy, et al., 1988).

Further research is required before firm claims can be made one way or another, but the majority of research tends to suggest impairments in emotional and social expression amongst individuals with DS.

Social Cognition

In contrast to the abovementioned social perceptual deficits reported in DS, most researchers suggest that social cognition or 'theory of mind' is intact in DS, or at least relatively preserved compared to social perceptual skills (Baron-Cohen, et al., 1985, 1986; Porter, 2008).

Like people with WBS and unlike autistic individuals, early signs of social cognition, including pretend play and joint attention, seem to be intact in DS, and individuals with DS show an interest in social interactions from a very early age. In addition, studies of early play in DS infants suggest no deficits in joint attention within this population (Sigman, 1999), and a sequence of early symbolic play that is *"markedly similar to that observed in normally developing children"* (Cicchetti, Beeghly, and Weiss-Perry, 1994 p. 211; Hill and McCune-Nicholich, 1981).

In addition, research suggests that people with DS display significantly higher frequencies of social interaction behaviors than typically developing mental age matched controls, and that individuals with DS show more empathy and sympathy toward another person's distress than typically developing individuals (Kasari, Freeman, and Bass, 2003; Kasari, Mundy, Yirmiya, and Sigman, 1990) and autistic individuals (Loveland and Belgin, 1991). Although, Kasari et al. (2003) noted some anomalies in the display of empathy by individuals with DS, namely, that individuals with DS were less likely to feel the same emotion as the protagonist in a hypothetical empathy situation (compared to typically developing controls).

Other research suggests that people with DS are less socially responsive than typically developing mental age matched peers (Mundy, Sigman, Kasari, and Yirmiya, 1988), and Beeghly (1998) argues that infants with DS show greater perseveration in their production of symbolic play relative to normally developing MA matched controls (Beeghly, 1998).

In older children and adults with DS, the typical tasks used to assess theory of mind development have included: classic false belief tasks such as the Sally and Anne Task[3] (Baron-Cohen, et al., 1985); classic vignettes assessing first order (Tager-Flusberg and Sullivan, 1994)[4] , advanced (Fletcher et al., 1995; Happé, Brownell, and Winner, 1999; Happé et al., 1996; Happé, Winner, and Brownell, 1998)[5] , and second order (Baron-Cohen, 1989; Bowler, 1992; Perner and Wimmer, 1985; Sullivan, Zaitchik, and Tager-Flusberg,

---

[3] The experimenter uses two dolls, "Sally" and "Anne". Sally has a basket; Anne has a box. Experimenters show their subjects (usually children) a simple skit, in which Sally puts a marble in her basket and then leaves the scene. While Sally is away and cannot watch, Anne takes the marble out of Sally's basket and puts it into her box. Sally then returns and the children are asked where they think Sally will look for her marble. Children are said to "pass" the test if they understand that Sally will most likely look inside her basket before realizing that her marble isn't there.

[4] First order theory of mind refers to the capacity to meta-represent the propositional content of one's own or another person's mental state (e.g. "I think x" or "she thinks y"); this develops around four years of age in typically developing individuals.

[5] Advanced theory of mind refers to a more sophisticated understanding of complex mental states such as deception, white lies, mistakes and double bluff as they typically occur in common social contexts.

1994)[6] theory of mind (e.g. see Porter, 2008); appreciation of humor (Porter, 2008; St James and Tager-Flusberg, 1994), and more indirect picture sequencing tasks (e.g. see Baron-Cohen, et al., 1986; Porter, 2008).

Using the Sally and Anne false belief task, Baron-Cohen, et al. (1985) found that their group of DS children performed similarly to mental age matched typically developing controls and significantly better than a group of children with autism; thus concluding that false belief understanding is intact in DS and impaired in autism.

Baron-Cohen, et al. (1986) and Porter (2008) used picture sequencing tasks to assess understanding of intentions, and, in the case of Porter, intentions, pretence and false beliefs in individuals with DS. Both research groups found no evidence to suggest impaired theory of mind capabilities in DS. Baron-Cohen, et al.'s DS group outperformed an autistic group of individuals on sequencing mental state stories, but not on physical or control stories, and we found that our DS group performed similarly to mental age matched controls and similar to (if not better than) individuals with WBS in their ability to sequence mental state stories (Porter, 2008).

In other related work, we found that our group of DS individuals showed a similar appreciation of humor (using picture jokes) to that of typically developing mental age matched controls and individuals with WBS , as well as a similar performance on first order, advanced and second order theory of mind, and the DS group actually outperformed the WBS group on certain aspects of second order theory of mind (more specifically on second order justification questions) once non-social cognitive capabilities were controlled (Porter, 2008).

It is well known that, due to the nature of theory of mind tasks, they rely heavily on non-social cognitive abilities such as mental age, language, short term memory and reasoning skills. When theory of mind impairments are documented in DS, this is typically because researchers have not adequately controlled for non-social cognitive variables likely to affect performance on theory of mind tasks (Porter, 2008; Yirmiya, Erel, Shaked, and Solomonica-Levi, 1998; Yirmiya, Solomonica-Levi, Shulman, and Pilowsky, 1996; Zelazo, Burack, Benedetto, and Frye, 1996).

In summary, research to date suggests impaired social perceptual abilities and intact social cognitive functioning in individuals with DS, thus supporting Tager-Flusberg and Sullivan's (2000) dissociative model of social functioning. There are, however, some limitations, as individuals can pass theory of mind tasks, but still demonstrate social cognitive deficits in day-to-day functioning (Klin, 2000). This suggests that theory of mind tasks may not be as ecologically valid as they were initially perceived to be.

[6] Second order theory of mind refers to a general capacity to recursively represent one person's mental state about a second person's mental state (e.g. "he thinks that she thinks"). Second order theory of mind abilities begin to develop around five to seven years of age in typically developing individuals.

Current Limitations of Research Exploring Social Functioning in DS

Klin (2000) suggests a discrepancy between theory of mind performance and level of social adaptation. Moreover, Klin suggests that there may be other social cognitive skills that are important for social adaptation that are not captured in existing tasks of social perception and social cognition, such as social attribution or the ability to anthropomorphize inanimate objects.

More specific limitations of existing social cognitive tasks, particularly theory of mind tasks, are outlined in Klin (2000); these include: (1.) the verbal nature of tasks; (2.) the explicit nature of tasks, and (3.) the dichotomous nature of tasks. First, the majority of theory of mind tasks are verbal in nature and rely heavily on language expression and verbal comprehension. Second, tasks typically overtly refer to a character's mental states, and third, performance on theory of mind tasks is generally scored as 'pass' or 'fail', with no quantitative continuum, yet, as Klin (2000) asserts, in naturalistic settings children with developmental delays are likely to display a continuum of social capabilities or incapabilities.

Because theory of mind tasks rely heavily on language capabilities, individuals with DS are typically matched to controls on verbal competence rather than global mental age when their performance on theory of mind tasks is compared to other populations. Because speech and language is typically a relative weakness in DS, however, this relative weakness in verbal abilities amongst individuals with DS also means that when groups are matched in this capacity, the DS group is likely to display an advantage over other groups in relation to general intellectual capabilities or general mental age. They may then use their intellect as an advantage to assist them in passing the tasks.

The explicit nature of the theory of mind tasks may also render these measures less sensitive to subtle social cognitive impairments in DS, although some indirect tasks such as the picture sequencing tasks (described above) have not proven more sensitive in detecting theory of mind impairments in DS (Baron-Cohen et al., 1996, Porter, 2008). Indirect tasks such as the picture sequencing task have, however, proven more sensitive than the classic verbal theory of mind tasks in detecting theory of mind deficits in some individuals with WBS, namely, those who used their good verbal capabilities to enhance their performance on the classic verbal theory of mind tasks (Porter, Coltheart, and Langdon, 2008).

Finally, the dichotomous nature of the theory of mind tasks (including the picture sequencing tasks) may fail to capture varying degrees of impairment amongst individuals with DS.

The Social Attribution Task

In order to overcome some of these limitations of existing social measures, Klin (2000) developed the Social Attribution Task (SAT, described in detail in Klin, 2000) for use with autistic individuals and individuals with Asperger's syndrome.

The SAT is a social cognitive procedure measuring a participant's ability to recognize visual stimuli as social phenomena and to then extract visual cues from a visual display in order to create a social context. The SAT utilizes Heider and Simmel's (1944) silent video display where a 'cast of characters' including a rectangle, a big triangle, a small triangle, and a small circle are displayed and move around the screen. The characters are designed to move in a contingent fashion (e.g. in synchrony, against each other), resulting in a compelling impact on the viewer that human actions are taking place (e.g. playing, fighting, kissing), and that human emotions are being portrayed (e.g. happiness, fear, frustration). This ability to anthropomorphize innate objects through structure and motion is present even in typically developing preschoolers aged 3 to 5 years (Berry and Springer, 1993).

The SAT reduces factors thought to facilitate theory of mind task performance without facilitating real-life social functioning. Moreover, the SAT has both an indirect and a more explicit measure of social understanding, and the task allows the researcher to quantify social understanding across a number of different dimensions.

The SAT has been used to document deficits in social understanding in children and adults with a range of developmental disorders including autism (Salter, Siegel, Claxton, Lawrence, and Skuse, 2008), Asperger's syndrome (Castelli, et al., 2002) and Prader-Willi syndrome[7] (Koenig, Klin, and Schultz, 2004), and even in individuals who have been shown to pass standard false belief and verbal theory of mind tasks (Abell, et al., 2000; Bowler and Thommen, 2000; Klin, 2000). To the best of my knowledge, the SAT had not been administered to children and adults with DS or WBS before.

In terms of Tager-Flusberg and Sullivan's (2000) model, the SAT is thought to predominantly measure social cognition or theory of mind (Klin, 2000; Siegal, and Varley, 2002), although it is also likely to measure some aspects of social perception. Neurologically, patients with amygdala impairments experience difficulties on the SAT (Heberlein and Adolphs, 2004), as well as patients with frontal lobe impairments (Castelli, et al., 2002). Some authors also suggest that this aspect of theory of mind, namely biological social attribution, is attributed particularly to the superior temporal gyrus (Castelli, et al., 2002; Siegal, and Varley, 2002).

Given the above, it is of interest to administer the SAT to individuals with DS, because the SAT is associated with abnormalities in those brain regions known to be impaired in DS (Castelli, et al., 2002; Siegal, and Varley, 2002).

Overview and Introduction to an Experiment Administering the SAT to Individuals with DS

The literature on social functioning in DS suggests that these individuals display a relative deficit in social perceptual skills compared to social cognitive or theory of mind abilities. However, there are some limitations to theory of mind measures, perhaps rendering

---

[7] PWS is identified by salient food-related characteristics including hyperphagia (overeating) and assiduous food seeking behaviors, facial features, hypogonadism, and short stature. PWS involves abnormalities on chromosome 15. People with PWS typically show higher intelligence than that seen in other genetic disorders, with a mean IQ around 70. There is no universal PWS cognitive profile, though some authors suggest strengths in spatial and visual processing and a weakness in short term memory (Dykens, 1998; Tager-Flusberg, 1999).

the conclusions somewhat premature. In addition, there are some aspects of social cognition, such as social attribution, which are not assessed using the classic theory of mind tasks.

Given these limitations, and given the overlap between those brain regions impaired in DS, and those regions important for the SAT, we decided to assess how DS individuals perform on the SAT.

Given what we have outlined above in terms of neurological regions involved during performance on the SAT, and given we know that individuals with DS display difficulties with social adaptation, one might expect the DS group to display impairments on this task.

On the other hand, given that the literature to date indicates relatively preserved social cognitive and theory of mind capabilities in DS, one might expect the DS group to display no impairments on the SAT.

The following section discusses an experimental study exploring performance on the SAT, comparing groups of individuals with DS, WBS, as well as chronological age matched and mental age matched controls.

Method

Participants

In the experiment to be described here, sixty-eight children and adults participated: 17 individuals with DS aged between 5 and 31 years; 17 individuals with WBS aged between 5 and 30 years; 17 typically developing individuals aged between 5 and 31 years (chronological age matched controls or CAC) and 17 typically developing individuals aged between 3 and 6 years (mental age matched controls or MAC). DS or WBS diagnoses were confirmed genetically. All DS participants had trisomy 21 (Antonarakis, 1991), and all WBS participants had genes deleted on the long arm of chromosome 7, including the elastin gene at 7q11.23 (Fryssira, Palmer, Hallidie-Smith, Taylor, Donnai, and Reardon, 1997). DS, WBS and CAC participants were individually matched on chronological age and gender. DS and WBS participants were also individually matched on mental age. Mental age was established using the Woodcock Johnson Test of Cognitive Ability – Revised (WJ-R COG, Woodcock and Johnson, 1989, 1990); the mental age of DS and WBS participants ranged from 3 to 6 years, consistent with the chronological age range of MAC. Individuals from the MAC group were individually matched to each pair of DS and WBS participants on (developmental/chronological) age and gender.

Descriptive statistics for these four groups are shown in Table 1. In addition to general mental age (an average mental age across the 7 core subtests from the WJ-R COG), verbal mental age, short term memory (STM) and nonverbal reasoning mental age scores are also displayed in Table 1. Verbal mental age is derived from an average performance across Test 6 'Picture vocabulary' and Test 20 'Listening Comprehension', STM is derived from an average performance across Test 2 'Memory for Sentences' and Test 9 'Memory for Words', and nonverbal reasoning mental age is derived from an average performance across Test 7 'Analysis-Synthesis' and Test 14 'Concept Formation' (see Woodcock and Johnson, 1989, 1990 and see the Appendix for a description of the WJ-R COG subtests). As can be appreciated from Table 1, WBS and DS participants displayed a similar cognitive capacity, not only in terms of their overall mental age, but also in terms of their language abilities, STM and nonverbal reasoning capabilities.

Table 1. Descriptive Statistics for the Four Groups

	DS	WBS	MAC	CAC	Sig. Group Comparisons
Mean chronological age (SD)	14.15 (6.52)	13.30 (7.47)	4.88 (0.85)	13.70 (6.80)	DS and MAC $[F(1, 32) = 33.77]^{**}$ WBS and MAC $[F(1, 32) = 21.35]^{**}$ MAC and CAC $[F(1, 32) = 22.05]^{**}$
Mean general mental age (SD)	4.81 (0.80)	4.73 (0.92)	n/a	n/a	NS
Mean verbal mental age (SD)	5.14 (1.20)	5.41 (1.16)	n/a	n/a	NS
Mean STM mental age (SD)	3.84 (0.72)	4.20 (0.52)	n/a	n/a	NS
Mean reasoning mental age (SD)	5.03 (0.76)	5.02 (0.92)	n/a	n/a	NS

Note: ** Significant at $p < .01$; NS = non-significant; chronological age and mental age are in years.

Overview of the Social Attribution Task (SAT)

On the SAT, participants view the Heider and Simmel (1944) video[8]. After viewing the video, as a part of the SAT, participants respond with a series of narratives. The first narrative (Narrative 1) is provided when the participant has viewed the 50 second video twice. Following this initial screening, the video is broken into six meaningful segments and these segments are shown serially to the participant. After each segment is shown, the viewer is asked "What happened here?" and, thus, produces a further six narratives (Narratives 2 to 7). Narratives 1 to 7 are described as spontaneous accounts of the visual display (Klin, 2000). Once Narratives 1 to 7 are obtained, explicit instructions are provided to the viewer. The viewer is told that the shapes are people and they are asked the following questions: "What kind of a person is the big triangle/small triangle/small circle?" (Narratives 8, 9, and 10, respectively). Finally, four short segments of the video are re-shown and the viewer is asked specific questions relating to a given social situation in each segment, such as "Why did the big triangle break the house? (Narratives 11 to 17; for details on all of the questions please see Klin, 2000).

[8] Heider and Simmel (1944) have established that the social attributions that relate to particular perceptual configurations are consistently conveyed by viewers and they have defined several perceptually based principles of social attribution. The video can be viewed at: http://www.metacafe.com/watch/152278/social_attribution_task/

The SAT Coding System

In order to provide reliable and quantifiable scores on the above Narratives, six indices of social cognition are provided, as well as two paralinguistic indices; these include:

Paralinguistic Indices

1) No. of propositions - Total number of propositions (verb + complement) in Narratives 1 – 7. Conversational words or sentences (e.g. "You know", "I think") are not included.
2) Pertinence Index - Percentage of non-pertinent propositions of total number of propositions (Narratives 1-7). Non-pertinent propositions are those which are not pertinent to the cartoon presented to the participant.

Social Cognitive Indices

1) Salience Index - Percentage of social elements identified in Narratives 1-7 (of the 20 elements most frequently identified by typically developing individuals, see Klin, 2000). This refers to the readiness with which a participant imposes a social interpretation to ambiguous visual stimuli.
2) ToM Cognitive Index - Percentage of pertinent propositions that contain cognitive mental state terms in Narratives 1-7 (e.g. belief, desire).
3) ToM Affective Index - Percentage of pertinent propositions that contain affective mental state terms in Narratives 1-7 (e.g. jealousy, pride).
4) Animation Index (0-6) - Level of social attribution on a scale from 0 (no social attribution) to 6 (very high level of social attribution) in Narratives 1-7. It measures the capacity for imposing a social frame of reference on the moving geometric shapes.
5) Person Index (0-6) - Ability to attribute personality features to shapes on a scale from 0 (no personality attributes, describes shapes in physical terms only) to 6 (high ability to impute psychological features to the shapes) in Narratives 8-10.
6) Problem-Solving Index - Percentage of questions answered correctly out of 10 (Narratives 11-17). This measures the extent to which the correct social attributions could be facilitated once the social problem was explicitly defined to the participant.

Each of these indices has objective criteria which is outlined in detail in Klin (2000), so this information is not repeated here.

Procedure

The procedure undertaken for the present study followed the procedure outlined in detail in Klin (2000). All administration instructions outlined in Klin (2000) were read verbatim. The only difference to Klin's procedure was that participants were asked to describe the video *during* rather than *after* the second viewing of the complete video. This altered procedure was undertaken in order to reduce the memory load for participants with an intellectual disability. Participants' responses were recorded and later transcribed by a research assistant who was blind to the purpose of the study. Briefly, the video was shown to each participant individually on a computer screen. The video was shown twice and Narrative 1 was obtained when participants explained what happened in the video (this was done during the second viewing). Following Narrative 1, the six short segments of the video were played serially and following each segment the participant was asked "What happened here?". Narratives 2 to 7 were obtained.

Once the participant provided Narrative 7, the participants were explicitly instructed as outlined in Klin (2000) that the shapes were people and they were asked to describe what kind of a person the big triangle/small triangle/small circle was. Narratives 8 to 10 were obtained. After Narrative 10, the final four short clips were shown serially and the appropriate questions were asked for each segment. Narratives 11 to 17 were obtained.

Administration of the SAT took less than half an hour. Following the SAT, the WJ-R COG was administered to DS and WBS participants; this took approximately one to one and a half hours to administer, with breaks.

Results

Inter-Rater Agreement

Two research assistants who were blind to the purpose of the study carefully read the coding criteria outlined in Klin (2000), and each independently coded all of the narratives and entered the eight index scores into an Excel spreadsheet. A third research assistant who was also blind to the purpose of the study then collated the two spreadsheets and checked for inter-rater disagreements. If the index scores from each coder were not 100% identical, the three research assistants discussed the areas of discrepancy, and together the research assistants decided on the appropriate code. All disagreements were discussed and resolved in the one meeting to ensure consistency. Following this meeting, participants were grouped (into DS, WBS, MAC or CAC groups), and descriptive and inferential statistics were conducted using the statistical analysis software SPSS.

SAT Index Scores

Table 2 displays average SAT index scores for each of the four groups. ANOVAs were performed on each of the indices across the four groups (second last column in Table 2).

Follow up analyses were then performed to compare each group to the other (far right column of Table 2). In line with Klin (2000), we set the alpha level at $p < .05$, with a Bonferoni adjustment for multiple (eight) comparisons at $p < .006$.

As illustrated in Table 2, the DS group performed similarly to the WBS group on all eight indices. Marked differences were obtained between the CAC group and the clinical groups, with the CAC outperforming the clinical groups on most indices ($p < .006$), apart from the ToM Cognitive Index ($p > .05$) and ToM Affective Index ($p > .1$). The DS group produced significantly fewer propositions (approximately half of the number made by the MAC group) and made double the number of impertinent propositions compared to the MAC group. Despite these differences between DS individuals and MAC on the paralinguistic indices, the DS group performed similarly to the MAC group on all six social cognitive indices ($p > .05$).

Table 2 also shows that no group benefited greatly from the explicit instruction that the shapes were people (Social Salience Index versus the Problem-Solving Index).

Associations between SAT Index Scores and Chronological Age, General Mental Age, Verbal Abilities, Short Term Memory, and Nonverbal Reasoning Skills

Table 3 shows the relationship between chronological age, general mental age, verbal abilities, short term memory and reasoning skills and performance on the different SAT index scores. Correlations are shown: i) averaged across all groups (top line); ii) for the DS group only (bolded numbers); and iii) for the WBS group only (italicized numbers).

All correlations are displayed, and maintaining the strict Bonferoni adjusted alpha level, those reaching significance at $p < .006$ are marked, although correlations reaching significance at $p < .05$ are also shown using a separate symbol. Because the sample size is small for DS and WBS groups alone, some correlations are moderate to high, but do not reach significance.

Averaged across groups, a number of significant correlations were obtained: (a.) global mental age, verbal mental age, short term memory and reasoning abilities all correlated significantly and positively with the number of propositions produced during the narratives (verbal mental age and short term memory were significant at $p < .006$, while global mental age and reasoning were significant at $p < .05$); (b.) general mental age, verbal abilities and reasoning skills correlated significantly and negatively with the production of *pertinent* propositions or the Pertinence Index (the former two cognitive abilities correlated at $p < .006$, the latter at $p < .05$); (c.) there was a significant and positive correlation between verbal mental age and the percentage of social elements identified or the Salience Index ($p < .05$); and (d.) there was a significant and positive correlation between verbal mental age and the level of social attribution made (once the explicit instruction was provided that the shapes were people) or the Problem-Solving Index ($p < .05$). The DS group alone (displayed in bold in Table 3) showed these same relationships, as well as some additional moderate to high positive correlations. For the DS group, in addition to the correlations outlined above, there was a moderate, positive (but non-significant) relationship between: (a.) reasoning skills and the Social Salience Index; (b) verbal abilities and attribution of affective mental states; (c.) general mental age and verbal mental age with the Person Index (personality attributions).

Table 2. Results of SAT Index Scores Obtained for the Four Groups

Mean SAT Index Scores	WBS	DS	MAC	CAC	Significance	Sig. Post-Hoc Group Comparisons
Paralinguistic Indices						
No. of propositions[a]	17.59	12.00	22.29	29.29	F (3, 64) = 11.38, p < .00	WBS and CAC ** DS and CAC** DS and MAC**
(SD)	(7.48)	(5.04)	(12.99)	(8.40)		
Pertinence Index[b]	32.28%	53.51%	23.46%	3.58%	F (3, 64) = 12.56, p < .00	WBS and CAC** DS and CAC** DS and MAC**
(SD)	(28.15)	(36.63)	(12.86)	(4.51)		
Social Cognitive Indices						
Salience Index[c]	13.82%	13.24%	23.82%	58.24%	F (3, 64) = 52.04, p < .00	WBS and CAC** DS and CAC** MAC and CAC**
(SD)	(7.19)	(10.60)	(12.81)	(16.10)		
ToM Cognitive Index[d]	11.56%	12.69%	23.23%	18.21%	F (3, 64) = 2.39, p > .08	
(SD)	(12.76)	(18.21)	(14.27)	(11.27)		
ToM Affective Index[e]	7.34%	5.85%	7.44%	.56%	F (3, 64) = 0.67, p > .1	
(SD)	(29.01)	(13.12)	(7.05)	(1.59)		
Animation Index (0-6)[f]	2.06	1.65	2.24	3.18	F (3, 64) = 10.75, p < .00	WBS and CAC** DS and CAC** MAC and CAC**
(SD)	(0.66)	(0.70)	(0.66)	(1.1)		
Person Index (0-6)[g]	1.71	.65	1.59	2.94	F (3, 64) = 5.94, p < .00	DS and CAC**
(SD)	(1.80)	(1.17)	(1.66)	(1.68)		
Problem-Solving Index[h]	19.41%	10.00%	21.76%	50.59%	F (3, 64) = 7.73, p < .00	WBS and CAC** DS and CAC** MAC and CAC**
(SD)	(17.49)	(9.35)	(19.76)	(20.76)		

Note: ** Significant at p < .006; [a] Total number of propositions in Narratives 1 – 7; [b] Percentage of non-pertinent propositions of total number of propositions (Narratives 1-7); [c] Percentage of the typical 20 social elements identified in Narratives 1-7; [d] Percentage of pertinent propositions containing theory of mind (ToM) cognitive terms in Narratives 1-7; [e] Percentage of pertinent propositions containing ToM affective terms in Narratives 1-7; [f] Level of social attribution on a scale of 0-6 in Narratives 1-7; [g] Ability to attribute personality features to shapes in a scale of 0-6 in Narratives 8-10; [h] Percentage of questions answered correctly (Narratives 11-17).

Table 3. Correlations between SAT Index Scores and Chronological Age, General Mental Age, Verbal Abilities, Short Term Memory, and Nonverbal Reasoning Skills

Number of propositions and SAT Index Scores	CA	MA°	VMA°	STM°	REAS°
Paralinguistic Indices					
No. of propositions[a]	.32	.41*	.57**	.56**	.35*
	.23	.52*	.54*	.68**	.57**
	_-.04_	_.45_	_.62**_	_.40_	_.29_
Pertinence Index[b]	-.24	-.50**	-.60**	-.30	-.34*
	-.30	-.64**	-.67**	-.30	-.39
	_-.26_	_-.47_	_-.50*_	_-.12_	_-.36_
Social Cognitive Indices					
Salience Index[c]	.07	.32	.43*	.08	.28
	.20	.32	.37	.01	.38
	_-.08_	_.35_	_.54*_	_.23_	_.19_
ToM Cognitive Index[d]	.29	.21	.20	.06	.16
	.15	.06	-.07	-.05	.09
	_.49*_	_.41_	_.62**_	_.16_	_.25_
ToM Affective Index[e]	-.15	.12	.30	.10	.06
	-.21	.06	.41	.09	.01
	_-.13_	_.29_	_.21_	_.46_	_.23_
Animation Index (0-6)[f]	-.09	-.02	.28	-.09	-.16
	-.01	-.04	.13	-.32	-.25
	_-.13_	_.04_	_.39_	_.11_	_-.10_
Person Index (0-6)[g]	.27	.41*	.31	.29	.23
	.16	.47	.35	.29	.35
	_.40_	_.44_	_.33_	_-.05_	_.19_
Problem-Solving Index[h]	-.01	.30	.34*	.25	.18
	.06	.77**	.59*	.45	.57*
	_-.01_	_.15_	_.21_	_.34_	_.03_

Note: * = significant at p < .05; ** = significant at .p < 006; ° = clinical groups only; **Bold** represents correlations for DS group only; *Italics* represents correlations for WBS group only; CA = chronological age; MA = mental age; VMA = verbal mental age; STM = short term memory (mental age equivalent); REAS = reasoning ability (mental age equivalent); [a] Total number of propositions in Narratives 1 – 7; [b] Percentage of non-pertinent propositions of total number of propositions (Narratives 1-7); [c] Percentage of the typical 20 social elements identified in Narratives 1-7; [d] Percentage of pertinent propositions containing theory of mind (ToM) cognitive terms in Narratives 1-7; [e] Percentage of pertinent propositions containing ToM affective terms in Narratives 1-7; [f] Level of social attribution on a scale of 0-6 in Narratives 1-7; [g] Ability to attribute personality features to shapes in a scale of 0-6 in Narratives 8-10; [h] Percentage of questions answered correctly (Narratives 11-17).

Finally, there were significant, moderate to high and positive relationships between mental age, verbal skills and reasoning abilities and the Problem-Solving Index for the DS group (mental age correlation $p < .006$, and verbal and reasoning skills correlations $p < .05$).

Correlations for the WBS group (displayed in italics in Table 3) were similar to the correlations averaged across groups, and to correlations for the DS group. In addition, for the WBS group: (a.) chronological age and verbal mental age were significantly and positively correlated with attribution of cognitive mental states ($p < .05$ and $p < .006$, respectively); (b.) short term memory was moderately and positively (but not significantly) correlated with attribution of affective mental states; and (c.) verbal mental age was moderately, positively (but not significantly) correlated with the Animation Index.

Conclusion

The study reported in this chapter used the Social Attribution Task (SAT) to measure social understanding in DS compared to individuals with WBS and mental age matched or chronological age matched typically developing controls. First, the DS group performed similarly to the WBS group and to mental age matched controls on all social cognition indices of the SAT. These three groups performed below the level of chronological age matched controls on most social cognition indices, apart from the theory of mind cognitive index (attribution of cognitive mental states) and the theory of mind affective index (attribution of affective mental states), where all four groups performed at a similar level. Results provide a clear sense that individuals with DS are able to attribute social meaning, mental states, and personality attributes to non-social and inanimate visual stimuli. Second, on the paralinguistic (narrative) indices, the DS group performed significantly below the level of mental age matched and chronological age matched controls, but commensurate with the performance of the WBS group, suggesting comparable narrative capabilities to the WBS group, but reduced narrative capabilities compared to typically developing controls. Finally, although the SAT is less reliant on non-social cognitive skills than classic theory of mind tasks, we found some moderate to high correlations between performance on the SAT and external measures of non-social cognition (such as global or verbal mental age). The above findings are discussed in more detail below.

The SAT and Social Cognitive Abilities in DS

The DS group showed a comparable performance to WBS individuals and MAC in terms of their ability to: (a.) identify common social elements in the video such as recognition that there is hostility between some of the shapes, and recognition that two of the shapes are friends; (b.) attribute meaningful cognitive and affective states to the shapes; (c.) see the shapes as animate and sociable beings; and (d.) attribute personality traits to the shapes. Moreover, DS individuals made these social interpretations even before the explicit direction was provided that the shapes were people. Of note, no group benefited from the explicit instruction, which is to be expected given that no group displayed a social attribution deficit.

This is similar to findings produced by Klin (2000) for their typically developing group of adults. Overall, results suggest no deficit in social attribution amongst individuals with DS.

Given that the SAT is thought to predominantly measure social cognition or theory of mind (Klin, 2000; Siegal, and Varley, 2002), the finding that individuals with DS performed similarly to WBS and MAC is consistent with the notion that social cognition is intact in DS, and with findings of relatively preserved theory of mind capabilities in DS. This is in contrast to the social perceptual deficits commonly reported within the syndrome (see above), and provides further support to suggest a dissociation between intact social cognition and impaired social perception amongst individuals with DS (e.g. see Porter, et al., 2008 and Porter, 2008). Findings, therefore, do not refute Tager-Flusberg and Sullivan's (2000) model of social functioning, which proposes that social cognitive and social perceptual functions can be selectively impaired.

On the other hand, the finding of intact social attribution (or intact performance on the SAT) in DS is perhaps inconsistent with neurological findings of impairments in the amygdala, frontal lobe and superior temporal sulcus amongst individuals with DS (see above); as these areas of the brain are reported to play a role in social attribution and in intact performance on the SAT (Adolphs, 1999; Castelli et al., 1999). This suggests that impairments in these 'social brain' regions may manifest differently in DS, not affecting social attribution, but (as discussed above) affecting other aspects of social understanding, including social perception and monitoring of appropriate social behaviors, as well as perhaps pragmatics (see below). It is also possible that the abnormalities in DS within these brain regions differ from those involved in social cognition and the SAT.

Paralinguistic and Narrative Competency in DS

In contrast to the DS group's intact social attribution skills, the SAT highlights the DS group's distinct difficulty with producing narratives, as previously documented by several other researchers (e.g. see Bellugi, et al., 1999; Reilly et al., 1995; Wang and Bellugi, 1993). The length of the DS individuals' narratives was, however, similar to that of the narratives produced by the WBS individuals; with both groups producing a similar number of propositions, on average. The reduced length of narratives for the DS group was indicated by the production of significantly fewer propositions compared to MAC. The quality of narratives was also compromised for the DS group, as evidenced by their significantly higher scores on the Pertinence Index compared to MAC (as well as, perhaps, a non-significant trend of higher scores compared to the WBS group). This means that individuals with DS produced a greater number of irrelevant propositions. Overall, half of the propositions produced by the DS group were irrelevant, compared to one third for the WBS group, and one quarter for MAC.

Example Narratives

Below are example narratives (see Example 1 and Example 2), obtained from DS, WBS, and typically developing individuals. The narratives highlight: (a.) that appropriate social attribution is demonstrated by all individuals, including those with DS or WBS, and (b.) the poorer linguistic quality of the narratives for both DS and WBS individuals, especially compared to CAC.

As Klin (2000) highlights in relation to similar deficits on the Pertinence Index for autistic adults, these linguistic deficits would very likely cause a series of communication breakdowns if individuals were interacting socially with another person (e.g. about the cartoon). Klin (2000) likens such deficits to pragmatic language impairments, a skill which is reportedly impaired in DS (e.g. see Berglund, Erikson, and Johansson, 2001; Sigman, 1999), and which is likely to impact on their day to day social functioning and social interaction capabilities.

Impairments in narrative, pragmatic language, and conversational abilities have also been reported in WBS (Bernicot, Lacroix, and Reilly, 2003; Laws and Bishop, 2004; Stojanovik, 2006).

SAT Narratives: Example 1

a) Narrative 1 produced by a 22 year old DS male (mental age 5 ½ years):

"Circle, triangle, triangle, and a square playing games. He broke the square."

b) Narrative 1 produced by a 22 year old WBS male (mental age 5 ½ years):

"The other part was playing with the other one. The circle was in the middle and going everywhere. More than likely they were playing games together..., like a friendly game. I think the other one was trying to say 'come on, let's play together and have fun'."

c) Narrative 1 produced by a 5 ½ year old typically developing male (MAC):

"The big triangle [is] locked in. The little triangle is hitting the big triangle. The big triangle hits the little triangle. The circle comes into the square and [then] comes out. The big triangle goes in. The little triangle is by himself and climbs up the wall. The circle is moving around. The little triangle and circle close it. The big triangle is stuck in there. The big triangle chases the others and then they go. The big triangle broke it."

d) Narrative 1 produced by a 22 year old typically developing male (CAC):

"It starts off with a larger triangle in a rectangle, and then the small triangle and circle enter on the screen. The larger triangle comes out of the rectangle and proceeds to attack...bump into the smaller triangle, and vice versa. The circle goes elsewhere, towards the box. The triangles continue to bump one another. The large triangle goes after the circle in the box. He chases it around the rectangle for a while; the circle escapes. The large triangle then comes into the rectangle and chases the small triangle and circle around the screen for a while. The larger triangle becomes trapped in the rectangle, and the small triangle and circle leave the screen. The larger triangle smashes the box up."

SAT Narratives: Example 2

e) Narrative 1 produced by a 10 year old DS female (mental age 5 years):

"Shapes, a triangle and a circle. Being kind. Being unkind. Fight that person. 'Get him!'. He breaks the square. He's angry."

f) Narrative 1 produced by a 10 year old WBS female (mental age 5 years):

"He breaks the thing up. He shuts the gate and smashes the thing up. The triangle and circle were circling him. The triangle went in. The circle went in, then the triangle went in. Then the circle came out and he shut the gate and smashed it."

g) Narrative 1 produced by a 5 year old typically developing female (MAC):

"They're fighting. The circle goes in [to the rectangle]. They're fighting. Big monster is coming into the circle. The circle can't get out now. They're fighting. The alarm is going on. It's about to crash..., he's crashing the home..... It's crashed."

h) Narrative 1 produced by a 10 year old typically developing female (CAC):

"There was one bully. It was locked in a cage and he broke out and attacked the people. He got the circle. He zoomed around with his friend. They went away and the bad person exploded.....bashed up the cage."

Heterogeneity

Another point of note is the heterogeneity observed amongst individuals with DS and individuals with WBS on the SAT, both in terms of their narrative competencies and, in particular, their social attribution. For example, some individuals with DS and some individuals with WBS failed to attribute social meaning to the shapes. Examples are shown below (see Example 3).

This heterogeneity in social cognitive skills is consistent with Porter et al.'s (2008) finding of heterogeneity in theory of mind capabilities amongst individuals with WBS, using another indirect measure of theory of mind understanding the - picture sequencing task (where participants must understand the mental states of story characters in order to sequence each story correctly). Future research should explore this heterogeneity in social cognitive abilities further, particularly in DS, but also in WBS, along with non-social cognitive correlates which might help explain the underlying cognitive (and neurological) cause of this heterogeneity.

SAT Narratives: Example 3

Narrative 1 produced by two 17 year old DS males (mental age 5 years), highlighting:

i) An example of impaired social attribution

"A diagram of a square, two triangles and a circle. The shapes go inside the rectangle. The triangle gets out of the diagram."

j) An example of intact social attribution

"It's a triangle and then the mother poking the triangle and the triangle thing went in the square and can't get out and the gap,...the mother got out the pointing bit and running around the square. Running around up the end and can't see it."

Narrative 1 produced by two 17 year old WBS males (mental age 5 years), highlighting:

k) An example of impaired social attribution

"A triangle was moving. The circle was moving with all the other triangles. The circle was in the big square. The triangle was in there [the big square]."

l) An example of intact social attribution

"Triangles, circles, and a square. Looks like they're playing a game.....cat and mouse. He's trying to get out. He's gonna try and help his mate. The triangle is trying to lock him out. The triangle is trying to get out of his little cage. Oh, he's breaking it. Naughty! Naughty!"

m) Narrative 1 produced by a 5 year old typically developing male (MAC)

"There was all kinds of different shapes. It looks like they were fighting because they were banging, ... and a little triangle, he looked like he bashed the house."

SAT Index Scores and Cognitive Correlates

Consistent with Klin (2000), our findings suggest no significant relationship between chronological age and performance on the SAT, apart from the WBS group, which displayed a significant correlation between chronological age and cognitive mental state attribution.

However, in contrast to Klin (2000), the current results suggest that the SAT may be more reliant on non-social cognitive skills than previously thought, at least for children and adults with developmental disabilities. While we found dissociations between paralinguistic and social cognitive indices of the SAT, some moderate to high correlations were observed between SAT social cognitive indices and verbal mental age, and global mental age. These correlations were not consistent across all social cognitive indices, however, which suggests that the SAT (or at least certain aspects of the task) may be less reliant on non-social cognition than some of the classic theory of mind tasks, such as the Sally and Anne task (described above).

Limitations and Future Research

One limitation of the study presented in this chapter is the small sample size, which, although comparable to sample sizes used in similar studies (e.g. Baron-Cohen et al., 1986; Castelli et al., 2002; Klin, 2000; Tager-Flusberg and Sullivan, 2000), causes low power. Although the current study had sufficient power for detecting group differences on the SAT, power issues arose when interpreting correlations between SAT and non-social WJ-R COG cognitive skills. This did not allow us to make solid claims regarding the possibility of different relationships between SAT indices and non-social cognitive abilities for DS versus WBS groups. Future research should attempt to use larger samples, thus providing the opportunity to explore these relationships for DS and WBS groups. Larger samples would also allow for the possibility of potentially sub-grouping DS individuals; for example, into those who perform well on social cognitive tasks and those who perform poorly (a method undertaken with our WBS cohort, see Porter et al., 2008, see also Porter, 2008).

Another limitation of the study presented here is that, because of this small sample size, we were unable to subgroup participants into children and adults. Although we failed to find significant correlations between chronological age and performance on the SAT, future research should attempt to directly compare children and adults with DS, to further explore the possibility of developmental differences in social cognitive capabilities, and to explore the possibility of different relationships between social and non-social cognition amongst children and adults with DS. Ideally, longitudinal studies should be conducted to explore these possibilities.

Finally, future research should explore the relationship between performance on the SAT and performance on classic theory of mind tasks, as well as correlations between these social cognitive measures and social adaptation or social difficulties experienced in day-to-day life. This would provide a direct exploration of the validity of these social cognitive measures.

Summary

The present chapter explored social functioning in DS, WBS and typically developing controls, focusing on an ability that had not yet been explored in DS or WBS – Social attribution. Social attribution is said to be a fundamental basis of human social interaction, which relates to social cognitive and theory of mind skills (Klin, 2000). Overall, findings suggest that social attribution is not impaired in DS or WBS, and, while below the level of their chronological age, is commensurate with their general cognitive capabilities (and commensurate with the performance of mental age matched typically developing controls). Findings provide further evidence to support the notion of intact social cognition in DS, and suggest that the day-to-day social difficulties experienced by individuals with DS are perhaps more likely to be the result of social perceptual abnormalities and more general non-social cognitive functions (e.g. pragmatic language skills), rather than social cognitive (or theory of mind) impairments. Results have implications with regard to Tager-Flusberg and Sullivan's (2000) model of social knowledge and with regard to the development of appropriate social intervention programs for individuals with DS. Moreover, the study demonstrates the viability of the SAT for children and people with a cognitive disability, and extends research on the SAT to children and adults with DS or WBS.

Acknowledgments

This study was funded by an Australian Rotary Health Research Fund Postdoctoral Fellowship, awarded to Dr Melanie Porter. A special thank you to participants and their families for their ongoing support in our research. Thank you also to my research assistants: Helen Dodd; Carly Black; Susan Van den Berg and Melissa Norris.

Appendix

Description of WJ-R COG Tests

Test	Description
Test 1: Memory for Names	Requires the participant to learn associations between unfamiliar auditory and visual stimuli. Measures learning and memory.
Test 2: Memory for Sentences	Requires the participant to hold and repeat verbatim single words, phrases, and sentences presented on a tape recorder. Measures immediate or working memory, comprehension, and expressive language ability.
Test 3: Visual Matching	Requires the participant to locate and circle two identical numbers within rows of six numbers for three minutes. Numbers begin as single digits and move to double then triple digit numbers towards the end. Measures speed of information processing, psychomotor speed, spatial perception, number recognition, and eye-hand co-ordination.
Test 4: Incomplete Words	Requires the participant to listen to words presented on a tape recorder. Each word is presented twice and has one or two phonemes missing. The participant is asked to produce the word without phonemes missing. Measures phonological awareness and auditory processing.
Test 5: Visual Closure	Requires the participant to identify distorted pictures. Pictures may have areas missing, may be silhouettes, or may have a superimposed pattern. Measures perceptual processing and global form recognition.
Test 6: Picture Vocabulary	This is a confrontation naming test and measures expressive language, general knowledge and perceptual processing.
Test 7: Analysis-Synthesis	Requires the participant to complete a logic puzzle by using the key provided. Measures nonverbal reasoning, the ability to monitor performance in response to feedback, working memory, online problem-solving and learning.
Test 9: Memory for Words	Requires the participant to repeat strings of unrelated words (from one to eight words) verbatim. Measures attention and verbal working memory (ability to hold information in mind and then repeat the information verbatim).
Test 14: Concept Formation	Involves learning concepts by viewing examples of the concept and non-instances of the concept. Feedback is provided for each response. Participants are not required to remember what happened over a series of items. Measures nonverbal reasoning and working memory.
Test 20: Listening Comprehension	Participants listen to tape recorded passages and supply the single missing word at the end of the passage. Passages increase in length. Measures comprehension, expressive vocabulary, semantic processing and attention.

References

Abell, F., Krams, M., Ashburner, J., Passingham, R., Friston, K., Frackowiak, R., et al. (1999). The neuroanatomy of autism: a voxel based whole brain analysis of structural scans. *Neuroreport, 10,* 1647-1651.

Adolphs, R. (1999). Social cognition and the human brain. *Trends in Cognitive Sciences, 3(12),* 469-479.

Adolphs, R., Tranel, D., Damasio, H., and Damasio, A. (1994). Impaired recognition of emotion in facial expressions following bilateral damage to the human amygdala. *Nature*, *372*, 669–672.

Antonarakis, S.E. (1991). Parental origin of the extra chromosome in trisomy 21 as indicated by analysis of DNA polymorphisms. *New England Journal of Medicine, 324,* 872-876.

Baron-Cohen, S. (1994). How to build a baby that can read minds: Cognitive mechanisms in mindreading. *Current Psychology of Cognition, 13,* 513-552.

Baron-Cohen, S. (1989). The autistic child's theory of mind: A case of specific developmental delay. *Journal of Child Psychology and Psychiatry, 30,* 285-287.

Baron-Cohen, S., Leslie, A. M., and Frith, U. (1985). Does the autistic child have a theory of mind? *Cognition, 21,* 37-46.

Baron-Cohen, S., Leslie, A. M., and Frith, U. (1986). Mechanical, behavioral, and intentional understanding of picture stories in autistic children. *British Journal of Developmental Psychology, 4*, 113-125.

Beeghly, M. (1998). Emergence of symbolic play: Perspectives from typical and atypical development. In E. Zigler (Ed.), *Handbook of mental retardation and development.* USA: Cambridge University Press.

Bellugi, U., Adolphs, R., Cassady, C., and Chiles, M. (1999). Towards the neural basis for hypersociability in a genetic syndrome. *NeuroReport, 10*, 1653-1657.

Bellugi, U., Korenberg, J. R., and Klima, E. S. (2001). Williams syndrome: An exploration of neurocognitive and genetic features. *Clinical Neuroscience Research, 1,* 217-229.

Bellugi, U., Lichtenberger, L., Jones, W., Lai, Z., and St. George, M. (2000). The neurocognitive profile of Williams syndrome: a complex pattern of strengths and weaknesses. *Journal of Cognitive Neuroscience, 12(Supplement),* 1-6.

Bellugi, U., Mills, D., Jernigan, T., Hickok, G., and Galaburda, A. (1999). In. H. Tager-Flusberg (Ed.), *Neurodevelopmental disorders* (pp. 111-136). Cambridge, Massachusetts: MIT Press.

Benton, A. L., Hamsher, K., Varney, N. R., and Spreen, O. (1983). *Benton test of facial recognition*. New York, NY: Oxford University Press.

Berger, J., and Cunningham, C.C. (1983). Development of early vocal behaviors and interactions in Down's syndrome and non-handicapped infant-mother pairs. *Developmental Psychology, 19,* 322-331.

Berglund, E., Erikson, M., and Johansson, I. (2001). Parental reports of spoken language skills in children with Down syndrome. *Journal of Speech, Language, and Hearing Research, 44 (1),* 179-191.

Bernicot, J., Lacroix, A., and Reilly, J. (2003). Narratives from children with Williams syndrome: Structural and pragmatic features. *Enfance, 55(3),* 265-281.

Berry, D., and Springer, K. (1993). Structure, motion, and preschoolers' perceptions of social causality. *Ecological Psychology, 5(4),* 273-283.

Bihrle, A. M., Bellugi, U., Delis, D., and Marks, S. (1989). Seeing either the forest or the trees: Dissociation in visuospatial processing. *Brain and Cognition,* 11, 37-49.

Bowler, D. M. (1992). "Theory of Mind" in Asperger's syndrome. *Journal of Child Psychology and Psychiatry, 33(5),* 877-893.

Bowler, D.M., and Thommen, E. (2000). Attribution of mechanical and social causality to animated displays by children with autism. *Autism, 4,* 141-147.

Brothers, L. (1990). The social brain: a project for integrating primate behavior and neurophysiology in a new domain. *Concepts in Neuroscience,1,* 27-51.

Castelli, F., Frith, C., Happè, F., and Frith, U. (2002). Autism, Asperger syndrome and brain mechanisms for the attribution of mental states to animated shapes. *Brain, 125(8),* 1839-1849.

Castelli, C., Vicari, S., Longobardi, E., Lami, L., Pizzoli, C., and Stella, G. (1998). Gestures and words in early development of children with Down syndrome. *Journal of Speech, Language, and Hearing Research, 41,* 1125-1135.

Carlesimo, G.A., Marotta, L., and Vicari, S. (1997). Long-term memory in mental retardation: Evidence for a specific impairment in subjects with Down's syndrome. *Neuropsychologia, 35,* 71-79.

Carvajal, F., and Iglesias, J. (2002). Face-to-face emotion interaction studies in Down syndrome infants. *International Journal of Behavioral Development, 26(2),* 104-122.

Carvajal, F., and Iglesias, J. (2006). Judgements of facial and vocal signs of emotion in infants with Down syndrome. *Developmental Psychobiology, 48(8),* 644-652.

Ciccetti, D., Beeghly, M., and Weiss-Perry, B. (1994). Symbolic development in children with Down syndrome and in children with autism: An organizational, developmental psychopathology perspective. In D. P. Wolf (Ed.), *Children at play: Clinical and developmental approaches to meaning and representation* (pp. 206-237). New York: Oxford University Press.

Conrad, N.J., Scmidt, L.A., Niccols, A., Polak, C.P., Riniolo, T.C., and Burack, J.A. (2007). Frontal electroencephalogram asymmetry during affective processing in children with Down syndrome: A pilot study. *Journal of Intellectual Disability Research, 51 (12),* 988-995.

Davis, M., and Whalen, P.J. (2001). The amygdala: vigilance and emotion. *Molecular Psychiatry, 6,* 13-34.

Dykens, E. M. (2003). Anxiety, fears, and phobias in persons with Williams syndrome. *Developmental Neuropsychology, 23(1 and 2),* 291-316.

Fletcher, P. C., Happé, F. G. E., Frith, U., Baker, S. C., Dolan, R. J., Frackowiak, R. S. J., and Frith, C. D. (1995). Other minds in the brain: A functional imaging study of "theory of mind" in story comprehension. *Cognition, 57,* 109-128.

Frangou, S., Aylward, E., Warren, A., Sharma, T., Barta, P., and Pearlson, G. (1997). Small planum temporal volume in Down's syndrome: A volumetric MRI study. *American Journal of Psychiatry, 154(10),* 1424-1429.

Frigerio, E., Burt, D.M., Gagliardi, C., Cioffi, G., Martelli, S., Perrett, D.I., and Borgatti, R. (2006). Is everybody always my friend? Perception of approachability in Williams syndrome. *Neuropsychologia, 44,* 254-259.

Fryssira, H., Palmer, R., Hallidie-Smith, K. A., Taylor, J., Donnai, D., and Reardon, W. (1997). Flourescent in situ hybridisation (FISH) for hemizygous deletion at the elastin locus in patients with isolated supravalvar aortic stenosis. *Journal of Medical Genetics, 34*(4), 306-308.

Galaburda, A.M. and Bellugi, U. (2000). Multi-level analysis of cortical neuroanatomy in Williams syndrome. *Journal of Cognitive Neuroscience, 12* (Suppl. 1), 74-88.

Gaser, C., Luders, E., Thompson, P.M., Lee, A.D., Dutton, R.A., Geaga, J.A., Hayashi, K.M., Bellugi, U., Galaburda, A.M., Korenberg, J.R., Mills, D.L., Toga, A.W., and Reiss, A.L. Increased local gyrification mapped in Williams syndrome. *Neuroimage, 33(1),* 46-54.

Golden, J.A., and Hyman, B.T. (1994). Development of the superior temporal neocortex is anomalous in trisomy 21. *Journal of Neuropathological Experimental Neurology, 55,* 513 - 520.

Gosch, A., and Pankau, R. (1994). Social-emotional and behavioral adjustment in children with Williams-Beuren syndrome. *American Journal of Medical Genetics, 53,* 335-339.

Happé, F. G. E. (1996). Studying weak central coherence at low levels: Children with autism do not succumb to visual illusions: A research note. *Journal of Child Psychology and Psychiatry, 37,* 873-877.

Happé, F. G. E., Brownell, H., and Winner, E. (1999). Acquired 'theory of mind' impairments following stroke. *Cognition, 70(3),* 211-240.

Happé, F. G. E., Winner, E., and Brownell, H. (1998). The getting of wisdom: Theory of mind in old age. *Developmental Psychology, 34,* 358-362.

Heberlein, A.S., and Adolphs, R. (2004). Perception in the absence of social attribution: selective impairment in anthropomorphizing following bilateral amygala damage. *Proceedings of the National Academy of Sciences,101(19),* 7487-7491.

Heider, F., and Simmel, M. (1944). An experimental study of apparent behavior. *The American Journal of Psychology, 57,* 243-259.

Hines, S., and Bennett, F. (1996). Effectiveness of early intervention for children with down syndrome. *Mental Retardation of Developmental Disabilities Research Reviews, 2,* 96-101.

Hill, P. M., and McCune-Nicholich, L. (1981). Pretend play and patterns of cognition in Down's syndrome children. *Child Development, 52,* 611-617.

Hippolyte, L., Barisnikov, K., and Van der Linden, M. (2008). Face processing and facial emotion recognition in adults with Down syndrome. *American Journal on Mental Deficiency, 113(4),* 292-306.

Hobson, R.P., Ousten, J., and Lee, A. (1989). Naming emotion in faces and voices: Abilities and disabilities in autism and mental retardation. *British Journal of Developmental Psychology, 7,* 237-250.

Jahromi, L., Gulsrud, A., and Kasari, C. (2008). Emotional competence in children with Down syndrome: Negativity and regulation. *American Journal of Mental Deficiency, 113 (1),* 32-43.

Jarrold, C., Baddeley, A. D., and Hewes, A. K. (1999). Genetically dissociated components of working memory: evidence from Downs and Williams syndrome. *Neuropsychologia, 37,* 637-651.

Jernigan, T. L., Bellugi, U., and Sowell, E. (1993). Cerebral morphological distinctions between William's and Down's syndromes. *Archives of Neurology, 50,* 186-191.

Jones, O. (1990). Prelinguistic communication skills in Down's syndrome and normal infants. In M. Beeghly (Ed.), *Children with Down syndrome: A developmental perspective* (pp. 1-28). Cambridge: Cambridge University Press.

Karrer, J., Karrer, K., Rathe, B., Chaney, L., and Davis, R. (1998). Event-related brain potentials during an extended visual recognition memory task depict delayed development of cerebral inhibitory processes among 6-month-old infants with Down syndrome. *International Journal of Psychophysiology, 29 (2),* 167-200.

Kasari, C., and Bauminger, N. (2000). Social and emotional development in children with mental retardation. In D. Elliott (Ed.), *Perceptual-Motor Behavior in Down Syndrome* (pp. 123-142). USA: Human Kinetics.

Kasari, C., Freeman, S.F., and Hughes, M.A. (2001). Task related social behavior in children with Down syndrome. *American Journal on Mental Retardation, 106,* 59-72.

Kasari, C., Freeman, S.F., Mundy, P., and Sigman, M. (1995). Attention regulation by children with Down syndrome: coordinated joint attention and social referencing. *American Journal on Mental Retardation,100,* 128-136.

Kasari, C., Freeman, S.F., and Bass, W. (2003). Empathy and response to distress in children with Down syndrome. *Journal of Child Psychology and Psychiatry, 44(3),* 424-431.

Kasari, C., Mundy, P., Yirmiya, N., and Signman, M. (1990). Affect and attention in children with down syndrome. *American Journal on Mental Retardation, 95(1),* 55-67.

Kasari, C., and Sigman, M. (1996). Expression and understanding of emotion in atypical development: Autism and Down syndrome. In M. W. Sullivan (Ed.), *Emotional development in atypical children* (pp. 109-130). Mahwah, NJ: Lawrence Erlbaum Associates.

Klin, A. (2000). Attributing social meaning to ambiguous visual stimuli in higher-functioning autism and Asperger syndrome: The Social Attribuition Task. *Journal of Child Psychology and Psychiatry, 41 (7),* 831-846.

Knieps, L., Walden, T., Tedra, A., and Baxter, A. (1994). Affective expressions of toddlers with and without Down syndrome in a social referencing context. *American Journal of Mental Deficiency, 99(3),* 301-312.

Koenig, K., Klin, A., and Schultz, R. (2004). Deficits in social attribution ability in Prader-Willi syndrome. *Journal of Autism and Developmental Disorders, 34(5),* 573-582.

Lacroix, A., Bernicot, J., and Reilly, J. (2004). Mental state expression in children with Williams syndrome: An analysis of mother-child collaborative interactions. *Psychologie Francaise, 49(2),* 161-176.

Landry, S.H. and Chapieski, M.L. (1990). Joint attention of six-month-old Down syndrome and preterm infacts: Attention to toys and mother. *American Journal on Mental Retardation, 94,* 488-498.

Laws, G., and Bishop, D.V. (2004). Pragmatic language impairment and social deficits in Williams syndrome: a comparison with Down's syndrome and specific language impairment. *International Journal of Language and Communication Disorders, 39(1),* 45–64.

Leonard, S., Msall, M., Bowler, C., Tremont, M., and Leonard, H. (2002). Functional status of school aged children with Down syndrome. *Journal of Paediatrics and Child Health, 38(2),* 160-165.

Leslie, A., and Frith, U. (1988). Autistic children's understanding of seeing, knowing, and believing. *British Journal of Developmental Pychology, 6,* 315-324.

Loveland, K. A., and Belgin, T. (1991). Social scripts for conversational interactions in autism and Down syndrome. *Journal of Autism and Developmental Disorders, 21(2),* 177-186.

Marui, W., Iseki, E., Kosaka, K., Kato, M., Adachi, Y., and Kenji, U. (1999). An autopsied case of Down syndrome with Alzheimer pathology and alpha-synuclein immunoreactivity. *Neuropathology, 19*(4), 410-416.

Mehler, J., and Dupoux, E. (1994). *What infants know: the new cognitive science of early development.* Oxford: Blackwell.

Mervis, C. (1988). Early lexical development: Theory and application. In L. Nadel (Ed.), *The psychobiology of Down syndrome* (pp. 101-143). Cambridge: MIT Press.

Meyer-Lindenberg, A., Hariri, A., Munoz, K., Mervis, C., Mattay, V., Morris, C. and Berman, K. (2005). Neural correlates of genetically abnormal social cognition in Williams syndrome. *Nature Neuroscience, 8*(8), 991-993.

Mobbs, D., Eckert, M.A., Mills, D., Korenberg, J., Bellugi, U., Galaburda, A.M., and Reiss, A.L. (2007). Frontostriatal dysfunction during response inhibition in Williams syndrome. *Biological Psychiatry, 62,* 256-261.

Mooney, C. M. (1957). Age in the development of closure ability in children. *Canadian Journal of Psychology, 11,* 219-226.

Mundy, P., Sigman, M., Kasari, C., and Yirmiya, N. (1988). Nonverbal communication skills in Down syndrome children. *Child Development, 59,* 235-249.

Murphy, G.M., Jr., and Ellis, W.G. (1991). The amygdala in Down's syndrome and familial Alzheimer's disease: Four clinicopathological case reports. *Biological Psychiatry, 30,* 92-106.

Nadel, L. (1999). Down syndrome in cognitive neuroscience perspective. In. H. Tager-Flusberg (Ed.), *Neurodevelopmental disorders* (pp. 197-221). Cambridge, Massachusetts: MIT Press.

Nowicki, S., and Duke, M. P. (1994). Individual differences in the nonverbal communication of affect: the diagnostic analysis of nonverbal accuracy scale. *Journal of Nonverbal Behavior, 18(1),* 9-35.

Pearson, G., Breiter, S., Aylward, E., Warren, A., Grygorcewicz, M., Frangou, S., Barta, P., and Pulsifer, M. (1998). MRI brain changes in subjects with Down syndrome with and without dementia. *Developmental Medicine and Child Neurology, 40(5),* 326-334.

Perner, J., Frith, U., Leslie, A., and Leekham, S.R. (1989). Exploration of the autistic child's theory of mind: knowledge, belief and communication. *Child Development, 60,* 689-700.

Pinter, J., Eliez, E., Schmitt, J., Capone, G., and Reiss, A. (2001). Neuroanatomy of Down's syndrome: A high-resolution MRI study. *American Journal of Psychiatry, 158,* 1659 – 1665.

Pitcairn, T. K., and Wishart, J. G. (2000). Face processing in children with Down syndrome. In D. Elliott (Ed.), *Perceptual-motor behavior in Down syndrome* (pp. 123-142). USA: Human Kinetics.

Porter, M.A. (2008). *Cognitive and social skills in neurodevelopmental disorders: An examination of Williams syndrome, Down syndrome and autism.* Saarbruecken, Germany: VDM Publishing.

Porter, M. A., and Coltheart, M. (2006). Global and local processing in Williams syndrome, autism, and Down syndrome: Attention, perception, and construction. *Developmental Neuropsychology, 30(3),* 771-789.

Porter, M.A., Coltheart, M., and Langdon, R. (2007). The neuropsychological basis of hypersociability in Williams and Down syndrome. *Neuropsychologia, 45(12),* 2839-2849.

Porter, M.A., Coltheart, M., and Langdon, R. (2008). Theory of mind in Williams syndrome assessed using a nonverbal task. *Journal of Autism and Developmental Disorders, 38,* 806-814.

Porter, M.A., Shaw, T.A., and Marsh, P. J. (Submitted). An unusual attraction to the eyes in Williams-Beuren syndrome: A manipulation of facial affect while measuring face scanpaths. (Submitted to *Cognitive Neuropsychiatry*).

Perner, J., and Wimmer, H. (1985). "John thinks that Mary thinks thay Y": Attribution of second order beliefs by 5- to 10-year-old children. *Journal of Experimental Child Psychology, 39,* 437-471.

Premack, D., and Woodruff, G. (1978). Does chimpanzee have a theory of mind? *Behavioral and Brain Sciences, 4,* 515-526.

Raz, N., Torres, I. J., Briggs, S. D., Spencer, W.D., Thornton, A.E., Loken, W.J., et al. (1995). Selective neuroanatomical abnormalities in Down's syndrome and their cognitive correlates: Evidence from MRI morphometry. *Neurology, 45*, 356-366.

Reilly, J. S., Harrison, D., and Klima, E. S. (1995). Emotional talk and talk about emotions. *Genetic Counseling, 6,* 158-159.

Riby, D. M., and Hancock, P. J. B. (2008). Do faces capture the attention of individuals with Williams syndrome or Autism? Evidence from tracking eye movements. *Journal of Autism and Developmental Disorders (Online First).*

Rondal, J.A. (1995). *Exceptional language development in Down syndrome: Implications for the cognitive-language relationship.* Cambridge: Cambridge University Press.

Risser, D., Lubec, G., Cairns, N., and Herrere-Marschitz, M. (1997). Excitatory amino acides and monoamines in parahippocampal gyrus and frontal cortical pole of adults with Down syndrome. *Life Sciences, 60 (15),* 1231-1237.

Rowe, J., Lavender, A., and Turk, V. (2006). Cognitive executive function in Down's syndrome. *British Journal of Social and Clinical Psychology, 45(1)* 5-17.

Salter, G., Seigal, A., Claxton, M., Lawrence, K., and Skuse, D. (2008). Can autistic children read the mind of an animated triangle? *Autism, 12 (4),* 349-371.

Sigman, M. (1999). Developmental deficits in children with Down syndrome. In. H. Tager-Flusberg (Ed.), *Neurodevelopmental disorders* (pp. 178-195). Cambridge, Massachusetts: MIT Press.

Serrano, J.M., Iglesias, J., and Loeches, A. (1995). Infants' responses to adult static facial expressions. *Infant Behavior and Development, 18,* 477-482.

Siegal, M., and Varley, R. (2002). Neural systems involved in 'theory of mind'. *Nature Reviews, 3,* 463-471.

Shapiro, M., Berman, K., Alexander, G., Weinberger, D., and Rapoport, S. (1999). Regional cerebral blood flow in Down syndrome adults during the Wisconsin Card Sort Test: Exploring cognitive activation in the context of poor performance. *Biological Psychiatry, 45 (9),* 1190-1196.

St James, P., and Tager-Flusberg, H. (1994). An observational study of humor in Autism and Down syndrome. *Journal of Autism and Developmental Disorders, 24 (5),* 603-617.

Stojanovik, V. (2006). Social interaction deficts and conversational inadequacy in Williams syndrome. *Journal of Neurolinguistics, 19,* 157-173.

Sullivan, K., Zaitchik, D., and Tager-Flusberg, H. (1994). Preschoolers can attribute second order beliefs. *Developmental Psychology, 30,* 395-402.

Tager-Flusberg, H. (1999). *Neurodevelopmental disorders*. Cambridge, Massachusetts: MIT press.

Tager-Flusberg, H., and Sullivan, K. (1994). Predicting and explaining behavior: A comparison of autistic, mentally retarded and normal children. *Journal of Child Psychology and Psychiatry, 35(6),* 1059-1075.

Tager-Flusberg, H., and Sullivan, K. (2000). A componential view of theory of mind: Evidence from Williams syndrome. *Cognition, 76,* 59-89.

Teipel, S.J., Alexander, G.E., Schapiro, M.B., Möller, H.J., Rapoport, S.I., and Hampel, H. (2004). Age-related cortical grey matter reductions in non-demented Down's syndrome adults determined by MRI with voxel-based morphometry. *Brain, 127*(4), 811-824.

Wang, P. (1996). A neuropsychological profile of Down syndrome: Cognitive skills and brain morphology. *Mental Retardation and Developmental Disabilities Reviews, 2(2),* 102-108.

Wang, P. P., and Bellugi, U. (1993). Williams syndrome, Down syndrome, and cognitive neuroscience. *Cognitive Neuroscience, 147,* 1246-1251.

Wang, P. P., and Bellugi, U. (1994). Evidence from two genetic syndromes for a dissociation between verbal and visual-spatial short-term memory. *Journal of Clinical and Experimental Neuropsychology, 16(2),* 317-322.

Warrington, E. K. (1984). *Warrington recognition memory test.* Windsor, England: Nfer-Nelson Publishing.

Weis, S. (1991). Morphometry and magnetic resonance imaging of the human brain in normal controls and Down's syndrome. *The Anatomical Record, 37,* 593-598.

Wellman, H. M., and Woolley, J. D. (1990). From simple desires to ordinary beliefs: The early development of everyday psychology. *Cognition, 13,* 103-128.

Williams, K., Wishart, J., Pitcairn, T., and Willis, D. (2005). Emotion recognition by children with Down syndrome: Investigation of specific impairments and error patterns. *American Journal on Mental Retardation, 110(5),* 378-392.

Woodcock, R. W., and Johnson, M. B. (Eds.). (1989, 1990). *Woodcock-Johnson psycho-educational battery - revised*: Itasca, IL: Riverside Publishing.

Yirmiya, N., Erel, O.Shaked, M., and Solomonica-Levi, D. (1998). Meta-analyses comparing Theory of Mind abilities of individuals with autism, individuals with mental retardation, and normally developing individuals. *Psychological Bulletin, 124(3),* 283-307.

Yirmiya, N., Pilowsky, T., Solomonica-Levi, D., and Shulman, C. (1999). Gaze behavior and theory of mind abilities in individuals with autism, Down syndrome, and mental retardation of unknown etiology. *Journal of Autism and Developmental Disorders, 29(4),* 333-341.

Yirmiya, N.Solomonica-Levi, D.Shulman, C., and Pilowsky, T. (1996). Theory of Mind abilities in individuals with autism, Down syndrome, and mental retardation of unknown etiology: The role of age and intelligence. *Journal of Child Psychology and Psychiatry, 37(8),* 1003-1014.

Ypsilanti, A., Grouios, G., Alevriadou, A., and Tsapkini, K. (2005). Expressive and receptive vocabulary in children with Williams and Down syndromes. *Journal of Intellectual Disability Research, 49(5),* 353-364.

Zelazo, P. D.Burack, J. A.Benedetto, E., and Frye, D. (1996). Theory of Mind and rule use in individuals with Down syndrome: A test of the uniqueness and specificity claims. *Journal of Child Psychology and Psychiatry, 37(4),* 479-484.

In: Handbook of Down Syndrome Research
Editors: Dominicus Jelinek and Gijs Dvorak
ISBN 978-1-60741- 690-6

Chapter 5

The Dysfunctional Gastro-Intestinal Tract in Down Syndrome – Congenital or Acquired?

S.W. Moore
University of Stellenbosch
South Africa

Down syndrome (DS) is associated with a number of associated additional clinical problems, in addition to its classical neurological and skeletal features [viz: decreased muscle tone (floppy baby), short stature, decreased intellectual capacity and brachycephaly and congenital heart disease]. Of these, gastro-intestinal tract (GIT) malfunction remains one of the most significant, but congenital hearing deficits are also not infrequent and there is an increased risk of certain tumours (i.e. Leukemia, retro-peritoneal teratomas [1]). On the other hand, certain other solid tumours have a decreased prevalence in DS (eg neuroblastoma, nephroblastoma, hepatoblastoma and medulloblastoma). [2].

GI malfunction has been reported in as many as 77% of DS affected individuals [3]but the true prevalence of functional GI disturbances in DS adults has been difficult to assess, as many DS individuals do not have access to regular healthcare checks [4].

From a genetic point of view, the genetic basis of DS is mostly either a Trisomy or a translocation of chromosome 21, and rarely involves a mosaic (often referred to as Partial trisomy). Essentially, this means that there is an extra copy of chromosome 21 is present in the majority of cases. It is currently thought that the resulting genetic imbalance plays a role in many of the debilitating Central Nervous system (CNS) associations of DS resulting in interest in the potential role of the 200-400 Chromosome 21 genes which may contribute to the phenotypic features of DS.

Two Hypotheses on Genetic Effects of Trisomy 21

The DS phenotype of is thought to result from the genetic imbalance which results from the overexpression of a gene or genes located on the triplicated chromosome 21 (a typical feature of the syndrome). Recent studies [5, 6] have demonstrated a dosage-dependent increase in chromosome 21 gene expression in trisomy 21, but it remains unclear whether this is a generalized or more local effect of the genetic disturbance.

There are two current hypotheses which attempt to explain the effects of the gene dosage imbalance in DS. The first hypothesis is that the "gene dosage effect" affects a critical region on chromosome 21 which contains a number of dosage-sensitive genes. The malfunction of these genes, in turn, then determines the final Downs phenotype. A second "amplified developmental instability" hypothesis suggests that the chromosome 21 Trisomy results in a generalized alteration of homeostasis during critical times during development which eventually account for typical the phenotype as well as the associated anomalies [7]. In this context, the natures of the gene products as well as their functional relationships are crucial as they may affect different aspects of neuronal development.

It is understood that where the gene dosage of affected genes exceeds 1.5 times the control values, they are likely to be involved in the DS phenotype [8] A recent microarray/ polymerase chain reaction study reported 29% of the expressed chromosome 21 transcripts being overexpressed in DS of which 22% were increased proportional to the gene-dosage effect, whereas 7% were amplified. [9] Of the remaining 71%, 56% of expressed sequences were compensated for increased gene-dosage (1.5) but a further 15% showed considerable individual variability. Current data , however, suggests that the DS phenotype cannot be fully explained by simple gene dosage effect [10], therefore implying that a number of relevant genes may be involved as gene modulators and the primary transcriptional effect of the disregulated chromosome 21, may lead to other disregulated signaling pathways thus influencing the eventual DS phenotypic expression

These 2 hypotheses are not necessarily mutually exclusive but as the genetic defect is germline, resulting from 3 copies of the gene, both could be valid. Study of the ENS could, therefore, provide clues as to the changes ongoing within the brain and ENS and vice versa. The crucial question is to identify the mechanisms by which the excessive gene products or defective genes influences neuronal maturation and development [11]

DS and Brain Development

As far as the Central Nervous system (CNS) associations of DS are concerned, it would appear that the DS-associated anomalous brain development, function and intellectual impairment is associated with the genetic imbalance resulting from the chromosome 21 trisomy. Although there is, as yet, no clear answer as to precisely which genes are involved, it is fairly clear that reduced cerebellar volume or cerebellar hypoplasia (or both) contribute to the overall congenitally acquired intellectual impairment in DS. The congenitally acquired cerebellar hypoplasia is also believed to contribute to decreased fine motor control in these individuals.

What is clear is that certain of these problems may become worse with time. An example of this is the ongoing degeneration of the brain which gives rise to early onset Alzheimer's disease in the majority. This deterioration of nerve function may also apply to certain other problems (eg. constipation) as these also appear to become progressively worse with time.

Despite the apparent lack of clarity as to the underlying pathogenic mechanisms for these phenomena, recently identified candidate genetic mechanisms provide (perhaps for the first time), unique insights into the genetic background into the neurological and cognitive disorders associated with DS. The development of murine trisomic and transgenic DS animal models, which, when coupled with powerful new micro anatomical technology, permit a novel understanding of the ongoing structural changes in the DS nervous system.

A critical area appears to be the Down Syndrome Critical Region 1 (DSCR1; MCIP1, Adapt78) region on the distal 10 Mb region of the long arm of chromosome 21 which is overexpressed in DS. This region has been associated with many of the DS phenotypic features but conclusive proof is lacking. It has recently been shown that DSCR1 is upregulated in endothelial cells in response to VEGF, TNF-alpha, and A23187 but is inhibited by inhibitors of the calcineurin-NFAT (nuclear factor of activated T cells) signaling pathway (12). The transcriptional regulation of Down syndrome critical region isoform 4 (DSCR1.4) is mediated by the calcineurin/nuclear factor of activated T cells (NFAT) pathway in neural cells [12, 13]. The calcineurin/Nuclear Factor of the Activated T cells (NFAT) pathway is thus dependent on DSCR1 overexpression in DS and is regulated by the inhibition of the calcineurin catalytic A subunit of the calcineurin-mediated signaling pathway.

Murine models of DS have contributed to the identification of 2 genes [DYRK1A and DSCR1] within in the Down syndrome critical region, which were initially thought to be possible candidate genes involved in the Down syndrome phenotype. The DYRK1A gene is particularly interesting as it is a key regulator of pluripotency and neuronal differentiation by encoding a dual-specificity proline-directed serine/threonine kinase. [14]. On current evidence, however, it would appear that the DYRK1A gene is more involved in the pathogenesis of cognitive deficits and the development of early onset Alzheimer's disease in DS [15] than in the GI malfunction associated with DS or other DS phenotypic features. The DYRK1A gene has also been shown to mediate the deregulation of REST with a 30%-60% reduced expression of Nrsf/Rest reported in transchromosomic DS models. Links between the early Alzheimer's disease occurring in DS patients and abnormal cholesterol metabolism remain speculative in terms of cognitive problems in DS, although the ABCG1 gene has been shown to play a possible role in maintaining cellular or tissue cholesterol homeostasis. [16]

Recent in vitro studies suggest that the DYRK1A mutation is related to phosphorylation of the tau protein thus contributing to enhanced neurofibrillary degeneration in patients with DS. [17]. In addition to being an important part of the pathogenesis of Alzheimer disease, the tau protein is usually not associated with an abnormal ENS and the ENS has been shown to be unaffected in Alzheimer's disease [18]. In fact, the tau microtubule-associated protein has been identified as a marker for normally innervated proximal bowel in HSCR [19, 20]

There is also a further relationship with folate metabolism with the combined MTHFR 677TT/MTR 2756AA genotype having been shown to be associated with increased DS risk

(P=0.034), whereas the MTHFR 1298AC/TYMS 2R/2R genotype has a reduced risk (P=0.003). [21].

The Link between Brain Development and the ENS

Central nervous system (CNS) development includes processes such as neural patterning, neuronal and axonal migration, as well as synaptic development. There appears to be a link between factors governing brain development and the development of the ENS. This is not surprising as both processes are largely controlled by the same or similar neural growth factors which are expressed at more or less in the same spatio-temporal manner.

The connection between brain development and the ENS is probably best illustrated by the established increased frequency of associated neuronal migration brain disorders (23.5%) (Including DS) in association with neurodevelopmental conditions such as Hirschsprungs disease (HSCR). [22]. This association may occur either as isolated defects or be associated with congenital malformation syndromes [22].

It is now understood that neocortical development arises from progenitor cells [mostly composed of radial glial cells [23]] which undergo neurogenesis under the influence of cell cycle signaling molecules.

The extent to which the defective signaling processes which affect the CNS also affect the Enteric Nervous system (ENS) is still not clearly understood. At the same time as CNS development is taking place, comparable processes take place in ENS neuroblast development, mostly under the control of similar signaling cascades. In addition to those factors influencing neural development, there is the critical issue of timing as the ENS develops in a tight spatio-temporal relationship. It is interesting to note that in the mouse model, neurogenesis of the cortex begins on day E11 [24, 24] which corresponds to a critical time in ENS development in mouse models of HSCR.

Associated Anomalies in DS and the GI Tract

Down syndrome (DS), with an estimated occurrence once every 500-700 live births, is relatively common and is the major genetic cause of mental retardation (MR) in humans. A number of other associated anomalies (e.g. cardiac, musculoskeletal, or multiple anomalies] are the next most common other anomalies associated with DS. In addition, the spectrum of other reported anomalies also includes increased relative risks for gastrointestinal malformations (OR 67.07), genitourinary (OR 3.62), orofacial (OR 5.63), and abdominal wall malformations (OR 3.25) [25].

Pathological studies on the DS brain demonstrate a decreased cerebellar volume, associated with a reduced granular cell count as well as abnormal lamination of the cortex. The resulting significant reduction in neurons shows abnormal dendritic trees and spines with abnormal synapses ("tree in winter appearance"). These neurological alterations are also fairly consistently expressed in experimental trisomic animals; appear to result from gene-dosage effects of the triplicated Human Chromosome 21 on critical developmental gene expression.

It would therefore appear that impaired gene transcription may result in variant signal transduction pathways during development which subsequently results in changes in neural patterning and development. As a result, dysfunctional neuronal circuits then result, which may be responsible for the associated anomalies seen in DS.

Our own series has reported a 24% occurrence of cardiac lesions in DS-HSCR patients [26], the most frequent being septation defects (Atrial/ ventricular septal defects). Cardiac anomalies may result from gene disruption during the critical window of the development of the heart A recently identified candidate for DS-related cardiac defects and skin abnormalities being the DSCOL6A1 gene on chromosome 21. [27]

An increased relative risk for gastrointestinal malformations (OR 67.07) therefore does exist.

Gastro-Intestinal (GI) Anomalies in DS

Up to 77% of DS affected individuals have experienced or develop associated GI abnormalities (3). These include both structural anomalies [resulting in a mechanical obstruction] and functional GI obstructions. Congenital abnormalities of embryologic development are not uncommon within the upper GIT (eg tracheo-esophageal fistula, duodenal stenosis/atresia, pyloric stenosis, annular pancreas, and Anorectal malformations. [28, 29]) and result in a mechanical, DS-related, neonatal intestinal obstruction. A large DS cohort reported an approximately 300 times increased risk for annular pancreas and duodenal atresia, and a 100 times increased risk for megacolon, esophageal, anal and small bowel atresia [30].

Clinically, there are clear motor disturbances of the oesophagus and colon in DS. A recent multifactorial study, reported a strong association between DS and pneumonia (OR 13.25) and Gastroesophageal reflux disease (GERD) (OR 4.28) [31]. A further review of 56 adult DS patients, reported chronic constipation (19%); unexplained chronic diarrhea (19%); GER (9%), cholelithiasis (4%), achalasia (2%) and unexplained abnormal liver function tests (2 %) as the most prominent symptoms encountered in DS in later years [32].

Genetic Links to GI Disease in DS

The possible causes for the structural changes encountered in DS, although still unclear, suggest a reduction in hedgehog signaling as a candidate pathway as current evidence suggests specific roles for the various Hedgehog ligands in GI development.

This is not entirely surprising as Hedgehog signaling [which controls the development of the endoderm within the surrounding mesoderm during embryogenesis] is essential for patterning the GI tract along anterior-posterior, dorsal-ventral, and radial axes, as well as in maintenance of stem cells. It is therefore thought to be responsible for much development of the gastrointestinal (GI) tract and associated viscera. Malfunction of this critical pathway has been reported in for a number of associated congenital conditions. (including GI anomalies) [33, 34, 35]. This effect has been shown to be a reversible using a small molecule agonist of the Hedgehog pathway [36].

Known Hedgehog pathways include the Sonic hedgehog (SHH), Indian hedgehog (IHH) and Desert hedgehog (DHH) pathways which then bind to PTCH1/PTCH or PTCH2 receptors. These complex signaling pathways may, in turn, control the stem cell signaling network and the subsequent Patched-dependent suppression releases the signal transducer Smoothened (SMO) which then activates STK36 serine/threonine kinase to stabilize the GLI family members and to phosphorylate SUFU for nuclear accumulation of GLI.

This then leads to GLI-dependent transcriptional activation of target genes, such as GLI1, PTCH1, CCND2, FOXL1, JAG2 and SFRP1. The transient proliferation of Hedgehog target cells arises from the GLI1-dependent positive feedback loop combined with PTCH1-dependent negative feedback. [37]

Other signaling pathways such as n MYC have also been implicated in the normal and abnormal downstream functioning of Shh [38]. Also linked to the Hedgehog pathways during embryogenesis are the BMP/TGFbeta, FGF, WNT and Notch signaling pathways. Fgf4 appears to be particularly important in duodenal development and early GIT patterning, being expressed early in the gastrulation and somite stages in the vicinity of origin of the posterior bowel. Its role is to establish gut tube domains along the A-P axis of the GIT by encouraging those posterior and inhibiting those anterior endoderm cells (39) The FGF-target genes [Sprouty1 and 2] are then expressed taking the endodermal response further [39]

The effect of DS on ENS development is more difficult to understand. Although a reduced mitogenic response to Hedgehog protein signaling has been reported in DS. [40,41,42], and Hedgehog protein signaling has been shown to be the probable cause of the granule cell precursor cell deficit observed the brain in early postnatal development, how exactly this works is as not yet clear.

Studies onTs65Dn mice [trisomic for orthologs of ± 50% of the chromosome 21 genes found on human] demonstrated DS-like craniofacial abnormalities (e.g. a small dysmorphic mandible) with an associated paucity of neural crest cells in the 1st pharyngeal arch derivatives of the experimental animals. Further study of the second pharyngeal arch (PA2), in these models, demonstrated deficits in delamination, migration, and mitosis of neural crest cells in DS animal models suggesting a neurocristopathy similar to that observed in GI maldevelopment. [42] This could potentially explain the deficient ENS observed in DS which is the probable cause of associated functional GI anomalies.

Evidence for ENS Dysplasia in DS

The normal development of the ENS is complex, involving cascades of signaling molecules that determine proliferation, migration, differentiation and survival of the enteric neuroblasts. It is generally accepted that developmental defects within the ENS are also likely to be the cause of significant functional disorders the pathological changes in the nervous system of patients with DS and probably underlie the physiological and neurological features of the associated anomalies of the GIT.

The gastrointestinal tract (GIT) is known to develop from the embryonic gut, which is an endodermally derived epithelium which is surrounded by cells of mesodermal origin. Cell signaling between these two layers appears to control the patterning and organogenesis and plays a critical role in coordinating GIT development. Vagal neural cells are thought to give rise to the majority of these ENS neuroblasts and the enteric nervous system develops from the colonization of neural crest cells which migrate down the developing GIT [43, 44]. Developmental defects within the ENS appear to be related either to defects in vagal cell migration or the development of the intermyenteric and submucosal plexuses.

Etiology of GI Anomalies in DS

The causes of the functional GI conditions associated with DS remain obscure, despite the detailed analyses of genetic influences on DS phenotypic features and a detailed analysis of the gene [45], but are most likely to result from disrupted signaling pathways in DS.

It is becoming clear that the decrease in normal development of the nervous system in DS may be either on the basis of decreased neuronal migration or a failure of the normal dendritic development within the nervous system.

Decreased neuronal migration has been reported in the cortex of the brain of animal DS models, under known chemotactic factors (viz: glutamate or N-methyl-D-aspartate (NMDA) stimulation, suggesting a defective NMDA receptor or (NMDAR-) signaling [46] There also appears to be a failure of the normal dendritic development in the brain of fetuses with DS, resulting in a "tree in winter" histological picture [47] due to the lack of branching. This is probably a reflection of the same processes which result in a reduced Cerebellar volume/ Cerebellar hypoplasia and the resultant intellectual impairment in DS patients.

Similar processes may simultaneously be occurring within the ENS. Evidence of distinct ENS variation in DS patients has included reduced numbers of esophageal plexus ganglia neurons In the histopathological study by Nakazato et al[48], DS patients had a mean of 69% the control number of neurons per ganglion of the deep submucous plexus and 75% in the Auerbach plexus. This decrease in the number of functional ganglia may go some way to explain the esophageal dysfunction commonly encountered in DS.

It would seem reasonable to extrapolate therefore that this decrease in ganglion cells reported in the oesophagus is also present throughout the GIT. In support of this, Leffler et al [49] have reported congenital Hypoganglionosis of the colon in the Trisomy 16-DS animal model. This is supported by other studies in the same animal [50] where the ENS was found to be abnormally developed with only some scattered neurons of altered density and size at ED14-16. On embryonic day (ED) 16+ there were only some scattered neurons with abnormal distribution, density and size as well as an absence of the colonic submucosal plexus plus an aganglionic segment observed in the ENS of these animals. These variations from normal ENS development appeared to be related to developmental delay or abnormal development which may parallel those changes found in DS. [26]

On the other hand, distinct histopathological differences have also been reported in the ENS ultrastructure in patients with DS-HSCR and other non-syndromic associations with HSCR. [51]. This study observed that the ENS of the rectosigmoid circular muscle layer was markedly reduced in patients with DS-HSCR whereas in other neurologically challenged individuals (eg Mowat-Wilson syndrome), the innervation appears to be much denser. Moreover, the myenteric ganglia in the rostral aganglionic bowel were found to be smaller in DS patients although not fulfilling criteria for hyper or Hypoganglionosis in the cases of syndromic HSCR. As a result of these associations, some of the most common functional GIT symptoms reported by DS patients are dysphagia for liquids and solids, vomiting/ Gastro-oesophageal reflux (GER) and heartburn as well as other oesophageal dysmotility symptoms [52]. An awareness of the clinical problems associated with oesophageal dysmotility is important in DS because of the significant incidence of associated complications. Motor disorders of the oesophagus such as achalasia of the lower esophageal sphincter also needs to be excluded in DS patients with dysphagia [53, 54]

It is also clear that the process affecting the nervous system in DS not only affects the microanatomy of nerve cells but also appears to modulate nerve function. Functional GI obstruction, on the other hand, most frequently results from achalasia, gastro-oesophageal reflux (GER) (Figure 1), Hirschsprung's disease (HSCR) and constipation. It is clear that other motor disorders of the GIT also appear among the most frequent complaints in DS and include unexplained chronic constipation (requiring differentiation from Hirschsprungs disease and anal stenosis, both of which have been shown to also have an increased incidence in DS(3)).

Physiological studies have shown significant differences in action potential and ionic current kinetics at the neuronal level [55]. Animal experimental models have also shown alterations of intracellular Ca2+ signaling pathways in DS in response to a number of other neurotransmitters studied (i.e. glutamate, acetylcholine, and GABA) [56] in these patients.

There appears to be an association between Hirschsprungs disease (HSCR), anorectal malformations and DS. A combination of all three has been reported on at least 2 occasions in the past [57, 58]. The aganglionic segment was reported as “distal” (short-segment) in one (58) whereas the other reported an aganglionic transition zone up to the descending colon [57].

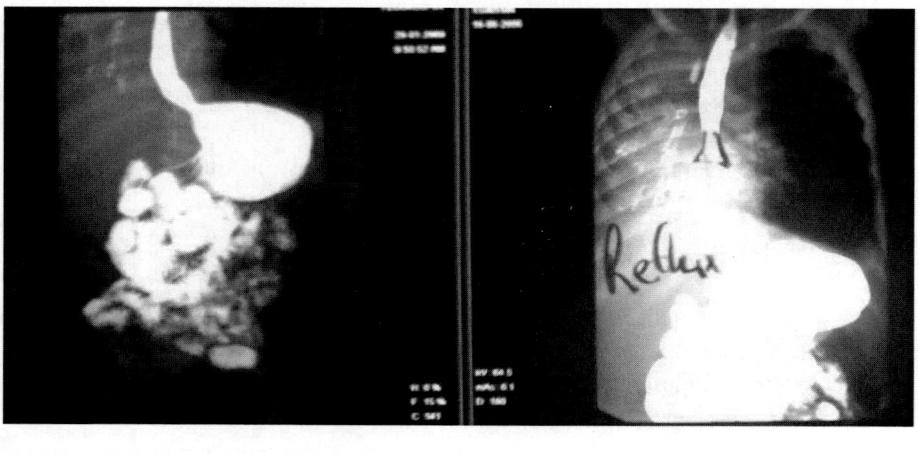

Figure 1. Severe GER in a Down’s patient.

It is possible that the genetic connection between these 2 conditions may lie in one of the major susceptibility genes common to all three conditions. Variation in the Endothelin/Sox 10 genes [59, 60] is a possible candidate as EDNRB gene variations have been observed in HSCR [61], ARM patients (59, 60) and DS-HSCR [62].

In addition to developmental defects, there may also be an ongoing loss/ degeneration of neural cells in the enteric nervous system (ENS), similar to that occurring in the brain of patients with DS [47], due to the same pathophysiological processes

Gastrointestinal Motor Disturbances in DS

A. Gastroesophageal Reflux (GER) In Down Syndrome

GER remains one of the most frequently encountered causes of oesophageal symptomatology in DS but runs the risk of being under reported because of its frequency of association. It is not only common but has an increase in the number of associated complications as demonstrated by the study by Hillemeier et al [63] who reported a 43% occurrence of serious complications arising from GER in DS patients. In addition, oro-pharyngeal aspiration may be associated with pneumonia and aspiration syndromes in dysphagic neurologically challenged children (eg DS).

In addition, CNS disease and gastrointestinal disease necessitating surgery have been independently associated with a poorer developmental outcome. [64]. In this context, oesophageal dysmotility (Figure 2) has been shown to complicate the postoperative course following surgical corrective procedures such as the anti-reflux procedure [65].

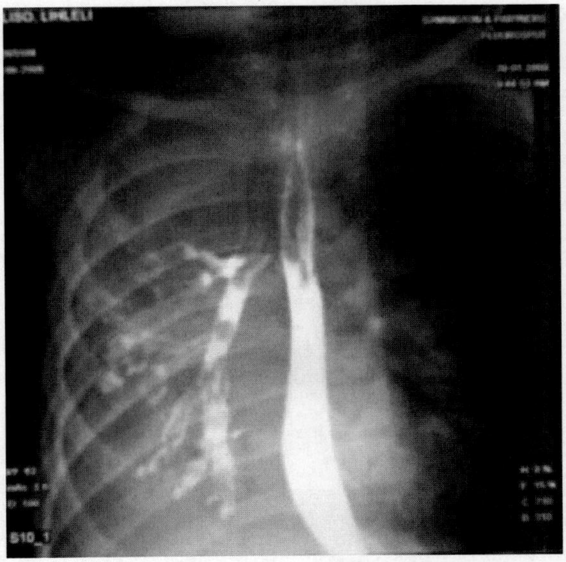

Figure 2. Respiratory aspiration of contrast due to an oesophageal motility problem.

B. Down Syndrome and Achalasia

Esophageal motor disorders, particularly achalasia, are not infrequent in DS and achalasia should be considered in any DS patient who presents with dysphagia. Achalasia remains a rare but important clinical entity [54] and should be differentiated from GER in this population in order to avoid complications

When the prevalence of both disorders is considered, it would appear that the prevalence of achalasia exceeds that expected in a normal population, occurring in approximately 2% of patients [32]. Symptoms may be subtle and whereas adult patients mainly present with dysphagia, the chief clinical features in children were respiratory symptoms and growth retardation [66].

C. Downs Syndrome and Chronic Constipation

Constipation remains one of the common symptoms experienced by DS children and adults although the true prevalence is probably underestimated. Unexplained severe constipation has been identified in 19 % of DS patients in a recent adult survey [32] but one suspects that the true incidence is somewhat higher and a prevalence in 56% was observed in our own series [26].What is not clear as to whether this is on a congenital or acquired basis. Experience suggests that it be a combination of the two.

D. Down Syndrome and Hirschsprungs Disease

DS children with constipation must be considered as potential candidates for Hirschsprungs disease (HSCR) because of the known, non-random association which exists between the two conditions. Hirschsprungs disease (DS-HSCR) (Figure 3) remains the most common of the congenital enteric nervous system dysganglionosis associated with DS [67, 68, 69] possibly due to a shared defect in neural crest cells (70). The reported incidence varies between 2% and 15%. [67, 71, 72, 73, 69, 74, 75, 76] and is higher than the 0.15-0.17% expected incidence in the normal population. Further comparison of the relative incidences of the two conditions (viz. 1:10000 and 1:600) shows an incidence of DS-HSCR approximately one in every 200-300 Downs syndrome patients [77].

In an early HSCR study Passarge [67] identified in 6 DS patients out of 63 probands (9.5%). Lower incidences have been reported, the reported prevalence varies between 2% and 15%. [67,71,72,73,69,74,75,76,78]}. In our own series of 408 HSCR patients, (79,80,81) , a 3.2% prevalence of Downs syndrome was reported with a female preponderance (66%) and an 85% association with other anomalies. This was in contrast to other series which show a distinct male preponderance [75, 76].

There was no family history of HSCR in any of the DS-HSCR patients. The length of the aganglionic segment in Down syndrome patients was limited to the rectosigmoid in 69%, the remainder having long colonic aganglionosis.

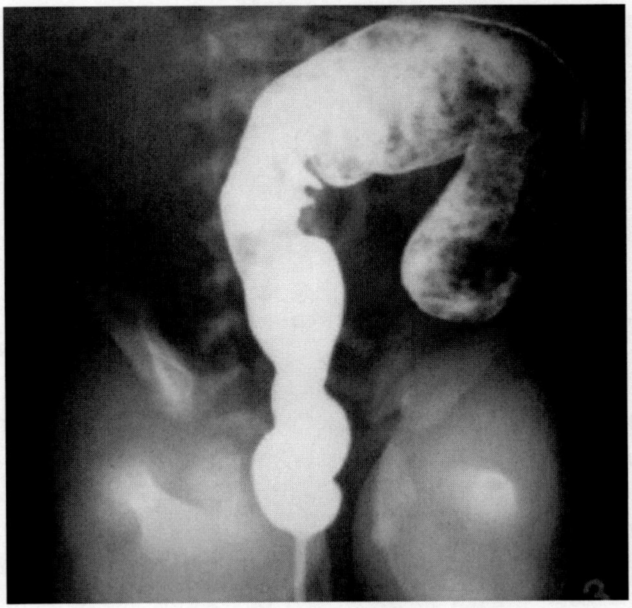

Figure 3. Contrast enema of DS with HSCR.

There were no patients with total colonic aganglionosis and DS but in 1 patient the transition zone was at the hepatic flexure indicating a very long segment.

Passarge [67] reported 83% mortality for Hirschsprung-associated enterocolitis (HAEC) in DS-HSCR patients in 1967. Up to 20 years later, Teitelbaum [82] still observed HAEC-related deaths in more than a third of DS-HSCR thus underlining the fact that there is a significantly higher overall incidence of pre and/or postoperative enterocolitis in DS-HSCR [83, 82]. It may also be a lethal combination in the setting of additional congenital abnormalities combined with an immunological response deficit. In our own series, Hirschsprung-associated enterocolitis (HAEC) occurred in 38% of the DS-HSCR patients as opposed to 16% of the 408 HSCR patients of our series [80, 84]. It was associated with a significant morbidity and mortality, accounting for the deaths of more than half of our DS-HSCR patients which is in keeping with other studies. [67, 82]

Outcome of DS-HSCR Surgery and Results

Despite significant improvement in diagnosis and postnatal care the incidence of enterocolitis, postoperative morbidity and mortality has been shown to be higher in patients with Trisomy 21 [67, 82, 85]. A possible explanation for this is an impaired immunological response resulting from an impaired humoral as well as T-lymphocyte immune functions [86, 87]

Surgical correction can be achieved in DS-HSCR but patients may require some form of ongoing help to facilitate acceptable bowel function. Long term functional results are influenced by a number of factors such as the ability to achieve normal toilet training, social background, overall ability of the individual child and the motivation to be socially acceptable. Although some may have a satisfactory result following surgical correction, patients with DS-HSCR are generally recognized as having a less confident prognosis [88].

Previous reports [75, 76] indicate that soiling (soiling and smearing) may continue beyond the 4th year of life in more than 60 percent of patients with Trisomy 21. Probable reasons for this include the failure to thrive attributed to their often abnormal stooling patterns as well as the type of definitive procedure performed [88]. Other factors such as the increased risk of associated anomalies, delay in diagnosis in DS and the risks of enterocolitis in an immunologic ally compromised child may also play a part.

E. Down Syndrome and the Uro-Genital System

The ENS and the innervation of the urological system are closely related and are often both affected by the same pathological processes. The genitourinary tract (GUT) is thus likewise involved in DS with associated defects being reported throughout the genitourinary tract (OR 3.62) [25]. The most frequent renal anomalies include renal hypoplasia, obstructive uropathy and glomerular microcysts as well as associated congenital ureteric defects such as megaureter and vesicoureteral reflux [89]. In addition, other functional defects include dysfunctional voiding and urinary retention and long-term bladder control is known to be difficult to achieve in many DS patients.

Genetic Links between DS, HSCR And Other Potential Candidate Genes

Current understanding is however that the phenotypic expression in DS and developmental defects most probably has a lot to do with the abnormal function of critical genes in a critical area [90]. It is widely accepted that many of the phenotypic features in DS result from the presence of an extra chromosome 21 [45, 12]. A DS critical area has been identified on chromosome 21 in the 21q22 position and although it may include parts of bands 21q22.2 and 21q22.3, it must exclude the genes S0D1 and APP and most of band 21q22.1 [91]. It is still not clear whether DS-HSCR results from an increased dose of specific genes affecting neural (and ENS) development (eg. the amyloid precursor protein gene, SOD-1) or, alternatively, results from abnormal proteins resulting from mutant chromosome 21 genes. The effective gene dosage of 1.5 times resulting from the extra chromosome 21 [12] may nevertheless influence gene penetrance of those genes involved in (ENS) development resulting in fairly widespread genetic effects

As the ENS is probably subject to similar genetic and signaling influences as the CNS during development, transcriptional genetic variations would affect the nature of gene products as well as their functional relationships by influencing different aspects of neuronal differentiation and metabolism [7].

Chromosome 21 has long been regarded as a potential candidate area for a modifying gene in HSCR [61, 92, and 78] as well as Hirschsprungs associated enterocolitis (HAEC) [78, 87]. Early linkage disequilibrium and identity-by-decent (IBD) analysis in a Mennonite HSCR kindred (61), suggested genetic modifier mapping to 21q22. Although the precise site of this “modifier” on chromosome 21 remains unknown, current data suggests a possible site just outside of the DS critical area, possibly in the flanking genes.

This area includes a number of genes known to be of potential importance in neuroblast development [eg. SOD-1, amyloid precursor protein (A :), Protein S-100 beta, and the ITGB2

(CD18) gene]. Of the remaining possible candidate genes, those lying within this critical area of the gene known to have an effect on neural development, include the ITGB2 (CD18) gene at 21q22.3 [93, 94, 95] and the SOD-1 gene localized to 21q22.1 [96]. These genes are known to be triplicated (91) and over expressed in DS (97, 98). It is therefore logical that the subsequent protein overexpression products may contribute to the abnormal development of the immune and nervous systems.

HSCR Major Susceptibility Genes in DS-HSCR

Major susceptibility genes associated with HSCR (viz: RET and EDNRB) are an obvious place to start in looking for connections with ENS deficits in DS. We identified RET gene variations in all but one case in a DS-HSCR cohort[26], the majority of which were missense mutations and SNP's. The most frequent RET allele variations identified were, in general, similar to those found in a sample of sporadic HSCR patients from the same ethnic groups (99) although the incidence of certain RET variations (eg A45) appeared more frequent in the DS-HSCR group [26] and was observed in conjunction with L769 in 12 of the 16 cases (75%) investigated. In a recent publication Arnold et al [(1)]showed differences in the common functional variant at chromosome 10q11. 2 (rs2435357; RET +9.7) between samples of HSCR alone, DS alone and DS-HSCR suggesting a link between the RET gene and chromosome 21 dosage.

Similarly a study of the EDNRB gene in these patients [100] demonstrated significant associations with 951+3A/G and 802-6C/T variations in exon 4 in HSCR patients. A further significant association with a novel EDNRB variant in exon 2 [561C/T (he)] ($p < .002$; x2 Yates correction 12.14) were identified in DS-HSCR. The nature of these variations suggests a low penetrance effect. for EDNRB in HSCR. Sakai et al [62], reported a patient with DS with point nucleotidic changes in both the RET and EDNRB genes [a de novo heterozygous (T→A) variation at the intron- related splicing donor site related to exon 10 of RET and a maternally derived (G→A) heterozygous substitution in the EDNRB exon 1 non-coding region].

The major susceptibility HSCR genes therefore remain important candidates for associations with HSCR and an abnormal ENS but there is little information as to how this is associated with chromosome 21.

DS and the SOD Gene

SOD-1 is a very likely candidate for neuroblast development, firstly due to its position as a flanking gene of the DS-critical region on chromosome 21. Secondly it plays a role in ENS function and neural cells within the oesophagus have been shown to express SOD1 in the myenteric, submucosal plexuses and interganglionic fibers [101]. It is also thought to influence RET gene function through the major susceptibility pathway of HSCR, GDNF [102] and GFR alpha (103). SOD1 plays a role to motor neuron degeneration in familial amyotrophic lateral sclerosis (ALS) [104,105], suggesting a possible common pathway in the etiology of a variety of neurodegenerative conditions. It remains, therefore, a primary target to explore in the role of chromosome 21 in DS-HSCR.

SOD1 is known to be overexpressed in the DS brain [97, 98]. There is also current evidence of SOD1 genetic variations occur in both HSCR and DS-HSCR patients more frequently than in the general population (106). These appear to occur particularly within the region that affects membrane folding in the molecule which would then prevent its stable integration [107].

Precisely how SOD (or lack thereof) affects the ENS is still not completely clear. It has been established that as one of the antioxidant enzymes found in the intramural oesophageal plexuses, it plays a role in nitric oxide neuroreglation of the neuromuscular junction by regulating NO-mediated neuromuscular communication [101]. Normally, Superoxide dismutase (SOD) prevents the deleterious effects of free oxygen radicals on tissue by converting the O2-. to H2O2. If these free radicals are not converted, the superoxide radical (O2-.) causes problems by combining with nitric oxide (NO) to create peroxynitrite, thus nullifying the biological activity of NO. As NO is the major neurotransmitter of the non-adrenergic, non-cholinergic (NACA) nervous system in the gut, neural transmission and GI function will be affected by both an increased Superoxide radical (O2-.) or a blocking of SOD activity. In addition, an increase in superoxide dismutase (SOD) catalytic activity (possibly due to increased gene dosage) may therefore alter hydrogen peroxide metabolism in trisomic cells in DS thus making them more sensitive to oxidative stress and vulnerable to ongoing damage [108]. Our own studies have identified 2 polymorphic SOD1 variations in 16 DS-HSCR patients. [109]. (table 1)

In addition to gene variations which will result in mutant proteins, it is possible that SOD1 overexpression may be the more powerful influence as a RET/GDNF expression/function modifier. This would, in turn, result in a decreased control of neural developing cells and consequently contribute to the abnormal development of the ENS [102].

Other Candidate Genes

Despite the detailed analyses of genetic influences on DS phenotypic features and a detailed analysis of the gene [45], the functional GI conditions associated with DS are still not clearly defined. These are nevertheless the most likely causes of the significant functional disorders of the GIT in DS.

These include amyloid precursor protein (A :), Protein S-100 beta, and the ITGB2 (CD18) gene] in addition to SOD-1.

ITGB2 is an important integrin whose gene is also over expressed in DS [110]. Integrins have a number of functions which include neutrophil adhesion, endothelial transmigration, and other adhesion-dependent neutrophil functions such as the clearance of pathogens and the regulation of apoptosis[111]Beta-1 integrins are widely expressed on developing neurons [112] and although they do not appear to have a significant role in the defective migration of neuroblasts in HSCR[113] it is well known that polarization of cells prior to migration requires absolute spatial organization of the Actin cytoskeleton as well as integrin activation.[114].

Among other functions, ITGB2 is responsible for the beta chain of the lymphocyte function-associated antigen (LFA-1) but it has been linked to HSCR via a previous reported association between leukocyte adhesion deficiency (LAD), (a 21q22.3 CD18/ITGB2 genetic mutation) and HSCR [115]. Although our studies have shown a link to HAEC possibly through LFA-1 [87], the effect of ITGB2 on developing ENS neuroblasts remains an open question. Our studies have shown a high number of polymorphisms and one mutation at D77N in 16 HSCR patients (Table 2) (Figure 4)

Table 1. Intronic variations SOD-1 gene in DS-HSCR patients

Exon	Variant	Patients	Controls	P-value
2	IVS2-20T→C	0.18	0.43	0.05
4	IVS3+124C→A	0.18	0.03	0.04

Table 2. ITGB2 gene variants in DS-HSCR patients

Exon/ Intron	Variant	Patients	Controls	P-value
5'	5'UTR-111T/C	0.14	0.01	<0.0001
2	24G/T	0.45	0.65	ns
4	295G/A	0.23	0.10	0.08
7	892A/G	0.27	0.12	0.07
10	1101C/A	0.36	0.03	0.0007
11	1323T/C	-	0.08	ns
3'	3'UTR+38T/C	-	0.08	ns
3'	3'UTR+122G/A	0.82	0.28	<0.0001
3'	3'UTR+145C/A	0.04	-	ns
3'	3'UTR+171G/C	0.04	-	ns
3'	3'UTR+268A/C	-	0.03	ns
3'	3'UTR+370G/T	0.23	0.05	0.04

The *S-100 beta* gene remains a candidate which has previously been explored in relation to other neural conditions (2, 76) as well as DS [116]. S100 beta is a calcium-binding protein expressed mainly by astrocytes in brain tissue and shown to be elevated in Down syndrome (DS) patients throughout their lives. It has been associated with neurodegenerative processes. [116]. Experiments whereby the disulfide-bonded dimeric form of S100 beta is added to primary neuronal and glial cultures of established cell lines show induction of axonal extension and alterations in astrocyte proliferation[117].

In keeping with this, the effect of extra copies of the S100B gene in murine animal models appears to affect dendritic development in the brain leading to a “tree in winter” appearance” [47]. It has also been shown that S100B overexpression correlates with Alzheimer pathology in post-adolescent Down syndrome patients suggesting an association between the two.

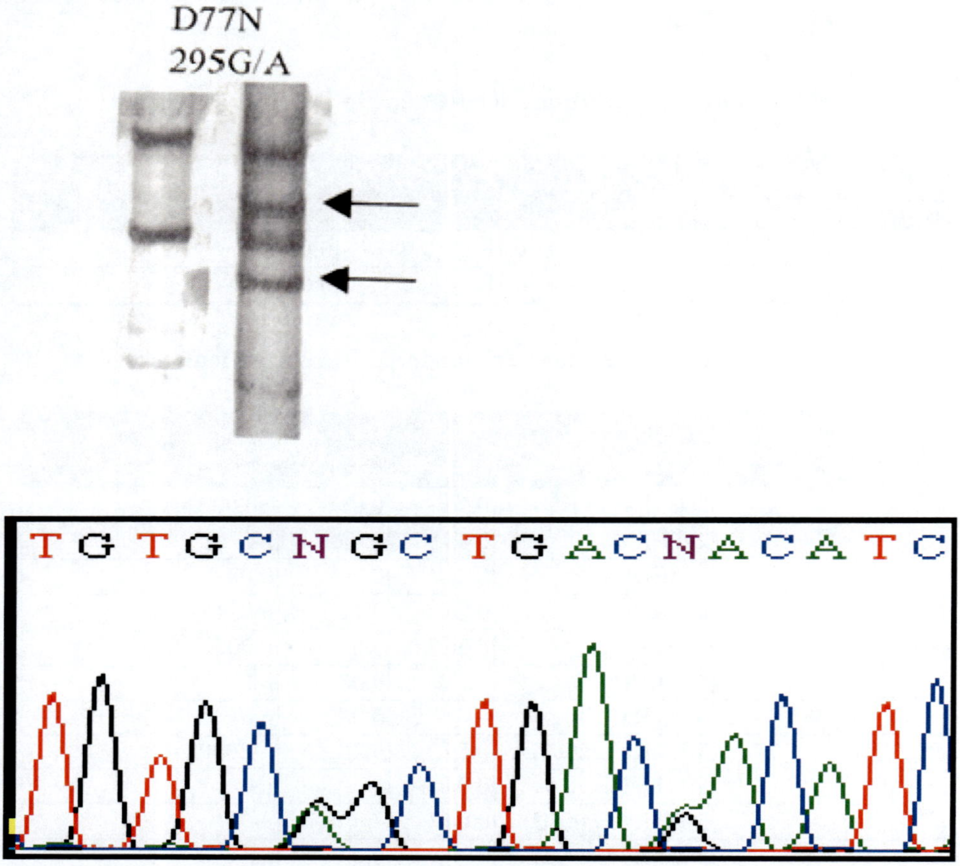

Figure 4. Mutation ITGB2 gene in DS.

The *Amyloid beta-peptide* (approximately 4 kDa-M(r)) is generated by the proteolytic cleavage of a larger beta-amyloid precursor protein (beta APP) encoded by a gene on chromosome 21. The abnormality in gene regulation of beta APP may be an important factor in the neuropathology of Alzheimer's disease no direct connection to HSCR has been described. More recently, the increased APP expression in a mouse model of Down's syndrome has been shown to disrupt NGF transport and result in cholinergic neuron degeneration.[118] There is some evidence against the overexpression of APP in DS[119] making it a less likely candidate for ENS maldevelopment, being mostly associated with Alzheimer's disease (AD). Furthermore although the full functions of the amyloid precursor protein (APP) gene are known to be required for the proper migration of neuronal precursors into the cortical plate during the development of the mammalian brain. [120], neurologic anomalies are not evident in APP knockout mice [121].

Other potential chromosome 21-related genes involved in neuronal development include Ets-2 transcription factors [122], the Down Syndrome Critical Region 1 gene (DSCR1) and the stress-inducible factor [123] as are the Down Syndrome Cell Adhesion Molecule (DSCAM) which maps to 21q22.2-->q22.3 (124), the DYRK1A protein (15) and TTC3 gene

[125]. DSCAM appears to be important as it is an axon guidance molecule mostly expressed in the developing neurons of the nervous system (both CNS and peripheral nerves) [126]. Interleukin-1 (a non-chromosome-21-based cytokine overexpressed in Down syndrome), situated in the 5'-flanking region of the beta APP gene appears to control transcription of beta APP [127]. Other growth factors in this region include nerve growth factor (NGF), basic fibroblast growth factor (bFGF), phorbol 12-myristate 13-acetate (PMA) and retinoic acid (RA). The association between ocular coloboma has been associated with a novel ZFHX1B missense mutation in a DS-HSCR patient also suggests a possible link [128]

In addition to all these potential genes influencing neuroblast development, animal studies in the trisomy 16 mouse (a DS animal model) have shown a marked decrease in nerve growth factor (NGF) sensitivity within trisomy 16 neurons ($P < 0.05$). This suggests that excess expression of genes on mouse chromosome 16 alters NGF-regulated adhesion to laminin. [129]. As laminin appears to be one of the most important components of the extracellular matrix in which enteric neuroblasts develop [130], and is affected in DS, this has interesting implications for the ENS in DS.

Laminin and Collagen

The synthesis of Laminin and its neurite outgrowth-controlling domain appears to be increased in brain tissue in DS. [131]. Premature neurite formation and inhibition of migration observed in an ls/ls murine model may have been promoted by the excessive secretion of laminin in the enteric mesenchyme[132,133] Down-regulation of the secretion of laminin-1, promotes neuron formation and has been linked to effects of endothelin-3 (ET-3) on smooth muscle[134]. This raises again the importance of the EDNRB / Endothelin 3 (ET-3) system in regulating enteric nervous system and melanocyte development.

Conclusion

The ENS in DS appears to be affected in a number of ways both by developmental defects and ongoing neuronal degeneration is also a factor to be bourne in mind. Disturbances of the GIT are not uncommon in DS and are probably related to an abnormal ENS. Functional GI disturbances may continue into adulthood in DS and require special counseling and follow-up.

References

[1] Altmann AE, Halliday JL, and Giles GG.Associations between congenital malformations and childhood cancer - a register-based case-control study. *Brit. J. Cancer* 1998; 78: 1244 -1249.

[2] Satge D, Sasco AJ, Carlsen NL, Stiller CA, Rubie H, and et al.A lack of neuroblastoma in Down syndrome: a study from 11 European countries. *Cancer Res*. 1998; 58 (3):448 -452.

[3] Spahis JK and Wilson GN.Down syndrome: perinatal complications and counseling experiences in 216 patients. *Am. J. Med. Genet.* 1999; 89 (2):96 -99.

[4] Henderson, A., Lynch, S. A., Wilkinson, S., and Hunter, M.Adults with Down's syndrome: the prevalence of complications and health care in the community. *Br.J Gen.Pract*. 2007; 57 (534):50 -55.

[5] Conti, A., Fabbrini, F., D'Agostino, P., Negri, R., Greco, D., Genesio, R., D'Armiento, M., Olla, C., Paladini, D., Zannini, M., and Nitsch, L.Altered expression of mitochondrial and extracellular matrix genes in the heart of human fetuses with chromosome 21 trisomyBMC.*Genomics* 2007; 8: 268

[6] Mao, R., Wang, X., Spitznagel, E. L., Jr., Frelin, L. P., Ting, J. C., Ding, H., Kim, J. W., Ruczinski, I., Downey, T. J., and Pevsner, J.Primary and secondary transcriptional effects in the developing human Down syndrome brain and heart. *Genome Biol.* 2005; 6 (13):R107

[7] Rachidi, M. and Lopes, C.Mental retardation in Down syndrome: from gene dosage imbalance to molecular and cellular mechanisms. *Neurosci. Res.* 2007; 59 (4):349 -369.

[8] Deutsch, S., Lyle, R., Dermitzakis, E. T., Attar, H., Subrahmanyan, L., Gehrig, C., Parand, L., Gagnebin, M., Rougemont, J., Jongeneel, C. V., and Antonarakis, S. E.Gene expression variation and expression quantitative trait mapping of human chromosome 21 genes. *Hum. Mol. Genet.* 2005; 14 (23):3741 -3749.

[9] it Yahya-Graison, E., Aubert, J., Dauphinot, L., Rivals, I., Prieur, M., Golfier, G., Rossier, J., Personnaz, L., Creau, N., Blehaut, H., Robin, S., Delabar, J. M., and Potier, M. C.Classification of human chromosome 21 gene-expression variations in Down syndrome: impact on disease phenotypes. *Am. J. Hum. Genet*. 2007; 81 (3):475 -491.

[10] Cheon, M. S., Bajo, M., Kim, S. H., Claudio, J. O., Stewart, A. K., Patterson, D., Kruger, W. D., Kondoh, H., and Lubec, G.Protein levels of genes encoded on chromosome 21 in fetal Down syndrome brain: challenging the gene dosage effect hypothesis (Part II). *Amino.Acids* 2003; 24 (1-2):119 -125.

[11] Benavides-Piccione, R., Ballesteros-Yanez, I., de Lagran, M. M., Elston, G., Estivill, X., Fillat, C., Defelipe, J., and Dierssen, M.On dendrites in Down syndrome and DS murine models: a spiny way to learn. *Prog.Neurobiol.* 2004; 74 (2):111 -126.

[12] Arron JR, Winslow MM, Polleri A, Chang CP, Wu H, Gao X, Neilson JR, and et al.NFAT dysregulation by increased dosage of DSCR1 and DYRK1A on chromosome 21. *Nature* 2006; 441 (7093):595 -600.

[13] Gwack Y, Sharma S, Nardone J, Tanasa B, Iuga A, Srikanth S, and et al.A genome-wide Drosophila RNAi screen identifies DYRK-family kinases as regulators of NFAT. *Nature* 2006; 441 (7093):646 -650.

[14] Canzonetta, C., Mulligan, C., Deutsch, S., Ruf, S., O'Doherty, A., Lyle, R., Borel, C., Lin-Marq, N., Delom, F., Groet, J., Schnappauf, F., De, Vita S., Averill, S., Priestley, J. V., Martin, J. E., Shipley, J., Denyer, G., Epstein, C. J., Fillat, C., Estivill, X., Tybulewicz, V. L., Fisher, E. M., Antonarakis, S. E., and Nizetic, D.DYRK1A-dosage imbalance perturbs NRSF/REST levels, deregulating pluripotency and embryonic stem cell fate in Down syndrome. *Am. J. Hum .Genet.* 2008; 83 (3):388 -400.

[15] Dowjat, W. K., Adayev, T., Kuchna, I., Nowicki, K., Palminiello, S., Hwang, Y. W., and Wegiel, J.Trisomy-driven overexpression of DYRK1A kinase in the brain of subjects with Down syndrome. *Neurosci Lett.* 2007; 413 (1):77 -81.

[16] Parkinson, P. F., Kannangara, T. S., Eadie, B. D., Burgess, B. L., Wellington, C. L., and Christie, B. R.Cognition, learning behaviour and hippocampal synaptic plasticity are not disrupted in mice over-expressing the cholesterol transporter ABCG1. Lipids Health Dis. 2009; 8 (1):5 E published 2-24-2009

[17] Wegiel, J., Dowjat, K., Kaczmarski, W., Kuchna, I., Nowicki, K., Frackowiak, J., Mazur, Kolecka B., Wegiel, J., Silverman, W. P., Reisberg, B., Deleon, M., Wisniewski, T., Gong, C. X., Liu, F., Adayev, T., Chen-Hwang, M. C., and Hwang, Y. W.The role of overexpressed DYRK1A protein in the early onset of neurofibrillary degeneration in Down syndrome. *Acta Neuropathol.* 2008; 116 (4):391 -407.

[18] Shankle, W. R., Landing, B. H., Ang, S. M., Chui, H., Villarreal-Engelhardt, G., and Zarow, C.Studies of the enteric nervous system in Alzheimer disease and other dementias of the elderly: enteric neurons in Alzheimer disease. *Mod.Pathol.* 1993; 6 (1):10 -14.

[19] Tam, P. K.An immunohistological study of the human enteric nervous system with microtubule-associated proteins. *Gastroenterology* 1990; 99 (6):1841 -1844.

[20] Deguchi, E., Iwai, N., Goto, Y., Yanagihara, J., and Fushiki, S.An immunohistochemical study of neurofilament and microtubule-associated Tau protein in the enteric innervation in Hirschsprung's disease. *J. Pediatr. Surg.* 1993; 28 (7):886 -890.

[21] Coppede, F., Migheli, F., Bargagna, S., Siciliano, G., Antonucci, I., Stuppia, L., Palka, G., and Migliore, L.Association of maternal polymorphisms in folate metabolizing genes with chromosome damage and risk of Down syndrome offspring. *Neurosci. Lett.* 2009; 449 (1):15 -19.

[22] Carrascosa-Romero MC, Fernandez-Cordoba MS, Gonzalvez-Pinera J, Gutierrez-Junquera C, and Pardal-Fernandez JM.[Neurocristopathies: a high incidence of cerebral dysgenesis in patients with Hirschsprung's disease.]. *Rev. Neurol.* 2007; 45 (12):707 -712.

[23] Tamamaki N, Nakamura K, Okamoto K, and Kaneko T.Radial glia is a progenitor of neocortical neurons in the developing cerebral cortex. *Neurosci. Res.* 2001; 41 (1):51 -60.

[24] Takahashi T, Nowakowski RS, and Caviness VS Jr.The cell cycle of the pseudostratified ventricular epithelium of the embryonic murine cerebral wall. *J. Neurosci.* 1995; 15: (9):6046 -6057.

[25] Cleves, M. A., Hobbs, C. A., Cleves, P. A., Tilford, J. M., Bird, T. M., and Robbins, J. M.Congenital defects among liveborn infants with Down syndrome. Birth Defects Res.*A Clin. Mol. Teratol. 2*007; 79 (9):657 -663.

[26] Moore SW.Downs syndrome and Hirschsprungs disease: a significant relationship? Int *J. Disabil. Hum. Dev.* 2006; 5 (4):369 -375.

[27] Xing, L., Salas, M., Lin, C. S., Zigman, W., Silverman, W., Subramaniyam, S., Murty, V. V., and Tycko, B.Faithful tissue-specific expression of the human chromosome 21-linked COL6A1 gene in BAC-transgenic mice. Mamm.*Genome* 2007; 18 (2):113 -122.

[28] Buchin PJ, Levy JS, and Schullinger JN.Down's syndrome and the gastrointestinal tract. *J. Clin. Gastroenterol.* 1986; 8 (2):111 -114.

[29] Levy J.The gastrointestinal tract in Down syndrome. *Prog. Clin. Biol. Res.* 1991; 373: 245 -256.

[30] Kallen, B., Mastroiacovo, P., and Robert, E.Major congenital malformations in Down syndrome. *Am. J. Med. Genet.* 10-16-1996; 65 (2):160 -166.

[31] Weir, K., McMahon, S., Barry, L., Ware, R., Masters, I. B., and Chang, A. B.Oropharyngeal aspiration and pneumonia in children. **Pediatr. Pulmonol**. 2007; 42 (11):1024 -1031.

[32] Wallace, R. A.Clinical audit of gastrointestinal conditions occurring among adults with Down syndrome attending a specialist clinic. *J. Intellect.Dev. Disabil.* 2007; 32 (1):45 - 50.

[33] Kim, JH, Kim PCW, and Hui, C-C.The VACTERL association: lessons from the Sonic hedgehog pathway. *Clinical Genetics* 2001; 59 (5):306 -315.

[34] Martinez-Frias ML, Bermejo E, and Frias JL.The VACTERL association: lessons from the Sonic hedgehog pathway. *Clin. Genet.* 2001; 60 (5):397 -398.

[35] Arsic, D., Qi, B. Q., and Beasley, S. W.Hedgehog in the human: a possible explanation for the VATER association. *J. Paediatr.Child Health* 2002; 38 (2):117 -121.

[36] Roper, R. J., Baxter, L. L., Saran, N. G., Klinedinst, D. K., Beachy, P. A., and Reeves, R. H.Defective cerebellar response to mitogenic Hedgehog signaling in Down [corrected] syndrome mice. Proc Natl.Acad.Sci.U.S A 2006; 103 (5):1452 -1456.

[37] Katoh, Y. and Katoh, M.Hedgehog signaling pathway and gastrointestinal stem cell signaling network (review). *Int. J. Mol. Med.* 2006; 18 (6):1019 -1023.

[38] Hatton, B. A., Knoepfler, P. S., Kenney, A. M., Rowitch, D. H., de, Alboran, I, Olson, J. M., and Eisenman, R. N.N-myc is an essential downstream effector of Shh signaling during both normal and neoplastic cerebellar growth. *Cancer Res.* 2006; 66 (17):8655 - 8661.

[39] Dessimoz, J., Opoka, R., Kordich, J. J., Grapin-Botton, A., and Wells, J. M.FGF signaling is necessary for establishing gut tube domains along the anterior-posterior axis in vivo. *Mech.Dev.* 2006; 123 (1):42 -55.

[40] Harmon, E. B., Ko, A. H., and Kim, S. K.Hedgehog signaling in gastrointestinal development and disease. *Curr.Mol. Med.* 2002; 2 (1):67 -82.

[41] Moldrich, R. X., Dauphinot, L., Laffaire, J., Rossier, J., and Potier, M. C.Down syndrome gene dosage imbalance on cerebellum development. *Prog.Neurobiol.* 2007; 82 (2):87 -94.

[42] Roper, R. J., Vanhorn, J. F., Cain, C. C., and Reeves, R. H.A neural crest deficit in Down syndrome mice is associated with deficient mitotic response to Sonic hedgehog. *Mech.Dev. E published* 11-21-2008;

[43] Gershon MD, Chalazonitis A, and Rothman TP.From neural crest to bowel: development of the enteric nervous system. *J. Neurobiol.* 1993; 24 (2):199 -214.

[44] Goyal RK and Hirano I.The enteric nervous system. *N.Engl.J. Med.* 4-25-1996; 334 (17):1106 -1115.

[45] Korenberg JR, Chen X, Schipper R, Sun Z, Gonsky R, Gerwehr S, and et al.Downs syndrome phenotypes: the consequence of chromosomal imbalance. *Proc. Natl. Acad. Sci.* 1994; 91: 4997 -5001.

[46] Behar, T. N. and Colton, C. A.Redox regulation of neuronal migration in a Down Syndrome model. Free Radic.Biol.Med 9-15-2003; 35 (6):566 -575.

[47] Mrak RE and Griffin WS.Trisomy 21 and the brain. *J. Neuropathol. Exp. Neurol.* 2004; 63 (7):679 -685.

[48] Nakazato Y and Landing BH.Reduced number of neurons in esophageal plexus ganglia in Down syndrome: additional evidence for reduced cell number as a basic feature of the disorder. *Pediatr. Pathol.* 1986; 5 (1):55 -63.

[49] Leffler A, Wedel T, and Busch LC.Congenital colonic hypoganglionosis in murine trisomy 16--an animal model for Down's syndrome. *Eur. J. Pediatr. Surg.* 1999; 9 (6):381 -388.

[50] Li, J., Busch, L. C., and Kuhnel, W.[PGP 9.5 immunohistochemical study on the development of the enteric nervous system of trisomy 16 mouse embryos and their normal littermates]. Zhongguo Yi.Xue.Ke.Xue.Yuan Xue.Bao. 2000; 22 (2):159 -164.

[51] Matsuda H, Hirato J, Kuroiwa M, and Nakazato Y.Histopathological and immunohistochemical study of the enteric innervations among various types of aganglionoses including isolated and syndromic Hirschsprung disease. *Neuropathology* 2006; 26 (1):8 -23.

[52] Zarate N, Mearin F, Hidalgo A, and Malagelada JR.Prospective evaluation of esophageal motor dysfunction in Down's syndrome. *Am. J. Gastroenterol.* 2001; 96 (6):1718 -1724.

[53] Preiksaitis HG, Miller L, Pearson FG, and Diamant NE.Achalasia in Down's syndrome. *J. Clin. Gastroenterol.* 1994; 19 (2):105 -107.

[54] Okawada M, Okazaki T, Yamataka A, Lane GJ, and Miyano T.Down's syndrome and esophageal achalasia: a rare but important clinical entity. *Pediatr. Surg. Int.* 2005; 21 (12):997 -1000.

[55] Caviedes, P., Caviedes, R., and Rapoport, S. I.Altered calcium currents in cultured sensory neurons of normal and trisomy 16 mouse fetuses, an animal model for human trisomy 21 (Down syndrome). *Biol.Res.* 2006; 39 (3):471 -481.

[56] Saud K, Arriagada C, Cardenas AM, Shimahara T, Allen DD, Caviedes R, and Caviedes P.Neuronal dysfunction in Down syndrome: contribution of neuronal models in cell culture. *J. Physiol.* Paris 2006; 99 (2-3):201 -210.

[57] Flageole H, Fecteau A, Laberge JM, and Guttman FM.Hirschsprung's disease, imperforate anus, and Down's syndrome: a case report. *J. Pediatr. Surg.* 1996; 31 (6):759 -760.

[58] Clarke SA and Van der Avoirt A.Imperforate anus, Hirschsprung's disease, and trisomy 21: a rare combination. *J. Pediatr. Surg.* 1999; 34 (12):1874

[59] Moore, S. W. and Zaahl, M. G.Association of endothelin-beta receptor (EDNRB) gene variants in anorectal malformations. *J. Pediatr. Surg.* 2007; 42 (7):1266 -1270.

[60] Stanchina L, Baral V, Robert F, Pingault V, Lemort N, Pachnis V, Goossens M, and Bondurand N.Interactions between Sox10, Edn3 and Ednrb during enteric nervous system and melanocyte development. *Dev. Biol.* 2006; 295(1):232-49

[61] Puffenberger E, Kauffman E, Bolk S, and et al.Identity-by-descent and association mapping of a recessive gene for Hirschsprung disease on human chromosome 13q22. *Hum. Mol. Genet.* 1994; 3: 1217 -1225.

[62] Sakai T, Wakizaka A, Nirasawa Y, and Ito Y.Point nucleotidic changes in both the RET proto-oncogene and the endothelin-B receptor gene in a Hirschsprung disease patient associated with Down syndrome. Tohoku *J. Exp. Med.* 1999; 187 (1):43. -47.

[63] Hillemeier, C., Buchin, P. J., and Gryboski, J.Esophageal dysfunction in Down's syndrome. *J. Pediatr. Gastroenterol. Nutr.* 1982; 1 (1):101 -104.

[64] van Trotsenburg AS, Heymans HS, Tijssen JG, de Vijlder JJ, and Vulsma T.Comorbidity, hospitalization, and medication use and their influence on mental and motor development of young infants with Down syndrome. *Pediatrics* 2006; 118 (4):1633 -1639.

[65] Bozinovski J, Poenaru D, Paterson W, and Kamal I.Esophageal aperistalsis following fundoplication in a patient with trisomy 21. *Pediatr.Surg .Int.* 2006; 15 (7):510 -511.

[66] Zarate, N., Mearin, F., Gil-Vernet, J. M., Camarasa, F., and Malagelada, J. R.Achalasia and Down's syndrome: coincidental association or something else?. *Am. J. Gastroenterol* .1999; 94 (6):1674 -1677.

[67] Passarge E.The genetics of Hirschsprungs Disease. *N. Engl. J. Med* . 1967; 276: 138 -143.

[68] Graivier L and Sieber WK.Hirschsprungs disease and mongolism. *Surgery* 1966; 60: 458 -461.

[69] Badner JA, Sieber WK, Garver KL, and Chakravarti A.A genetic study of Hirschsprung disease. *Am. J. Hum. Genet.* 1990; 46: 568 -580.

[70] Besson WT, Kirby ML, Van Mierop LHS, and Teabeaut JR.Effects of the size of lesions of the cardiac neural crest at various embryonic ages on incidence and type of cardiac defects. *Circulation* 1986; 73: 360 -364.

[71] Garver K, Law J, and Garver B.Hirschsprung disease: a genetic study. *Clin. Genet.* 1985; 28: 503 -508.

[72] Ikeda K and Goto S.Additional anomalies in Hirschsprungs disease: an analysis based on a nationwide survey in Japan. Z Kinderchir 1986; 41: 279 -281.

[73] Spouge D and Baird PA.Hirschsprungs Disease in a large birth cohort. *Teratology* 1985; 32: 171 -177.

[74] Goldberg EL.An epidemiological study of Hirschsprung's disease. *Int. J. Epidemiol.* 1984; 13: (4):479 -485.

[75] Caniano DA, Teitelbaum DH, and Qualman SJ.Management of Hirschsprungs disease in children with Trisomy 21. *Am. J. Surg.* 1990; 159: 402 -404.

[76] Quinn FM, Surana R, and Puri P.The influence of trisomy 21 on outcome in children with Hirschsprung's disease. *J. Pediatr. Surg.* 1994; 29: 781 -783.

[77] Omenn GS and McKusick VA.The association of Waardenburgh syndrome and Hirschsprungs megacolon. *Am. J..Med. Genet.* 1979; 3: 217 -223.

[78] Moore SW.The contribution of associated congenital anomalies in understanding Hirschsprung's disease. *Pediatr. Surg. Int.* 2006; 22 (4):305 -315.

[79] Moore SW, Rode H, Millar AJ, Albertyn R, and Cywes S.Familial Aspects of Hirschsprungs Disease. *Eur. J. Pediat. Surg.* 1991; 1: 97 -107.

[80] Moore SW and Johnson GA.Hirschsprung's disease: Genetic and functional associations of Downs and Waardenburghs Syndromes. Seminars in Paediatric Surgery (USA) 1998; 7 (3):156 -161.

[81] Moore SW.Congenital anomalies and genetic associations in Hirschsprungs Disease. chapter9 in Hirschsprungs disease and Allied Disorders Holschneider AM, Puri P eds, 3rd Edition, 2008; Springer Verlag, Berlin pp 115-131.

[82] Teitelbaum DH, Qualman SJ, and Caniano DA.Hirschsprungs disease: Identification of risk factors for enterocolitis. *Ann. Surg.* 1988; 207: 240 -244.

[83] Morabito A, Lall A, Gull S, Mohee A, and Bianchi A.The impact of Down's syndrome on the immediate and long-term outcomes of children with Hirschsprung's disease. *Pediatr. Surg. Int*.2006; 22 (2):179 -181.

[84] Moore SW.The contribution of associated congenital anomalies in understanding Hirschsprung's disease. *Pediatr. Surg. Int.* 2006; 22 (4):305 -315.

[85] Grosfeld J, Ballantine T, and Csicsko J.A critical evaluation of the Duhamel operation for HSCR. *Arch. Surg.* 1978; 113: 454 -459.

[86] Wilson-Storey WD, Scobie WG, and Raeburn JA.Defective white blood cell function in Hirschsprungs disease: a possible predisposing factor for enterocolitis. *J. Roy. Coll. Surg. Edin.* 1988; 33 (4):185 -188.

[87] Moore SW and Zaahl MG.The *ITGB2* immunomodulatory gene (CD18), enterocolitis and Hirschsprung's disease (HSCR). *J. Pediatr. Surg.* 2008; 43(8):1439-44

[88] Catto-Smith AG, Trajanovska M, and Taylor RG.Long-term continence in patients with Hirschsprung's disease and Down syndrome. *J. Gastroenterol. Hepatol.* 2006; 21 (4):748 -753.

[89] Mercer ES, Broecker B, Smith EA, Kirsch AJ, Scherz HC, and A Massad C.Urological manifestations of Down syndrome. *J. Urol.* 2004; 171 (3):1250 -1253.

[90] Epstein CJ.Down's syndrome: critical genes in a critical region. *Nature* 2006; 44 (7093):582 -583.

[91] Korenberg, J. R., Kawashima, H., Pulst, S. M., Ikeuchi, T., Ogasawara, N., Yamamoto, K., Schonberg, S. A., West, R., Allen, L., Magenis, E., and .Molecular definition of a region of chromosome 21 that causes features of the Down syndrome phenotype. *Am. J. Hum. Genet.* 1990; 47 (2):236 -246.

[92] Bolk-Gabriel S, Salomon R, Pelet A, and et al.Segregation at three loci explains familial and population risk in Hirschsprung disease. Nat Genet 2002; 1: 89 -93.

[93] Marlin SD, Morton CC, Anderson DC, and Springer TA.LFA-1 Immunodeficiency disease. *J. Exp. Med.* 1986; 164: 855 -867.

[94] Solomon, E., Palmer, R. W., Hing, S., and Law, S. K.Regional localization of CD18, the beta-subunit of the cell surface adhesion molecule LFA-1, on human chromosome 21 by in situ hybridization. *Ann. Hum. Genet.* 1988; 52 (Pt 2):123 -128.

[95] Petersen MB, Slaugenhaupt SA, Lewis JG, Warren AC, Chakravarti A, and Antonarakis SE.A genetic linkage map of 27 markers on human chromosome 21. *Genomics* 1991; 9 407 -419.

[96] Crapo, J. D., Oury, T., Rabouille, C., Slot, J. W., and Chang, L. Y.Copper,zinc superoxide dismutase is primarily a cytosolic protein in human cells. *Proc. Natl.Acad.Sci.U.S A* 1992; 89 (21):10405 -10409.

[97] Meguid NA, Kholoussi NM, and Afifi HH.Evaluation of superoxide dismutase and glutathione peroxidase enzymes and their cofactors in Egyptian children with Down's syndrome. *Biol. Trace Elem. Res.* 2001; 81 (1):21 -28.

[98] Netto CB, Siqueira IR, Fochesatto C, Portela LV, da Purificacao Tavares M, Souza DO, Giugliani R, and Goncalves CA.S100B content and SOD activity in amniotic fluid of pregnancies with Down syndrome. *Clin. Biochem.* 2004; 37 (2):134 -137.

[99] Julies MG, Moore SW, Kotze MJ, and du Plessis L.Novel *RET* mutations in Hirschsprung's disease patients from the diverse South African population. *Eur. J. Hum. Genet.* 2001; 9 (6):419 -423.

[100] Arnold, S., Pelet, A., Amiel, J., Borrego, S., Hofstra, R., Tam, P., Ceccherini, I., Lyonnet, S., Sherman, S., and Chakravarti, A. Interaction between a chromosome 10 RET enhancer and chromosome 21 in the Down syndrome-Hirschsprung disease association 2009; Hum Mutat. 30 (5): 771-775

[101] Zaahl MG, du Plessis L, Warnich L, Kotze MJ, and Moore SW.Significance of novel endothelin-B receptor gene polymorphisms in Hirschsprung's disease: Predominance of a novel variant (561C/T) in patients with co-existing Down's syndrome. *Mol. Cell. Probes.* 2003; 17 (1):49 -54.

[102] Thomas, R. M., Fang, S., Leichus, L. S., Oberley, L. W., Christensen, J., Murray, J. A., Ledlow, A., and Conklin, J. L.Antioxidant enzymes in intramural nerves of the opossum esophagus. *Am. J. Physiol.* 1996; 270 (1 Pt 1):G136 -G142.

[103] Manabe Y, Nagano I, Gazi MS, Murakami T, Shiote M, Shoji M, Kitagawa H, and Abe K.Glial cell line-derived neurotrophic factor protein prevents motor neuron loss of transgenic model mice for amyotrophic lateral sclerosis. *Neurol. Res.* 2003; 25 (2):195 -200.

[104] Zhang J and Huang EJ.Dynamic expression of neurotrophic factor receptors in postnatal spinal motoneurons and in mouse model of ALS. *J. Neurobiol.* 2006; 66 (8):882 -895.

[105] Siddique T, Figlewicz DA, Pericak-Vance MA, Haines JL, Rouleau G, Jeffers AJ, Sapp P, Hung WY, Bebout J, McKenna-Yasek D, and et al.Linkage of a gene causing familial amyotrophic lateral sclerosis to chromosome 21 and evidence of genetic-locus heterogeneity. *N. Engl. J. Med.* 1991; 24 (20):1381 -1384.

[106] Vlug AS, Teuling E, Haasdijk ED, French P, Hoogenraad CC, and Jaarsma D.ATF3 expression precedes death of spinal motoneurons in amyotrophic lateral sclerosis-SOD1 transgenic mice and correlates with c-Jun phosphorylation, CHOP expression, somato-dendritic ubiquitination and Golgi fragmentation. *Eur. J. Neurosci.* 2006; 22 (8):1881 -1894.

[107] Zaahl MG, van Huyssteen B, Strickland N, Panton NA, and Moore SW.Hirschsprung's disease (HSCR) and Chromosome 21: Investigating two possible modifier loci, superoxide dismutase (*SOD1*) and integrin-beta2 gene (*ITGB2*) . in press;

[108] Julien JP and Kriz J.Transgenic mouse models of amyotrophic lateral sclerosis. *Biochim. Biophys. Acta* 2006; 1762 (11-12):1013 -1024.

[109] Ordonez, F. J. and Rosety-Rodriguez, M.Correlation between glutathione peroxidase activity and anthropometrical parameters in adolescents with Down syndrome. *Res.Dev. Disabil.* 2007; 28 (1):105 -108.

[110] Moore SW and Zaahl MG.Exploring aspects of Chromosome 21 genes ITGB2 and SOD-1 in Downs syndrome (DS) Hirschsprungs disease. Abstract 23: Development of the Enteric Nervous System: Cells, Signals and GenesUCL Institute of Child Health London 22-25 Feb 2009

[111] Taylor, G. M., Haigh, H., Williams, A., D'Souza, S. W., and Harris, R.Down's syndrome lymphoid cell lines exhibit increased adhesion due to the over-expression of lymphocyte function-associated antigen (LFA-1). *Immunology* 1988; 64 (3):451 -456.

[112] Ross GD.Regulation of the adhesion versus cytotoxic functions of the Mac-1/CR3/alphaMbeta2-integrin glycoprotein. *Crit. Rev. Immunol.* 2000; 20 (3):197 -222.

[113] Clegg DO, Wingerd KL, Hikita ST, and Tolhurst EC.Integrins in the development, function and dysfunction of the nervous system. *Front Biosci*. 2003; 8: d723 -750.

[114] Tanyel FC, Muftuoglu SF, Dagdeviren A, Unsal I, Buyukpamukcu N, and Hicsonmez A.Expression of beta-1 integrins in ganglionic and aganglionic segments of patients with Hirschsprung's disease. *Eur. J. Pediatr. Surg.* 1997; 7 (1):16 -20.

[115] Jones SL and Sharief Y.Asymmetrical protein kinase A activity establishes neutrophil cytoskeletal polarity and enables chemotaxis. *J. Leukoc. Biol.* 2005; 78 (1):248 -245.

[116] Rivera-Matos I, Rakita R, Mariscalco M, Elder F, Dreyer S, and Cleary T.Leukocyte adhesion deficiency mimicking Hirschsprung disease. *J. Pediatr.* 1995; 127 (5):755 -757.

[117] Netto CB, Portela LV, Ferreira CT, Kieling C, Matte U, Felix T, da Silveira TR, Souza DO, Goncalves CA, and Giugliani R.Ontogenetic changes in serum S100B in Down syndrome patients. *Clin. Biochem.* 2005; 38 (5):433 -435.

[118] Reeves, R. H., Yao, J., Crowley, M. R., Buck, S., Zhang, X., Yarowsky, P., Gearhart, J. D., and Hilt, D. C.Astrocytosis and axonal proliferation in the hippocampus of S100b transgenic mice. *Proc.Natl.Acad.Sci.U.S A* 1994; 91 (12):5359 -5363.

[119] Salehi A, Delcroix JD, Belichenko PV, Zhan K, Wu C, Valletta JS, Takimoto-Kimura R, Kleschevnikov AM, Sambamurti K, and et al.Increased App expression in a mouse model of Down's syndrome disrupts NGF transport and causes cholinergic neuron degeneration. *Neuron* 2006; 51 (1):29- -42.

[120] Argellati, F., Massone, S., d'Abramo, C., Marinari, U. M., Pronzato, M. A., Domenicotti, C., and Ricciarelli, R.Evidence against the overexpression of APP in Down syndrome. *IUBMB.Life* 2006; 58 (2):103 -106.

[121] Young-Pearse, T. L., Bai, J., Chang, R., Zheng, J. B., LoTurco, J. J., and Selkoe, D. J.A critical function for beta-amyloid precursor protein in neuronal migration revealed by in utero RNA interference. *J. Neurosci.* 2007; 27 (52):14459 -14469.

[122] Heber, S., Herms, J., Gajic, V., Hainfellner, J., Aguzzi, A., Rulicke, T., von, Kretzschmar H., von, Koch C., Sisodia, S., Tremml, P., Lipp, H. P., Wolfer, D. P., and Muller, U.Mice with combined gene knock-outs reveal essential and partially redundant functions of amyloid precursor protein family members. *J. Neurosci.* 2000; 20 (21):7951 -7963.

[123] Engidawork, E., Baiic, N., Fountoulakis, M., Dierssen, M., Greber-Platzer, S., and Lubec, G.Beta-amyloid precursor protein, ETS-2 and collagen alpha 1 (VI) chain precursor, encoded on chromosome 21, are not overexpressed in fetal Down syndrome:

further evidence against gene dosage effect. *J. Neural. Transm.Suppl.* 2001; (61):335 - 346.

[124] Lott, I. T., Head, E., Doran, E., and Busciglio, J.Beta-amyloid, oxidative stress and down syndrome. *Curr.Alzheimer Res.* 2006; 3 (5):521 -528.

[125] Barlow, G. M., Lyons, G. E., Richardson, J. A., Sarnat, H. B., and Korenberg, J. R.DSCAM: an endogenous promoter drives expression in the developing CNS and neural crest. *Biochem.Biophys.Res.Commun.* 2002; 299 (1):1 -6.

[126] Berto, G., Camera, P., Fusco, C., Imarisio, S., Ambrogio, C., Chiarle, R., Silengo, L., and Di, Cunto F.The Down syndrome critical region protein TTC3 inhibits neuronal differentiation via RhoA and Citron kinase. *J. Cell Sci.* 2007; 120 (Pt 11):1859 -1867.

[127] Baumann, J. Down syndrome cell adhesion molecule--a common determinant of brain and heart wiring. *Pediatr. Res.* 2007; 62 (1):1

[128] Donnelly RJ, Friedhoff AJ, Beer B, Blume AJ, and Vitek MP.Interleukin-1 stimulates the beta-amyloid precursor protein promoter. *Cell Mol. Neurobiol.* 1990; 10 (4):485 - 495.

[129] Gregory-Evans CY, Vieira H, Dalton R, Adams GG, Salt A, and Gregory-Evans K.Ocular coloboma and high myopia with Hirschsprung disease associated with a novel ZFHX1B missense mutation and trisomy 21. *Am. J. Med. Genet.* A 2004; 131 (1):86 - 90.

[130] Pearce R, Galdzicki Z, and Rapoport SI.Decreased sensitivity to nerve growth factor of dorsal root ganglion neurons cultured from mouse trisomy 16, a model of Down's syndrome. *Brain Res.* 1995; 680 (1-2):108 -116.

[131] Rothman TP, Chen J, Howard MJ, Costantini F, Schuchardt A, Pachnis V, and Gershon MD.Increased expression of laminin-1 and collagen (IV) subunits in the aganglionic bowel of ls/ls, but not c-ret -/- mice. *Dev. Biol.* 1996; 178 (2):498 -513.

[132] Murtomaki S, Risteli J, Risteli L, Koivisto UM, Johansson S, and Liesi P.Laminin and its neurite outgrowth-promoting domain in the brain in Alzheimer's disease and Down's syndrome patients. *J. Neurosci. Res.* 1992; 32 (2):261 -273.

[133] Rothman TP, Goldowitz D, and Gershon MD.Inhibition of migration of neural crest-derived cells by the abnormal mesenchyme of the presumptive aganglionic bowel of ls/ls mice: analysis with aggregation and interspecies chimeras. *Dev. Biol.* 1993; 159 (2):559 -573.

[134] Wright TC, Orkin RW, Destrempes M, and Kurnit D.Increased adhesiveness of Down syndrome fetal fibroblasts *in vitro.* Proc Natl Acad Sci USA 1984; 81: 2426 -2430.

[135] Gershon MD.Endothelin and the development of the enteric nervous system. *Clin. Exp. Pharmacol. Physiol.* 1999; 26 (12):985 -988.

In: Handbook of Down Syndrome Research
Editors: Dominicus Jelinek and Gijs Dvorak
ISBN 978-1-60741- 690-6

Chapter 6

Infectious Diseases of Respiratory System During Pregnancy

Andrew E. Czeizel[1], Nándor Ács[2], and Ferenc Bánhidy[2]
[1] Foundation for the Community Control of Hereditary Diseases, Budapest, Hungary
[2] Second Department of Obstetrics and Gynecology, Semmelweis University, School of Medicine, Budapest, Hungary

Abstract

Infectious diseases of respiratory system frequently complicate pregnancy. This review is to evaluate the possible association between maternal infectious diseases of respiratory system during pregnancy and preterm birth or structural birth defects, i.e. congenital abnormalities (CAs), in addition their pregnancy complications based on the data set of the Hungarian Case-Control Surveillance of Congenital Abnormalities.

At the evaluation of *common cold*, it is necessary to differentiate the usual common cold (with short duration and without fever) and common cold with secondary complications (i.e. with longer duration and frequently high fever). Pregnant women with common cold mainly with secondary complications had not a higher incidence of pregnancy complications. The gestational age at delivery was 0.1 week shorter with a somewhat higher rate of preterm birth, but these differences had no real clinical importance. However, an association of common cold (mainly with secondary complications) in the second and/or third gestational month of pregnancy with a higher rate of newborns with congenital cataract, cleft lip ± palate and possible some other specific congenital abnormalities was found and these association was preventable with antifever drug treatments.

Acute infectious diseases of respiratory system cover a wide spectrum of diseases from sinusitis to pneumonia. These diseases during pregnancy have no obvious effect for pregnancy complications. Severe lower category of these infectious respiratory diseases associated with a higher risk for preterm birth, but their mild upper category seems to reduce indirectly the rate of preterm birth. Acute infectious diseases of respiratory system during the second and third gestational months of pregnancy did not associate with a higher risk for the total group or any specific group/entity of congenital abnormalities. However, the frequently high fever related tonsillitis in pregnant women associated with a higher risk for congenital cataract, neural-tube defects, cleft lip $\pm$ palate and unclassified multiple congenital abnormalities. We may suppose that the association between these fever sensitive defect groups and tonsillitis may be caused by high fever, because the parallel antifever treatment was able to prevent this risk.

Finally the *influenza* during pregnancy was evaluated. The short duration of influenza in pregnant women did not increase the risk for pregnancy complications. Our study showed that the appropriately treated pregnant women affected with influenza in the first and second trimester of pregnancy have no higher risk for preterm birth. However, the high fever related influenza in the second and/or third gestational month of pregnancy may associate with a higher risk of some - hyperthermia sensitive – CAs such as neural-tube defects, congenital cataract, cleft lip $\pm$ palate, cleft palate only, cardiovascular CAs, and unclassified multiple CAs. The main finding of our study is that this higher risk for these major CA can be prevented by the parallel use of antifever drugs.

Introduction

Infectious diseases of respiratory system frequently complicate pregnancy. Here we focus the two main adverse pregnancy outcomes of pregnant women affected with infectious diseases of respiratory system: *preterm birth* and structural birth defects, *congenital abnormalities*, in addition we evaluate their pregnancy complications.

In Hungary practically all deliveries took place in inpatients obstetric clinics and birth attendants were obstetricians during the study period. Thus both *birth weight* and *gestational age* at delivery were medically documented in the discharge summary of mothers after delivery. Gestational age was calculated from the first day of the last menstrual period. The definition of *preterm birth* was less than 37 completed weeks (less than 259 days), while the definition of low birth weight newborns was less than 2,500 gram.

Three groups of preterm birth are worth differentiation (I). spontaneous (about 50%), (II) preterm premature membrane rupture (30%) and (III) medically induced preterm birth due to maternal and genital complications (20%) [1].

Birth defects – or by according to the World Health Organization's (WHO) term: congenital anomalies – are structural, functional and/or biochemical-molecular defects present at birth whether detected at that time or not. Among different categories of birth defects, *congenital abnormalities* (CAs), i.e. structural-morphological defects represent the largest one. CAs have two main medical characteristics: (i) defect conditions with a limited chance for complete recovery, and (ii) the earliest (fetal-birth) onset. Thus, there is only one optimal medical solution and it is the prevention.

The causes of CAs can be classified into three groups:

1 *Genetic* which includes chromosomal aberrations (e.g. Down syndrome) and Mendelian single-gene defects (e.g. achondroplasia).

2 *Environmental* which includes infectious agents (e.g. rubella virus), maternal diseases (e.g. diabetes mellitus), teratogenic drugs, alcohol, smoking and environmental pollutants.
3 *Complex* (multifactorial) origin caused by gene-environmental interaction when the so-called polygenic liability (predisposition) is triggered by environmental "risk" factors.

This review is to evaluate the possible association between *maternal infectious diseases of respiratory system* in pregnant women and preterm birth or CAs on their offspring, in addition the pregnancy complications of mothers during the study pregnancy based on the data set of the Hungarian Case-Control Surveillance of Congenital Abnormalities (HCCSCA).

Hungarian Case-Control Surveillance of Congenital Abnormalities

The HCCSCA was established in 1980 and at present it is the largest population-based data set of cases with different CAs and their matched controls in the world [2]. *Cases* with CA were identified from the Hungarian Congenital Abnormality Registry [3] while *controls* without CA from the National Birth Registry. In general two or three controls were matched to each case on the basis of three criteria: (i) same sex, (ii) same birth week and (iii) same district of parents' residence. In addition, a *malformed control group* including cases with Down syndrome caused by non-disjunction before conception was also selected from the Hungarian Congenital Abnormality Registry to estimate better the recall bias.

Three sources of information were used to obtain exposure data in the mothers of cases, controls and malformed controls:

- Prospective medically recorded data. The mothers were asked to send us prenatal care logbook and all other medical records (mainly discharge summaries). Prenatal care was mandatory for pregnant women in Hungary (if somebody did not visit prenatal care clinic, she did not receive a maternity grant and leave), thus nearly 100% of pregnant women visited prenatal care clinics, an average 7 times in their pregnancies. The task of obstetricians in the prenatal care is to record all pregnancy complications, maternal diseases and related drug prescriptions in the prenatal care logbook.
- Retrospective maternal self-reported information. A structured questionnaire, a list of maternal diseases and drugs as memory aid and informed consent were mailed to the mothers immediately after the selection of cases, controls and malformed controls. Mothers were asked to read the enclosed list of maternal diseases and drugs in order to refresh their memory, after this to complete the structured questionnaire, and to send them back with signed informed consent in our prepaid envelop.
- Supplementary information from non-respondent mothers. Regional nurses were asked to visit all non-respondent case and malformed control mothers, in addition

200 control mothers and to help mother fill-in the same questionnaire, to evaluate available medical records and to obtain lifestyle data through a personal interview. Unfortunately the Ethics Committee did not allow visiting all non-respondent control mothers because – according to their opinion – this visit might disturb these families.

- Most chronic diseases were prospectively and medically recorded mainly in prenatal logbooks. The proportion of medically recorded acute diseases depended on the severity of diseases. As our validation study [4] showed mainly severe acute diseases were recorded medically in prenatal logbook.

At the evaluation of pregnancy complications and birth outcomes, preterm birth was evaluated only controls in the data set of the HCCSCA. Cases with CA were excluded because CAs may have a more drastic effect for the incidence of pregnancy complications and birth outcomes (e.g. rate of preterm birth) than the maternal diseases studied.

The evaluation of possible association of maternal diseases with the higher risk for different CAs was based on the comparison of cases with CA and their matched controls without CA in the data set of the HCCSCA. The diagnosis of CAs is based on the report of medical doctors in the Hungarian Congenital Abnormality Registry, in addition the quality of CA-diagnosis is improved and specified better due to the results of recent medical examination in the HCCSCA. CAs are evaluated in the so-called *informative offspring*: live-born babies, stillborn fetuses and electively terminated pregnancies in the second and/or trimester after the prenatal diagnosis of fetal defect.

At the evaluation of CAs we follow the following principles:

1 CA cannot be regarded as a single homogeneous birth outcome because teratogenic factors such as maternal diseases (e.g. diabetes mellitus) or chemical teratogens such as drugs (e.g. retinoid acid-isotretinoin, hydantoin-phenytoin, valproate, warfarin) do not uniformly increase the rates of all CAs but rather tends to increase the occurrence of one or a limited number of specific CAs, therefore we have to evaluate CA-entities or CA-groups separately. First, the so-called isolated CAs (e.g. cleft lip) and multiple-syndromic CAs (e.g. cleft lip with cardiovascular CAs and hypospadias) are differentiated because their severity and etiology differ significantly. Second, 25 groups of isolated CAs are classified according to well-defined diagnostic criteria. Third, multiple CAs are classified as CA-syndromes and CA-associations while the group of unclassified multiple CAs includes unidentified (though previously delineated) and undelineated CA-syndromes and CA-associations, in addition random combinations of CAs.

2 Different CAs have different critical periods [5]. Previously the critical period of CAs was considered during the first 3 months of gestation, i.e. in the first trimester. However, *gestational time* is calculated from the first day of the last menstrual period and it is worth differentiating three time windows: (i) First month of gestation because it is before the organogenesis. The first two weeks are before conception while the third and fourth weeks comprise the pre- and implantation period of zygotes and blastocysts including omnipotent stem cells. Thus CAs cannot be induced by environmental agents in the first month of gestation and it explains the

"all-or-nothing effect" rule, i.e. total loss or normal further development. (ii) The most sensitive, the so-called critical period for CAs. (iii) The "postcritical period" of CAs, i.e. pregnancy after the organ-forming period. These facts explain why the previous use of first trimester concept is misleading, thus outdated [6]. The critical period of most major CAs occurs in the second and third gestational months; we used therefore this time window as the critical period of CAs in our population-based case-control studies [7-9]. However, it is well-known that human teratogens can induce CAs after the third gestational month, i.e. after the first trimester (e.g. hypospadias, undescended testis). This methodological problem encourages us to introduce a new critical time approach based on the specified critical periods of different CAs separately and our study showed that this is feasible [5], but we have to wait for the international consensus [10].

3 In general maternal diseases cannot be regarded homogeneous pathological conditions, e.g. pneumonia may have different etiology, thus we have to do our best to work homogeneous disease entities as much as possible.

4 At the evaluation of maternal diseases we have to consider related drug treatments, but we have to avoid the usual methodological errors in previous studies when drugs were combined as antibiotics, penicillins, tetracyclines, sulfonamides, etc because different drugs have different chemical structures, indications and routes of administration.

5 The validity of diagnosis of CAs and maternal diseases, in addition drug treatment can be improved with multiple sources of data, in addition extra validation studies.

6 Confounders such as maternal age, parity, socioeconomic status of pregnant women, etc. may modify the association studied, thus we have to calculate adjusted risk figures.

7 Among confounders the possible folic acid and/or multivitamin supplementation in the periconceptional period or in early pregnancy have some preventive effect of some CA, thus we have to consider this recently recognized effect as well [11-15].

8 We have to consider recall bias at the comparison of cases and controls. The birth of an infant with CA is a serious traumatic event for most mothers who therefore try to find a causal explanation such as diseases or drug uses during pregnancy for CA of their babies. This does not occur after the birth of a healthy newborn infant. Thus recall bias might inflate an increased risk for CAs. Our previous analysis showed that a case-control surveillance of this type may cause spurious association between drugs and CAs with biased risk (odds ratio) up to a factor of 1.9 [16]. There are three possibilities to restrict or exclude recall bias. (i) The evaluation of exposures only during the critical period of CAs because we expect an underreporting of exposure in both the critical and non-critical periods of CAs in the control group. (ii) The use of prospectively and medically recorded data as a gold standard. (iii) Comparison between cases with CA and malformed control (cases affected with Dow syndrome caused by numerical chromosomal aberration in the preconceptional period) because the mothers of malformed controls have similar recall.

9 Multiple comparisons may produce a non-causal association because a significant difference is expected in every 20th estimation as a result of chance.

10 The first thought after the recognition of an association should be the exclusion of all possible biases and chance.

Here we evaluate the data set of the HCCSCA, 1980-1996 because after 1996 the collection of data has been changed (all mothers are visited at home by regional nurses) but the data have not been validated. Thus our previous publications were based on the data set of 17 years between 1980 and 1986.

Table 1 shows the number and percentage rate of more frequent maternal infectious diseases of respiratory system (which occurred in 10 or more mothers in either group) in the group of cases (including 22,843 informative offspring) and controls (containing 38,151 newborn infants).

Non-infectious diseases of respiratory system such as allergic rhinitis (hay fever), asthma bronchiale, emphysema, pneumothorax, epistaxis (from nose), in addition tuberculosis are excluded from this analysis. Influenza is the disease of the whole human body, but the predominance of symptoms is connected with the respiratory system, thus we evaluate this viral disease here.

Table l. The number and rate (%) of more frequent maternal infectious diseases of respiratory system during pregnancy in the case and control groups of the HCCSCA

Infectious diseases of respiratory system	Case group		Control group	
	No.	%	No.	%
Acute respiratory infections				
Common cold (nasopharyngitis)	3,827	16.8	5,475	14.4
Acute sinusitis	141	0.6	250	0.7
Acute pharyngitis	641	2.8	1,048	2.8
Acute tonsillitis	674	3.0	1,165	3.1
Acute laryngitis-tracheitis	404	1.8	804	2.1
Acute bronchitis-bronchiolitis	339	1.5	398	1.0
Pneumonia	116	0.5	182	0.5
Others (pleurisy)	8	0.0	12	0.0
Influenza	1,328	5.8	1,838	4.8
Chronic infectious diseases				
Chronic bronchitis	13	0.1	16	0.1

Respiratory System and Function During Pregnancy

The proper function of respiratory system in collaboration with cardiovascular system is extremely important to achieve adequate oxygenation of the fetus therefore there are significant changes in the maternal cardiorespiratory system during pregnancy.

First the anatomic changes of the respiratory system in pregnant women are summarized [17]. The level of the diaphragm rises by 4 cm and the transverse diameter of the chest increases by 2 cm, in addition the so-called subcostal angle increases from 68 to 103 degrees. These changes together the enlarging uterus result in a decrease in residual volume because lungs are somewhat compressed. However, the decrease of residual lung volume does not associate with decreased ventilation because the excursion of the diaphragm in respiration increases by 1.5 cm.

Though there is no increase in respiratory rate, maternal minute ventilation is increased due to an increase of tidal volume (about 500 to 700 ml in each breath). This hyperventilation results in a compensatory alkalosis and an increase in arterial oxygenation tension in the third trimester of pregnancy. The residual volume is reduced by 20% during pregnancy, but the vital capacity (i.e. the maximum volume of gas that can be expired after a maximum inspiration) does not change during pregnancy [17]

Second, the oxygen delivery and consumption in pregnancy are also changed partly due to the physiological anemia of pregnancy because it results in a reduction in the hemoglobin concentration and arterial oxygen content. Oxygen consumption increases steadily during pregnancy.

Third, at the evaluation of infectious diseases of respiratory diseases we have to consider the immunology of pregnancy. In general, immune function is similar in pregnant and non-pregnant women. However, both T-cell and NK-cell function shows a decrease in pregnant women. Nevertheless there is no clear trend toward either the suppression or enhancement of systematic immune function during gestation [18].

Common Cold

The common cold is a conventional term for mild upper respiratory illnesses caused by different microorganisms mainly from the virus family of picornoviridae (rhinoviruses, echoviruses, coxsackie viruses) influenza, parainfluenza, metapneumovirus, adeno- and respiratory syncytial viruses [19]. The common cold is manifested such as acute coryza or nasopharingitis with the symptoms of nasal stuffiness and discharge, sneezing, sore throat, and cough, in general without fever [20]. However, common cold is frequently followed by secondary complications including fever.

The common cold is the most frequently reported maternal disorders during pregnancy in Hungary (Table 1). The data set of the HCCSCA included 3,827 cases with CA, 5,475 controls without CA and 144 malformed controls affected with Down syndrome (the total group includes 834 malformed controls). The seasonal monthly distribution of common cold showed a higher occurrence between October and February with a peak in December. The usual duration of common cold was one week without secondary complications. However, about two-third of our pregnant women affected with common cold had a longer duration due to secondary complications including sinusitis, otitis media, laryngitis, tracheitis, bronchitis, etc and in general these mothers had fever (and antifever therapy).

At the analysis of our data in the HCCSCA [7, 21, 22] showed that about 50% of common cold was medically recorded in the prenatal care logbook. Major part of these pregnant women had secondary complications on the basis of longer duration of diseases and high fever (over 38.5 degree Celsius) in 57% of pregnant women. Thus, data shown here may reflect mainly pregnant women with more severe common cold with secondary complications.

Common cold was diagnosed in all gestational months with the somewhat higher prevalence in third-fifth gestational months.

Table 2 shows the incidence of pregnancy complications in pregnant women with or without common cold as a reference group. The proportion of anemia was larger, while the rate of threatened preterm delivery was smaller in mothers with common cold than in the reference group. The higher rate of anemia was in agreement with the lower intake of iron in pregnant women with common cold.

Table 3 summarizes the birth/pregnancy outcomes of pregnant women with or without common cold. There was no difference in the sex ratio and in the rate of twins between the two study groups. Mean gestation age was 0.1 week shorter and this finding was agreement with the somewhat higher rate of preterm birth in the babies of pregnant women with common cold compared to the reference group. However, the mean birth weight was larger by 34 gram and the rate of low birth weigh newborns was lower in babies of mothers with common cold during pregnancy.

Table 2. Incidence of pregnancy complications in pregnant women with or without common cold during pregnancy

Pregnancy complications	Pregnant women with common cold %	Pregnant women without %	Comparison OR (95% CI)
Nausea and vomiting, severe	9.1	10.3	0.9 (0.8 – 1.0)
Threatened abortion	16.2	17.2	0.9 (0.9 – 1.0)
Pre-eclampsia – eclampsia	8.4	8.5	1.0 (0.9 – 1.1)
Threatened preterm delivery	10.4	15.0	0.7 (0.6 – 0.7)
Placental disorders	1.2	1.6	0.7 (0.6 – 1.0)
Poly/oligohydramnios	0.6	0.5	1.1 (0.7 – 1.5)
Gestational diabetes	0.5	0.7	0.7 (0.5 – 1.0)
Anemia	18.9	16.3	1.2 (1.1 – 1.3)

Table 3. Data of birth outcomes of newborn infants born to mothers with or without common cold

Birth outcomes	Newborn infants born to mothers with common cold	Newborn infants born to mothers without common cold	Comparison
Quantitative	Mean (S.D.)	Mean (S.D.)	t-test
Gestational age at delivery	39.3 (2.0)	39.4 (2.1)	p=0.01
Birth weight	3,305 (487)	3,271 (51)	p=0.01
Categorical	%	%	OR (95% CI)
Preterm birth	9.6	9.1	1.2 (1.1 – 1.5)
Low birth weight	4.2	5.9	0.8 (0.7 – 0.9)

On the one hand the somewhat shorter gestational age at delivery and higher rate of preterm birth were in agreement with the symptoms of pregnant women with the fever related common cold with secondary complications though a lower rate of threatened preterm delivery was recorded among these females. On the other hand there was a somewhat larger birth weight and lower rate of low birth weight in newborn infants born to mothers with common cold, in general with secondary complications. These surprising findings need confirmation or rejection in further studies. At present our hypothesis is that the anxiety caused by the severe but relatively short (2 weeks) common cold resulted in an improved lifestyle (a higher rate of smoking cessation and vitamin use) in the further part, mainly during the third trimester of pregnancy, when there is the most intensive fetal growth.

Antifever drugs (acetylsalicylic acid, paracetamol and dipyrone) and antimicrobial drugs (such as ampicillin, penamecillin, clotrimazole) were used more frequently by pregnant women with common cold. However, there was no significant difference in the use of these drugs between case and control mothers with common cold.

Among pregnancy supplement, the use of folic acid was somewhat lower in case mothers than control mothers with common cold (48.6% vs. 52.1%, OR with 95% CI: 0.9, 0.8-1.0). The intake of vitamin C was much more frequent in mother with common cold than in mothers without common cold.

Our main aim was to study the possible association of maternal common cold with a higher risk for CAs.

First, the possible association of maternal common cold (mainly with secondary complications) in the second and/or third gestational month with 25 isolated CA groups and 1 unclassified multiple CA group was evaluated in the cases-all matched control analysis and a higher risk for 8 CA-groups were found (Table 4). However, this risk disappeared in the group of neural-tube defect at the evaluation of only medically recorded common cold. At the comparison of all cases with malformed controls (i.e. Down syndrome) with similar recall (bias), only congenital cataract and cleft lip ± palate showed a higher risk.

These analyses clearly demonstrated the importance of methodology in the human studies of teratogenic and maternal effects, e.g. the exclusion of recall bias by the comparison of case and malformed controls.

Table 4. Estimation of the association of maternal common cold (in general with secondary complications) in the second and/or third gestational month of pregnancy with 7 CA groups/entities in all cases-matched control analysis with or without antifever drug treatments, in cases and their matched controls with only medically recorded common cold, finally in all cases-malformed control analysis

CA groups / entities	Cases-all matched controls OR (95% CI)	Antifever drugs* with OR (95% CI)	without	Medically recorded OR (95% CI)	Comparison with malformed controls OR (95% CI)
Isolated					
Neural-tube defects	1.7 (1.3 –2.4)	1.0 (0.6 – 1.7)	2.4 (1.9 – 3.0)	1.5 (0.9 – 2.4)	1.3 (0.9 – 1.9)
Congenital hydrocephaly	6.3 (2.7 – 14.8)	2.1 (0.7 – 6.8)	2.6 (1.7 – 4.0)	3.6 (1.3 – 9.7)	1.5 (0.9 – 2.5)
Congenital cataract**	4.0 (1.7 – 9.2)	0.6 (0.1 – 4.0)	11.1 (5.3–23.3)	3.6 (1.6 – 8.2)	4.0 (2.6 – 6.2)
Cleft lip ± palate	3.2 (2.3 – 4.3)	1.4 (0.9 – 2.2)	2.9 (2.4 – 3.6)	2.3 (1.5 – 3.6)	1.7 (1.2 – 2.5)
Cleft palate only	2.0 (1.3 – 3.3)	1.2 (0.6 – 2.4)	1.7 (1.2 – 2.5)	2.3 (1.2 – 4.1)	1.1 (0.7 – 1.8)
Cardiovascular CAs	1.5 (1.3 – 1.8)	1.0 (0.7 – 1.3)	1.5 (1.3 – 1.8)	1.5 (1.2 – 2.0)	1.0 (0.7 – 1.3)
Limb deficiencies	1.7 (1.1 – 2.7)	1.2 (0.6 – 2.3)	1.8 (1.2 – 2.6)	2.2 (1.1 – 4.1)	1.2 (0.8 – 1.9)
Unclassified multiple CAs	2.1 (1.6 – 2.9)	1.3 (0.8 – 2.0)	2.0 (1.6 – 2.6)	2.0 (1.4 – 2.9)	1.3 (0.9 – 1.9)
Grand total	1.5 (1.4 – 1.6)	-	-	1.4 (1.3 – 1.6)	1.0 (0.8 – 1.2)

*unmatched analysis

**common cold and influenza were combined

However, our study showed an association of maternal common cold with congenital cataract and cleft lip + palate if maternal disease occurred in the critical period of this CA. The explanation for this association may be the high fever, because this association was prevented by the parallel antifever drug treatment (Table 4). We cannot exclude the possible association between maternal common cold with secondary complications and the previously mentioned other CAs but these possible associations were also prevented with antifever drug treatments.

At the evaluation of the association of maternal severe complicated common cold with congenital cataract and cleft lip ± palate, in addition possible others CAs we have to differentiate the possible teratogenic effect of microbial agents of common cold, secondary complications with fever, medications and malnourishment. We did not find any report regarding the teratogenic effect of microbial agents having a role in the origin of common cold [23]. Antifever drugs used for the treatment of common cold did not show teratogenic effect [24, 25]. Severe malnourishment may cause folate deficiency thus indirectly predisposition for some CAs [26], but most common colds are not so severe and long that can induce real malnourishment. Thus we may suppose that fever may be the causal factor similar to influenza in the origin of "hyperthermia sensitive" CAs. The importance of high fever will be discussed in the Discussion part of this paper.

Previously Kruppa et al [27] found a possible association between anencephaly (the most severe form of neural-tube defects) and maternal common cold, while Zhang and Cai [28] reported an association between common cold and neural-tube defects, hydrocephalus and cleft lip ± palate.

In conclusion, at the evaluation of common cold, it is necessary to differentiate the usual common cold (with short duration and without fever) and common cold with secondary complications (i.e. with longer duration and frequently high fever). Pregnant women with common cold mainly with secondary complications had not a higher incidence of pregnancy complications. The gestational age at delivery was 0.1 week shorter with a somewhat higher rate of preterm birth, but these differences had no real clinical importance. However, an association of common cold with secondary complications in the second and/or third gestational month of pregnancy with a higher rate of newborns with congenital cataract, cleft lip $\pm$ palate and possible some other specific congenital abnormalities was found and these associations were preventable with antifever drug treatments

Acute Infectious Diseases of Respiratory System

Acute infectious diseases of respiratory system (AIDRS) represent a wide spectrum, and according to International Classification of Diseases, WHO, we differentiate sinusitis, pharyngitis, tonsillitis, laryngitis-tracheitis, bronchitis-bronchiolitis and pneumonia. As it appeared at the analysis of our data, it is worth separating upper/mild category of AIDRS including sinusitis, pharyngitis, tonsillitis, laryngitis-tracheitis and lower/severe category of AIDRS comprising of bronchitis-bronchiolitis, pneumonia.

AIDRS, particularly uncontrolled or poor controlled, may cause both maternal and fetal morbity and mortality [29], nevertheless the possible associations of AIDRS with birth outcomes and CAs, in addition pregnancy complications have not been frequently studied [30].

The data set of the HCCSCA included 2,118 cases, 3,455 controls and 92 malformed controls born to mothers with AIDRS during the study pregnancy [8, 22, 31]. The duration of AIDRS was 1.2 $\pm$ 0.4 week in our pregnant women, though the duration of AIDRS and the proportion of medically recorded diseases depended on the severity of AIDRS (e.g. the latter was nearly 100% in the group of pneumonia). Hospitalization occurred only in pregnant women with pneumonia. AIDRS were recorded more frequently in the 3rd gestational month followed by 4th and 5th month. The monthly distribution of AIDRS showed some seasonality, the maximum was found in January followed by February, while the minimum occurred in July followed by August.

First the incidence of pregnancy complications in pregnant women with or without AIDRS as reference group was compared (Table 5).

The occurrence of pre-eclampsia was lower in pregnant women with AIDRS than in pregnant women without AIDRS. On the other hand the rarely occurred poly/oligohydramnios was somewhat higher among pregnant women with AIDRS.

In the second step we evaluated the incidence of pregnancy complications in different groups of AIDRS.

Table 5. Incidence of pregnancy complications in pregnant women with different groups of acute infectious diseases of respiratory system and the reference group (pregnant women without these diseases)

Pregnancy complications	Sinusitis (N=250)	Pharyngitis (N=1,048)	Tonsillitis (N=1,165)	Laryngitis-tracheitis (N=804)	Bronchitis-broncholitis (N=308)	Pneumonia (N=182)	Total (N=3,455)*		Reference (N=34,696)		Comparison OR (95% CI)
							No.	%	No.	%	
Nausea/vomiting	53.2	50.9	53.6	52.5	48.0	49.5	1,994	51.3	18,175	52.4	1.0 (0.9 – 1.1)
medically recorded	8.8	11.2	10.3	11.6	5.0	8.8	329	9.9	3,540	10.2	0.9 (0.8 – 1.0)
Threatened abortion	20.4	17.5	14.7	18.3	13.1	23.1	573	16.6	5,939	17.1	1.0 (0.9 – 1.1)
Pre-eclampsia	9.6	7.5	5.9	7.5	8.0	9.3	254	7.4	2,904	8.4	0.8 (0.7 – 0.9)
Threatened preterm Delivery	20.0	12.6	14.5	14.9	5.8	10.4	455	13.2	4,992	14.4	0.9 (0.8 – 1.0)
Placental disorders	2.0	2.4	1.6	2.0	0.3	1.6	58	1.7	535	1.5	1.1 (0.8 – 1.4)
Poly/oligohydramnios	0.0	1.2	0.9	0.7	0.3	0.1	2.6	0.8	179	0.5	1.2 (0.8 – 1.2)
Gestational diabetes	1.2	0.9	0.9	0.5	0.3	0.0	22	0.6	248	0.7	0.9 (0.6 – 1.4)
Anemia	14.4	19.1	14.2	19.5	11.3	18.7	55.3	16.0	5,803	16.7	0.5 (0.8 – 1.0

Nausea and vomiting in pregnancy was evaluated in the whole groups (based on both medically recorded and maternal reported information) and in the subgroups based only on medically recorded nausea and vomiting in the prenatal logbook. The latter group represented the severe form with medical treatment. The groups of upper AIDRS category showed a somewhat higher value (52.4%) than the groups of lower AIDRS category (48.4%), and this trend occurred in the prevalence of severe nausea and vomiting as well (10.7% vs. 6.2%). These findings are worth mentioning because nausea and vomiting in pregnancy seems to have a protective affect of fetal death [32] and CAs [33].

The occurrence of both threatened abortion and pre-eclampsia reflected a U-shaped severity curve; they showed the highest prevalence in the groups of pneumonia and sinusitis. Threatened preterm delivery and gestational diabetes occurred most frequently in the group of sinusitis. The occurrence of placental disorders and poly/oligohydramnios was found most frequently in the group of pharyngitis. However, these differences can be explained mainly by the chance.

Table 6 summarizes the birth/pregnancy outcomes of pregnant women with or without AIDRS.

Table 6. Birth outcomes of pregnant women with different manifestations of AIDRS and without AIDRS as reference

Different AIDRS	Gestational age at delivery (wk)		Preterm births		Birth weight (g)		Low birth weight newborns	
	Mean	S.D.	No.	%	Mean	S.D.	No.	%
Sinusitis	39.6	1.7	14	5.6	3,348	489	13	5.2
Pharyngitis	39.6	1.7	61	5.8	3,364	476	36	3.4
Tonsillitis	39.7	1.9	63	5.4	3,340	500	56	4.8
Laryngitis – tracheitis	39.8	1.7	32	4.0	3,349	512	39	4.9
Bronchitis – bronchiolitis	39.1	2.3	49	12.3	3,271	534	26	6.5
Pneumonia	38.9	2.2	28	15.4	3,217	525	16	8.8
Total	39.6	1.9	233	6.7	3,328	503	172	5.0
Mild/upper	39.7	1.8	161	5.5	3,343	496	134	4.6
Severe/lower	39.1	2.3	75	13.0	3,255	528	40	6.9
Total	39.6	1.9	233	6.7	3,328	503	172	5.0
Comparison	<0.0001		0.7 (0.6 – 0.8)		<0.0001		0.9 (0.8 – 1.0)	
Reference (without AIDRS)	39.3	2.1	3,263	9.4	3,271	512	1,195	5.8

There was no difference in the sex ratio and in the rate of twins between the study groups. Mean gestational age was 0.3 week longer of pregnant women with AIDRS and this finding was agreement with the lower rate of preterm birth in their babies compared to the reference group. However, the mean birth weight was also by 57 gram larger and the rate of low birth weigh newborns was somewhat but not significantly lower in newborn infants born to mothers with AIDRS during pregnancy. However, the larger mean birth weight can be explained by the longer mean gestational age at delivery.

The detailed analysis of these variables in the different groups of AIDRS showed a different and interesting pattern. There was a significantly shorter mean gestational age at delivery and higher rate of preterm birth in lower AIDRS category while upper AIDRS category associated with a longer mean gestational age at delivery and lower rate of preterm birth compared to the reference group, i.e. pregnant women without AIDRS. We did not find significant differences in the mean birth weight and the rate of low birth weight newborns between upper and lower AIDRS categories at the calculation of adjusted risk figures, i.e. considered confounders (among them gestational age).

We repeated these calculations based on only medically recorded AIDRS, and similar associations were found

Among drugs, antimicrobial (ampicillin, penamecillin) and antifever (acetylsalicylic acid, paracetamol, aminophenazone) drugs had a more frequent use in mothers with AIDRS, but there was no significant difference in their use between case and control mothers affected with AIDRS. The use of pregnancy supplements such as folic acid and multivitamins was similar in pregnant women with or without AIDRS, only vitamin C was used more frequently by pregnant women affected with AIDRS.

The association between severe lower category of AIDRS and higher rate of preterm birth is plausible due to the pathological condition of mothers related to fever, drug treatments, etc. However, the association between mild upper category of AIDRS and lower rate of preterm birth would need further explanation. On the one hand we may hypothesize that pregnant women with mild AIDRS later may be more health consciousness. On the other hand most pregnant women were treated by antimicrobial drugs, and some of them (e.g. ampicillin) may have a beneficial effect for the parallel existing sexually transmitted infections/diseases [34] which can induce preterm birth.

The prevalence of AIDRS in the second and/or third gestational months of pregnant women who later delivered cases with 26 CA-groups and their matched controls did not show significant difference in the total groups of CAs or any CA-entities or groups (Table 7).

Table 7. Estimation of association of maternal acute infectious diseases of respiratory system and tonsillitis in the second and/or third gestational month of pregnancy with or without antifever treatment

CA groups / entities	Cases-all matched controls OR (95% CI)	Tonsillitis OR (95% CI)	Antifever with treatment OR (95% CI)	Antifever without treatment OR (95% CI)
Isolated CAs				
Neural-tube defects	0.8 (0.6 – 1.2)	1.9 (1.4 – 2.7)	1.2 (0.6 – 2.3)	2.0 (1.4 – 2.8)
Congenital cataract	3.0 (0.8 – 12.0)	4.4 (1.3 – 14.0)	0.6 (0.1 – 4.0)	8.6 (4.0 – 15.1)
Cleft lip ± palate	1.2 (0.9 – 1.7)	1.6 (1.1 – 2.4)	0.6 (0.3 – 1.2)	1.8 (1.3 – 2.4)
Unclassified multiple CAs	1.0 (0.8 – 1.4)	2.2 (1.3 – 3.9)	1.9 (0.8 – 7.5)	2.5 (1.9 – 3.7)
Total	0.9 (0.8 – 1.0)	1.2 (0.6 – 1.4)	-	-

However, at the analysis of different groups of AIDRS separately, tonsillitis in the second and/or third gestational months of pregnancy did not show an association with the total group of CAs, but 4 CA-groups/entities showed an association with this fever related maternal diseases. Our validation study showed that 47.7% of pregnant women with tonsillitis had high fever. (The proportion of pregnant women with high fever was lower than

20% in other groups of AIDRS.) The highest OR was found in the group of cases affected with congenital cataract, followed by cases with unclassified multiple CA. The other two CA-groups represented the "hyperthermia sensitive" neural-tube defects and cleft lip ± palate. Again we checked these data in the subgroups with and without antifever drug treatments, and the previously found associations disappeared in the subgroups of pregnant women with antifever drug treatment while these risks increased in the subgroups without this treatment.

Previously mainly pneumonias in pregnant women were reported in the international literature. Pneumonia is rare during pregnancy, occurring in 1 per 118 to 2,288 [17], our figure 1 in 210 is nearer to the upper limit of this range. In most cases pathogens were not identified, however, other studies showed that pneumococcus and *Haemophilus influenza* are the most common identifiable causes of pneumonia in pregnant women [35, 36]. In the lack of comprehensive serologic testing, the true incidence of viral pneumonia, *Legionella* and mycoplasma pneumonia is difficult to estimate. In our material aspiration and varicella pneumonia, in addition HIV patients with pneumonia caused by *Pneumocystis carinii* or other agents did not occur.

Preterm delivery was found as a common complication (up to 43%) in pregnant women with pneumonia after the introduction of antibiotic therapy as well [35-37] with lower mean birth weight (2,770 ± 224 vs. 3,173 ± 99 g) in one study [35]. Our recent experiences were better in Hungarian pregnant women affected with pneumonia.

In conclusion, in general AIDRS during pregnancy have no obvious effect for pregnancy complications. However, severe lower category of AIDRS associated with a higher risk for preterm birth, but the mild upper category of AIDRS seems to reduce indirectly the rate of preterm birth. The latter finding needs further studies whether this association is causal or can be explained by unevaluated confounders. Finally AIDRS during the second and third gestational months of pregnancy did not associate with a higher risk for the total group of CAs or any group of specific CA-groups/entities. However, the frequently high fever related tonsillitis associated with a higher risk for congenital cataract, neural-tube defects, cleft lip ± palate and multiple CAs. We may suppose that the association between these fever sensitive CA-groups and tonsillitis may be caused by high fever, because the parallel antifever treatment was able to prevent this risk.

Influenza

Influenza is an acute infectious disease caused by influenza A, B and C viruses which occurs as an epidemic, in general winter [38, 39]. Most epidemic infections are due to influenza A, and influenza epidemics were recorded in Hungary between December and April. The latency period is about 2 (1-5) days, the usual duration of influenza is 5 days in general with high fever, coryza, headache, malaise and cough. However, if symptoms persist longer than 5 days, in general secondary bacterial infections of the respiratory system occur [40].

Pregnant women may have a higher risk for influenza pneumonia, partly in new pandemics [41, 42]. For example mortality rate of pregnant women with influenza pneumonia was about 50% in 1918-1919 [43, 44].

The data set of the HCCSCA included 1,328 cases with CA and.1,838 controls without CA, in addition 36,313 pregnant women without influenza were considered as reference group [9, 22, 45]. All pregnant women were affected with influenza during the epidemic periods, and 72% of them were recorded in the prenatal care logbook. The onset of influenza according to gestational months did not show any obvious difference with the exception of low prevalence in the 9th month. In our study 91.5 % of pregnant women had fever over 38.5 Celsius degree according to our validation study.

First we evaluated pregnancy complications (Table 8). These pregnancy complications did not show a higher incidence in pregnant women affected with influenza.

The birth outcomes of newborn infants without CA born to mothers with influenza or without influenza as reference group during the study pregnancy were analyzed in the second step, and the results of this evaluation showed unexpected results (Table 9).

There was no difference in the sex ratio and in the rate of twins between the two study groups. Mean gestational age at delivery was 0.1 week longer, and in agreement with this finding, the rate of preterm birth was somewhat lower in newborn infants born to mother with influenza during pregnancy compared with the reference group, i.e. pregnant women without influenza.

Table 8. Incidence of pregnancy complications in pregnant women with or without influenza during pregnancy

Pregnancy complications	Pregnant women with influenza	Pregnant women without influenza	Comparison OR (with 95% CI)
	No.	%	
Nausea and vomiting, severe	9.4	10.2	0.9 (0.8 – 1.1)
Threatened abortion	19.0	17.0	1.1 (0.9 – 1.3)
Pre-eclampsia (hypertension, edema, proteinuria)	10.6	12.2	0.9 (0.7 – 1.1)
Threatened preterm delivery (incl. cervical incompetence)	15.2	15.8	1.0 (0.9 – 1.1)
Placental disorders (placenta previa, premature separation of placenta, antepartum hemorrhage)	1.7	1.5	1.1 (0.8 – 1.6)
Poly/oligohydramnios	0.7	0.5	1.3 (0.7 – 1.6)
Gestational diabetes	0.9	0.7	1.3 (0.7 – 2.4)
Anemia	17.0	16.6	1.0 (0.9 – 1.2)

Mean birth weight was 37 g larger in live-born babies of pregnant women with influenza during pregnancy and this difference was reflected in the lower rate of low birth weight newborns as well. However, these differences were explained partly by the somewhat longer gestational age, partly maternal variables. The proportion of professionals was somewhat higher among pregnant women with influenza (14.2% vs. 11.3%), in addition pregnant women with influenza used more frequently vitamins (e. g.: C. 9.1% vs. 4.2% and multivitamins: 7.6% vs. 6.5%). On the other hand, it is necessary to mention that influenza occurred rarely in the third trimester of pregnancy, thus our data are not appropriate to study the possible association of maternal influenza during the third trimester with higher risk for preterm birth.

Table 9. Data of birth outcomes of newborn infants born to pregnant women with influenza or without influenza

Birth outcomes	Newborn infants born to pregnant women with influenza	without influenza	Comparison
Quantitative	Mean (S.D.)	Mean (S.D.)	Adjusted t
Gestational age at delivery	39.5 (1.9)	39.4 (2.1)	p=0.12
Birth weight	3,311 (492)	3,274 (512)	p=0.08
Categorical	%	%	Adjusted OR (95% CI)
Preterm birth	8.0	9.2	0.9 (0.8 – 1.1)
Low birth weight	4.7	5.7	0.9 (0.7 – 1.1)

Thus, the short duration of usual maternal influenza during the first and second trimesters of pregnancy does not induce a higher prevalence of unsuccessful birth/pregnancy outcomes. In fact we found a somewhat but significantly lower rate of preterm birth.

The major objective of our study was the evaluation of prevalence of maternal influenza in the second and/or third months of pregnancy, i.e. in the critical period of most major CAs (Table 10).

Of 26 CA-entities, 5 showed an association with maternal influenza. The higher risk for congenital cataract, cleft lip ± cleft palate, neural-tube defects and cardiovascular CAs was significant, while cleft palate was near to the level of significance (and unmatched analysis resulted in a significant association).

In the next step we attempted to differentiate cases with the above five "candidate" CAs according to maternal influenza in the second and/or third months of gestation with or without antifever treatment. We did not find this association if maternal influenza was treated by antifever drugs (Table 9).

Our studies showed the importance of specificity of teratogens as one of the important rule of human teratology. At the evaluation of the possible association between maternal influenza and 26 different CAs, 5 showed a higher risk. Another important rule in human teratology is the time factor, i.e. critical period of different CAs.

The previously mentioned association of maternal influenza with cleft lip ± cleft palate, neural-tube defects, cardiovascular CAs and cleft palate was found if this maternal disease occurred in the critical period of these CAs.

However, an obvious association was found between the maternal influenza and congenital cataract not only during the critical period of lens but during the entire pregnancy. Thus, congenital cataract is not only a defect of embryogenesis but it may be connected with the developmental disturbance of lens in the second and third trimesters of pregnancy.

Table 10. Estimation of the association (risk) of maternal influenza during the second and/or third gestational months of pregnancy with 5 CA groups in the cases-matched control analysis

Isolated CA-groups / entities	Case-all matched controls	Antifever drugs	
		with	without
	OR (95% CI)	OR (95% CI)	OR (95% CI)
Neural-tube defect	1.9 (1.1 – 3.3)	0.7 (0.3 – 1.6)	2.7 (1.8 – 4.0)
Cong. cataract*	4.0 (1.7 – 9.2)***	0.6 (0.1 – 4.0)	11.1 (5.3 – 23.3)
Cleft lip ± palate	3.2 (2.0 – 5.3)	1.4 (0.8 – 2.5)	3.3 (2.4 – 4.7)
Cleft palate only	2.2 (0.9 – 5.1)*	1.3 (0.6 – 2.9)	2.5 (1.4 – 4.5)
Cardiovascular CA	1.7 (1.3 – 2.3)	1.4 (0.9 – 2.1)	1.7 (1.3 – 2.2)
Total	1.4 (1.3 – 1.6)	-	-

*Unmatched analyses showed OR (95% CI): 2.5 (1.6 – 4.0)
**Influenza and common cold were combined
***During entire pregnancy OR (95% CI): 7.4 (3.9 – 14.0)

At the evaluation of possible association between maternal influenza and neural-tube defects, cleft lip ± cleft palate, cleft palate only, cardiovascular CAs, and congenital cataract, it is necessary to consider and differentiate the possible effect of pathogens (i.e. influenza viruses), symptoms of the disease, particularly high fever, medications and the secondary complications such as malnourishment. In the study by Shien et al [46] influenza viruses did not cross the placenta until late in gestation period, i.e. after the critical period of CAs. In addition, influenza viruses caused fetal death in pregnant animals but not specific CAs. Thus, we may suppose that influenza viruses are not teratogenic. The different drugs used for the treatment for maternal influenza were evaluated in detail but these medications did not indicate any teratogenic effect [25]. In fact they showed an "anti-teratogenic" effect in our studies. The hazards of secondary complications of maternal influenza are difficult to exclude, but they exist in fetuses of all pregnant women and only 5 CAs showed association with maternal influenza. The common factor may be the high fever in the origin of these 5 CA-groups, and this hypothesis is confirmed by the protective effect of antifever drugs.

Hyperthermia-induced CAs were detected first in animal investigations [47, 48], however, later the evidences for human teratogenicity of high fever have been continuing to accumulate. Here only those CAs are mentioned which were found in our study associated with high fever related influenza.

The association between high fever and isolated neural-tube defects was shown [48-60]. The spectrum of high fever related CAs was expanded for cleft palate [61], cleft lip ± palate [62] and cardiovascular CAs [63, 64]. However, to our best knowledge, the association of high fever with congenital cataract [22] and multiple CAs [65] were found by us, in addition we delineated the typical pattern of component CAs in high fever related MCA-syndrome [66].

Previously Botto et al [67] showed that the association of maternal fever with some CAs can be reduced by folic acid containing multivitamins. Our previous studies confirmed that the periconceptional high dose folic acid or folic acid containing multivitamin supplementation can also contribute to the prevention of neural- tube defects, oral clefts and cardiovascular CA due to influenza related hyperthermia [9, 68].

In conclusion, the short duration of influenza in pregnant women did not increase the risk for pregnancy complications. Our study showed that the appropriately treated pregnant women affected with influenza in the first and second trimester of pregnancy have no higher risk for preterm birth. However, the high fever related influenza in the second and/or third gestational month of pregnancy may associate with a higher risk of some - hyperthermia sensitive – CAs such as neural-tube defects, congenital cataract, cleft lip $\pm$ palate, cleft palate only, cardiovascular CAs, and multiple CAs. The main finding of our study is that this higher risk for major CA can be prevented by the parallel use of antifever drugs.

Discussion

The evaluation of acute infectious diseases of respiratory system in pregnant women was differentiated in three approaches.

The first approach included pregnancy complications and our data did not detect any characteristic and clinically important association between maternal common cold, AIDRS, influenza and different pregnancy complications.

The second approach was connected with birth outcomes of newborn infants without CA born to mother with common cold, AIDRS, and influenza during the study pregnancy. Our results were controversial, therefore unexpected. Pregnant women with common cold (mainly with secondary complications), mild upper category of AIDRS and influenza associated with a lower risk for preterm birth. Only the severe lower category of AIDRS associated with a higher risk of preterm birth.

The third and main approach was the estimation the possible association of acute infectious diseases of respiratory system in pregnant women (exactly in the second and/or third gestational months, i.e. the critical period of most major CA) with CAs. Our studies showed some association of certain similar CA with these maternal diseases, namely common cold with secondary complications, tonsillitis and influenza. We suppose that this CA pattern may be associated with the common denominator of these maternal diseases, i.e. high fever.

High temperature may result in arrest of mitotic activity and immediate death of cells in mitosis with threshold elevations (1.5-2.5 Celsius degree) and a delayed death of cells probably in S phase with higher elevation (3.5 or more Celsius degree). Apoptosis is also affected by hyperthermia, in addition high fever may cause micro-vascular disturbances leading to leakage, edema and hemorrhage. These pathological processes may be more obvious in embryos with extreme intensive development, particularly in certain critical locations, such as neural-tube, eyes, face and cardiovascular system .

Of course, the teratogenic effect of maternal fever depends on the severity, duration and timing [68]. Over 40 degrees Celsius, the teratogenic effect of fever is no doubt; however, it is worth calculating a 38.5 degrees Celsius threshold. One or more days seem to be the critical duration of high fever. The timing of high fever determines the risk of specific CAs. If the neuronal cell population cannot recover from the antimitotic insult and heat stress response of high fever, mainly the development of brain is affected. For example if it occurs during the time of neural tube closure (i.e. between 21th and 28th postconceptional days, i.e. third postconceptional week), there is a higher risk for neural-tube defects [68].

"The prevention is better than cure" and we can translate this slogan for the prevention of CA due to high fever related acute infectious diseases of respiratory system in pregnant women. Thus, it is worth recommending the vaccination against influenza for women who are planning their pregnancy during the expected epidemic period. In addition it is necessary to start the antifever therapy as soon as possible in pregnant women with fever related acute infectious diseases of respiratory system. This treatment may include both old-fashioned but not inefficient physical treatment (compress or Priessnitz method) and antifever drugs immediately after the diagnosis of fever related respiratory diseases particularly influenza in pregnancy to prevent the teratogenic hyperthermia. Finally, the periconceptional high dose folic acid or folic acid containing multivitamin supplementation can also contribute to the prevention of neural-tube defects, oral clefts and cardiovascular CA due to fever related hyperthermia [9, 68].

General Conclusions

Maternal diseases are common during pregnancy and some of them (e.g. diabetes mellitus, phenylketonuria) are well-known teratogenic. However, we have to widen the spectrum of these diseases with high fever related maternal diseases such as influenza, tonsillitis, common cold with secondary complications.

In the past the possible teratogenic effect of drugs has been studied frequently but the potential hazards of underlying diseases were rarely evaluated. Our preliminary calculation is that the attributable risk of fever related maternal diseases in the origin of CAs is obviously larger (about 5%) [68] while the attributable risk of all human teratogenic drugs used during pregnancy (2%) [25].

Thus, an important task is to study systematically the teratogenic and/or fetotoxic effect of all maternal diseases during pregnancy.

The teratogenic potential of high fever related maternal diseases is preventable by the reduction or avoidance of teratogenic effect of hyperthermia by the antifever therapy.

References

[1] Goldenberg RL, Culhane JF, Iams JD, Romero R. Epidemiology of preterm birth. *Lancet* 2008; 371: 75-84.

[2] Czeizel AE, Rockenbauer M, Siffel Cs, Varga E. Description and mission evaluation of the Hungarian Case-Control Surveillance of Congenital Abnormalities, 1980-1996. *Teratology* 2001; 63: 176-185.

[3] Czeizel AE. The first 25 years of the Hungarian Congenital Abnormality Registry. *Teratology* 1997; 55: 299-305.

[4] Czeizel AE, Petik D, Vargha P. Validation studies of drug exposures in pregnant women. *Pharmacoepid Drug Safety*. 2003; 12: 409-416.

[5] Czeizel AE, Puho HE, Ács N, Bánhidy F. Use of specified critical periods of congenital abnormalities instead of the first trimester concept. *Birth Def Res Part A* 2008; 82: 139-146.
[6] Czeizel AE. The first trimester concept is outdated. *Cong Anom (Kyoto)* 2001; 41: 204.
[7] Ács N, Bánhidy F, Puho HE, Czeizel AE. Population-based case-control study of the common cold during pregnancy and congenital abnormalities. *Eur J Epidemiol* 2006; 21: 65-75.
[8] Ács N, Bánhidy F, Puho HE, Czeizel AE. Acute respiratory infections during pregnancy and congenital abnormalities. A population-based case-control study. *Cong Anom (Kyoto)* 2006; 46: 86-96.
[9] Ács N, Bánhidy F, Puho HE, Czeizel AE. Maternal influenza during pregnancy and rijk of congenital abnormalities in offspring. *Birth Defects Res Part A* 2005; 73: 989-996.
[10] Czeizel AE. Specified critical period of different congenital abnormalities: A new approach fro human teratological studies. *Cong Anom (Kyoto)* 2008; 48: 103-109.
[11] Czeizel AE, Dudás I. Prevention of the first occurrence of neural-tube defects by periconceptional vitamin supplementation. *N Engl J Med* 1992; 327: 1832-1835.
[12] Czeizel AE. Prevention of congenital abnormalities by periconceptional multivitamin supplementation. *Br Med J* 1993; 306: 1645-1648.
[13] Czeizel AE. Reduction of urinary tract and cardiovascular defects by periconceptional multivitamin supplementation. *Am J Med Genet* 1996, 62: 179-183.
[14] Czeizel AE, Dobó M, Vargha P. Hungarian two-cohort controlled study of periconceptional multivitamin supplementation to prevent certain congenital abnormalities. *Birth Defects Res Part A.* 2004; 70: 853-861.
[15] Botto LD, Olney RS, Erickson JD. Vitamin supplements and the risk for congenital anomalies other than neural tube defects. *Am J Med Genet Part C* 2004; 125C: 12-21.
[16] Rockenbauer M, Czeizel AE, Olsen J et al. Recall bias in a case-control study on the use of medicine during pregnancy. *Epidemiology* 2001; 12: 461-466.
[17] Whitty JE, Dombrowski MP. Respiratory disease in pregnancy. In: Creasy RK, Resnik MD (eds.): *Maternal-Fetal Medicine.* 5th ed. Saunders, Philadelphia, 2004.pp. 953-974.
[18] Silver RM, Peltier MR, Branch DW: The immunology of pregnancy. In: Creasy RK, Resnik MD (eds.): *Maternal-Fetal Medicine.* 5th ed. Saunders, Philadelphia, 2004.pp.89-109.
[19] Makele MJ, Puhakka T, Ruskanen O et al. Viruses and bacteria in the etiology of common cold. *J Clin Microbiol* 1998; 36: 539-542.
[20] Heikkinen T, Jarvinen A. The common cold. *Lancet* 2003; 361: 51-59.
[21] Bánhidy F, Ács N, Puho HE, Czeizel AE. Pregnancy complications and delivery outcomes of pregnant women with common cold. *Cent Eur J Publ Health* 2006; 14: 12-16.
[22] Vogt G, Puhó E, Czeizel AE. Population-based case-control study of isolated congenital cataract. 2005. *Birth Defects Res Part A* 2005; 73: 997-1005.
[23] Roulston A, Marcellus RC, Branton PE. Viruses and apoptosis. *Ann Rec Microbiol* 1999; 53: 577-628.
[24] Heinonen OP, Slope D, Shapiro S. Birth Defects and drugs in Pregnancy. Publishing Sciences Group, Littleton, MA., 1977

[25] Bánhidy F, Lowry RB, Czeizel AE. Risk and benefit of drug use during pregnancy. *Int J Med Sci* 2005; 2: 100-106.

[26] Huang RF, Ho YH, Lin HL et al. Folate deficiency induces a cell-cycle-specific apoptosis in Hep62 cells. *J Nutr* 1999; 129: 25-31.

[27] Kruppa K, Holmberg PC, Kousma E et al. Anencephaly and maternal common cold. *Teratology* 1991; 44: 51-55.

[28] Zhang J, Cai WW. Association of the common cold in the first trimester of pregnancy with birth defects. *Pediatrics* 1993; 92: 559-563.

[29] Remington JS, Klein JO (eds.) Infectious Diseases in the fetus and newborn Infant. 4th ed., W. B. Saunders, Philadelphia.

[30] Hartert TV, Nenzil KM, Mitchel EE et al. Maternal morbidity and perinatal outcomes among pregnant women with respiratory hospitalization during influenza season. *Am J Obstet Gynecol* 2003; 189: 1705-1712.

[31] Bánhidy F, Ács N, Puho HE, Czeizel AE. Maternal acure respiratory infectious diseases during pregnancy and birth outcomes. *Eur J Epidemiol* 2008; 23: 29-35.

[32] Weigel MM, Weigel R. Nausea and vomiting o early pregnancy and pregnancy outcome. An epidemiological study. *Br J Obstet Gynaecol* 1989; 96: 1304-1311.

[33] Czeizel AE, Puho E, Ács N, Bánhidy F. Inverse association between severe nausea and vomiting in pregnancy and some congenital abnormalities. *Am J Med Genet* 2006; 140A: 453-462.

[34] Kazy Z. Puho HE, Czeizel AE. The possible preterm birth preventive effect of ampicillin during pregnancy. *Arch Gynecol* 2006; 274: 215-221.

[35] Madinger NE, Greenspoon JS, Gray-Ellrodt A. Pneumonia during pregnancy: Has modern technology improved maternal and fetal outcome? *Am J Obstet Gynecol* 1989; 161: 657-

[36] Berkovitz K, LaSala A. Risk factors associated with the increasing prevalence of pneumonia during pregnancy. *Am J Obstet Gynecol* 1990; 163: 981-

[37] Benedetti TJ, Valle R, Ledger W. Antepartum pneumonia in pregnancy. *Am J Obstet Gynecol* 1982; 144: 412-

[38] Roberts RB. Infectious Diseases: Pathogenesis, Diagnosis and Therapy. Years Book *Medical Publ, Chicago*, 1986.

[39] Parker MT, Collier LH. Topley Wilson Principle of Bacteriology, *Virology and Immunity.* Decker BC, Hamilton, Ontario, 1990.

[40] Berkow R, Fletchert AJ. The Merck Manual of Diagnosis and Therapy. 16th ed. *Merck and Co Inc*, Rahury, NY, 1992.

[41] Kort BA, Cefalo RC, Baker VV. Fatal influenza A pneumonia in pregnancy. *Am J Perinatol* 1986; 3: 179-

[42] Mullooly JP, Barker WH, Nolan TF Jr. Risk of acute respiratory disease among pregnant women during influenza A epidemics. *Publ Health Rep* 1986; 101: 205-

[43] Harris JW. Influenza occurring in pregnant women. *Am J Med Ass* 1919; 72: 978-

[44] Freeman DW, Barno A. Death from Asian influenza associated with pregnancy. *Am J Obstet Gynecol* 1959; 78: 1172-

[45] Ács N, Bánhidy F, Puho E, Czeizel AE. Pregnancy complications and delivery outcomes of pregnant women with influenza. *J Mat-Fetal Neonat Med* 2006; 19: 135-140.

[46] Shien JH, Shiota K. Folic acid supplementation of pregnant mice suppresses heat-induced neural-tube defects in offspring. *J Nutr* 1999; 129: 2070-2073.

[47] Edwards MJ. Hyperthermia as a teratogen: A review of experimental studies and their clinical significance. *Terat Carcinog Mutag* 1986; 6: 563-582.

[48] Edwards MJ, Shiota K, Walsh DA, Smith MS. Hyperthermia and birth defects. *Reprod Toxicol* 1995; 411-425.

[49] Chance PF, Smith DW. Hyperthermia and meningomyelocele and anencephaly. *Lancet* 1978; 1: 769-770

[50] Halperin LR, Wilroy RS Jr. Maternal hyperthermia and neural-tube defects. *Lancet* 1978; 212-213.

[51] Miller P, Smith DW, Shepard TH. Hyperthermia as one possible etiology of anencephaly. *Lancet* 1978; 1: 519-521.

[52] Clarren SK, Smith DW, Harvey MAS, et al. Hyperthermia: A prospective evaluation of a possible teratogenic agent in man. *J Pediatr* 1979; 95: 81-83.

[53] Layde PM, Edmonds LD, Erickson JD. Maternal fever and neural tube defects. *Teratology* 1980; 21: 105-108.

[54] Fisher NL, Smith DW. Occipital encephalocele and early gestational hyperthermia. *Pediatrics* 1981; 68: 480-483.

[55] Shiota K. Neural-tube defects and maternal hyperthermia in early pregnancy. Epidemiology in a human embryo population. *Am J Med Genet* 1982; 12: 281-288.

[56] Hunter AGW. Neural tube defects in eastern Ontario and western Quebec: Demography and family data. *Am J Med Genet* 1984; 19: 45-63.

[57] Milunsky A, Ulcickas M, Rothman KJ et al. Maternal heat exposure and neural-tube defects. *J Am Med Ass* 1992; 268: 882-885.

[58] Lynberg MC, Khoury MJ, Lu X, Cocian T. Maternal flu, fever and the risk of neural-tube defects: a population-based case-control study. *Am J Epidemiol* 1994; 140: 244-255.

[59] Shaw GM, Todoroff K, Velie EM, Lammer EJ. Maternal illness, including fever, and medication use as risk factors of neural-tube defects. *Teratology* 1998; 57: 1-7.

[60] Medveczky E, Puhó E, Czeizel AE. The evaluation of maternal illnesses in the origin of neural-tube defects. *Arch Obstet Gynec* 2004, 207: 244-251.

[61] Smith DW, Clarren SK, Harrey MA. Hyperthermia as a possible teratogenic agent. *J Pediatr* 1978; 92: 878-883.

[62] Métneki J, Puhó E, Czeizel AE. Maternal diseases and isolated orofacial clefts in Hungary. *Birth Defects Res Part A* 2005; 73: 617-623.

[63] Tikkanen J, Heinonen OP. Maternal hyperthermia during pregnancy and cardiovascular malformations in the offspring. *Eur J Epidemiol* 1991; 7: 628-635.

[64] Botto LD, Lynberg MC, Erickson JD. Congenital heart defects, maternal febrile illness, and multivamin use: a population-based study. *Epidemiology* 2001; 12: 485-490.

[65] Czeizel AE, Puho HE, Ács N, Bánhidy F. High fever-related maternal diseases as possible cause of multiple congenital abnormalities: A population-based case-control study. *Birth Defects Res Part A* 2007; 79: 544-551.
[66] Czeizel AE, Puho HE, Ács N, Bánhidy F. The delineation of a multiple congenital abnormality syndrome in the offspring of pregnant women with high fever related disorders – a population-based study. *Cong Anom (Kyoto)* 2008; 48: 158-166.
[67] Botto LD, Erickson JD, Mulinare J et al. Maternal fever, multivitamin use and selected birth defects: evidence or interaction. *Epidemiology* 2002; 13: 620-621.
[68] Czeizel AE, Ács N, Bánhidy F et al. Primary prevention of congenital abnormalities due to high fever related maternal diseases by antifever therapy and folic acid supplementation. *Current Woman's Health* 2007; 3: 1-12.

In: Handbook of Down Syndrome Research
Editors: Dominicus Jelinek and Gijs Dvorak

ISBN 978-1-60741- 690-6

Chapter 7

Mitochondrial Function in Down Syndrome

Anna Gvozdjáková*[*1], Jarmila Kucharská[1], Zuzana Sumbalová[1], Richard Kvetňanský[2], Miroslav Mikulecký[3], Boris Mravec[2,4], and Ram B Singh[5]

[1]Comenius University, Medical Faculty, Pharmacobiochemical Laboratory of Third Medical Clinic, Bratislava, Slovakia
[2]Institute of Experimental Endocrinology, Slovak Academy of Sciences, Bratislava, Slovakia
[3]Department of Statistics and Biometry, Neuroendocrinology Letters, Stockholm-Sweden and Bratislava-Slovakia;
BioCos, University of Minnesota, Minneapolis, MN, USA
[4]Comenius University, Medical Faculty, Institute of Pathophysiology, Bratislava, Slovakia
[5]Halberg Hospital and Research Institute, Moradabad UP, India

Abstract

This chapter guides readers through mitochondrial physiology, mitochondrial medicine and possible adjunctive therapy in Down syndrome (DS), and generally in neurodegenerative diseases. DS is an inherited disease with an extra copy of chromosome 21, and the onset of Alzheimer's disease by middle age. Mitochondrial dysfunction and oxidative damage have been implicated in the pathogenesis of DS, ageing and generally in neurodegenerative diseases.

Brain mitochondrial coenzyme "Q-CLOCK" as well as circadian cascade of oxidative phosphorylation presented in this chapter can contribute to the explanation of brain mitochondrial diseases.

* Corresponding address: Anna Gvozdjáková Comenius University, Medical Faculty, Pharmacobiochemical Laboratory of Third Medical Clinic, Hlboká 7, 811 05 Bratislava, Slovakia, Email: anna.gvozdjakova@stonline.sk, Q10@Q10.sk, Phone/fax: +421 2 5249 1422.

Documented bioavailability of liposomal coenzyme Q_{10} in rats brain nuclei, tissue and mitochondria could be beneficial for the adjunctive therapy at the condition of damaged brain mitochondrial energy production and oxidative stress in patients with Down syndrome.

1. Mitochondrial Physiology

Mitochondria are small granules in cells, similar in their shape and size to bacteria. The quantity of cell mitochondria depends on the function of the cell and the energy demand of the organs. Thrombocyte contain between two and six mitochondria, most organs contain between 500 and 2,000 mitochondria/cell, however the oocyte possesses close to 100,000 mitochondria. Brain mitochondria are the main energy producer for neuronal cells function. Dysfunction of brain mitochondria is one of the major factors participating in the mitochondrial diseases of central and peripheral nervous systems.

1.1. Mitochondrial Architecture

Mitochondria consist of four compartments:

1 *Outer mitochondrial membrane (OMM)* separates cytosol from intermembrane space. The OMM participates in the import protein from cytosol to the mitochondrial interior. Smaller molecules can diffuse to the intermembrane space, larger molecules are transported into the intermembrane space and matrix [1]. Proteins from the matrix are transported across the inner and outer mitochondrial membrane through two complexes: *TIM* (complex of transport inner membrane) *TOM* (complex of transport outer membrane) [2, 3] via the TIM/TOM complex located at contact sites [4]. Contact sites are called the *mitochondrial permeability transition pore (MPTP),* their activation leads to membrane depolarization. Mitochondria move within a cell and this mobility is essential for the distribution and function of mitochondria within a cell as well as during cells division and differentiation [5]. Mitochondrial fusion is mediated by guanosine triphosphatases (GTPases). Mitochondrial fission requires a large GTPase, named the dynamic-like protein (DLP1), [6].

2 *Inner mitochondrial membrane (IMM)* separates the intermembrane space from the matrix. The folding of the IMM increase the surface area of this membrane. Inner mitochondrial membrane represent five complexes of the electron transport respiratory chain (Complex I-IV), and ATP-synthase complex (Complex V – F_1F_o-ATP-ase).

3 *Intermembrane space* contains a mobile electron carrier for the mitochondrial respiratory chain – cytochrome c. The release of cytochrome c into the cytosol iniciates caspase-dependent apoptosis activation.

4 *Matrix* contains the machinery necessary to transcribe and translate the 13 proteins of oxidative phosphorylation. Several metabolic pathways are located in the matrix: pyruvate dehydrogenase complex (PDHC) - oxidation of pyruvate to acetyl CoA,

further oxidation to ketone bodies, amino acids, initiation of the urea acid cycle, fatty acid oxidation, Krebs cycle, import of proteins, heme synthesis as well as suppression of free radical damage through manganese-superoxide dismutase (Mn-SOD).

1.2. Mitochondrial Genetics and Energy Metabolism

Mitochondria serve as centers of genetic information. They have own double-stranded circular mitochondrial deoxyribonucleic acid (mtDNA), encoding 13 compounds of the four respiratory chain Complexes (I, II, IV, and V).

Mitochondria serve as central of intermediary metabolism: oxidative phosphorylation, fatty acid oxidation, Krebs cycle, gluconeogenesis, urea cycle, ketogenesis. Mitochondria are one of the main sites of the reactive oxygen radicals production, they play a crucial role in apoptosis.

Mitochondria are the main energy producers in the body from carbohydrates, fats and proteins. Five protein complexes (Complex I – V) of the respiratory chain are located in the inner mitochondrial membrane. Mobile components of the respiratory chain are coenzyme Q and cytochrome c. Coenzyme Q can occur in oxidized form (ubiquinone - Q), reduced form (ubiquinol - QH_2) and radical form ($Q^{\cdot}$), called "Q-CYCLE". Complexes I – IV receive electrons from the catabolism of carbohydrates, fats and proteins. Complex I and II collect these electrons, transfer them to coenzyme Q_{10}, Complex III and Complex IV. The redox energy released during the electron transfer process in Complex I, III and IV is utilized to actively pump out H^+ from the mitochondrial matrix to the intermembrane space, generating the *electrochemical gradient of* H^+ ($\Delta\mu H^+$) across the inner membrane and is utilized by Complex V (ATPase) to produce ATP [7, 10]. $\Delta\mu H^+$ is known as proton-motive force, which includes *the membrane potential* ($\Delta\Psi$) and *proton gradient* (ΔpH). The produced ATP is translocated from the mitochondria into cytoplasm by adenine nucleotide translocase [8, 9]. Flow electrons and protons are translated from the matrix into the intermembrane space.

1.3. Mitochondrial ROS, NOS and Antioxidants

A small portion (up to 2%) of electrons passing through the electron transport chain, mostly at complex I and III react with molecular oxygen and yield superoxide anion ($O_2^{\cdot -}$), which occurs on the outer mitochondrial membrane, in the matrix and on the both sides of the inner mitochondrial membranes. In the brain under physiological conditions, mitochondrial Complex I appears to be a primary source of $O_2^{\cdot -}$ and hydroxyl radical ($OH^{\cdot}$). Superoxide anion can be converted into other *reactive oxygen species (ROS)* such as hydrogen peroxide (H_2O_2), which is produced by activity of the mitochondrial matrix enzyme manganese-dependent superoxide dismutase (MnSOD) or by cuprum- and zinc-dependent superoxide dismutase (CuZnSOD) in the intermembrane space.

The amount of produced ROS in physiological and pathological conditions is regulated by Ca^{2+}. These radicals are normal products of oxidative processes and it is believed that they have physiological function as signaling molecules. However, radicals may be harmful when they are produced in increased amounts, when a dynamic balance between ROS production and endogenous antioxidants systems function is disturbed. They can potentially damage various types of macromolecules, including lipids, proteins and nucleic acids. These damages are referred as "oxidative stress", and have been implicated in ageing and various pathological processes.

Nitric oxide (NO) regulates several systems in the organism, e.g. the central nervous system, cardiovascular system, immune system. Mitochondria are important targets of NO, contribute to its several biological functions. It is suggested that NO play an important role in Aβ - induced mitochondrial dysfunction cell death. NO is produced in vivo in the oxidation of L-arginine to L-citruline in a reaction catalyzed by NADPH-dependent enzymes called *nitric oxide synthases (NOS).* Four isoforms of NOS were discovered. Two of them are constitutive or normally present: *neuronal NOS (nNOS), endothelial NOS (eNOS), inductible NOS (iNOS),* typical of macrophages. The fourth isoform is *mitochondrial NOS (mtNOS).*

Mitochondria produce NO through Ca^{2+}-sensitive mitochondrial NO synthase (mtNOS). The NO produced by mtNOS regulates mtiochondrial oxygen consumption and transmembrane potential via reversible reaction with cytochrome c oxidase. NO decreases mitochondrial oxygen consumption, the electrochemical gradient, proton gradient, resulting in decreased ATP formation. MtNOS activity in the brain is modulated by hypoxia. Modulated coordination of mtNOS and mitochondrial Mn-superoxide dismutase (SOD2) activity, localized in matrix, contributes to establish the rat brain redox status and participate in the normal physiology of brain development [11]. MtNOS is a crucial biochemical regulator of mitochondrial function [10, 12, 13, 14].

Several *antioxidants* prevent mitochondria from oxidative stress.

a/ Coenzyme Q (QH – ubiquinol) – as antioxidant interferes with the propagation of free radical-mediated chain reactions, eliminates various peroxides in the presence of succinate.

b/ Cytochrome c, respiratory chain electron carrier, has detoxifying role against ROS.

c/ Superoxide dismutase (SOD): Superoxide anion is enzymatically converted to H_2O_2 by a family of metalloenzymes – superoxide dismutases (SODs). The role of SODs is to increase the rate of the reaction of a diffusion-controlled process. The mitochondrial matrix contains a specific form of SOD, MnSOD, which eliminates $O_2^{\cdot -}$ formed in the matrix or on the inner side of the inner membrane. Steady-state concentration of superoxide radical in the intermembrane space is controlled by Cu/ZnSOD, by cytochrome c and by the lower pH [15].

1. 4. Brain Mitochondrial Coenzyme "Q-CLOCK"

Coenzyme Q_{10} (CoQ_{10}, ubiquinone) is a crucial mobile component of the respiratory chain of the inner mitochondrial membrane. The dominant human form of coenzyme Q is CoQ_{10}, the dominant rats form is CoQ_9. The central role of human form of CoQ_{10} is the electron transport and proton transfer between Complex I and Complex III, and between Complex II and Complex III. The global functions of CoQ_{10} are in cellular ATP production, "redox poise" (ratio reduced to oxidized form), metabolic flux modulation, gene regulation and oxygen radicals production [16]. CoQ_{10} levels in plasma, tissues and heart mitochondria show biological circadian or circasemidian rhythms [17, 18, 19, 20, 21].

The mechanisms of brain physiological and pathological function that show circadians or circasemidians are not fully known. In our experimental study were used three-months-old Wistar rats. They were synchronized during 60 days to 12 hours dark spans vy Halberg's antiphasic lighting regimens. One regimen LD 12:12 was shifted to sample in the dark during waking hours. 24- and 12-hours periodicities were tested by Halberg's cosinor [73] with the presentation of results based on the confidence and tolerance estimates [74, 75]. Original software [76] was used for the calculations and drawings. In isolated brain mitochondria, CoQ_{10} and CoQ_9 levels were estimated by HPLC with UV detection. The activity of oxidative phosphorylation for Complex I and II of respiratory chain function was determined using Clark oxygen electrode.

This pilot study shown brain mitochondrial circasemidian (12 h) or circadian (24 h) rhythms showed maximum - PEAKS for $CoQ_{10\text{-}OX}$ at 19:24 h and 7:28 h, minimum – NADIRS at 14: 04 h and 1:03 h. PEAKS for $CoQ_{9\text{-}OX}$ were at 18:48 h and 7:57 h, minimum – NADIRS at 14:14 h and 1:03 h. Nocturnal activity of rats was between 22:00 – 10:00 h, diurnal inactivity was between 10:00 – 22:00 h. It is known that biorhythms in humans are opposite to those in rats, due to the inverted day-time regimen of life. "Q-CLOCK" in brain mitochondria of control rats is shown in Fig 1, table 1.

Table 1. Circadian variations of coenzyme Q in mitochondria of control rat brain

Hours	08:00	12:00	16:00	20:00	24:00	04:00
$CoQ_{10\text{-}ox}$ (nmol/mg prot.)	0.518	0.279	0.344	0.346	0.255	0.338
$CoQ_{9\text{-}ox}$ (nmol/mg prot.)	1.188	0.669	0.719	0.773	0.631	0.803
$CoQ_{10\text{-}ox} + CoQ_{9\text{-}ox}$ (nmol/mg prot.)	1.706	0.948	1.063	1.119	0.886	1.141

Brain mitochondrial "Q-CLOCK" changes may play an important role in the pathogenesis of altered brain function and in mitochondrial diseases of the brain.

1. 5. Circadian Cascade of Brain Mitochondrial Oxidative Phosphorylation

Circadian variations of oxidative phosphorylation showed different times of oxidative phosphorylation parameters at Complex I and Complex II: ADP:O – coefficient of oxidative phosphorylation, OPR – rate of ATP production, S_3 – ADP-stimulated respiration, S_4 – basal respiration, RCI – respiratory control index. These variations exhibited two circadian maxima and two minima of oxidative phosphorylation activity of brain mitochondria of control rats (Table 2).

Table 2. Circadian variations of oxidative phosphorylation in mitochondria of control rat brain

	Hours	08:00	12:00	16:00	20:00	24:00	04:00
Complex I:							
ADP:O (nmol ADP/nAtO)		2.89	2.89	2.53	2.54	2.77	2.51
OPR (nmol ATP/mg prot./min)		167.83	112.62	101.91	105.00	105.00	100.80
S_3 (nAtO/mg prot.)		75.19	54.85	46.08	52.10	48.93	52.35
S_4 (nAtO/mg prot.)		38.80	27.12	24.19	24.00	25.06	24.72
RCI (S_3/S_4)		1.94	2.02	1.90	2.17	1.95	2.18
Complex II:							
ADP:O (nmol ADP/nAtO)		1.29	1.27	0.00	1.29	1.49	0.00
OPR (nmol ATP/mg prot./min)		166.00	101.12	0.00	105.07	125.61	0.00
S_3 (nAtO/mg prot.)		165.00	105.10	123.84	105.23	131.56	145.43
S_4 (nAtO/mg prot.)		141.20	86.55	123.84	86.08	115.22	145.43
RCI (S_3/S_4)		1.17	1.22	1.00	1.22	1.15	1.00

Complex I: Maximum OXPHOS activity (circasemidian PEAK I – 12 hours) is between 5:36 and 10:45 hours (lasting 5.09 hours) – rat inactivity, and (circadian PEAK II – 24 hours) between 20:00 and 23:04 hours (lasting 3.04 hours) – rat activity. Minimum of OXPHOS activity NADIR I is between 12:48 and 17:40 hours (lasting 4.08 hours) and NADIR II between 0:05 and 4:35 hours (lasting 4.30 hours).

Table 3. Complex I: Circasemidian (12 hours) and circadian (24 hours) cascade of oxidative phosphorylation of control brain rats

PEAK I (12 hours):	PEAK II (24 hours):
RCI at 5:36 hours	RCI at 20:00 hours
OPR at 8:14 hours	S_4 at 20:01 hours
S_3 at 8:25 hours	S_3 at 20:11 hours
S_4 at 8:43 hours	OPR at 20:29 hours
ADP:O at 10:45 hours	ADP:O at 23:04 hours

Complex II: Maximum of OXPHOS activity of circasemidian (PEAK I – 12 hours) is between: 10:02 and 18:55 hours (lasting 8.53 hours) – rat inactivity and circadian (PEAK II – 24 hours) from 22:02 to 5:36 hours (lasting 7.34 hours) – rat activity. Minimum (NADIR I and II) of OXPHOS activity is between 12:30 and 16:09 hours (lasting 3.39 hours) and between 22:13 and 4:24 hours (lasting 6.11 hours).

Table 4. Complex II: Circasemidian (12 hours) and circadian (24 hours) cascade of oxidative phosphorylation of control rat brain

PEAK I (12 hours)	PEAK II (24 hours):
RCI at 10:02 hours	OPR at 22:02 hours
ADP:O at 10:02 hours	RCI at 22:03 hours
OPR at 10:38 hours	ADP:O at 22:17 hours
S_4 at 16:53 hours	S_3 at 23:29 hours
S_3 at 18:55 hours	S_4 at 5:36 hours

Decreased 12-hour brain mitochondrial respiratory chain function and ATP production between 16:00 and 20:00 hours and uncoupling effect in Complex II at 16:00 and 4:00 hours, as well as "Q-CLOCK" changes, may be important in the pathogenesis of altered brain function. Understanding of the brain mitochondrial "Q-CLOCK" and ATP production during circasemidian and circadian rhythms can contribute to the explanation of mechanisms triggering an acute brain and heart attack [17-21].

2. Mitochondrial Medicine

Mitochondrial Medicine includes clinical, biochemical, electron microscopy and genetic evaluation important for diagnosis and treatment of mitochondrial diseases. The first mitochondrial disorder was demonstrated by Luft in 1959 – 1962, and it was termed Luft's disease. In isolated mitochondria of human subject striated muscle uncoupling of oxidative phosphorylation was found. The high level of cytochrome c oxidase, relatively low level of coenzyme Q_{10}, and high content of RNA in muscle homogenate was evidence for mitochondrial protein synthesis. Electron microscopy showed large accumulations of mitochondria, with highly variable size and with paracrystalline inclusions, possibly composed of lipofuscin granules [22]. An outline of the development of mitochondrial medicine was for the first time published by Luft in 1994 [23].

2.1. Mitochondrial Diseases

Mitochondrial diseases are associated with low energy production, increased free radical production and lactic acidosis. Some mitochondrial diseases affect only one tissue, most often skeletal muscle, brain, heart, liver, kidneys or endocrine glands. Other organs may be involved secondarily. Mitochondrial diseases of central nervous system include: sometimes dementia, seizures, ataxia, myoclonus, psychomotor retardation, psychomotor regression, hemiparesis/hemianopia, cortical blindness, migraine-like headaches, dystonia, short stature. In peripheral nervous system was documented neuropathy. In skeletal muscle: fatigue, myopathy, weakness, exercise intolerance, loss of coordination and balance, in skeletal muscle biopsy ragged-red fibers are present. In eyes: ptosis, external ophthalmoplegia, cataracts, retinis pigmentosa with visual loss, optic atrophy, in ear – hearing loss. In blood:

sideroblastic anemia. Other clinical features involved in mitochondrial diseases are e.g. gastrointestinal (constipation, acid reflux, vomiting), hepatopathies, liver failure, kidneys – Fanconi's syndrome (loss of essential metabolites in urine), pancreatic diseases – diabetes, sperm defects – mitochondrial "spermatopathy" [8, 24].

Causes of Mitochondrial Diseases are Primary or Secondary

A primary cause of mitochondrial diseases is in a genetic level. It is a defect in nuclear DNA (nDNA*)* encoding for mitochondrial protein (defects of respiratory chain subunits, mitochondrial motility and importation, mitochondrial transcription or translation) or in mitochondrial DNA (mtDNA) mutations (mitochondrial protein synthesis, protein-coding genes). A number of diseases with mutations in the mtDNA have been linked to dysfunction of mitochondrial respiratory chain function and ATP production, of fatty acid oxidation and other metabolic pathways [25]. Mutation of mtDNA was first documented in neurodegenerative disorders [26].

Secondary causes of mitochondrial diseases are brought on by factors such as ischemia, reperfusion, cardiovascular diseases, renal failure, pancreatic and hepatic damage, diabetes, infectious agents, gastrointestinal diseases, oncological diseases, alcohol, smoking, stress, drugs and aging.

The following syndromes are important for the understanding of mitochondrial medicine: *KSS – (Kearns-Sayre Syndrome*) with ophthalmoplegia, retinal pigmental degeneration, sometimes heart block, ataxia, hyperparathyroidism and short stature. There is a defect in coenzyme Q metabolism in KSS and it becomes manifest before the age of 20 years. *MERRF* – (myoclonic epilepsy and ragged red fibers syndrome) with intense myoclonus, epilepsy, progressive ataxia, muscle weakness and wasting, deafness, and dementia. Maternal inheritance and reduced activities of Complexes I and IV are established in MERRF. *MELAS* – (mitochondrial myopathy, encephalomyopathy, lactic acidosis, and stroke-like episodes) with episodic vomiting, lactic acidosis, and myopathy with ragged red fibers, sometimes dementia, generalized seizures, deafness, and short stature. Reduced activities in Complexes I and IV are established. *CPEO* – (chronic progressive external ophthalmoplegia) with signs and symptoms similar to those in KSS but in addition there is retinitis pigmentosa and CNS dysfunction. *LHON* – (Leber's hereditary optic neuropathy) with optic atrophy and retinal microangiopathy, and in some patients movement disorders, bulbar dysfunction, EEG abnormalities and short stature. Maternal inheritance and reduced activity of Complex I are well established in LHON. The manifestations appear at the age of 12 – 30 years. *Leigh´s syndrome* with subacute necrotizing encephalomyopathy and early childhood degeneration (with respiratory abnormalities, weak cry, impaired feeding, vision, and hearing, ataxia, weakness, and hypotension). Reduced activities of Complexes I or IV are established in Leigh's syndrome and may be associated in some cases with pyruvate dehydrogenase complex deficiency. *Pearson's syndrome*, a systemic disorder of oxidative phosphorylation in infants, predominantly affecting the bone marrow and pancreas, with death early in the course of the disease from complications of bone marrow failure and repeated transfusions. *Alpers´syndrome* or progressive infantile poliodystrophy, with seizures, dementia, spasticity, blindness and liver dysfunction accompanied by specific cerebral degeneration [65].

2.2. Mitochodrial Dysfunction of the Brain

Mitochondria contribute near 90% of the required energy for cellular functions by two linked metabolic processes: the citric acid cycle (anaerobic) and electron respiratory chain (aerobic). Under physiological conditions the brain has low levels of stored glycogen and is highly dependent on oxidative metabolism. Glucose is the primary energy substrate and brain cells metabolize ketones during fasting reductions of blood glucose. Ketone bodies (acetoacetate, and β/hydroxybutyrate) are derived from fatty acids oxidation in the liver. Fatty acid oxidation in brain is limited. They are transported into the brain through the blood-brain barrier via monocarboxylic transporters. The basal rate of glucose utilization in astrocytes is higher than in neurons. Glucose taken up by astrocytes is high than in neurons, is metabolized to lactate glycolytically, which is then released in the extracellular space to be utilized by neurons. Lactate, which is characteristically found in the brain, can serve as an energy source of the brain function through pyruvate by lactate dehydrogenase. Pyruvate is another important energy substrate abundantly distributed in brain synapses. Most of the brain energy production in form of ATP via oxidative phosphorylation is located in neuronal cells. Other brain glial cells and vascular endothelial cells active participate in the flux of energy substrates to neuron [14].

Mitochondrial dysfunction plays a crucial role in neurology. Causes of brain mitochondrial disorders can be found on molecular level. Mutations can be in mitochondrial DNA (mtDNA) or nuclear DNA (nDNA) - inherited disease. Brain mitochondrial disorders on metabolic level can be associated with aging. Pathogenesis of mitochondrial diseases involves dysfunction of ATP production, which is important for life and death, apoptosis, reactive oxygen species production and for calcium homeostasis. Brain mitochondrial oxidative phosphorylation dysfunction and genetic disorders have major deleterious effects on mitochondrial dynamics, such as motility, fission, fusion and distribution. In the nervous system, mitochondrial dynamics are crucial for long distance distribution of energy [24].

2.3. Mitochondrial Dysfunction of Down Syndrome and Neurodegenerative Diseases

Down´s syndrome (DS) or trisomy 21 is the most common chromosomal abnormality, the most common genetic cause of mental retardation, it is an inherited disease with onset prior to birth. Children with Down syndrome have an extra copy of chromosome 21, results in an extra gene for cytoplasmic superoxide dismutase (Cu/Zn SOD), with excessive activity of Cu/Zn SOD [27]. This extra chromosome causes "over expression" of genes that change metabolism and function of antioxidants, amino acids, digestive enzymes, and other essential nutrients [28].

The neuropathology of DS is complex and includes decreased brain weight, decreased neuronal number, abnormal neuronal differentiation, and structural changes in dentritic spines. DS caused by trisomy 21 is associated with an increased incidence of congenital anomalies, neurodevelopmental impairment and accelerated ageing. DS include several deficiencies, such as immune deficiencies and dysfunction, cataract formation, hearing-loss, skin atrophy and Alzheimer s type –neuropathology [29].

The gene associated with collagen (connective tissue) overexpression is located on the 21st chromosome and may be responsible for the presence of hypotonia issues common in Down syndrome. By the third decade, subjects with DS manifest neuronal pathology resembling Alzheimer's disease, with developing dementia. Although the gene(s) responsible for the neuropathology associated with DS have not yet been fully characterized, the development of AD in DS may be related to the over expression of the amyloid beta precursor protein (Aβ PP) due to increased gene dosage, leading to increased Aβ generation.

Aging is a biological complex of progressively decreasing metabolic processes, decreasing energy production and physiological functions of the organism. In aging also ultrastructural mitochondrial changes are involved. Mitochondria become larger and less numerous with vacuolization, crystal rupture and the accumulation of intramitochondrial paracrystalline inclusions. Cytochrome c oxidase deficiency in cardiomyocytes of the aged human heart was first demonstrated in 1989 [30]. Histochemical analysis of muscle fibers from elderly subjects has been shown to be associated with very high levels of mutant mtDNA. Free radical accumulation contributes to the progression of changes during aging. Accumulated oxidative damage of mtDNA, proteins and lipids could play a causal role in the aging process. As biomarker of oxidative damage 8-hydroxy-2′-deoxyguanosine (OH_8dG) is used, which is accumulated with age in mtDNA of the human brain and heart [31].

Mitochondrial dysfunction and free radical-induced oxidative damage have been implicated in the pathogenesis of several different neurodegenerative diseases such as Alzheimer's disease, Parkinson's disease, Huntington's disease, amyotrophic lateral sclerosis. The defective ATP production and increased oxygen radicals may induce cell death, therefore mitochondria are not able to maintain energy demand of the cell [32].

Alzheimer´s Disease

Alzheimer's disease (AD) is a neurodegenerative disorder characterized by an age-dependent loss of memory and impairment of multiple cognitive functions. AD is inherited only in 2% of cases, genetic mutations are responsible for causing "familial AD", early-onset AD. In *early-onset* AD, genetic mutations are in genes, concerning beta-amyloid precursor protein (βAPP), which accelerates the disease process, or the proteins preselinin 1 (PS1) or presenilin 2 (PS2) are involved. Presenilins interact with β-catenin to form presenilin complexes. The role of presenilins leading to AD development is not quite clear [33]. Mutations in the human presenilin gene probably play a role in oxidative stress. Increased expression of presenilins increases DNA fragmentation and produces apoptotic changes, which are important consequences of oxidative damage. Oxidative stress plays an important role in AD pathogenesis [34, 69, 71]. Most AD cases are "sporadic", *late-onset* AD. In familiar form of AD have been identified three genes: amyloid precursor protein (APP), presenilin 1 (PS1) and presenilin 2 (PS2). Recently have been found a neuronal sortilin-related receptor (SORL1), which is genetically associated with Alzheimer disease [35]. During progression of AD, brain energy metabolism is impaired. Increased production of free radicals induces interruption of brain mitochondrial oxidative phosphorylation and impairs energy homeostasis. Mitochondrial dysfunction in neurodegenerative disorders may contribute to the pathogenesis of Alzheimer's disease [1, 3, 68, 70].

AD is associated with the accumulation of intracellular neurofibrilary tangles (NFTs), consisting mainly of hyperphosphorylated forms of the microtubule-associated protein tau [36, 37] and extracellular accumulation of β-amyloid protein (Aβ). Accumulation of Aβ proteins increase the accumulation of ROS, especially H_2O_2, induce membrane lipid peroxidation [29] and impairs of mitochondrial respiratory chain, which leads to mitochondrial membrane depolarization and mitochondrial permeability transition pore (MPTP) induction. Opening of MPTP could contribute to Ca^{2+} and cytochrome c release from mitochondria. Cytochrome c release supports activation of the caspase cascade and can thus induce cell death (apoptosis). Decline of mitochondrial enzyme activity was reported in AD patients: the pyruvate dehydrogenase complex, the alpha-keto glutarate dehydrogenase complex, and cytochrome c oxidases are affected.

Aβ also interacts with glia cells. Elevation of Ca^{2+} concentration increases the activity of nitric oxide synthase (NOS), resulting in nitric oxide radical ($NO^{\cdot}$) production, which interacts with superoxide radical ($O_2^{\cdot-}$). Elevation of Ca^{2+} concentration and of free radicals contributes to the damage of proteins, lipids and DNA. Aβ proteins may be a trigger in mitochondrial energy dysfunction via increasing ROS production.

The exact mechanisms of how Aβ damages the neurons are still unknown. Petersen at al., 2008 [3] showed that presequence protease (PreP) is responsible for the degradation of the accumulated Aβ in mitochondria. Accumulation of Aβ has been detected in mitochondria. Authors presented an unique import mechanism for Aβ in mitochondria and demonstrated that Aβ is located to the mitochondrial cristae. Authors suggest that Aβ can be internalized by cells, imported into mitochondria via the TOM complex, and accumulated in the cristae. Mitochondrial function can be negatively affected by Aβ.

Deficit in mitochondrial function cause selective neuronal degeneration and may be involved in a number of neurodegenerative disorders [25]. Mitochondrial DNA repair is impaired after oxidative damage in DS fibroblasts. DS cortical neurons in culture exhibit intracellular accumulation of ROS and increased lipid peroxidation leading to neuronal apoptosis.

Alterations in mitochondrial energy metabolism may be directly associated with oxidative stress and apoptosis in DS. Energy depletion and oxidative stress can also induce amyloidogenic changes in AβPP processing, suggesting a potential link between mitochondrial dysfunction, oxidative stress and Aβ production. Dysfunction of mitochondrial electron transport proteins and close relationship between mitochondrial abnormalities and oxidative damage have been described in AD brains [38]. Other cause of mitochondrial dysfunction in the human AD brain was presented as the progressive blockade protein import channels by APP [66]. Morphometric analysis showed that mitochondria are significantly reduced in AD. Authors findings show major abnormalities in mitochondrial vulnerable neurons, suggesting an intimate relationship between mitochondria and oxidative damage in AD. Findings suggest that mitochondrial dysfunction may play a significant role in the development of AD neuropathology in DS patients by promoting aberrant AβPP processing and intracellular accumulation of Aβ [38]. Chronic AβPP over expression in DS may impair mitochondrial function. Which in turn increases intracellular accumulation of Aβ and reduces secretion of neuroprotective AβPPs. Impaired mitochondrial function could result from direct toxic effects of Aβ or from metabolic cost of clearing aggregated proteins through chaperones and degradative apparatus, processes that are highly energy dependent. Chronic protein aggregation in these diseases may lead to a state impaired mitochondrial function and ATP depletion [28].

Parkinson´s Disease

Parkinson's diseases (PD) is a neurodegenrative disorder characterized by the loss of dopaminergic neurons of the substantia nigra, with reduction of dopamine in the striatum. At 60% depletion of dopaminergic neurons in the substantia nigra and 80% dopamine content in the striatum, symptoms of PD appear (tremor, abnormal movements, instability, rigidity) [40]. The implication of oxidative stress as a major factor in the pathogenesis of PD is accepted. Abnormally high levels of brain tissue iron of PD patients may serve as an important generator of reactive oxygen species [25]. The etiology and metabolism in Parkinson's disease progression is unknown. In early-onset PD, mutations of various genes were documented, which may damage mitochondrial function and stimulate neurodegeneration. In platelet mitochondria of PD patients, Complex I activity was reduced [41]. Inhibition of Complex I activity may play a pathogenic role in some patients with PD [42]. Mitochondrial abnormalities contribute to the initiation and progression of PD.

Huntington´s Disease

Huntington's disease (HD) is a hereditary neurodegenerative disorder, characterized by degeneration of basal ganglia. Symptoms of HD include chorea, gradual inability to control movements, psychological, cognitive impairment and dementia. The age of onset is variable but usually in the fourth decade of life, with death within 10 – 15 years. Strong evidence from studies suggests the involvement of oxidative stress, energy metabolism defects, which can contribute to the altered gene regulation [43, 44]. The mutant gene – huntingtin – was identified. The exact function of huntingtin is not yet known, but mutant protein may interfere with mitochondrial energy production. Mitochondrial dysfunction has been identified as a pathologic factor in HD, impairment of Complexes II and III was found in basal ganglia homogenates from HD patients [45].

Pretreatment with coenzyme Q_{10} and vitamin E in the experimental model of HD prevented elevation of creatine kinase activity in cytosol. This positive CoQ_{10} and vitamin E pretreatment effect could contribute to non-mitochondrial activity of CoQ_{10} in trans-plasma membrane electron transport, mediated by cytosolic $NADH/NAD^+$ ratio [19].

Multiple Sclerosis

Multiple sclerosis (MS) is generally considered to be an inflammatory disease with a substantial autoimmune contribution. Impairment of Complex I in chronic plaque zone was associated with oxidative damage to mitochondrial DNA. In 2005, mitochondrial Complex I gene variants were found to be associated with MS.

Amyotrophic Lateral Sclerosis

Mitochondrial dysfunction is a primary feature of amyotrophic lateral sclerosis (ALS). Mitochondrial pathology was observed in an early stage in the degeneration of motor neurons. Muscle mitochondria from ALS patients exhibit impaired mitochondrial electron transport and elevated free radical production.

Friedreich´s Ataxia

Friedrich's ataxia (FA) is an autosomal recessive neurodegenerative disease, characterized by cerebral ataxia and other CNS defects. The most marked pathological changes include loss of large sensory neurons in the dorsal root ganglia and degeneration of the dorsal columns of the spinal cord. The disease is associated with an expanded trinucleotide repeat in the frataxin gene, mitochondrial protein with iron-sulphur regulation. Mitochondrial oxidative phosphorylation abnormalities, increased free radical generation and iron accumulation in cardiac and skeletal muscle were found [47].

2. 4. Oxidative Stress and Antioxidants in Down Syndrome

Mitochondria are the major endogenous source of ROS. In normal ageing ROS production increases, whereas antioxidant capacity fails. The role oxidative stress in the pathogenesis of AD was documented [48]. Age is the major risk factor for AD development, characterized by the accumulation of Aβ in mitochondrial membranes, which inhibits enzymatic activity of respiratory chain complexes (III and IV), causes reduction in the rate of oxygen consumption and enhanced of ROS production. Impaired intramitochondrial metabolism associated with respiratory chain dysfunction and the consequent oxidative stress are being considered as a possible pathogenic mechanism in a number of neurodegenerative disorders, including AD [14].

In Down syndrome patients plasma biomarkers of oxidative stress (protein carbonyls and 4-hydroxy-2-nonenal) and allantoin (non-enzymatic oxidative product of uric acid in human) were significantly increased [49, 50]. The main enzyme defense mechanism against harmfull effect of reactive oxygen species are activities of superoxide dismutase, glutathione peroxidase, glutathione reductase, myeloperoxidase and catalase [51].

DS patients have an extra copy of chromosome 21, resulting in an extra gene for cytoplasmic superoxide dismutase (Cu/Zn SOD), with excessive activity of Cu/Zn SOD [27]. Oxidative imbalance in trisomic cells is age-dependent and depends on the relationship between SOD and (CAT+GPx) [51]. Disturbance of antioxidant enzyme balance in patients with DS was documented and can be a key to DS pathogenesis [52].

3. Possible Adjunctive Therapy for Brain Mitochondrial Diseases

Oxidative stress and damage of brain mitochondrial abnormalities participate in the early neuronal cell death, in the pathogenesis of Down syndrome and Alzheimer´s disease. Possible therapeutics for mitochondrial energy dysfunction is coenzyme Q_{10} (antioxidant and crucial part of mitochondrial respiratory chain), α-lipoic acid (antioxidant and mitochondrial co-factor), carnitine (antioxidant and participants in mitochondrial fatty acids transport) as well as nicotinamide (electron donor for Complex I).

α-lipoic acid scavenges superoxide radical, hydroxyl radical, peroxyl radical, singlet oxygen and hydrochlorous acid. It can remove heavy metals by chelation, regenerates other antioxidants like coenzyme Q_{10}, vitamin E, vitamin C, glutathione. α-lipoic acid is a part of the pyruvate dehydrogenase complex, located in mitochondrial matrix. Therapy with α-lipoic acid shown to be beneficial effect in neurodegeneration, in oxidative stress, diabetes, in cataract formation [53, 55].

Carnitine is a naturally occurring compound in the body, belongs to a group like vitamin nutrients. It is a necessary component for fatty acid oxidation, plays an important role in many physiological metabolic pathways in the human body. In patients with neuromuscular diseases carnitine supplementation is able to improve ankle and knee function and handgrip strength. Supplementation with carnitine improved myocardial fatty acids utilization in patients with hypertension. Beneficial effect of carnitine supplementation was proved in chronically hemodialyzed patients, in HIV disease and in patients with immunodeficiency [54].

Several data of successful supplementary antioxidant therapy in AD were published recently. CoQ_{10} supplementation in children with Down syndrome was published recently. Children were supplemented with reduced form of CoQ_{10} ubiquinol$_{10}$), during 3-month, in daily dose 10 mg/kg body weight. Authors showed normalization of pro-oxidative state after ubiquinol supplementation [56]. Therapy with exogenous antioxidants, as coenzyme Q_{10}, selenium (co-factor for glutathione peroxidase), alpha-lipoic acid or zinc (part of SOD1), could play an important role in prevention or at least delaying the progression of AD and perhaps of Down syndrome [57].

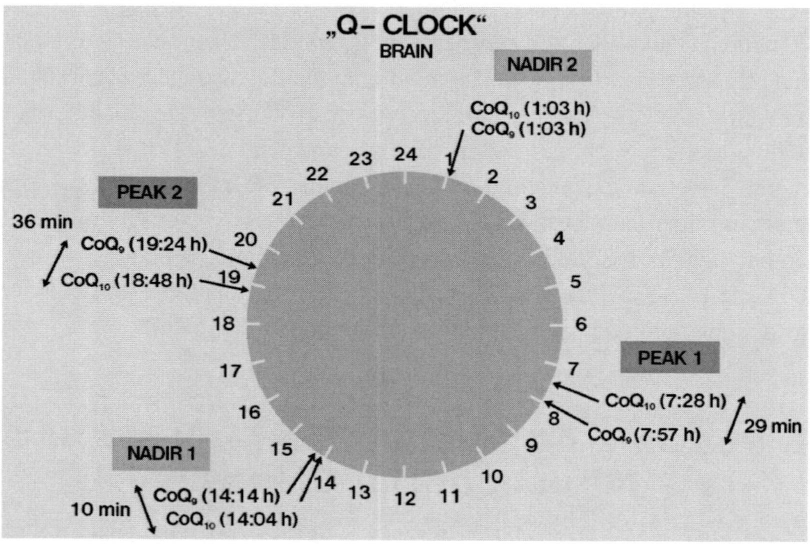

Figure 1. "Q-CLOCK" in brain mitochondria of control rats.

Coenzyme Q_{10} (ubiquinone) is a key component of the mitochondrial respiratory chain. Its reduced form (ubiquinol) has strong antioxidant properties. Synthesis of CoQ_{10} decreased with ageing, with mitochondrial diseases of various organs. Supplementation with CoQ_{10} has potentially neuroprotective effects on neurodegenerative diseases such as Parkinson's disease, Huntington´s disease, amyotrophic lateral sclerosis. Neuroprotective effect of administrated CoQ_{10} on the transgenic mice reduced Aβ42 overproduction, its intracellular accumulation and decreased oxidative stress [58]. Water-soluble CoQ_{10} stabilized the mitochondrial membrane when neuronal cell were subjected to oxidative stress, prevented the collapse of the mitochondrial membrane potential, decreased ROS production. Authors suggest that CoQ_{10} has the potential to be used as a therapeutic intervention for neurodegenerative diseases [64].

Supplementation with CoQ_{10} stimulates mitochondrial energy production. Based on the role of CoQ_{10} in various tissues and mitochondrial function, incorporation, bioavailability of liposomal CoQ_{10} in brain nuclei compartments has been presented [59]. Experimental animals, control rats were supplemented with liposomal CoQ_{10} (Li-Q-Sorb®, Tishcon Corp., USA) during 30 days in daily doses 200 mg CoQ_{10}/kg body weight by oral gavage. In brain nuclei were determinate $CoQ_{9\text{-}OX}$, $CoQ_{10\text{-}OX}$, compared with levels of CoQ in control animals. Bioavailability of liposomal CoQ_{10} supplementation in brain nuclei compartments has been shown, that CoQ_{10} supplementation can participate in regulation of: circadian rhythmus (brain, heart, liver), (SCHN, DMN), decreased stress in PVN, DMN, food intake (PVN), in regulation of digestion (DMN), movement (SN). These results contribute to the basic information for supplementary therapy with CoQ_{10} in AD perhaps in DS patients (Figure 2).

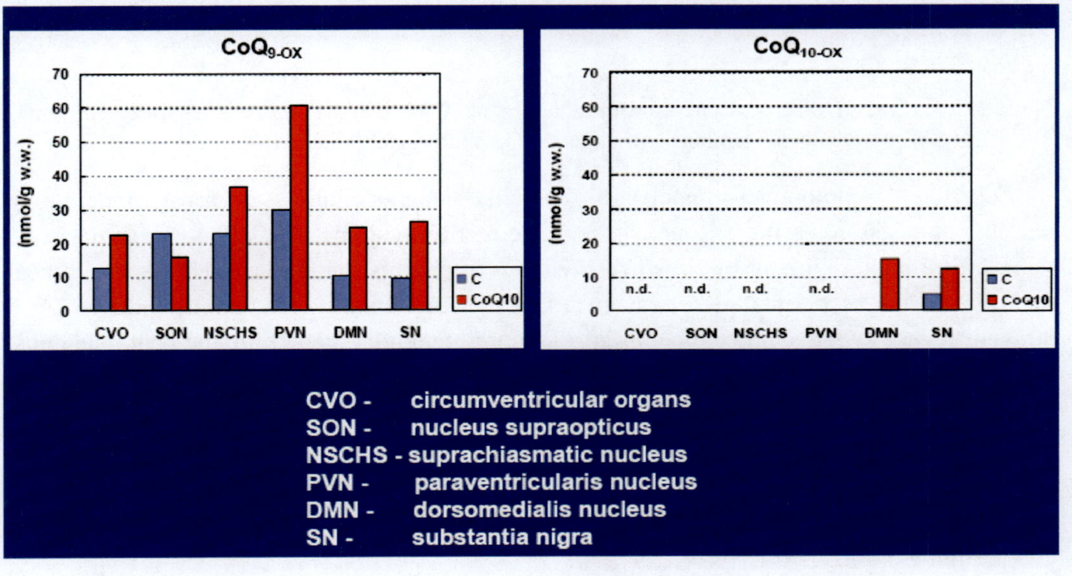

Figure 2. Bioavailability of liposomal coenzyme Q10 - Li-Q-Sorb® in tissue brain – nuclei.

Authors found that CoQ_{10} supplementation: a/ stimulated CoQ_9 concentration, CoQ_{10} was not detectable in CVO. b/ decreased CoQ_9 concentration in SON, CoQ_{10} – was not detectabe. c/ Increased CoQ_9 concentration in NSCHS, CoQ_{10} was not detectable. d/

Increased CoQ_9 in PVN, CoQ_{10} was not detectable. e/ Stimulated endogenous level of CoQ_9 and CoQ_{10} in DMN and SN.

Schematic brain structures show figures 3-5.

Sensory circumventricular organs (*CVOs*) –include subfornical organum (SFO), organum vasculosum laminae terminalis (OVLT), and area postrema (AP). This brain structures are enable to monitor chemical composition of circulating plasma (figure 3).

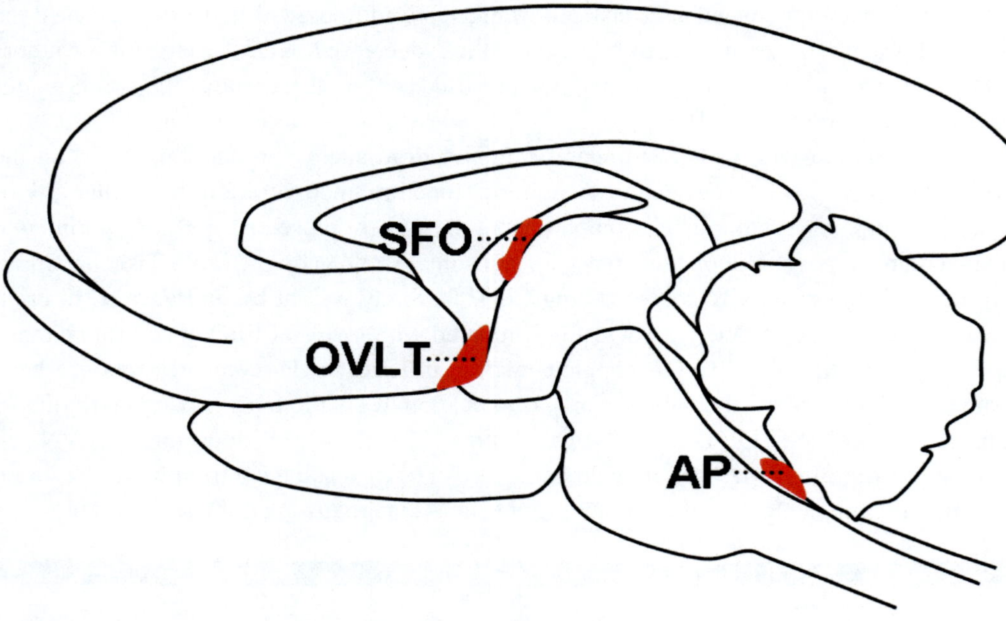

Figure 3. Localization of sensory circumventricular organs (CVOs) in the rat brain. AP - area postrema, OVLT - organum vasculosum laminae terminalis, SFO - subfornical organum

SON – supraopticus nucleus: contain magnocellular neurons innervating neurohypophysis –releasing vasopresin, regulate of fluid volume. *NSCHS* – suprachiasmatic nucleus: is a main regulator of circadian rhythmus in organism, innervates (indirectly) pineal glands, as well as peripheral organs (heart, liver) modulates circadian rhythms. *PVN* – paraventricular hypothalamic nucleus is a major integratory center in the hypothalamus, enables maintain homeostasis, participates in regulation of autonomic nervous system, cardiovascular function, response to stress, food intake, metabolic rate (figure 4).

DMN – dorsomedialis hypothalamic nucleus is involved in: regulation of digestion, fluid balance, reproduction, circadian rhythm, thermoregulation and response to stress.

SN – substantia nigra participates in modulation of motor activities via regulation of extrapyramidal systems (figure 5).

An experimental model of Alzheimer's disease was developed [60]. In an experimental model of mitochondrial Alzheimer's disease (MAD) we found damage of brain and heart mitochondrial respiration at Complex I and II and ATP production at Complex V, Figure 6 [61].

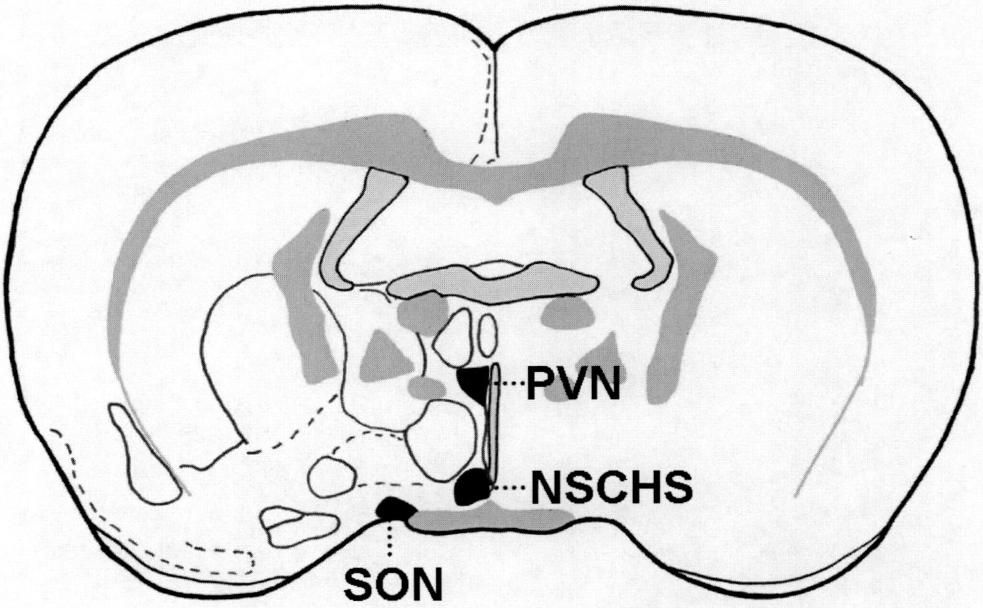

Figure 4. Localization of SON, PVN, NSCHS.

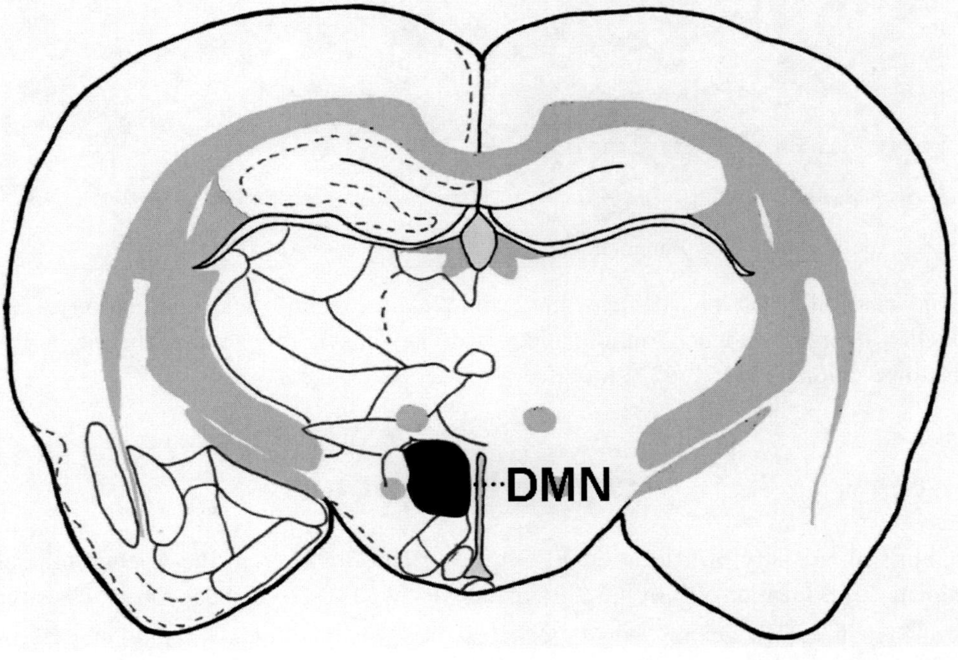

Figure 5. Localization of DMN, SN.

Supplementation with liposomal CoQ_{10} in animal model of Alzheimer´s diseases decreased oxidative stress, increased brain mitochondrial CoQ_9 concentration, increased activity of brain mitochondrial respiratory chain function and ATP production. These findings are of potential significance in the liposomal CoQ_{10} treatment in AD patients [62].

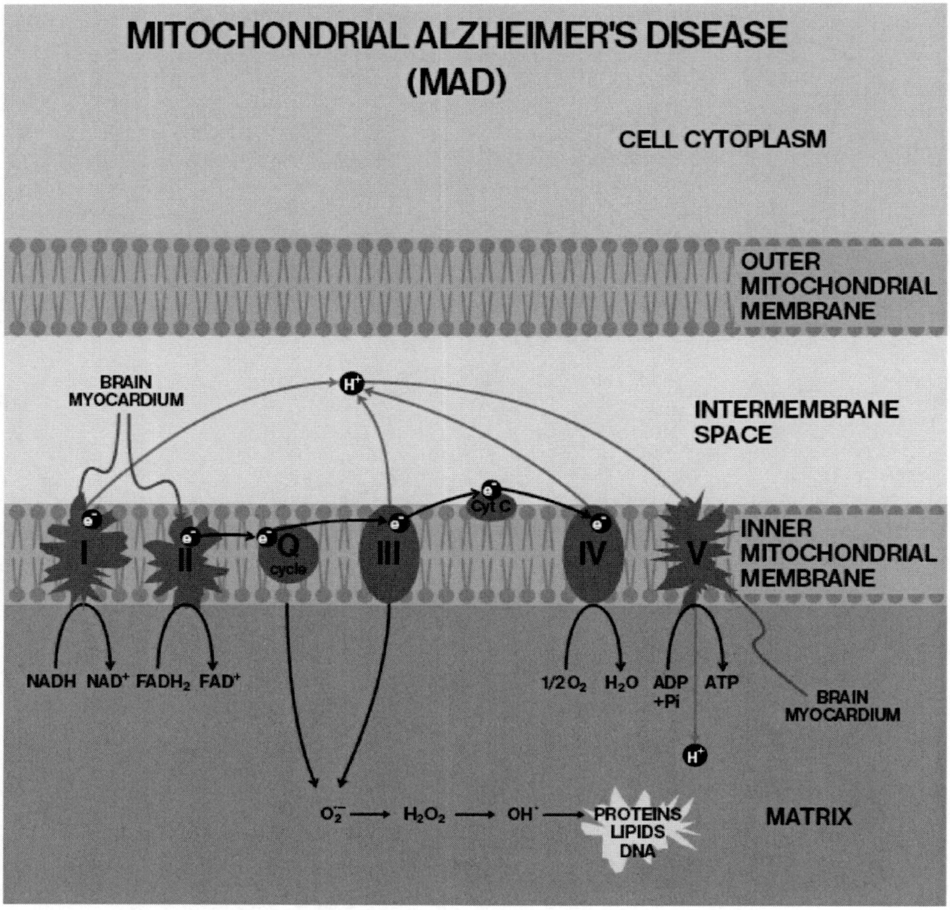

Figure 6. Experimental model of mitochondrial Alzheimer´s diseases (MAD).

The possibility of the supplementary antioxidants therapy and stimulation of energy production in brain mitochondria, in patients with Down syndrome and Alzheimer's diseases seems to be rational [58, 61, 62, 64, 67].

Acknowledgments

Grants of Ministry of Education VEGA 3442/06,Grants from the Agency for Science of Ministry of Education VEGA 1/3442/06 and APVV 0148-06, Tishcon Corp., USA for (Li-Q-Sorb®) is gratefully acknowledged, technical assistance: A. Štetková and Peter Gvozdják, architect, MSc. (Atelier 2) for his great help in preparing the colour figures.

References

[1] Yaffe MP (1999). The machinery of mitochondrial inheritance and behviour, *Science* 283: 1493-1497

[2] Neupert W, Herrmann JM. (2007) Translocation of proteins into mitochondria. *Annu Rev Biochem* 76:723-749

[3] Petersen CAH, Alikhani N, Behbahani H, Wiehager B, Pavlov PF, Alafuzoff I, Leinonen V, Ito A, Winblad B, Glaser E, Ankarcrona M. (2008) The amyloid β-peptide in imported into mitochondria via the TOM import machinery and localized to mitochondrial cristae. *http://pnas.org/content/105/35/13145.full, 5.11.2008.*

[4] Ziegelhoffer-Mihalovičová B, Kolár F, Jacob W, Tribulová N, Uhrík B, Ziegelhoffer A. (1980) Modulation of mitochondria contact sites formation in immature rat heart. *Gen Physiol Biophys* 17:385-390

[5] Capetanaki Y.(2002) Desmin cytoskeleton: potential regulator of muscle mitochondrial behavior and function. *Trend Cardiovasc Med* 12:339-348

[6] Brookes PS, Yoon Y, Robotham J, Anders MW, Sheu SS. (2004) Calcium, ATP, and ROS: a mitochondrial love-hate triangle. *Am J Physiol Cell Physiol* 287:C817-C833.

[7] Fukui H, Moraes CT. (2008) The mitochondrial impairment, oxidative stress and neurodegeneration connection: reality or just an attractive hypothesis? *Trends in Neurosciences* 31(5):251–256.

[8] Gvozdjáková A.(2008). Mitochondrial physiology. In: Gvozdjáková A. (Ed). *Mitochondrial Medicine*, Springer (Netherlands), pp 1-17.

[9] Fleury CH, Mihnotte B, Vayssiere JL. (2001) Mitochondrial reactive oxygen species and apoptosis. In: Ebadi M, Marwah J, Chopra R (Eds) *Mitochondrial Ubiquinone (Coenzyme Q_{10}.)* Prominent Press, pp 361 – 398.

[10] Grafourifar P, Cadenas C. (2005) Mitochondrial nitric oxide synthase. *TRENDS in Pharmacol Sciences* 26(4):190-195.

[11] Riobo NA, Melani M, Sanjuan N, Fiszman L, Gravielle MC, Carreas MC, Cadenas E, Poderoso JJ. (2002) The modulation of mitochondrial nitric-oxide synthase activity in rat brain development. *J Biol Chem* 277(45): 42447–42455.

[12] Bruckdorfer R.(2005) The basics about nitric oxide. *Molec Aspects of Medicine* 26:3-31.

[13] Ghafourifar P, Richter C.(1997) Nitric oxide synthase actvitiy in mitochondria. *FEBS Lett* 418:291-296.

[14] Parihar MS, Brewer GJ.(2007) Mitoenergetic failure in Alzheimer diseases. *Am J Physiol Cell Physiol* 292: C8 – C23.

[15] Gvozdjáková A. (2008) Mitochondrial free radicals and antioxidants. In: Gvozdjáková A. (Ed). *Mitochondrial Medicine*, Springer (Netherlands), pp 50-54.

[16] Linnanne AW, Eastwood H. (2004) Cellular redox poise modulation; the role of coenzyme Q_{10}, gene and metabolic regulation. *Mitochondrion* 4:779–789.

[17] Gvozdjáková A, Kucharská J, Cornélissen G., Mikulecký M, Singh RB, Halberg F. (2004) Variation in cardiac mitochondrial coenzyme Q_{10} and oxidative phosphorylation. *Int J Cardiol* 97(2):S15, *Third International Congress on Cardiovascular Disease, Taipei, Taiwan*, 26 – 28 November 2004.

[18] Gvozdjáková A, Kucharská J, Cornélissen G., Mikulecký M, Singh RB, Halberg F. (2005) Circadian and semicircadian variations of heart mitochondrial coenzyme Q in relationship to oxidative phosphorylation. *Fourth Conference of the Intenrational Coenzyme Q_{10} Association, Los Angeles, USA*, 14 – 17 April 2005, Abstract Book pp113 –115.

[19] Singh RB, Weydahl A, Otsuka k, Watanabe Y, Yano S, Mori H, Ichimaru Y, Mitsutake G, Sato Y, Fanghong L, Zhao ZY, Karlik C, Gvozdjakova A. (2001) Can nutrition influence circadian rhythm and heart variability? Biomed Pharmacol 2001, 55: 115 – 124

[20] Halberg F, Cornélissen G, Singh RB, Gvozdjáková A, Otsuka K, Beaty L, Katinas G, Hermida R, Ayala D, Czaplicki J. (2008) Chronobiology, chronomics and N-of-1 tests of timing coenzyme Q_{10}. In: Gvozdjáková A. (Ed). *Mitochondrial Medicine*, Springer (Netherlands), pp 55-92.

[21] Mikulecký M, Gvozdjáková A, Kucharská J, RB Singh. (2008) Circa(semi)dian periodicity of coenzyme „Q_{10}-CLOCK" and cascade of oxidative phosphorylation in control and diabetic rat heart mitochondria. In: Gvozdjáková A. (Ed). *Mitochondrial Medicine*, Springer (Netherlands), pp 151-160.

[22] Luft R, Ikkos D, Palmieri G, Ernster L, Afzelius B. (1962) A case of severe hypermetabolism of nonthyroid origin with the defect in the maintenance of mitochondrial respiratory control: a correlated clinical, biochemical and morphological study. *J Clin Invest* 41:1776-1804.

[23] Luft R. (1994) The development of mitochondrial medicine. *Proc Natl Acad Sci USA* 91:9831-9838.

[24] DiMauro S, Schon EA. (2008) Mitochondrial disorders in nervous system. *Annu Rev Neurosci* 31:91–123.

[25] Beal MF. (2005) Mitochondria take center stage in ageing and neurodegeneration.*Ann Neurol* 58(4):495–505.

[26] Wallace DC, Singh G, Lott MT, Hodge JA, Schurr TG, Lezza AM, Elsas LJ, Nicoskelainen EK. (1988) Mitochondrial DNA mutation associated with Leber's hereditary optic neuropathy. *Science* 24:21427–21430.

[27] Epstein CJ. (1995) Down's syndrome (trisomy 21). In: Scriver CR, Beaudet AL, Sly WS et al. (eds). *The Metabolic and Molecular Bases of Inherited Diseases.* New York, NY:McGraw-Hill.

[28] Busciglio J, Pelsman A, Wong C, Pigino G, Yuan M, Yanker BA. (2002) Altered metabolism of the amyloid β precursor protein is associated with mitochondrial dysfunction in Down's syndrome. *Neuron* 33(5):677– 688.

[29] Capone GT. (2003) Evidence for increased mitochondrial superoxide production in Down syndrome. *New Orleans 2003 Trisomy 21 Research Conference* Abstracts, September 13 – 14, 2003, p.5.

[30] Muller-Hocker J. (1989) Cytochrome – c –oxidase deficient cardiomyocytes in the human heart – an age-related phenomenon. A histochemical ultracytochemical study.*American Journal Pathology* 134(5):1167–1173.

[31] Hayakawa M, Katsumata K, Yoneda M, Tanaka M, Sugyiama S, Ozawa T. (1996) Aged-related extensive fragmentation of mitochondrial DNA into minicircles.*Biochem Biophys Res Coommun* 226(2):369–377.

[32] Zhu X, Lee HG, Casadesus G, Avila J, Drew K,, Perry G, Smith MA. (2005) Oxidative imbalance in Alzheimer's disease. *Mol Neurobiol* 31(1-3):205-217.

[33] Fraser PE, Yang DS, Yu G, Lovesque L, Nishimura M, Arawaka S, Serpell LC, Rogaeva E, Hyslop PG. (2000) Presenilin structure, function and role in Alzheimer's disease. *Biochim Biophys Acta* 1502:1-15.

[34] Smith MA, Rottkamp CA, Nunomura A, Raina AK, Perry G. (2002) Oxidative stress in Alzheimer's disease. (Review). *Biochim Biophys Acta* 1502:139–144.

[35] Rogaeva E, Meng Y, Lee JH, Gu Y, Kawarai T , Zou F et al. (2007) The neuronal sortilin-related receptor SORL1 is genetically associated with Alzheimer diseases. *Nat Genet* 39(2):167–177.

[36] Goerdet M, Spilantini MG. (2006) A sentury of Alzheimer's disease. *Science* 314:777-781.

[37] Robertson ED, Scearce-Levie K, Palop JJ, Yan F, Cheng IH, et al. (2007) Teducing endogenous tau ameliorates amyloid β-induced deficits in Alzheimer's disease mouse model. *Science* 316:750-754.

[38] Hirai K, Aliev G, Nunomura A, Fujioka H, Russel RL, Atwood CS, et al. (2001) Mitochondrial abnormalities in Alzheimer's disease. *J Neurosci* 21(9):3017-3023.

[39] Valla J, Berndt JD, Gonzalez-Lima F. (2001) Energy hypometabolism in posterior cingulate cortex of Alzheimer's patients: superficial laminar cytochrome oxidase associated with disease duration. *J Neurosci* 21:4923-4930.

[40] Dauer W, Przedborski S. (2003) Parkinson's disease: mechanisms and models. *Neuron* 39:889–909.

[41] Haas RH, Nasirian F, Nakano K et al. (1989) Low platelet mitochondrial complex I and complex II/III activity in early untreated Parkinson's disease. *Ann Neurol* 37: 714– 722.

[42] Vila M, Przedborski S. (2004) Genetic clues to the pathogenesis of Parkinson's disease. *Nat Med* 10 (Suppl): S58-S62.

[43] Browne SE, Beal MF. (2004) The energetics of Huntington's disease. *Neurochem Res* 29 (3):531–546.

[44] Browne SE, Ferrante RJ, Beal MF. (1999) Oxidative stress in Huntington's disease.*Brain Pathology* 9:147-163.

[45] Gardian G, Vecsei L. (2004) Huntington's disease: pathomechanism and therapeutic perspectives. *J Neural Transm* 111:1485–1494.

[46] Kašparová S, Sumbalová Z, Bystrický P, Kucharská J, Liptaj T, Mlynárik V, Gvozdjáková A. (2006) Effect of coenzyme Q_{10} and vitamin E on brain energy metabolism in the animal model of Huntington's disease. *Neurochem International* 48:93–99.

[47] Cooper JM, Schapira AH. (2003) Friedrich's ataxia: disease mechanisms, antioxidant and coenzyme Q_{10} therapy. *Biofactors* 18:163–171.

[48] Filipcik P, Cente M, Ferencik M, Hulin I, Novak M. (2006) The role of oxidative stress in the pathogenesis of Alzheimer's diseases. *Brat Med J* 107(9-10): 384-394.

[49] Žitňanová I., Korytár P., Aruona OI, Šustrová M., Garaiová I., Muchová J., Kalnovičová T., Pueschel S., Ďuračková Z.(2004) Uric acid and allantoin in Down Syndrome: antioxidant and oxidative stress mechanisms? *Clin Chim Acta* :139-146.

[50] Žitňanová I, Korytár P, Sobotová H, Horáková Ľ, Šustrová M, Pueschel S, Ďuračková Z. (2006) Markers of oxidative stress in children with Down Syndrome. *Clin Chem Lab Med* 44(3):306-310.

[51] Muchová J, Šustrová M, Garaiová I, Liptáková A, Blažíček P, Kvasnička P, Pueschel S, Ďuračková Z (2001) Influence of age on activities of antioxidant enzymes and lipid peroxidation products in erythrocytes and neutrophils of Down dyndrome patients. Free Rad Biol Med, 31(4) : 499-508.

[52] Remacle J, Lambert D, Raes M, Pigeolet E, Michiels C, Toussaint D. (1992) Importance of various antioxidant enzymes for cell stability. *Biochem J* 286:41–46.

[53] Packer L, Tritschler HJ, Wessel K. (1997) Neuroprotection by the metabolic antioxidant alpha-lipoic acid. *Free Radic Biol Med* 22(1-2):359-378.

[54] Sinatra ST (2005) The Sinatra solution. Metabolic cardiology. Basic Health 231 pp.

[55] Cadenas E, Packer L (1996) (eds) Handbook of Antioxidant. Marcel Dekker, NY, pp. 545-591.

[56] Miles MV, Patterson BJ, Chalfonte-Evans ML, Horn PS, Shapiro MB, Steele PE, Tang H, Hotze SL. (2007) Coenzyme Q_{10} (ubiquinol-10) improves oxidative balance in children with trisomy 21. Pediatr Neurol 2007, http://raysahelian.com/ downsyndrome.html].

[57] [57] Zana M, Janka Z, Kalman J. (2007) Oxidative stress: A bridge between Down´s syndrome and Alzheimer´s diseases. *Neurobiology of Ageing* 28:648-676).

[58] Yang X, Yang Y, Li G, Wang J, Yang ES. (2008) Coenzyme Q_{10} attenuates β-amyloid pathology in the aged transgenic mice with Alzheimer presenilin 1 mutation. *J Mol Neurosci* 34:165-171.

[59] Gvozdjáková A, Kucharská J, Vančová O, Sumbalová Z, Kvetňanský R, Mravec B, Singh RB, Horecký J. (2008) Bioavailability of liposomal coenzyme Q_{10} in brain nuclei and its effect on mitochondrial function in an animal model of Alzheimer s disease. *International Conference „Oxidative stress in ageing", Bratislava, Slovakia*, April 23 – 25, 2008, abstract book, p. 15.

[60] Horecký J, Bačiak L, Vančová O, Wimmerová S, Kašparová S. (2006) Effect of transient ischemia on rat brain energy metabolism assessed in vivo by 31P MRS and in vitro by mitochondrial OXPHOS. *Biochim Biophys Acta* – Bioenergetics, Suppl. S:178-179.

[61] Horecký J, Vančová O, Kucharská J, Gvozdjáková A. (2008) Coenzyme Q_{10} supplementation in mitochondrial Alzheimer's disease (experimental model). . In: Gvozdjáková A. (Ed). *Mitochondrial Medicine*, Springer (Netherlands), pp 335-339.

[62] Gvozdjáková A, Vančová O, Kucharská J, Horecký J (2007) Coenzyme Q_{10} supplementation in an experimental model of Alzheimer's disease. *5th Conference of the International Coenzyme Q_{10} Association, Kobe, Japan,* November 9 – 12, 2007, abstract book 177 – 179.

[63] [63] Somayajulu M, McCarthy S, Hung M, Sikorska M, Borowski B, Pandey S. (2004) Role of mitochondria in neuronal cell death induced by oxidative stress; neuroprotection by coenzyme Q_{10}. *Neurobiol Dis* 18(3):618-627.

[64] Li G, Zou L, Cao CM, Yang ES. (2005) Coenzyme Q_{10} protect SHSY5Y neuronal cells from beta amyloid toxicity and oxygen-glucose deprivation by inhibiitng the opening of the mitochondrial permeability transition pore. *Biofactors* 25(1-4):97-107.

[65] Luft R, Landau BR. (1995) Mitochondrial medicine. *J Intern Med* 238:405-421.

[66] Devi L, Prabhu BM, Galati DF, Avadhani NG, Anandatheerthavarada HK. (2006) Accumulation of amyloid precursor protein in the mitochondrial import channels of human Alzheimer's diseases nrain is associated with mitochondrial dysfunction. *J Neuroscience* 26(35):9057–9068.

[67] Li G, Zou L, Jack CR, Yang Y, Yang ES. (2007) Neuroprotective effect of coenzyme Q_{10} on ischemic hemisphere in aged mice with mutations in the amyloid precursor protein. *Neurobiology in Ageing* 28(6):877-882.

[68] Moreira PI, Santos MS, Oliviera CR. (2007) Alzheimer's diseases: a lession from mitochondrial dysfunction. *Antioxid Redox Signal* 9(10):1621–1630.

[69] Onyango IG, Khan SM. (2006) Oxidative stress, mitochondrial dysfunction, and stress signaling in Alzheimer's disease. *Curr Alzheimer Res* 3(4):339–349.

[70] Crouch PJ, Cimdins K, Duce JA, Bush AI, Trounce IA. (2007) Mitochondria in ageing and Alzheimer's diseases. *Rejuvenation Res* 10(3):349–357.

[71] Sastre J, Pallardo FV, Assuncion GJ, Vina J. (2000) Mitochondria, oxidative stress and ageing. *Free Rad Res* 32:189–198.

[72] uckley F. (2008) Modelling Down syndrome. *Down syndrome research and practice* 12(2):98–102.

[73] Bingham Ch, Arbogast B, Cornélissen GG, Lee JK, Halberg F. (1982) Inferential statistical methods for estimating and comparing cosinor parameters. *Chronobiologia* 9:397-439.

[74] Kubáček L. (1988) *Foundation of estimation theory*. Elsevier, Amsterdam, Oxford, New York, Tokyo.

[75] Kubáčková L. (1992) *Foundation of experimental data analysis*. CRC Press, Boca Raton, Ann Arbor, London, Tokyo.

[76] Kubáček L, Valach A, Mikulecký M. (2000) Time series analysis with periodic components. Computer programme. *ComTel*.

In: Handbook of Down Syndrome Research
Editors: Dominicus Jelinek and Gijs Dvorak
ISBN 978-1-60741- 690-6

Chapter 8

Informed Choice in Antenatal Screening of Down's Syndrome

***Kleanthi Gourounti*[1] *and Jane Sandall*[2]**
[1]Elena Benizelou Hospital, Departmemt of Midwifery,
Technological Educational Institution of Athens, Greece
[2]Department of Midwifery and Nursing,
King's College London, UK

Abstract

The importance of making an informed choice in a medical field depends on the specific clinical context. When patients refer minor everyday problems to health care professionals and there is a routine and simple treatment or benefit there is no need to initiate a process of informed decision making. In this case informed consent is enough. However, several of choices in pregnancy, such as how to give birth and whether or not to undergo screening test for Down's syndrome, have important implications for women and her family and thus informed choice has fundamental importance. Screening doesn't have only benefits but also has risks. Harms from screening arising mainly from the false negative and false positive results because of their medical, psychological and legal consequences. Therefore, the choice to undergo screening for Down's syndrome should be based on a full understanding of the likely benefits, harms and limitations. Many definitions have been given for informed choice but all these definitions have two core characteristics: a) relevant, good quality information and b) consistency between attitudes and behaviour. "An informed decision could be defined as a reasoned choice which is made by a reasonable individual using relevant information about the advantages and disadvantages of all possible courses of action in accord with the individual's belief". The conclusions that have been drawn from this chapter mainly concern the measurement, the determinants and the factors that may impact on informed choice. In general, there is a lack of standardized measures that assess the multidimensionality of informed choice, as the majority of the existent measures are either single dimensioned or measures of self report. According to the findings of relevant original studies, the majority of women have a relatively poor level of knowledge and understanding about the Down's syndrome screening and the vast majority of women have a positive attitude towards screening for Down's syndrome. In general, the rates of informed choice about screening for Down' syndrome have been found low. Since informed choice is determined by knowledge and by attitude-behaviour consistency of participants, the factors that may influence the knowledge and the attitudes of women could impact on informed choice rate. The factors that may impact on the informed choice of women by affecting their level of knowledge and their degree of understanding of information given, could be the way of presentation of information (special leaflets, video, computer systems), and the level of knowledge and the communication skills of health care professionals. Factors that may influence women's attitudes could be the attitudes of health care professionals, social influences and organizational factors such as the way of offering screening. Health care professionals (midwives and obstetricians) should dedicate more time to discussing with women and should provide information which is understandable and suitable to their learning ability. Moreover, it could be concluded that attitude is a stronger predictor of informed choice than level of knowledge since the majority of women who attend screening for Down syndrome have positive attitude and not good level of knowledge. Therefore, the attempt to increase attitude-behavior consistency could be more successful in increasing informed choice in screening for Down syndrome than increasing the level of knowledge.

Introduction

This chapter explores relevant literature to informed choice in antenatal screening for Down's syndrome and includes 6 sections. The first section describes presents the models of decision making, the terminology of informed choice and describes the various definitions that have been given for informed choice. Section 2 describes the development of the informed choice in maternity and section 3 describes the importance of informed choice in screening for Down's syndrome. The fourth, fifth and sixth sections describe the determinants and the measurement of informed choice. And the seventh section reviews the factors that may impact on informed choice. The conclusion of the chapter is presented in the section 8.

1. Terminology

Decision making in health care has been described on a continuum from paternalism to informed choice through shared decision making (Charles *et al*, 1999).

For many years, the main approach to making decisions in the medical field has been this of paternalism (Emanuel and Emanuel, 1992). In the purest form of the paternalistic model, the patient passively consents to professional authority by agreeing with the doctor's decision. Paternalism or making decisions on behalf of others is based on the assumption that health care professionals 'know best' and can make the 'correct' choice because of their training and education (Brown *et al*, 1992). In a paternalistic model the doctor will make a decision for the patient without involving him or her in the decision making process. Thus, in this model there is no doctor-patient partnership, there is only a passive doctor and a dominant doctor.

In a shared decision making model there is an interaction between the patient and the doctor in all the stages of the decision making process (Charles *et al*, 1999). In this model there is a two way exchange of information, both patient and health care professionals reveal preferences and both agree on the decision.

In an informed choice model the patients receive information by their health care professional and then make their own decisions about the treatment they want to receive without reference to the health care professional (Charles *et al*, 1999). In this model the health care professional communicate to the patients information concerning all the available options but are not involved in the decision making process. The amount and the type of information must be sufficient in order to enable patients to make an informed choice.

Although there is a debate and often a confusion concerning the terminology (shared decision making, informed choice or informed consent) it can be concluded that there are obvious borders between shared decision making and informed choice. Also there are obvious differences between informed consent and informed choice because informed consent implies agreement with a suggested or recommended way of action but informed choice implies choice of the most suitable course of action.

In the case of antenatal screening for Down's syndrome there is no recommended course of action (Marteau *et al*, 2005). Therefore the term of informed consent is not enough in the context of Down's syndrome screening because couples make choices rather than simply agree with a proposed course of actions.

Many definitions have been given for informed choice but from all these definitions emerge that informed choice has two core characteristics:

- Informed choice should be based on relevant, good quality information.
- Informed choice should reflect the decision makers' values or attitudes.

Some of the definitions of informed choice that have been given are:

"An informed decision is one where a reasoned choice is made by a reasonable individual using relevant information about the advantages and disadvantages of all possible courses of action in accord with the individuals belief" (Beker et al, 1999).

"If people are to participate in an informed way they need information about the relevant options, skills or assistance to understand and interpret the information, to recognize their personal values, to engage in decision making and to communicate their decision to health care professionals" (Entwistle et al, 1998a).

"An important goal of informed consent is to present information to patients so that they can decide which medical option is best for them, according to their values" (Ubel and Loewenstein, 1997).

"An effective decision will be defined as those that are informed, consistent with values and congruent with behaviour" (O' Connor et al, 1997).

The definition of informed choice by O'Connor *et al* (1997) includes a third key characteristic, this of consistent behaviour. In the case of antenatal screening for Down's syndrome the consistent behaviour could be expressed as the uptake or non uptake of screening.

Thus, in the case of antenatal screening for Down's syndrome it can be concluded that there are two types of informed choice: an informed choice to decline screening, where the individuals with good knowledge and negative attitudes toward screening don't undergo for screening and an informed choice to accept screening, where individuals with good knowledge and positive attitudes toward screening accept to undergo screening (Marteau *et al*, 2001). The choices that occur when individuals do not have relative, good knowledge or when their attitudes are not reflected in their behaviour, are uninformed (Marteau *et al*, 2001).

2. Development of Informed Choice in Maternity

It is known that maternity care policies from 1904 to 1990 suffered from paternalism (Kirkham, 2004).

Evidence has existed for many years concerning the importance of childbearing women being provided with information in order that they make an informed choice (Green *et al*, 1988). Research also has demonstrated that women's satisfaction from their pregnancy and their childbearing is related to whether or not they feel that they have received enough information (Shapiro *et al*, 1983).

Definitions of informed choice and measures of effective decision making have only been available since the mid to late 1990s (Beker *et al*, 1999, O' Connor, 1995). The UK NHS started in mid 1990s to promote partnership between health care professionals and patients when making decisions about individual clinical care, basing these decisions on research evidence (Entwistle *et al*, 1998b).

In 1993, *Changing Childbirth,* a policy document for England, has acted as a catalyst for this movement in maternity care, promoting care which is women -centred and the provision of choice and information in order to enable women to feel in control of their care (Department of Health, 1993). In response to this movement, the Department of Health funded the Midwives Information and Resource Service (MIDIRS) and the NHS to produce evidence-based leaflets on ten 10 decision points which were related to pregnancy issues. This collaboration resulted in the production of 10 evidence-based leaflets, which are known as MIDIRS Informed Choice Leaflets (www.infochoice.org).

Since the development of the informed choice concept in maternity care many studies have been conducted in order to investigate the percentage of women who exercise informed choice during their maternity care. In a study that was conducted in Wales in 1996-97 was found that 72% of women felt that they have made informed choices regarding their antenatal care (Churchill and Benbow, 2000). In a study by Wyke *et al* (2001) that was conducted in UK was found that 50% of women felt that they were encouraged to make informed decisions about their antenatal care. In large study by O'Cathain *et al* (2002) was found that approximately half of women felt that they had exercised informed choice in maternity care.

In this study was found that the perception of informed choice differed by decision point and was higher for the screening for Down's syndrome (73%). It was also found that women who felt that they made informed choices about ultrasound scans were more likely to feel that they had made informed choices overall during their antenatal care.

3. Importance of Informed Choice in Antenatal Screening for Down's Syndrome

The importance of making an informed choice in a medical field depends on the specific clinical context. When patients refer minor everyday problems to health care professionals and there is a routine and simple treatment or benefit there is no need to initiate a process of informed decision making (Charles *et al*, 1999). In this case informed consent is enough. The need for exercising informed choice is most compelling when different courses of actions exist, with different benefits and risks, and outcomes are uncertain. Since the individual will bear the consequences of whatever action is taken, it is important that his or her values and preferences are known and respected.

Several of choices in maternity, such as how and where to give birth and whether or not to undergo screening test for Down's syndrome, have important implications for women and her family (Levy, 1999) and thus informed choice has fundamental importance.

As it has been referred in the previous chapter, screening doesn't have only benefits but also has risks. Harms from screening arising mainly from the false negative and false positive results because of their medical, psychological and legal consequences (Petticrew *et al,* 2000). The initial decision to enter a screening procedure can result in the individual feeling that they have boarded a train from which they cannot alight (Emery, 2001). Antenatal screening for Down's syndrome provides a clear example of this process. In the case of antenatal screening for Down's syndrome a pregnant woman and her partner have a series of decision to face (Jepson *et al,* 2001). Although certain cut off levels of risk are used to define a high-risk or 'positive' result the couple must decide what an acceptable risk is for them and balance this risk with the risk of a miscarriage that may rise by invasive procedures of prenatal diagnosis (amniocentesis or chorionic villus sampling (CVS)). In this procedure the couple must be aware of the false positive rate of screening. Finally, if the fetus is found to have Down's syndrome the couple must make a decision whether to terminate the pregnancy or not. Also the couples that accept to undergo screening for Down's syndrome must be aware of the false negative results and their consequences. It is therefore important that the initial choice about issues such as screening for Down's syndrome be fully informed. Of course the majority of women that undergo screening for Down's syndrome will receive negative results and thus the understanding of their knowledge and their choice will not be tested (Green *et al*, 2004).

The choice to undergo screening for Down's syndrome should be based on a full understanding of the likely benefits, harms and limitations. Raffle (2001) warns that 'harm to uninformed participants of screening leads to anger, bitterness and potentially litigation'.

4. Determinants and Measure of Informed Choice in Antenatal Screening for Down' S Syndrome

Operationalizing the majority of definitions of informed choice, as a measure, requires the measurement of two core characteristics: knowledge and attitudes toward the screening for Down's syndrome.

As it was referred above achieving informed choice in screening programmes and especially in screening for Down's syndrome is very important because screening carries not only benefits but also harms. Although this achievement may be obstructed by the lack of a standardized measure of informed choice because it is not possible to assess the percentage of women who make informed choices if there are no means of measuring informed choice. In a study by Bekker *et al* (1999) it was found that often studies assess the knowledge of participants but few (fewer than a third of 547 articles) include a measure of informed choice. Existing measures of informed choice either use items to assess just a single dimension (such as a measure of knowledge) of informed choice (Kirkham and Stapleton, 2001) or use items on whether women thought that had exercised informed choices (O' Cathain *et al*, 2002). These types of measures have many weaknesses. Single dimension measures (measure of knowledge only) are unable to reflect the multidimensionality of the construct of informed choice (Marteau *et al*, 2001) and self-assessment of information and self-report of informed choice is not a reliable measure of actual informed choice (Green *et al*, 2004). Self-assessment of information is reasonable when the main interest is in anxiety but is less useful if the interest is in informed choice, since women may be satisfied with very little information and they may think that understand something fully when in fact they haven't correct or sufficient understanding (Green *et al*, 2004). For example, in the study by O'Cathain *et al* (2002) it was found that women with lower educational status and women from manual occupations were more likely to perceive that they exercised informed choices although it would be expected less educated women to have difficulties making informed choices. Most often only knowledge is assessed in order to measure informed choice. A measure of informed choice (Multidimensional Measure of Informed Choice) for use in antenatal screening for Down's syndrome that assesses both knowledge and individuals' attitudes was developed by Marteau *et al* (2001). The Multidimensional Measure of Informed Choice (MMIC) has been used in many studies so far (Jacques et al, 2005, Rowe et al, 2006, Gourounti and Sandall, 2008) and has been translated and validated in Greek (Gourounti and Sandall, 2009).

5. Informed Choice: Measure of Information and Knowledge

There is an assumption that if women are provided with appropriate information they will make a choice which is based on this information and this choice will be informed. The question that raises is "what is appropriate" in terms of amount, context, type and frame of given information concerning the antenatal screening for Down's syndrome. Knowledge assesses the individuals' ability to recall information (Bekker *et al*, 1999) and thus the type and the presentation of the information could influence the level of knowledge and consequently the informed choice. To facilitate the transformation of the information into knowledge, the health care professionals must act on some occasions as a filter, on other occasions as a conduit and on some other occasions simply as a reservoir (Berger, 2003).

The definition that was given by Bekker *et al* (1999) required that individuals must use all the available information in order to make an informed choice. Individuals, however, have different needs and interest in information when facing decision (Miller *et al*, 1983). Courts in United Kingdom do not accept that 'informed choice' means 'all the information that is available' because this might confuse or alarm the patients (Kircham, 2004).

According to Michie *et al* (2003) there are three approaches in order to quantify the needed information concerning the antenatal screening for Down's syndrome. The first approach would be to ask people that have been offered screening what information they think is necessary for women in order to enable them to make an informed choice. This approach would involve asking individuals that have undergo screening and received different outcomes (true negative results, true positive results, false negative and false positive results). The problems in this approach would be firstly that the perception of necessary information before undergo screening varies among individuals and secondly the provision of amount and type of information varies among individuals that received different outcomes. The second approach would be to determine the needed information for an informed choice by comparing the psychological outcomes (satisfaction, anxiety, and regret) of screening with different types and amounts of knowledge. By using this approach the knowledge that would associated with the better psychological outcomes would be defined as good knowledge. The third approach would be to use professional guidelines about the needed information. Although there is no "gold standard" for good knowledge in some areas, such as in the area of prenatal screening for Down's syndrome, professional guidelines outline areas of which participants should be aware when making informed choices. Three sets of professional guidelines have been issued in UK in the last decade that all clearly identify the information that should be provided to women in order to enable them to make an informed choice about Down's syndrome screening (Royal College of Obstetricians and Gynaecologists, 1993, UK National Screening Committee, 2003, General Medical Council, 1999). According to the above guidelines, the information provided to women considering antenatal screening for Down syndrome is mainly focused on the likelihood of detection, the meaning of a negative result, the meaning of a positive result, the options following after a screen positive result, the condition screened for and the risks that attached to screening.

It could be noticed that there is a tendency of the above guidelines to provide information that is essential from the maternity services perspective rather than from that of the pregnant women (Green *et al*, 2004). This led to an emphasis on procedural aspects of screening rather than the characteristics of children with Down's syndrome. In study by Bryant *et al* (2001) a critical evaluation of leaflets given to pregnant women in the UK prior to undergoing serum screening was conducted. Bryant et al described that the majority of given information (89%) was of a medico-clinical nature, with 11% addressing other issues associated with the condition of Down syndrome. Hall et al (2007) recently described the presentation of choice and information about the condition of Down's syndrome and Down's syndrome screening in written information given to women in five European (UK, Netherlands, Italy, Spain, Chech Republic) and in two Asian (India, China) countries. Hall et al concluded that leaflets contained relatively little information about Down's syndrome condition and the majority of statements concerning Down's syndrome condition were negative. In a study by Williams *et al* (2002) was found that practitioners tend to focus more on the process of screening for Down's syndrome rather than the condition that is being screened. The lack of providing information concerning the condition of Down's syndrome has been demonstrated in study by Chilaka *et al* (2001) and in study by Mulvey and Wallace (2000) that observed that only 33% and 44% of women respectively knew about the condition of Down's syndrome. Furthermore, in a study by Murray *et al* (2001) that assessed the quality of written information (leaflets) used in 64 UK units that offered Down's syndrome screening was found that only 11% of the leaflets included the basic items of recommended information by the RCOG (1993).

Additionally, it could be noticed that the above guidelines commonly recommend the offering of information concerning the positive and the negative results of screening by using likelihoods and probabilities. Although, there is evidence that suggests that interpretation of numerical information by lay people is problematic (Gigerenzer and Edwards, 2003, Edwards *et al*, 2002). The fact that antenatal screening for Down's syndrome does not offer definite results, but instead gives probabilities raises many concerns concerning the women's understanding of screening results (Ettore, 2000). In a study by Smith *et al* (1994a) it was found that only 36% of women that have been offered serum screening for Down's syndrome understood that a negative result would not guarantee that the fetus is normal. Additionally, only 32% of women understood that most women with positive results would have a normal fetus. In another study by Grewal *et al* (1997) was found that half women did not realise that positive results could occur without fetal abnormality, or negative results could be falsely reassuring. It has been also found that knowledge questionnaires that contain a lot of simple procedural items, such as the fact that the Down's syndrome screening uses scanning and blood sample, are likely to generate much higher scores than those that include items concerning risk or other numerical material (Green *et al*, 2004). In study by De Vigan *et al* (2002) was stated that it was avoided to include in the knowledge scale questions about risks and meaning of risk, as earlier surveys have shown that many women have difficulty understanding this kind of concepts (Julian-Reynier *et al*, 1993). In studies that questions regarding meaning of high and low risk were included in the knowledge scale, the correct rate was low (Gekas et al, 1999, Jacques et al, 2005, Gourounti and Sandall, 2008). In a study by Pilnick *et al* (2003) was found that a way of improving women's understanding of risk in screening for Down's syndrome was to present the same information in several ways, such as: there is a possibility that the baby would be affected, the screening is not a diagnostic test thus cannot give a certain result, the outcome cannot be guaranteed. The duties of the health care professionals towards the patients are to give information in a way that they can understand and to respect their rights in order to be fully involved in their case (Godolphin, 2003). The aim of having an effective risk communication is not only the decrease of risk but is also the empowerment of the patients and the promotion of their autonomy in order for them to make an informed-sharing decision (Gourounti and Lykeridou, 2005).

For many years, the aim of giving information about screening was the achievement of high uptake but now the goal isn't everyone to have positive attitudes toward undergoing screening but to make an informed choice. By giving information not only about the benefits but also about the implications of screening both women and health care professionals will be benefit because the women' autonomy will be respected, women will make informed choices and health care professionals will not carry the blame for problems that are inherent in screening. There is evidence that giving information that emphasizes only the positive aspect of screening leads to less methodical and systematic cognitive process of decision making (Dunegan, 1993). In a study by Michie *et al* (1997) it was found that women who didn't accept to undergo screening for Down's syndrome made their decisions more systematically than those who accepted to undergo screening. This result may indicate that the more women make systematic decisions by weighing up the advantages and disadvantages of having and not having screening, the more likely women decide against having screening. Also decisions may change when the same factual information is presented in different ways, for example, by presenting the information either positively or negatively (Bekker *et al*, 1999). This means that the way in which the information about the prenatal screening for Down's syndrome is presented may affect the decision making and inevitably the informed choice of women (Michie *et al*, 1999).

On the other hand if we adopt an approach that makes explicit the limitations and the implications of screening then another set of problems will be encountered (Raffle, 2001). It will be a risk of decrease in screening uptake and subsequently population's benefits may reduce (cost-effectiveness could be reduced if uptake falls as low as to make services barely viable). Although it is inappropriate to continue to use information about antenatal screening purely for encouraging high uptake (Raffle, 2001) because antenatal screening for Down's syndrome carries many medical, psychological and legal implications.

Information is a key component in the provision of informed choice and thus the effective presentation of information may improve the women's knowledge and subsequently increase the rate of informed choice (Jepson *et al*, 2001). Oral and written information therefore needs to be comprehensive, clear and accurate (Murray *et al*, 2001). Many attempts have been made to increase women's knowledge concerning the antenatal screening for Down's syndrome by using different media (special leaflets, videos and computer-based systems). In some studies was found that these attempts have had limited success (Michie *et al*, 1997, Graham *et al*, 2000) but in some others was found the opposite (Thornton *et al*, 1995, Browner *et al*, 1996, Hewison *et al*, 2001). Therefore it can be concluded that the presentation type of information may impact on the level of knowledge and subsequently can facilitate the informed choice in antenatal screening for Down's syndrome.

Although many attempts have been made to increase women's knowledge and understanding of information concerning antenatal screening for Down's syndrome, many studies have shown that women have a poor level of knowledge and understanding about the Down's syndrome screening and the Down's syndrome condition (Gourounti and Sandall, 2008, Rowe et al, 2006, Jacques et al, 2005, Chilaka *et al*, 2001, Mulvey and Wallace, 2000, Freda *et al*, 1998, Grewal *et al*, 1997). In a recent study by Gourounti and Sandall (2008) that was conducted in Greece and MMIC was used, only 46% women were classified as having good level of knowledge. In two previous studies that were conducted in Australia (Rowe et al, 2006, Jacques et al, 2005) and MMIC was also used, only 48% and 68% of women respectively were classified as having good level of knowledge. Nevertheless, in the study by van den Berg *et al* (2005) that was conducted in Netherlands, it was found that 83% of women were sufficient knowledgeable about prenatal screening. This finding may be due to the situation in which prenatal screening in Netherlands is not offered routinely as it is offered in other countries. Therefore the women that participated in the study by van den Berg and colleagues perhaps made their decision more consciously than women who participated in other studies. This is supported by research from countries where prenatal screening is offered routinely which suggest that the making of a deliberate decision is no longer necessary for prenatal screening (Green and Statham, 1996, Press and Browner, 1997). The 'routinization' of prenatal screening may lead to lower level of knowledge and subsequently to less informed-choices.

If informed choice is a priority, it follows that women's knowledge and understanding must be measured after efforts have been made to inform them, but before any decision has been performed (Green *et al*, 2004). Finally, if measuring of knowledge is to be examined the question that arises is how and when to measure the understanding of information and the knowledge. If knowledge is measured before decision making it may create a picture of lay understanding. If knowledge is measured after screening has been made, then knowledge is likely to be increased because of the direct experience of women and the extra information that women took by the professionals who performed the screening test. Therefore, measurement of knowledge must be performed before screening performance because measurement of knowledge after screening cannot predict the women's knowledge at the time of decision making (Green *et al*, 2004).

6. Informed Choice: Measure of Attitudes

In order for a choice to be truly informed should be based not only on knowledge but should be also consistent with values and attitudes of individuals. Attitude toward a concept can be defined as a person's general feeling of 'favourableness' or 'unfavourableness' for that concept (Ajzen and Fishbein, 1980). Thus, in the case of antenatal screening for Down's syndrome, the attitude of relevance is the attitude towards undergoing the screening test (Marteau *et al*, 2001).

According to the 'theory of reasoned action' the attitude toward the behaviour is determined by the person's feelings, intentions, subjective norms (social influence) and person's evaluation of the outcomes associated with the behaviour (Ajzen, 1988). The theory of reasoned action could be implemented in the case of prenatal screening for Down's syndrome. Therefore, in the case of antenatal screening for Down's syndrome the subjective (social) norms represent the perception of a woman regarding what other people (partner, family, and friends) think about her accepting or declining the screening test. For example, a woman may feel persuaded to accept screening when it proposed by a doctor or a midwife or may feel forced to accept screening if her partner has a negative attitude to children with Down's syndrome. The outcomes that are associated with the decline or the acceptance of screening for Down's syndrome may be the possible option of a termination of an affected by

Down's syndrome pregnancy and the birth of a child with Down's syndrome. In a study by Moyer *et al* (1999) was found that factors that influenced women's decision concerning prenatal screening included moral beliefs, family and social influences (subjective norms), feelings about having a child with Down's syndrome and willingness to put the fetus at elevated miscarriage risk (associated outcomes).

It is unlikely that choices are based solely on the given information, and other factors including individuals' beliefs and social, religious and cultural background are likely to influence decision making and informed choice (Jepson *et al*, 2001). Although knowledge is seen as the key component of informed choice, a study by Michie *et al* (2003) found that knowledge didn't play very important role whether women would undergo screening for Down's syndrome and attitudes towards undergoing screening was a strong predictor of uptake. The findings of studies that used MMIC and specifically measured women's attitudes showed that the vast majority of women were categorized as having a positive attitude towards screening for Down's syndrome. In studies by Jaques *et al* (2005) and by Rowe et al (2006) that were conducted in Australia, 99% and 87% of women respectively that attended screening for Down's syndrome, were classified as having a positive attitude towards screening. In study by Gourounti and Sandall (2008) that was conducted in Greece, 96% of participants were classified as having a positive attitude towards screening. These findings indicate that attitudes towards screening are a strong predictor of uptake.

In the area of prenatal screening for Down's syndrome a woman is likely to use her knowledge according to her attitude (Michie *et al*, 2003). Thus, women with a negative attitude towards termination of pregnancy and knowing that the screening test may result in offering of a termination of the pregnancy, is likely to use their knowledge in order to reject the test. By contrast for a woman with a negative attitude towards the birth of a child with Down's syndrome, information about the performance of screening test will be important. Therefore, it could be concluded that interventions that aim to improve informed choice by enabling people to act consistently with their attitudes may be more successful than interventions that aim to improve knowledge.

7. Informed Choice Rate and Factors that Impact on Informed Choice

Measurement of informed choice requires the measurement of knowledge and attitudes towards antenatal screening for Down's syndrome. According to Marteau and colleagues (2001) choices may be classified as informed when women have simultaneously good level of knowledge and positive attitudes towards Down's syndrome screening. Choices may be classified as uninformed when women have poor level of knowledge and negative attitudes towards Down's syndrome screening or when women have poor level of knowledge and positive attitudes or when they have good level of knowledge and inconsistent attitudes with their behaviour. In general, the rates of informed choice about screening for Down' syndrome have been found low. In the preliminary study by Marteau *et al* (2001) only 43% of women had made informed choice about Down's syndrome screening. In the studies by Rowe et al (2006) and by Gourounti and Sandall (2008) the rates of informed choice were 37% and 44%

respectively. In the validation study of the multidimensional measure of informed choice (Michie *et al*, 2002) it was found that the rate of informed choice was 59%. In the study by Michie *et al* (2002) the questionnaires were filled in after screening, therefore it could be concluded that experience of screening may accounted for the higher percentage of informed choice of their population. Unfortunately, Michie and colleagues didn't refer the percentages of women with good and poor level of knowledge and women with positive and negative attitudes. Thus, it is impossible to know if the higher percentage of informed choice is due to the higher knowledge or to the more positive attitudes of women in their sample. In the studies by van den Berg *et al* (2005) and by Jaques *et al* (2005) it was found that the rates of informed choice were even higher (68%). The higher percentages of informed choice in the above studies were mostly due to the increased level of knowledge. In a study that measured the women's perceptions of informed choice in maternity (O'Cathain *et al*, 2002) was found that 73% of women had the perception of having made an informed choice about screening for Down's syndrome. This finding may not reflect the actual rate of informed choice because it was found that the less educated women were more likely to perceive that they had exercised informed choice. This was a surprising finding because it is usually expected that less educated women will have difficulties seeking information and making choices (O' Cathain *et al*, 2002). There is also evidence that suggest that people with lower levels of education are less likely to be knowledgeable about medical issues (Santalahti *et al*, 1998).

Since informed choice is determined by knowledge and by attitude-behaviour consistency of participants, the factors that may influence the knowledge, the attitudes and the consistency between attitudes and behaviour of women could impact on informed choice. Shakespeare (1999) has written that 'in hundred of small ways, the choice of to have or not to have prenatal screening is unfree, with women complying with suggested 'routine' obstetric measures and being influenced by directive health professionals without full and adequate information'.

The factors that may impact on the informed choice of women by affecting their knowledge and understanding of given information could be the presentation of information (special leaflets, video, computer systems), knowledge and the communication skills of health care professionals. Health care professionals who lack knowledge themselves will be unable to give accurate and complete information to the women (Smith *et al*, 1994b, Sadler, 1997, Tyzack and Wallace, 2003). Rowe et al (2006) stated that the considerable low rate of informed choice in their study could be attributed to the fact that health providers themselves in Australia are not well informed about the tests, and may lack the skills necessary to convey complex information in the context of an antenatal visit.

Factors that may impact on informed choice by influencing women's attitudes could be the attitudes of health care professionals, social influences and organizational factors such as the way of offering screening. There is evidence that women who undergo screening for Down's syndrome are influenced by the attitude of the health care professionals, of their family and of their partner (Jaques *et al*, 2004, Moyer *et al*, 1999). Thus health care professionals that have more positive attitudes towards Down's syndrome are more likely to emphasize the benefits of screening and to conduct screening tests in a combination with other antenatal tests. On the other hand, health care professionals with more negative attitudes are more likely to emphasize the negative aspects of screening and to conduct screening separately from other tests (Dormandy and Martaeu, 2004). Although, a study by Dormandy and Marteau (2004) found that attitudes of health care professionals didn't influence women's attitudes toward screening for Down's syndrome. A study by Dormandy *et al* (2002a) found that when the screening is combined with other tests results in higher uptake. In a study by Dormandy *et al* (2002b) was found that the proportion of women who made an informed choice to accept screening for Down's syndrome was higher at the routine (screening combined with other tests) hospital visit than the separate (screening separately from other tests) hospital visit. A possible explanation of this finding may be that when screening tests are offered in combination with other tests lead to higher levels of informed choice by removing practical barriers to uptake, such as the extra hospital visit. Health care systems appear to facilitate informed choice in the context of screening for Down's syndrome by the routine offering of test.

8. Conclusion

This literature review has described the development of informed choice in maternity and has showed the fundamental importance of informed choice in screening for Down's syndrome. It has also described the determinants of informed choice and the factors that may impact on informed choice. The conclusions that have been drawn from this literature review concern mainly the measurement, the determinants and the factors that may impact on informed choice. Concerning the knowledge which is one of the determinants of the informed choice, has been concluded that: a) levels of knowledge adequate for informed decision making have not achieved, b) women's knowledge is influenced by the way of presentation of information and by the knowledge of healthcare professionals, c) a considerable amount of given information concerning the results of screening is not easily understandable by women because of the numerical approach of information and thus d) knowledge is not the same as understanding. It has been also concluded that the professional recommendation concerning the given information about screening for Down's syndrome may be inadequate because they don't include information about the condition of Down's syndrome. Moreover, concerning the women's attitude which is another determinant of informed choice could be concluded that attitude is a stronger determinant of informed choice than knowledge. Therefore, the attempt to increase attitude-behavior consistency, could be more successful in increasing informed choice in screening for Down's syndrome than increasing the level of knowledge (Dormandy *et al*, 2005). Finally, it is has also been described that external factors that may influence the knowledge, the attitudes and the consistency between attitudes and behaviour of women could impact on informed choice.

References

Ajzen I. and Fishbein M. (1980) *Understanding Attitudes and Predicting Social Behaviour.* Englwood Cliffs, New Jersey: Prentice Hall.

Ajzen I. *Attitudes, Personality and Behaviour*. (1988) Open University Press, Bristol.

Bekker H., Thornton J., Aire M., et al. (1999) Informed decision making : an annotated bibliography and systematic review. *Health Technology Assessment*. 3: 1

Berger K. (2003) Informed choice: information or knowledge? *Med Law*. 22(4): 743-50

Brown J., Kitson A., McKnight T. (1992) *Challenges in caring*. Chapman and Hall, London.

Browner C., Preloran M., Press N. (1996) The effects of ethnicity, education and an information video on pregnant women's knowledge and decision about a prenatal diagnostic screening test. *Patient Education Counseling*. 27: 135-46

Bryant LD. Murray J. Green JM. Hewison J. Sehmi I. Ellis A. (2001) Descriptive information about Down syndrome: a content analysis of serum screening leaflets. *Prenatal Diagnosis*. 21(12):1057-63

Charles C., Whelan T., Gafni A. (1999) What do we mean by partnership in making decisions about treatment? *British Medical Journal*. 319: 780-782

Chilaka V., Konje J., Stewart C., Narayan H., Taylor D. (2001) Knowledge of Down syndrome in pregnant women from different ethnic groups. *Prenatal Diagnosis*. 21: 159-164

Churchill H. and Benbow A. (2000) Informed choice in maternity services. *British Journal Midwifery*. 8(1): 41-47

Department of Health. *Changing Childbirth*. (1993) Report of the Expert Maternity Group. HMSO, London.

De Vigan C., Vodovar V., Goujard J., Garel M., Vayssiere C., Goffinet F. (2002). Mothers' knowledge of screening for trisomy 21 in 1999: a survey in Paris maternity units. 104: 14-20

Donegan K. (1993) Framing, cognitive modes, and image theory: toward an understanding of a glass half full. *J Appl Psychology*. 78: 491-503

Dormandy E., Hooper R., Michie S., Marteau T. (2002b) Informed choice to undergo prenatal screening: a comparison of two hospitals conducting testing either as part of a routine visit or requiring a separate visit. *J Med Screening*. 9: 109-114

Dormandy E., Michie S., Weinman J., Marteau T. (2002a) Variation in uptake of serum screening: the role of service delivery. *Prenatal Diagnosis*. 22: 67-9

Dormandy E. and Marteau T. (2004) Uptake of a prenatal screening test: the role of healthcare professionals' attitudes towards the test. *Prenatal Diagnosis*. 24: 864-868

Edwards A., Elwyn G., Mulley A. (2002) Explaining risks: turning numerical data into meaningful pictures. *British Medical Journal*. 324: 827-324

Emanuel E. and Emanuel L. (1992) Four models of the physician-patient relationship. *JAMA* 267: 2221-6

Emery J. (2001) Is informed choice in genetic testing a different breed of informed decision making? A discussion paper. *Health Expectations*. 4: 81-86

Entwistle V., Sowden A., Watt I. (1998a) Evaluating interventions to promote patient involvement un decision making: by what criteria should effectiveness be judged? *Journal of Health Services Research and Policy*. 3: 100-7

Entwistle V., Sheldon T., Sowden A., et al. (1998b) Evidence-informed patient choice. *International Journal of Technology Assessment in Health Care*. 14: 215-225

Etore E. (2000) Reproductive genetics, gender and the body: 'please doctor, may I have a normal baby' *Sociology*. 34(3): 403-420

Freda M., DeVore N., Valentine-Adams N., Bombard A., Merkatz I. (1998) Informed consent for maternal serum alpha-phetoprotein screening in an inner city population: how informed is it? *J Obstetr Gynecol Neonat Nursing*. 27: 99-106

Gekas J., Gondry J., Mazur S., Cesbron P., Thepot F. (1999). Informed consent to serum screening for Down syndrome: are women given adequate information? Prenat. Diagnosis 19: 1-7

General Medical Council. (1999) *Seeking patients' consent: the ethical considerations*. London.

Gigerenzer G. and Edwards A. (2003) Simple tools for understanding risks: from innumeracy to insight. *British Medical Journal*. 327: 741-4

Godolphin W. (2003) The role of risk communication in shared decision making. *British Medical Journal.* 327:692-3

Gourounti K. and Lykeridou K. (2005) The risk in public health. *Review of clinical pharmacology and pharmacokinetics*. 19 (2): 93-97

Gourounti K. and Sandall J. (2008) Do pregnant women in Greece make informed choices about antenatal screening for Down's syndrome? A questionnaire survey. Midwifery 24, 153–162

Gourounti K. and Sandall J. The validation and translation of Multidimensional Measure of Informed Choice in Greek. Midwifery 2009 April 16 (epud ahead of print)

Graham W., Smith P., Kamal A., Fitzmaurice A., Smith N., Hamilton N. (2000) Randomized controlled trial comparing effectiveness of touch screen system with leaflet for providing women with information on prenatal tests. *British Medical Journal*. 320: 155-60

Green J. and Coupland V. (1988) *Great expectations: a prospective study of women's expectations and experiences of childbirth.* Centre for Family Research, Cambridge.

Green J., Hewison J., Bekker H., Bryant L., Cuckle H. (2004) Psychological aspects of genetic screening of pregnant women and newborns: a systematic review. *Health Technology Assessment.* 8 (33).

Grewal GK. Moss HJ. Aitken DA. Bjornsson S. Cameron AD. Pell JP. (1997) Factors affecting women's knowledge of antenatal serum screening. *Scottish Medical Journal.* 42(4):111-3

Green J. and Statham H. Psychological aspects of prenatal screening and diagnosis. In: Marteau T., Richards M, editors. (1996) The troubled helix: social and psychological implications of the new genetics. Cambridge University Press

Hall S., Chitty L., Dormandy E., Hollywood A., Wildschut H., Fortuny A., Masturzo B., Santavy J., Kabra M., Mas R. and Marteau T. (2007) Undergoing prenatal screening for Down's syndrome: presentation of choice and information in Europe and Asia. *European Journal of Human Genetics*. 15: 563–569

Hewison J., Cuckle H., Baillie C., Sehmi I. Lindow S. et al. (2001) Use of videotapes for viewing at home to inform choice in Down syndrome screening : a randomized conrolled trial. *Prenatal Diagnosis*. 21: 146-9

Jaques A., Bell R., Watson L., Halliday J. (2004) People who influence women's decisions and preferred sources of information about prenatal testing for birth defects. *Aust N Z J Obstet Gynecol*. 44: 233-238

Jepson R., Forbes C., Sowden A., Lewis R. (2001) Increasing informed uptake and non-uptake of screning: evidence from a systematic review. *Health Expectations*. 4: 116-130

Julian- Reynier C., Marquart-Moulin G., Moatti J., et al. (1993). Attitudes of women of childbearing age towards prenatal diagnosis in south-eastern France. Prenatal Diagnosis 13: 6

Kirkham M. (2004) *Informed choice in maternity care*. Palgrave Macmillan.

Kirkham M. and Stapleton. (2001) *Informed choice in maternity care: an evaluation of evidence based leaflets.* York NHS Centre for Reviews and Dissemination.

Levy V. (1999) Mainting equilibrium: a grounded theory study of the process involved when women make informed choices during pregnancy. *Midwifery*. 15: 109-119

Marteau T., Dormandy E., Crockett R. (2005) Informed choice: why measuring behaviour is important. *Arch Dis Child* . 90: 546

Marteau T., Dormandy E., Michie S. (2001) A measure of informed choice. *Health expectations*. 4: 99-108

Midwives Information and Resource Service (MIDIRS). Informed Choice Leaflets [online] available: www.infochoice.org. [accessed 25.6.05]

Michie S., Smith D., McClennan A., Marteau T. (1997) Patient decision making : an evaluation of two different methods of presenting information about a screening test. *Br J Health Psychol.* 2: 317-26

Michie S., Smith D., Marteau T. (1999) Prenatal tests: how are women deciding? *Prenatal Diagnosis* 19: 743-8

Michie S., Dormandy E., Marteau T. (2002) The multi-dimensional measure of informed choice: a validation study. Patient Education and Counselling 48: 87-91

Michie S., Dormandy E., Marteau T. (2003) Informed choice : understanding knowledge in the context of screening uptake. *Patient Education Counseling.* 50: 247-253

Miller S., Mangan C. (1983) Interacting effects of information and copying style in adapting to gynaecologic stress: should the doctor tell all? *Journal of Personal and Social Psychology*. 45: 223-236

Moyer A., Brown B., Gates E., Daniels M., Brown H., Kuppermann M. (1999) Decisions about prenatal testing for chromosomal disorders: perceptions of a diverse group of pregnant women. *J Womens Health Gend Based Med.* 8(4): 521-31

Mulvey S. and Wallace E. (2000) Women's knowledge and attitudes to first and second trimester screening for Down's syndrome. *Br J Obstet Gynaecol* 107: 1302-5

Murray J., Cuckle H., Sehmi I., Wilson C., Ellis A. (2001) Quality of written information used in Down syndrome screening. *Prenatal Diagnosis.* 21: 138-42

National Screening Committee UK. (2003) *Antenatal Screening for Down's Syndrome-policy and quality issues*, London, Department of Health

O' Cathain A., Thomas K., Walters S., Nicholl J., Kirkham M. (2002) Women's perceptions of informed choice in maternity care. *Midwifery.* 18: 136-44

O' Connor A. (1997) Decisional conflict, In *Nursing diagnosis and intervention: Planning for patient care*, ed McFarland G. and McFarlane E., Mosby.

Petticrew M., Sowden A., Lister-Sharp D., Wright K. (2000). False-negative results in screening programmes: a systematic review of impact and implications. *Health Technology Assessment* 4(5).

Pilnick A., Fraser D., James D. (2004) Presenting and discussing nuchal translucency screening for fetal abnormality in UK. *Midwifery*. 20: 82-93

Press N. and Browner C. (1997). Why women say yes to prenatal diagnosis. Soc. Sci. Med. 45 (7): 979-989

Raffle A. (2001) Information about screening- is it to achieve high uptake or to ensure informed choice? *Health Expectations*. 4: 92-98

Royal College of Obstetricians and Gynaecologists. (1993) *Report of the RCOG Working Party on Biochemical markers and the Detection of Down's syndrome*, London, RCOG.

Rowe H., Fisher J., Quinlivan J. (2006) Are pregnant Australian women well informed about prenatal genetic screening? A systematic investigation using the Multidimensional Measure of Informed Choice. *Australian and New Zealand Journal of Obstetrics and Gynaecology* 46: 433–439

Sadler M. (1997) Serum screening for Down's syndrome: how much do health professionals know? *Br J Obstet Gynaecol*. 104: 176-9

Santalahti P., Aro A., Hemminki E., Helenius H., Ryynanen M. (1998). On what grounds do women participate in prenatal screening? Prenatal Diagnosis. 18: 153-165

Shakespeare T. (1999) Losing the plot? Medical and activist discourses of contemporary genetics and disability. *Sociology of Health and Illness* 21: 669-688

Sharpino M., Najman J., Chang A., Keeping J., Morrison J., et al. (1983) Information control and the exercise of power in the obstetrical encounter. *Soc Sci Med.* 17(3): 139-46

Smith D., Shaw R., Marteau T. (1994a) Informed consent to undergo serum screening for Down's syndrome: the gap between policy and practice. *British Medical Journal.* 309: 776

Smith D., Shaw R., Marteau T. (1994b) Lack of knowledge in health professionals: a barrier to providing information to patients. *Quality in Health Care*. 3: 75-78

Thornton J., Hewison J., Lilford R., Vail A. (1995) A randomized trial of three methods of giving information about prenatal testing. *British Medical Journal.* 311: 1127-30

Tyzack K. and Wallace E. (2003) Down syndrome screening: what do health professionals know? *Aust N Z J Obstet Gynecol*. 43: 217-221

Ubel P., Loewenstein G. (1997) The role of decision analysis in informed consent: choosing between intuition and systematic. *Social Science and Medicine.* 44: 647-656

Williams C., Alderson P., Farsides B. (2002) What constitutes 'balanced information' in the practitioners' portrayals of Down's syndrome? *Midwifery*. 18: 230-237

Wyke S., Hewison J., Elton R., et al. (2001) Does general practitioner involvement in commissioning maternity care makes a difference? *Journal Health Services Research Policy*. 6: 99-104

van den Berg M., Timmermans D., ten Kate L., van Vugt J., van der Wal G. (2005). Are pregnant women making informed choices about prenatal screening? Genetics in Medicine. 7(5): 332-338

In: Handbook of Down Syndrome Research
Editors: Dominicus Jelinek and Gijs Dvorak
ISBN 978-1-60741- 690-6

Chapter 9

Mother-Child and Father-Child Interaction in Families of Children with Down Syndrome

Simona de Falco[a], Paola Venuti[a], Gianluca Esposito[a], and Marc H. Bornstein[b]

[a]Department of Cognitive Science and Education, University of Trento, Italy
[b]Child and Family Research, *Eunice Kennedy Shriver* National Institute of Child Health and Human Development, National Institutes of Health, Department of Health and Human Services, USA

Abstract

Healthy parent-child interaction is as essential to the early development of children with Down Syndrome as it is for typically developing children. In early childhood, this transaction is largely regulated by reciprocal emotional exchanges between partners. Through their caregiving, parents supply their children with the experiences they need for both physical and psychological growth. Contemporary opinion is that positive emotional sharing is an indispensable frame to effective caregiving of children with an intellectual disability, but at the same time specific cognitive and/or motor impairments may short-circuit the child's ability to understand and exchange emotions.

In this chapter we first outline the current findings about parent-child interaction in children with Down Syndrome. Then we report in details the results of two studies about children with Down Syndrome in which we compared mother-child and father-child dyads with respect to some pivotal aspects of parent-child interaction, namely affective quality and play behaviours; for each study, the differences and similarities between mothers and fathers as well as the children's contribution to relationship functioning are presented. The discussion of the findings refer to the theoretical perspective according to which dyadic interactions based on emotional involvement may lead to enhanced cognitive functioning in children with Down Syndrome. Finally, the clinical implications of this framework are discussed.

Introduction

Parent-child interaction plays a crucial role in the development of children with special needs (Greenspan, 1997). Empical findings support the idea that the development of children with Down Syndrome (DS), as the development of children with other intellectual disabilities, depends remarkably on the cognitive and social stimulation provided by the "good enough" parents (Pino, 2000; Venuti, de Falco, Giusti and Bornstein, 2008; de Falco, Esposito, Venuti and Bornstein, 2008). However, the atypical features displayed by a child with DS may influence dyadic parent-child interactions resulting in dyadic interaction styles that differ from those of typically developing children for many reasons. First, parental interaction style may be affected by the diminished children's responsiveness and involving abilities: children with DS make fewer initiations and engage in less structured turn-taking social games compared to typically developing children (Beeghley, Weiss-Perry, and Cicchetti, 1989; Cielinski, Vaughn, Seifer, and Contreras, 1995; Mundy, Sigman, Kasari, and Yirmiya, 1988; Landry and Chapieski, 1990; Richard, 1986; Slonims and McConachie, 2006). Moreover, parental interaction behaviours may also reflect their feelings and perceptions, namely their worries for children's health and future, the delusion of their expectations (of a healthy child) and the difficulties in accepting their child's condition (Drotar, Baskiewitz, Irvin, Kennel, and Klaus, 1975; Solnit and Stark, 1961).

The quality of mother-child interaction has been a recurrent topic in the literature about families of children with DS. Several studies have concentrated on one aspect which differentiates mothers of children with DS children from mothers of typically developing children, namely directiveness (Beeghly and Cicchetti, 1987; Cielinski et al., 1995; Landry and Chapieski, 1989; Marfo et al., 1998). This directive attitude consists in a tendency to intensely structure and organize the child's activities and it has been sometimes associated with over-controlling or intrusive behaviors and with a lack of sensitivity (Berger and Cunningman, 1983). However, when accurately distinguishing between maternal directiveness and intrusiveness, investigators have often attributed to the former an adaptive and functional role (Cielinski et al. 1995; Crawley and Spiker 1983; Marfo, 1990).

Despite the evidence for the risk of difficulties in parent-child interaction for families of children with DS versus typically developing children (Brooks-Gunn and Lewis, 1984), this families may benefit from a specific condition known as the "Down syndrome advantage" (Seltzer and Ryff, 1994; Hodapp et al., 2001). This phenomenon was described on the bases of several empirical studies that found that mother-child relationship quality is better with children with DS compared to children with other intellectual disabilities (Marcheschi, Millepiedi, and Bargagna, 1990), perhaps because children with DS generally display more cheerful, sociable personalities (Hodapp, 2002) relative to children with other special needs. Moreover, parents of DS children have been found to suffer lower levels of stress compared with parents of children with intellectual disabilities of different etiologies (Fidler, Hodapp, and Dykens, 2000). Accordingly, some studies on mother-child play interaction on children with DS compared to children with typical development, highlighted substantial similarities in terms of maternal sensitivity and dyadic harmony, despite the directiveness shown by mothers (Beeghly et al., 1989; Crawlay and Spiker, 1983).

Although both parents may be practically and emotionally involved in childrearing, most of these studies on interactions between parents and their children with DS have been conducted with mothers (Cielinski *et al.*, 1995; Marcheschi *et al.*, 1990; Ruskin *et al.*, 1994;). Only recently, the role of the father in parenting a child with intellectual disability has come to the investigators' attention (Olsson and Hwang 2001; Shin *et al.*, 2006; Glidden *et al.* 2006). Paternal stress and coping skills are becoming interesting issues and there is a growing body of literature on fathers of children with DS (Ricci and Hodapp 2003; Hodapp 2007; Stoneman, 2007; Senese *et al.* 2008). Specifically, it seems that fathers of children with DS perceive them as having fewer maladaptive behaviours and more positive personality traits when compared to fathers of children with other intellectual disabilities (Ricci and Hodapp 2003). Moreover, they have been found to perceive the relationship with their children as more harmonious (Hornby, 1996) compared to fathers of children with other intellectual disabilities. Indeed, these studies seem to show that the "Down syndrome advantage" may be true for fathers as for mothers.

However, to date there is a lack of studies on observed interactions between fathers and children with DS. Yet, there are significant reasons to extend to fathers the investigation of parent-child interaction with DS children (Ricci and Hodapp, 2003). First, theorists and researchers agree that paternal involvement in childrearing exerts a unique positive influence on several domains of growth and adaptation (Parke, 2002; Venuti, and Giusti, 1996; Booth and Crouter, 1998). Different aspects of paternal involvement have been associated to positive outcomes in child social development, cognitive competence and academic achievement (Cabrera *et al.*, 2000; Tamis-LeMonda and Cabrera, 2002).. Another reason to investigate the actual interactions between fathers and children with DS is that, although both parents of children with DS, compared to parents of typically developing children, show decreased levels of well-being (Roach *et al.* 1999: Hodapp 2002), several studies comparing fathers to mothers of children with other intellectual disabilities found that fathers experience less stress (Goldberg *et al.* 1986; Bristol *et al.* 1988; Damrosch and Perry 1989; Olsson and Hwang 2001; Shin *et al.*, 2006). No specific studies to date have clarified if this is true also in families of children with DS but it might be the case that the maternal and paternal contributions to the development of children with DS may differ as a result of differences in feelings and emotional reactions.

Empirical Studies

In this paragraph we summarize the results of a series of empirical studies about children with Down Syndrome. In these studies, we compared mother-child and father-child dyads with respect to some pivotal aspects of parent-child interaction, namely emotional availability and play behaviours.

Dyadic Emotional Availability

The parent-child relationship is not unidirectional with only parents affecting their children. It is, rather, a fluid two-way exchange where signals and behaviors from both partners constantly affect one another in bidirectional transaction (Bornstein, 2003, 2008; Sander, 2000; Stern, 1985; Trevarthen and Aitken, 2001; Van Egeren, Barratt, and Roach, 2001; Venuti et al., 2008). In early childhood, this transaction is largely regulated by reciprocal emotional exchanges between partners (Emde and Easterbrooks, 1985; Greenspan, 1997; Trevarthen, 2003; Tronick, 2005). Expressing emotions through their voices, faces and gestures, parents engage their children, direct and maintain child attention, and build the rhythm of expectable dyadic interaction (Bornstein, Gini, Leach, Haynes, Painter, and Suwalsky, 2006a; Martin, Clements, and Crnic, 2002; Weinberg and Tronick, 1996). Reciprocally, even young children use multiple signals that convey their emotional states and needs to their parents (Barnard, Hammond, Booth, Bee, Mitchell, and Spieker, 1989; Bornstein, Gini, Suwalsky, Leach, and Haynes, 2006b; Trevarthen, 1993, 2003).

Contemporary opinion is that positive emotional sharing is an indispensable frame to effective caregiving of children with a developmental disability. At the same time, it is recognized that specific cognitive and/or motor impairments may short-circuit the child's ability to understand and exchange emotions (Greenspan, 1997; Trevarthen and Aitken, 2001; Venuti et al., 2008).

Emotional availability (EA; Biringen, 2000; Biringen and Robinson 1991) is a relational construct that refers specifically to emotional transactions between children and their parents (Aviezer, Sagi, Joels, and Ziv, 1999; Biringen and Robinson, 1991; Bretherton, 2000; Emde, 1980). This construct, based on attachment theory (Ainsworth, Blehar, Waters, and Wall, 1978) integrated with Emde's (1980) emotions perspective, refers to parental attitudes and behaviors (sensitivity, structuring, nonintrusiveness, and nonhostility) and to children's ability to respond and involve the parent, highlighting the role of emotion understanding and expression as barometers of dyadic functioning. Given the significant and meaningful associations between EA and many discrete affective indices of parent-child interaction (Kogan and Carter, 1996; Robinson, Little, and Biringen, 1993; Zimmerman and McDonald, 1995), EA can be considered a global index of the overall quality of the parent-child affective relationship (Biringen, 2000). Studies of emotional availability suggest that the construct not only plays a role in the prediction of attachment (Easterbrook and Biringen, 2000, 2005) but also in developmental phenomena as far ranging as sleep patterns and language gains in typically and atypically developing children (Pressman, Pipp-Siegel, Yoshinaga-Itano, and Deas, 1999; Sagi, Tirosh, Ziv, Guttman, and Lavie, 1998).

To date, the majority of studies of EA have involved typically developing children mainly interacting with their mothers. Very few studies have involved children with special needs (Venuti, et al 2008; Wiefel et al., 2005) or fathers. The present study aimed to investigate EA in children with Down syndrome (DS) interacting separately with their mothers as well as their fathers. To reach this aim we coded 10-min free-play interactions of 22 children with DS (*M* chronological age = 35.32 mo) separately with each parent using the Emotional Availability Scales (EAS; Biringen, Robinson, and Emde, 1998, 3rd edition). Specifically, we explored EA levels in families of children with DS and compared dimensions of EA between the parents of children with DS to evaluate if fathers show similar or different levels of EA than mothers, as suggested by the literature in typically developing children (Lovas, 2005; Volling et al., 2002). Moreover, we investigated if EA in mothers and fathers were associated. Finally, starting from the systems view of parent-child interaction in general (Bornstein, 2003; Sander, 2000; Stern, 1985; Trevarthen and Aitken, 2001; Venuti et al., 2008) we to investigated the extent to which children with DS show different levels of responsiveness and involving with the two parents, and if these levels are associated.

Table 1. Emotional Availability Scales in Mother-Child and Father-Child Dyads

		Mother-Child	Father-Child	$t(21)^a$	r^b
Parent					
Sensitivity (1 = highly insensitive; 9 = highly sensitive): assesses the parent's contingent responsiveness to child signals, appropriate affectivity, acceptance, flexibility, affect regulation, conflict resolution, and variety and creativity in play	*M* *Range* *SD*	5.75 3-8 1.28	5.73 3.5-8.5 1.15	.09	.54**
Structuring (1 = nonoptimal; 5 = optimal): assesses the degree to which the parent appropriately scaffolds or organizes the child's activities and exploration, by providing rules and a supportive framework without compromising the child's autonomy	*M* *Range* *SD*	3.64 2-4.5 .74	3.77 2.5-5 .63	-1.06	.63**
Nonintrusiveness (1 = intrusive; 5 = nonintrusive): measures the degree to which the parent is able to support the child's play and exploration, without interrupting the child by being overdirective, overstimulating, overprotecting, and/or interfering.	*M* *Range* *SD*	4.09 2.5-4.5 .80	4.11 2.5-5 .65	-.12	.25
Nonhostility (1 = markedly hostile; 5 = nonhostile): measures the degree to which the parent is able to talk to or behave with the child in a way that is generally patient, pleasant, and harmonious and not rejecting, abrasive, impatient, or antagonistic.	*M* *Range* *SD*	4.59 3.5-5 .48	4.64 4-5 .41	234	.60**

Table 1. (Continued)

		Mother-Child	Father-Child	$t(21)^a$	r^b
Child					
Responsiveness (1 = nonoptimal; 7 = optimal): focuses on the child's age- and context-appropriate ability and interest in in responding to the parent's bids (i.e., the balance between connection and autonomy) as well as the extent of the child's enjoyment of the interaction	*M*	4.95	5.21	-1.12	.39
	Range	2.5-6.5	3.5-6.5		
	SD	1.06	.78		
Involving (1 = nonoptimal; 9 = optimal): assesses the child's ability and willingness to engage the parent in interaction	*M*	4.72	5.11	-1.43	.46*
	Range	2.5-6.5	3.5-6.5		
	SD	1.08	.72		

* $p < .05$; ** $p < .01$

Because mother age, child chronological and child developmental age were associated with the EAS, we used as scores the standardized residuals of a regression with these 3 variables as predictors.

[a] Dependent *t*-test values are reported; for Nonhostility, paired Wilcoxon signed-ranks test value is reported.

[b] Pearson product–moment *r* coefficients values are reported; for Nonhostility, Spearman's rank order coefficient value is reported.

Results showed that the mean level reached by the dyads in this study was slightly above the midpoint for Sensitivity and Structuring, close to the optimal level for Nonintrusiveness, even closer for Nonhostility, and "good enough" for the child scales of Responsiveness and Involving. As for Sensitivity, the scores of this sample are similar to those reported in the other studies of children with special needs or at-risk children (Easterbrooks et al., 2005; Wiefel et al., 2005). Moreover, scores accord with the results of some investigators who found, using a different assessment of maternal sensitivity, no differences between mothers of children with DS and typical development (Beeghly et al., 1989; Crawlay and Spiker, 1983).

Both parents in this study showed high levels of Nonintrusiveness, in contrast with the directive style often described in the literature about mothers of children with DS. Moreover no associations were found between Nonintrusiveness and Structuring scales, indicating that higher intrusiveness is not always associated with lower structuring. This finding accords with the idea that, when interacting with children with DS, parents may need to use a more directive style to successfully promote sophisticated play, without necessarily being intrusive.. The optimal level of Nonhostility observed in this sample shows that, although interacting with children who have objective impairments, parents of children with DS do not display a rejecting, abrasive, or impatient attitude. On average, children with DS reached a "good enough" level in Responsiveness, as described in the manual; indicating that they were generally positive and emotionally available, even even if they showed less clear joy or appropriateness in their affective responsiveness than expected by the optimal level (Biringen et al., 1998). Similarly, for Involving, children with DS showed clear, although not optimal, tendencies to engage a parent in play. These findings are consistent with the idea that children with DS generally display more cheerful, sociable personalities compared to children with other types of disability (Hodapp, 2002).

As for the comparisons between mothers and fathers in their EA, results show substantial similaries. In the literature about children with typical development, mothers are often reported as more sensitive compared to fathers (Lamb et al., 1982; Nakamura, Stewart, and Tatarka, 2000). This idea has been confirmed by the two existing studies that aimed to compare parents with regard to EA (Lovas, 2005; Volling et al., 2002). Yet, in a study where the EAS were applied to a child psychiatric population, Wiefel et al. (2005) reported no differences between parents' EAS ratings. To help interpret this finding, Some other cues may derive from the literature about emotional reactions and parental stress in fathers of children with disabilities. Although it has been found that both parents of children with disabilities suffer from more parenting stress and and lower levels of well-being compared to parents of children with typical development (Hodapp, 2002; Lamb and Billings, 1997), some scholars argue that fathers feel themselves more in control of the situation and experience less stress , compared to mothers (Bristol, Gallagher, and Shopler, 1988; Damrosch and Perry, 1989; Goldberg, Marcovitch, MacGregor, and Lojkasek, 1986; Hodapp, 2002). Another possible interpretation could be that, in families of children with special needs, fathers may reach the same levels of emotional availability as mothers for compensation. In other words, it could be that, perceiving the special parenting needs of their children, fathers pay more attention to their own and their children's emotional exchanges during interaction.

Corresponding EA dimensions of one parent tended to be positively associated with those of the other parent for all but Nonintrusiveness scales. It could could be that, consistently with the process of "assertive mating", EA encompasses general features of empathy and socioemotional competence, which tend to be similar in married couples and is. Or it could be that children's own ways of interacting exert similar influences on their two parents' EA (see below).

With respect to child EA dimensions, both continuity and stability across children's interactions with their two parents were found. Continuity means that the mean levels of mother- and father-child EA were comparable, and this finding is consistent with the general similarity with regard to EA between mother- and father-child dyads; it also reveals that there were no general quantitative or qualitative differences in the ways children were responsive to or involving of their mothers compared to their fathers. Stability tells us about the consistency of individual differences in the group. On the one hand, these findings accord with the bidirectional nature of parent-child interaction and specifically with the idea of the child's contribution to dyadic exchanges, telling us that each child brings to the interaction with both parents the child's own ways of being responsive and involving. On the other hand, the moderate degree of stability confirms that child EA is also related to individual parental interactive style and probably to the history of the parent-child relationship.

Play Behaviors

Many of children's first experiences of the world and much of their first learning take place during play (Bornstein 2007; Tamis-LeMonda and Bornstein, 1996; Piaget 1962;

Vygotsky 1978).While children grow up, more mature cognitive skills emerge which in turn allow for more sophisticated play. The development of play follows universal progression both for typically developing children and for children with DS, as extensively reported by the literature, (Hill and McCune-Nicolich, 1981; Cunningham *et al.* 1985; Beeghly and Cicchetti 1987; Mundy *et al.* 1987). Simple sensorimotor object exploration and manipulation tend to progressively diminish during the first years of life, whereas more complex and hierarchically integrated forms of play, such as combinatorial and symbolic play, increase. This universal trends have been associated with the emergence of new cognitive skills in the child, a reason why maturity in play is traditionally thought to index children's overall cognitive level (Piaget 1962; Hill and McCune-Nicolich 1981; Beeghly and Cicchetti 1987). Although these developmental tendencies in children's play, there are significant dyadic effects. The role of caregiver in the development of play in typically developing children is a recurrent topic in the literature about both typically developing children and in children with intellectual disabilities (Fiese 1990; Bornstein *et al.*, 1996; Noll and Harding 2003; Bornstein *et al.* 1996, 2002; Cielinski *et al.*, 1995; Venuti *et al.* 1997; 2008). The presence of the parent during play and his/her specific behaviours exert a powerful influence on the amount, duration, and complexity of child play. By providing adequate scaffolding during collaborative play, parents help their children to practice more sophisticated behaviours (and underlying mental skills) they can potentially reach. Concerning DS children specifically, Cielinski and colleagues (1995) found that child play sophistication was higher during collaborative play with mother than during solitary play, but the authors did not address the quantity of exploratory and symbolic play activities separately. Venuti and colleagues (2008), who considered the amounts of both exploratory and symbolic play, found that the presence of the mother during play resulted in more child exploratory, but not symbolic play. Moreover, a positive link between the affective quality of parent-child interaction and the play skills of children with DS have been found; that is, within interactions of higher affective quality, children with DS display more sophisticated play behaviours (Marcheschi *et al.* 1990; Venuti *et al.* 2008; de Falco *et al.* 2008).

To date the role of caregiver in the play development of children with DS is still an under-investigated topic. Moreover, the majority of studies have been conducted with mothers (e.g., Marcheschi *et al.*, 1990; Cielinski *et al.*, 1995; Roach *et al.*, 1998), and very few studies have directly compared father- with mother-child play in children with DS. Therefore the main aim of the study we present was to compare the play of DS children with their two parents as well as the two parents' play behaviours. Data were collected during 3 consecutive 10-min sessions. A set of standard, age-appropriate toys was used. During the first session (solitary play), the child played with the toy set on his or her own; during the second and third sessions (collaborative play), the mother or the father were asked to play with the child. The order of the mother and father collaborative play sessions was counterbalanced. The same play code was applied to child play in solitary and collaborative sessions and to mother and father play. The play code used consisted of a mutually exclusive and exhaustive category system that included 8 levels and a default (no play) category. Levels 1-4 constitute the macro-category Exploratory play, and Levels 5-8 constitute the macro-category Symbolic play. For each level four measures were calculated: the absolute frequency, the proportion frequency, the absolute duration, and the proportion duration. Their mean standard score was used as a summary index representing the amount of each play level and each macro-category.

Results show that DS children with both fathers and mothers, increase in their exploratory activity from solitary to collaborative play. Exploratory play represents a specific challenge for children with DS as reported in the literature.

Table 2.Maternal and paternal play in collaborative play sessions

	Mother play		*Father play*		*t(19)*	*r(18)*
Play duration (in sec)	*M*	*SD*	*M*	*SD*		
Exploratory play	59.81	46.58	45.85	44.01	2.33	-.29
Symbolic play	33.05	26.52	63.70	48.73	-2.45	.12

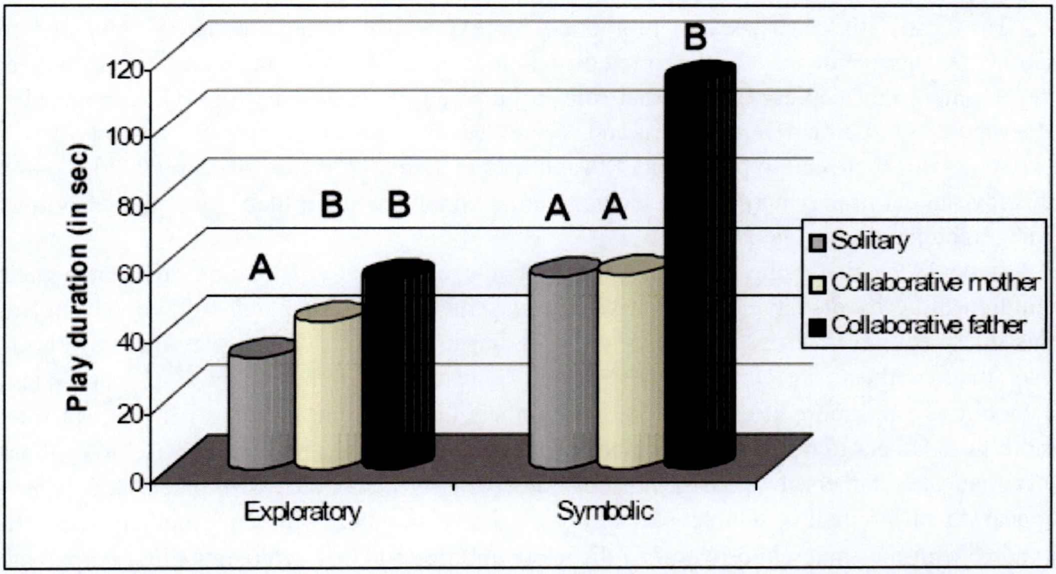

Note. Bars with different letters represent significant mean differences in summary indexes at Tukey HSD *post-hoc* tests for $p < .05$.

Figure 1.Child exploratory and symbolic play by situation.

Several studies demonstrated that children with DS show poor exploratory play even when compared to mental age-matched control children, and this deficit could be related to other basilar deficits of children with DS, such as movement or instrumental thinking, attention and objct mastery (Ruskin *et al.* 1994; Landry and Chapieski 1989). The findings of this study suggest that both parents are able to help their children to improve in what they specifically lack. By participating in their play, both parents provide the adequate support children with DS need to overcome their basilar difficulties in solitary exploration.

By contrast, children increased in symbolic activity from solitary to collaborative play only with their fathers. Symbolic play includes the use of representations and pretense which underscore more complex cognitive skills compared to exploratory behaviours. Previous studies of children with DS have highlighted that their symbolic play skills are substantially linked to their general intellectual impairment, rather than to a specific deficit and are therefore similar to those of metal age-matched typically developing children. Therefore, the results of this study show that fathers, unlike mothers, were able to promote a kind of play that is cognitively advanced although not specifically compromised in this population.

Altogether these results expand the literature on parent-child play in children with DS by extending to fathers the influential role on their children's play that has been previously highlighted mostly by studies involving mothers. Moreover, from the direct comparison of child play with the two parents, we found that children with their fathers displayed the same amount of exploratory, but a higher amount of symbolic activity than with mothers. Therefore, children played more during the collaborative session with their fathers and the extra-time consisted of a more advanced kind of play. Thus, this study offers some evidence that children with DS might benefit more from their fathers' than from their mothers' play during joint play in terms of their increased play sophistication.

How did fathers succeed in promoting more pretense in their children compared to mothers? This result may be interpreted in light of the literature on fatherhood in typical development that depicts the paternal role in parenting as largely carried out through play (Hewlett 1992; Lamb 1997; Caneva and Venuti 1998). Fathers are reported as more active playmates for their children compared to mothers (Lamb 1977; Tamis-Lemonda 2004), and this investment in play may be conducive to children advancing in their symbolic behaviours when in collaborative play.

It could be that fathers in this sample in the collaborative situation stimulated their children more by displaying more symbolic play themselves compared to their wives. But this interpretation is not supported by these findings; fathers did not display more symbolic play than mothers. By contrast, these results indicate that fathers play significantly less symbolically and more at exploration than mothers did. Thus, it appears as if mothers tried more than fathers to demonstrate symbolic play to their children but children followed them less than their fathers. Moreover, not only did the play behaviours of mothers and fathers appear to differ in this sample but they were not associated with one another; although playing with the same child, who has the same abilities and characteristics, the two parents engaged in different behaviours when joining him/her in play.

A possible explanation for the unique paternal influence on child symbolic play may concern parent-child attunement. Perhaps fathers tried to promote pretense mostly when there was a joint focus on this kind of play and they did not over-demonstrate symbolic play to their children. The correlation analyses partially support this hypothesis; when playing together, fathers and children in the sample showed a high degree of mutual attunement. Therefore, fathers may tailor their behavior to their children's abilities and interests, and at the same time DS children respond to their fathers' bids. The associations between fathers and their DS children's play were strong both for exploratory and symbolic play, highlighting attunement that represents an essential social frame for cognitive development (Vygotsky 1978; Greenspan 1997; Venuti 2007;). By contrast the degree of mutual attunement was somewhat lower for mother-child play.

Conclusion

Healthy parent-child interaction is as essential to the early development of children with special needs as it is for children with typical development and among the prominent factors that lead to effective parent-child interaction, Emotional Availability is crucial (EA; Biringen, 2000; Easterbrooks and Biringen 2000, 2005). Parents and their children with Down Syndrome (DS) show adequate levels of EA in average and this is equally true for both mother-child and father-child dyads. Moreover, taking a closer look to the effect of parent-child interaction on one important indicator of child cognitive development, namely play, we found that maternal and paternal contributions to child play skills are both positive but different. During collaborative play children with DS received specific and non overlapping scaffolding from their two parents and fathers seemed to provide a unique contribution. Especially through their play, fathers may exert a unique and supplementary role in successfully parenting a child withDS. For this reason, we think it is important to involve fathers in early intervention programs for children with DS.

More in general, we think that early intervention programmes may enhance their effectiveness by promoting parental EA as well as children's responsiveness to and involvement with the parent. Furthermore, the Emotional Availability Scales (Biringen, Robinson and Emde, 1998) could be a useful tool for assessing specific strengths and problems in the parent-child relationship with special needs children, and may be helpful in defining and evaluating specific intervention goals concerning the emotional quality of dyadic interaction. Being able to assess higher levels of EA in clinical practice would mean uncovering an important strength to support interventions focused on other weak areas of child development; indeed, there is empirical evidence that both mother-child and father-child EA can influence cognitive performance in children with DS during joint play (Venuti et al., 2008; de Falco, Esposito, Venuti, and Bornstein, 2008). On the other hand, revealing a specific profile of low parent-child EA would enable to implement (and evaluate afterwards) intervention programs focused on the parent-child relationship aimed to prevent secondary deficits that originate from or are comorbid with dysfunctional dyadic interactions. Moreover, the association we found between the two parents' EA may be relevant from a clinical stand point too. Whatever the reason, it suggests that, when problems in mother-child relationship are encountered by a clinician, special attention has to be paid to father-child relationship, as it is likely to be impaired as well. In other words, at least in families with DS, low EA of one parent should be considered a risk factor for the child's relationship with the other parent, and calls for therapeutic support to the whole family. On the other side, the presence of a "good enough" pattern of dyadic EA with the mother would suggest that father-child EA is healthy too, which does not mean it should be excluded from intervention, but, in contrast, that it should be targeted in the intervention as an important and unique resource to assure the development of the whole potentialities of children with DS.

References

Ainsworth, M.D.S., Blehar, M.C., Waters, E., and Wall, S. (1978). *Patterns of attachment: A psychological study of the strange situation*. Hillsdale, NJ: Lawrence Erlbaum.

Aviezer, O., Sagi, A., Joels, T., and Ziv, Y. (1999). Emotional availability and attachment representations in kibbutz infants and their mothers. *Developmental Psychology, 35*, 811-821.

Barnard, K. E., Hammond, M. A., Booth, C. L., Bee, H. L., Mitchell, S. K., and Spieker, S. J. (1989). Measurement and meaning of parent-child interaction. In F. J. Morrison, C. Lord, and D. P. Keating (Eds.), *Applied developmental psychology, Vol. 3* (pp. 40-80). New York: Academic Press.

Beeghly M., Weiss-Perry B.W. and Cicchetti D. (1989) Structural and affective dimensions of play development in young children with Down syndrome. *International Journal of Behavioral Development* 12, 257-277.

Beeghly M. and Cicchetti D. (1987) An organizational approach to symbolic development in children with Down syndrome. *NCMJ Directions in Child Development* 36, 5-29.

Berger, J., and Cunningham, C.C. (1983). Development of early vocal behaviors and interactions in Down's syndrome and nonhandicapped infant-mother pairs. *Developmental Psychology, 19,* 322-331.

Biringen, Z. (2000). Emotional Availability: Conceptualization and Research Findings. American *Journal of Orthopsychiatry, 70,* 104-114.

Biringen, Z. (2005). Training and reliability issues with the emotional availability scales. *Infant Mental Health Journal, 26*, 404-405.

Biringen, Z., and Robinson, J. (1991). Emotional availability in mother-child interactions: A reconceptualization for research. American Journal of Orthopsychiatry, 61, 258-271.

Biringen, Z., Robinson, J.L., and Emde, R.N. (1998). Emotional Availability Scales (3rd Ed.), Unpublished manual, Department on Human Development and Family Studies, Colorado State University, Fort Collins, CO.

Biringen, Z., Damon, J., Grigg, W., Mone, J., Pipp-Siegel, S., Skillern, S., and Stratton, J. (2005). Emotional availability: differential predictions to infant attachment and kindergarten adjustment based on observation time and context. *Infant Mental Health Journal, 26,* 295–308.

Biringen, Z., Fidler, D.J., Barrett, K.C., and Kubicek, L. (2005). Applying the emotional availability scales to children with disabilities. *Infant Mental Health Journal, 26,* 369-391.

Booth A. and Crouter A. C. (1998) *Men in families*. Mahwah: Erlbaum.

Bretherton, I. (2000). Emotional availability: An attachment perspective. Attachment and Human Development, 2, 233-241.

Bornstein, M.H., (2003). Parenting e sviluppo infantile: Considerazioni intraculturali ed interculturali. In C. Poderico, P. Venuti, R. Marcone (Eds.), Diverse culture: bambini diversi? (pp. 31-56). Roma: Unicopli.

Bornstein M. H. (2007) On the significance of social relationships in the development of children's earliest symbolic play: An ecological perspective. In: *Play and development:*

Evolutionary, sociocultural, and functional perspectives (eds A. Gönçü and S. Gaskins), pp. 101-129. Mahwah, NJ: Erlbaum.

Bornstein, M.H (2008). Toward a model of culture-parent-child transactions. In A. Sameroff (Ed.), *Transactions* (pp. xx-xx). Washington, DC: American Psychological Association.

Bornstein M.H., Venuti P. and Hahn C. (2002) Mother-child play in Italy: regional variation, individual stability, and mutual dyadic influence. *Parenting: Science and Practice* 2, 273-301.

Bornstein M.H., Haynes O.M., O'Reilly A.W. and Painter K. (1996) Solitary and collaborative pretense play in early childhood: Sources of individual variation in the development of representational competence. *Child Development* 67, 2910-2929.

Bornstein, M. H., Gini, M., Putnick, D. L., Haynes, O. M., Painter, K. M., and Suwalsky, J. T. D. (2006a). Short-term reliability and continuity of emotional availability in infant-mother dyads across contexts of observation. *Infancy, 10,* 1-16.

Bornstein, M. H., Gini, M., Suwalsky, J. T. D., Leach, D. B., and Haynes, O. M. (2006b). Emotional availability in mother-child dyads: Short-term stability continuity from variable and person points of view. *Merrill-Palmer Quarterly, 52,* 547-571.

Bristol M., Gallagher J. and Shopler E. (1988) Mothers and fathers of young developmentally disabled and nondisabled boys: Adaptation and spousal support. *Developmental Psychology* 24, 441–451.

Brooks-Gunn J. and Lewis M. (1984) Maternal Responsivity. *Interactions with handicapped infants Child Development* 55, 782-793.

Cabrera N. J., Tamis-LeMonda C. S., Bradley R. H., Hofferth S. and Lamb M. E. (2000) Fatherhood in the twenty-first century. *Child Development* 71, 127 – 136.

Caneva L. and Venuti P. (1998) Stile materno e stile paterno nel gioco con i figli: uno studio osservativo a tre e tredici mesi. *Psicologia Clinica dello Sviluppo* 2, 303-326.

Cielinski K.L., Vaughn B.E., Seifer R. and Contreras J. (1995) Relations among sustained engagement during play, quality of play, and mother-child interaction in samples of children with Down syndrome and normally developing toddlers. *Infant Behaviour and development* 18, 163-176.

Crawley, S.B., and Spiker, D. (1983). Mother-child interaction involving two-years olds with DS: A look at individual differences. *Child Development, 54,* 1312-1323.

Cunningham C.C., Glenn S.M, Wilkinson P. and Sloper P. (1985) Mental ability, symbolic play and receptive and expressive language of young children with Down's syndrome. *Journal of Child Psychology and Psychiatry* 26, 255-265.

Damrosch S. and Perry L. (1989) Self-reported adjustment, chronic sorrow, and coping of parents of children with Down Syndrome. *Nursing Research* 38, 25–30.

de Falco S., Esposito G., Venuti P. and Bornstein M.H. (2008) Father's play with their Down Sindrome children. *Journal of Intellectual Disability Research* 52 (6), 490-502.

Drotar, D., Baskiewitz, A., Irvin, N., Kennel, J., and Klaus, M. (1975). The adaptation of parents to the birth of an infant with a congenital malformation: A hypothetical model. *Pediatrics, 56,* 710–717.

Easterbrooks, M.A., and Biringen, Z. (2000). Guest editors' introduction to the special issue: Mapping the terrain of emotional availability and attachment. *Attachment and Human Development, 2,* 123–129.

Easterbrooks, M.A., and Biringen, Z. (2005). The emotional availability scales: methodological refinements of the construct and clinical implications related to gender and at-risk interactions. Infant Mental Health Journal, 26(4), 291-294.

Emde, R.N. (1980). Emotional availability: A reciprocal reward system for infants and parents with implications for prevention of psychosocial disorders. In. P.M. Taylor, (Ed.), Parent-infant relationships. Orlando, FL: Grune and Stratton.

Emde, R.N., and Easterbrooks, M.A. (1985). Assessing emotional availability in early development. In D. K. Frankenberg, R. N. Emde, and J. W. Sullivan (Eds.), Early identification of children at risk: An international perspective (pp. 79-101). New York: Plenum Press.

Fidler, D.J., Hodapp, R.M., and Dykens, E.M. (2000). Stress in families of young children with DS, Williams syndrome, and Smith-Magenis syndrome. Early Education and Development, 11, 395–406.

Fiese B.H. (1990) Playful relationships: A contextual analysis of mother-toddler interaction and symbolic play. *Child Development* 61, 1648-1656.

Glidden L.M., Billings F.J. and Jobe B.M. (2006) Personality, coping style and well-being of parents rearing children with developmental disabilities. *Journal of Intellectual Disability Research* 50, 949-62.

Goldberg S., Marcovitch S., MacGregor D. and Lojkasek M. (1986) Family responses to developmentally delayed preschoolers: Etiology and the father's role. *American Journal on Mental Retardation* 90, 610–617.

Greenspan S.J. (1997) *Developmentally Based Psychotherapy.* Madison, CT: International University Press.

Hewlett B. (1992) *Father–child relations: Cultural and biosocial contexts*. New York: Aldine de Gruyter.

Hill P.M. and McCune-Nicolich L. (1981) Pretend play and patterns of cognition in Down's syndrome. *Child Development* 52, 611-617.

Hodapp R.M. (2007) Families of persons with Down syndrome: New perspectives, findings, and research and service needs. *Mental Retardation and Developmental Disabilities Research Reviews* 13:3, 279-287.

Hodapp R.M. (2002) Parenting children with mental retardation. In: *Handbook of Parenting* 2nd edn. *Volume I, How Children Influence Parents* (ed. M.H. Bornstein), pp. 355-381. Hillsdale, Erlbaum, NJ.

Kogan, N., and Carter, A.S. (1996). Mother-infant reengagement following the still-face: The role of maternal emotional availability in infant affect regulation. Infant Behavior and Development, 19, 359-370.

Lamb M. E. (ed.) (1997) *The role of the father in child development*, 3rd edn. Wiley, New York.

Lamb M. E. (1977) Father-infant and mother-infant interaction in the first year of life. *Child Development* 48(1), 167-181.

Lamb M.E. and Billings L.L.A. (1997). Fathers of children with special needs. In M. E. Lamb (Ed.), *The role of the father in child development,* 3rd ed. New York: John Wiley and Sons, 179-190.

Lamb, M. E., Frodi, A. M., Frodi, M., and Hwang, C. P. (1982). Characteristics of maternal and paternal behavior in traditional and nontraditional Swedish families. *International Journal of Behavioral Development, 5,* 131–141.

Landry S.H. and Chapieski M.L. (1989) Joint attention and infant toy exploration effects of DS and prematurity. *Child Development* 60, 103-1 18.

Landry, S.H., and Chapieski, M.L, (1990). Joint attention of six-month old DS and preterm infants: Attention to toys and mother. American Journal on Menial Retardation, 94, 488-498.

Lovas, G. S. (2005). Gender and patterns of emotional availability in mother-toddler and father-toddler dyads. *Infant Mental Health Journal, 26,* 327-353.

Marcheschi M., Millepiedi S. and Bargagna S. (1990) Lo sviluppo del gioco e l'interazione madre-bambino nel bambino Down. *Psichiatria dell'Infanzia e dell'Adolescenza* 3, 645-652.

Marfo, K. (1990). Maternal directiveness in interactions with mentally handicapped children: An analytical commentary. *Journal of Child Psychology and Psychiatry, 31,* 531-549.

Marfo, K., Cynthia, F.D., Dedrick, F. and Barbour, N. (1998). Mother-child interactions and the development of children with mental retardation. In A.B., Burack, R.M., Hodapp, E.F. Zigler, (Eds.), Handbook of Mental Retardation and Development (pp. 637-668). Cambridge: Cambridge University Press.

Martin, S. E., Clements, M. L., and Crnic, K. A. (2002). Maternal emotions during mother-toddler interaction: Parenting in affective context. *Parenting: Science and Practice, 2,* 105-126.

Mundy P., Sigman M., Ungerer J. and Sherman T. (1987) Nonverbal communication and play correlates of language development in autistic children. *Journal of Autism and Developmental Disorders* 17, 349-364.

Mundy, P., Sigman, M., Kasari, C, and Yirmiya, N. (1988). Nonverbal communication skills in DS children. Child Development, 59, 235-249.

Nakamura, W.M., Stewart, K.B., and Tatarka, M.E. (2000). Assessing father–infant interactions using the NCAST Teaching Scale: A pilot study. *American Journal of Occupational Therapy, 54,* 44–51.

Noll L.M. and Harding C.B. (2003) The relationship of mother-child interaction and the child's development of symbolic play. *Infant Mental Health* 24, 557-570.

Notaro, P.C., and Volling, B.L. (1999). Parental responsiveness and infant-parent attachment: A replication study with fathers and mothers. *Infant Behavior and Development, 22,* 534-352.

Olsson M.B. and Hwang C.P. (2001) Depression in mothers and fathers of children with intellectual disability. J*ournal of Intellectual Disability Research* 45, 535-543.

Parke R.D. (2002) *Mahwah.* Parke fathers and families. In: *Handbook of Parenting Volume 3, Being and Becoming a Parent (2e)* (ed. M.H. Bornstein) pp. 27-73, Erlbaum, Mahwah, NJ.

Parke, R. D., and Tinsley, B. J. (1987). Family interaction in infancy. In J. D. Osofsky (Ed.), Handbook of infant development (2nd ed., pp.579– 641). New York: Wiley.

Piaget J. (1962) *Play, dreams and imitation in childhood.* New York: Norton.

Pino, O. (2000). The effect of context on mother's interaction style with Down's syndrome and typically developing children. *Research in developmental disabilities, 21,* 329-346.

Pressman, L.J., Pipp-Siegel, S., Yoshinaga-Itano, C., and Deas, A. (1999). Maternal sensitivity predicts language gain in preschool children who are deaf and hard of hearing. Journal of Deaf Studies and Deaf Education, 4, 294-304.

Ricci L.A. and Hodapp R.M. (2003) Fathers of children with Down's syndrome versus other types of intellectual disability: perceptions, stress and involvement. *Journal of Intellectual Disability Research* 47, 273-284.

Richard, N.B. (1986). Interaction between mothers and infants with DS: Infant characteristics. Topics in Early Childhood Special Education, 6, 54-71.

Roach, M.A., Barratt, M.S., Miller, J.F., Leavitt, J.A. (1998). The structure of mother-child play: young children with Down syndrome and tipically developing children. *Developmental Psychology, 34,* 77-87.

Roach M.A., Orsmond G.I. and Barratt M.S. (1999) Mothers and fathers of children with Down syndrome: Parental stress and involvement in childcare. *American Journal on Mental Retardation* 104, 422-436.

Robinson, J.L., Little, C., and Biringen, Z. (1993). Emotional communication in mother-toddler relationships: Evidence for early gender differentiation. Merrill-Palmer Quarterly, 39, 496-517.

Ruskin E., Mundy P., Kasari C. and Sigman M. (1994) Object mastery motivation in children with DS. *American Journal of Mental Retardation* 98, 499-509.

Sagi, A., Tirosh, E., Ziv, Y., Guttman, S., and Lavie, P. (1998). Attachment and sleep patterns in the first year of life. Paper presented at the International Conference on Infant Studies, Atlanta.

Sander, L. (2000). Where are we going in the field of infant mental health? *Infant Mental Health Journal, 21,* 1–18

Senese V. P., La Femina F., Buro L., Saladino G. and Di Lucia G. (2008) Effetti dello sviluppo atipico sulla relazione genitori-figli: uno studio preliminare. *Congresso Nazionale della Sezione di Psicologia Dinamico-Clinica* Padova.

Shin J., Nhan N.V, Crittenden K.S.,. Hong H.T.D., Flory M. and Ladinsky J. (2006) Parenting stress of mothers and fathers of young children with cognitive delays in Vietnam. *Journal of Intellectual Disability Research* 50, 748-760.

Slonims, V., and McConachie, H. (2006). Analysis of mother–infant interaction in infants with down syndrome and typically developing infants. *American Journal on Mental Retardation,* 111, 273-289.

Solnit, A., and Stark, M. (1961). Mourning and the birth of a defective child. The Psychoanalytic Study of the Child, 16, 523–537.

Stern, D. (1985). The Interpersonal World of the Infant. New York: Basic Books.

Stoneman Z. (2007) Examining the Down syndrome advantage: Mothers and fathers of young children with disabilities. *Journal of Intellectual Disability Research* 51(12).

Tamis-LeMonda C. S. (2004) Conceptualizing Fathers' Roles: Playmates and More. *Human Development* 47(4), 220-227.

Tamis-LeMonda C. S. and Bornstein M. H. (1996) Variation in children's exploratory, nonsymbolic, and symbolic play: An explanatory multidimensional framework. In:

Advances in infancy research, Volume I0 (eds C. R. Rovee-Collier and L. P. Lipsitt), pp. 37-78. Ablex, Norwood, NJ.

Tamis-LeMonda C. S. and Cabrera C. S. (2002) *Handbook of father involvement: Multidisciplinary perspectives*. Erlbaum, Mahwah, NJ.

Trevarthen, C. (1993). The function of emotions in early infant communication and development. In J. Nadel and L. Camaioni (Eds.), New perspectives in early communicative development (pp. 48±81). New York: Routledge.

Trevarthen, C. (2003). Conversations with a two month-old. In J. Raphael-Leff (Ed.), Parent-infant psychodynamics: Wild things, mirrors and ghosts (pp. 25–34). Philadelphia: Whurr Publishers.

Trevarthen, C., and Aitken, K.J. (2001). Infant intersubjectivity: research, theory and clinical applications. Journal of Child Psychology and Psychiatry. 42, 3-48.

Tronick, E.Z. (2005). Why is connection with others so critical? The formation of dyadic states of consciousness and the expansion of individuals' states of consciousness: coherence governed selection and the co-creation of meaning out of messy meaning making. In J. Nadel and D. Muir (Eds.), Emotional development: Recent research advances. New York, NY, US: Oxford University Press, 2005. pp. 293-315.

Van Egeren, L.A., Barratt, M.S., and Roach, M.A. (2001). Mother–infant responsiveness: Timing, mutual regulation, and interactional context. *Developmental Psychology, 37,* 684–697.

Venuti P., de Falco S., Giusti Z. and Bornstein M.H. (2008) Play and Emotional Availability in Young Children with Down Syndrome. *Infant Mental Health Journal* 29-2.

Venuti P. (2007) *Percorsi evolutivi: Forme Tipiche e Atipiche*. Carocci, Roma.

Venuti P. and Giusti F. (1996) *Madre e Padre: antropologia, scienze dell'evoluzione e psicologia*. Giunti: Firenze.

Venuti P., Rossi G., Spagnoletti M.S., Famulare E. and Bornstein M. H. (1997) Gioco non simbolico e simbolico a 20 mesi: comportamenti di gioco del bambino e della madre. *Età Evolutiva* 10, 25-35. Volling, B.L., McElwain, N.L., Notaro, P.C., and Herrera, C. (2002). Parents' Emotional Availability and Infant Emotional Competence: Predictors of Parent–Infant Attachment and Emerging Self-Regulation. *Journal of Family Psychology, 16,* 447–465.

Vygotsky L. (1978) *Mind in society*. Cambridge, MA: Harvard University Press.

Weinberg, M. K., and Tronick, E. Z. (1996). Infant affective reactions to the resumption of maternal interaction after the still-face. *Child Development, 67,* 905-914.

Wiefel, A., Wollenweber, S., Oepen, G., Lenz, K., Lehmkuhl, U., and Biringen, Z. (2005). Emotional availability in infant psychiatry. *Infant Mental Health Journal, 26,* 392-403.

Zimmerman, L., and McDonald, L. (1995). Emotional availability in infants' relationships with multiple caregivers. American Journal of Orthopsychiatry, 65, 147-152.

In: Handbook of Down Syndrome Research
Editors: Dominicus Jelinek and Gijs Dvorak
ISBN 978-1-60741- 690-6

Chapter 10

Ultrasound Screening for Down Syndrome

***M. Sami Walid*[1] *and Nadezhda V. Zaytseva*[2]**
Medical Center of Central Georgia, Macon, GA, USA
Kuban State Medical University, Krasnodar, Russian Federation

Abstract

The introduction of the ultrasound imaging technology in the second half of the 20th century has revolutionized prenatal care. The ultrasound-based diagnostic medical imaging technique is now an indispensable component of the screening system of every pregnant woman. It is used to confirm the gestational age of the fetus and detect problems of serious medical nature, such as blockage of the small intestine, heart defects and chromosomal abnormalities. Knowing about the existence of these fatal anomalies as early in pregnancy as possible helps parents in decision-making regarding the future of the fetus.

Studies in the mid-1990s have shown a strong association between the size of the collection of fluid at the back of the fetal neck, called nuchal transluceny (NT), and the risk of Down syndrome. Early attempts to use measurement of NT thickness were limited by a wide variety in measurement discrepancies. Ultrasound NT measurement is usually done between 10 and 14 weeks gestation. It is highly dependent on the experience of the ultrasonographer. Small differences -- less than one tenth of a millimeter -- in NT measurements can make the designation of "normal" or "abnormal" result. Recognizing the potential importance of the problem that would arise from the performance of NT measurement by untrained ultrasonographers, many authoritative organizations have recommended that first trimester screening not be made widely available until a national program of quality review and oversight is established for the United States. Thus, NT measurements should only be offered in the setting of an accredited sonography center. Recently, standardized guidelines on measuring NT thickness along with specific training and certification have been instituted, making this ultrasound measurement a useful marker as part of first trimester screening. Correct performance of NT measurement is critical to the accuracy, safety, and effectiveness of the non-invasive prenatal screening system.

Introduction

The ultrasound imaging technology was one of the greatest inventions in the 20th century. Quickly it became an indispensable component in the prenatal care of every pregnant woman. It is used to confirm the gestational age and to screen for fetal malformations and abnormalities, such as intestinal atresia, heart defects and Down syndrome (trisomy 21). Knowing about the existence of these fatal anomalies early in pregnancy helps parents decide the future of the pregnancy. Since having a child with Down syndrome is a traumatizing and disruptive outcome to the family and the financial burden, including health care expenditures, physical therapy and special education, may be enormous prenatal detection of affected fetuses is of great importance in order that parents can be prepared for the birth of an affected child or consider pregnancy termination.

Antenatal Screening for Down Syndrome

In the beginning, it is worth noting that different types of prenatal testing exist that can be performed to evaluate the chance of a fetus having Down syndrome or determine the diagnosis of Down syndrome. A screening test establishes the chance of a fetus having Down syndrome. It does not provide a definite diagnosis. A diagnostic test studies the chromosomes of the fetus. If there are three copies (trisomy) of chromosome 21, then the fetus is confirmed to have Down syndrome.

Down syndrome has been traditionally screened for in the second trimester using laboratory and ultrasound techniques. The Triple Test is usually performed between the 15th and 18th weeks of pregnancy, but it can be done as late as the 20th week. The test measures the levels of three components in the maternal serum: alpha-fetoprotein (AFP), human chorionic gonadotropin (hCG), unconjugated estriol (uE3). If inhibin A is added this is then called the Quadruple Test. Low AFP, low estriol, high hCG, and high inhibin A levels are associated with a higher risk of Down syndrome. Low levels of the first three components mean the fetus has an increased risk of having trisomy 18, a more severe but less common chromosomal abnormality than Down syndrome. High levels of AFP point to neural tube defects like spina bifida, abdominal wall defects like omphalocele or gastroschisis, or multiple gestation like twins or triplets. To determine the fetus's chances of having a neural tube defect, the patient's level of AFP is plugged into a formula along with the fetus's gestational age, the mother's age, and other factors. To determine the fetus's chances of having Down syndrome or trisomy 18, the patient's levels of the three or four components are plugged into a formula along with the fetus's gestational age and the mother's age. The patient's age is factored in because although anyone can have a baby with a chromosomal abnormality, the risk increases as the mother ages. For example, the likelihood of carrying a baby with Down syndrome ranges from about 1 in 1,295 at age 20 to about 1 in 82 at age 40. Using advanced maternal age and low maternal serum AFP levels as criteria, only 40% of fetuses with Down syndrome are identified.[1] The triple test can detect approximately 60% of the pregnancies affected by trisomy 21, with a false-positive rate of about 5%.[2,3,4] In women older than 35 years, the triple test fails to detect 10% to 15% of pregnancies affected by trisomy 21.[4,5] An estimate of gestational age by ultrasound examination improves the accuracy of the triple test due to better reliability than the last menstrual period. A Double test consisting of AFP and hCG is less sensitive. First-trimester hCG and pregnancy-associated plasma protein A (PAPP-A) screening for Down syndrome can achieve detection rates as high as those associated with AFP and hCG or AFP, hCG and E3 screening in the second trimester.[6] These tests provide the patient with an assessment of the baby's risk, not a diagnosis. If positive, they guide the physician and the patient to proceed with an invasive diagnostic test — amniocentesis or chorionic villus sampling.

The efficacy of Down syndrome screening by combining second trimester maternal serum analytes and ultrasound findings has been shown in a 2002 study. By ultrasound findings alone, sensitivity was 79.9% with a false-positive rate of 6.7%. The blood quadruple test alone showed 81.5% sensitivity and 6.9% false-positive rate. However, when ultrasound findings (nuchal translucency and long-bone measurements) were combined with the quadruple test, sensitivity of 90% detection was achieved, with a 3.1% false-positive rate.[7] Thus, this combined modality of screening is substantially more effective than either serum screening or ultrasound alone. Even so, 90% sensitivity means 10% of Down syndrome cases will be missed. At this stage, a genetic counselor can help the patient understand the results and her options. The patient may want to discuss the pros and cons of undergoing amniocentesis to confirm whether the fetus has a chromosomal problem or not.

Ultrasound Screening for Down Syndrome

There are two levels of ultrasound scanning that are performed in a pregant woman. Level I ultrasound scan documents the basic information of pregnancy. In the first trimester this includes the location of the gestational sac, the crown-rump length, the presence or absence of fetal life, evaluation of the uterus, cervix and adnexa. Second and third trimester scan includes the documentation of fetal life, the number of fetuses, and their presentation, an estimate of amniotic fluid volume, the location of the placenta, the gestational age, the biparietal diameter (BPD), femur length (FL), abdominal circumference (AC) and other fetal measurements, and visualization of basic fetal anatomy including a 4 chamber view of the heart, the spine, stomach, kidneys, bladder, umbilical cord insertion, etc.

A level II ultrasound examination is a 'targeted' examination. This is usually performed at a credentialed perinatal center where more expertise in ultrasound scanning is available. Situations when a level II scan is ordered include: suspected fetal anomaly, severe IUGR, elevated maternal-serum AFP, oligohydramnios, polyhydramnios, two-vessel umbilical cord, fetal cardiac arrhythmia, exposure to drugs or chemicals in the first trimester, and increased risk of Down syndrome, etc. In a level II scan the sonographer tries as hard as possible to look for and assess any abnormality that is present in the fetus. There is no level III or level IV scans.

Level II or targeted ultrasound screening gives the physician and patient additional information about the status of the fetus. For the most accurate results, the study should be done by a sonographer certified by the American Registry for Diagnostic Medical Sonography (ARDMS) in a specialized center that is certified and accredited by the

American Institute of Ultrasound in Medicine (AIUM). Practices accredited by the AIUM have demonstrated competency in every aspect of their operation, including education and training of physicians and sonographers, ultrasound equipment maintenance, document storage, policies safeguarding patients and personnel, and accuracy in diagnosis.

Traditional biometry used in screening for Down syndrome consists of measuring the actual to expected FL ratio, the BPD/FL ratio, and the nuchal translucency (NT) thickness. In Down syndrome both the femur and humerus tend to be shortened. When available, an estimate of gestational age based on ultrasound measurement should be used in the risk estimation formula instead of the approximation based on the patient's last menstrual period. The biparietal diameter provides the best gestational age estimate. Femur length and composite estimates derived from it should not be used for this purpose, because this parameter underestimates the gestational age of fetuses with trisomy 21.

The formulation of femur measurement for the identification of fetuses at risk for Down syndrome has been done two decades ago. In a 1989 study, a regression analysis performed to compare biparietal diameter (BPD) to femur length (FL) in 709 control fetuses yielded the following formula: Expected FL = 0.9028 × BPD -9.3105. Compared with 20 Down syndrome fetuses, a ratio of measured-to-expected femur length of 0.91 or lower indicated Down syndrome with a sensitivity of 40%, a specificity of 95%, and a positive predictive value of 3.1%. Eight of the 20 fetuses with Down syndrome (40%) also had a thickened nuchal fold (6 mm or larger). The authors said that if the nuchal fold measurements had been considered with the femur length findings, two more of the fetuses with Down syndrome would have been identified, yielding a sensitivity of 45% and a positive predictive value of 4.3%.[8]

The nuchal translucency thickness is the thickness of the skin fold behind the nape of the neck (Figure 1). In chromosomal abnormalities this may be increased due to venous or lymphatic engorgement. The neck is the area where the lymphatics are last to develop. Skin of the neck is bulged outward when there is a fluid load that the lymphatics are unable to drain. Studies in the mid 1980s have suggested that ultrasound measurement of the NT thickness between 10 and 13 weeks of pregnancy (beginng of second trimester) can be used to predict Down syndrome.[9] However, nuchal thickening can sometimes be found in normal fetuses. In addition, early attempts to use this dimention were limited by wide differences in measurement techniques. In reaction to this, standardized guidelines on measuring NT thickness along with specific training and certification requirements have been set up, making this ultrasound measurement useful as part of the antenatal screening scheme.

Percentage of Down syndrome fetuses with an NT of 6 mm or more between 14 and 20 weeks' gestation vary from 69% to as low as 38%.[1,10] The AFDPHE (Association Française pour le Dépistage et la Prévention des Handicaps de l'Enfant) study found that the NT was 6 mm or more in 8.5% of chromosomally normal fetuses and in 38% of those with trisomy 21 with a false-positive rate below 5%.[10]

Among pregnancies with nuchal translucencies above the 99th percentile – corresponding to a measurement of 3.5 mm or greater –an increasing risk of major chromosomal abnormalities is noted. Similarly, the risk of fetal structural anomalies increases among chromosomally normal fetuses with NTs above the 99th percentile. The risk of major fetal malformation was estimated at 10% with nuchal translucencies from 3.5 - 4.4 mm, 19%

for NTs from 4.5 - 5.4 mm, 24% for NTs of 5.5 - 6.4 mm, and 46% for NT greater than 6.5 mm.[11] Overall, 15% of fetuses with NT greater than 6.5 mm went on to have normal pediatric outcomes whereas 95% of those with normal karyotype and normal anatomy went on to have normal outcomes. The presence or absence of septations cannot be used to distinguish between increased NT and cystic hygromas; outcomes are determined primarily by the thickness of the NT.[12]

The Nicolaides group, basing on their findings in 1015 fetuses at 10-13 weeks, estimated the risk for chromosomal abnormalities (trisomies 21, 18 and 13) with NT thicknesses of 3 mm, 4 mm, 5 mm and ≥ 6 mm. They were respectively 3 times, 18 times, 28 times and 36 times higher than the respective numbers expected on the basis of maternal age alone.[13]

The incidence of Down syndrome at age 35 is around 1 out of 270. If the fetus has an NT thickness of 6mm the risk of Down syndrome becomes 36/270 or 1 out of 7.5. Neck findings are best sought between 10 and 14 weeks gestation. Afterwards, there is sufficient lymphatic development that NT is not often found, even when there is aneuploidy. Amniocentesis should always be done when there is question or worry about aneuploidy, whether there are neck findings or not. Absence of NT does not exclude chromosomal problems.

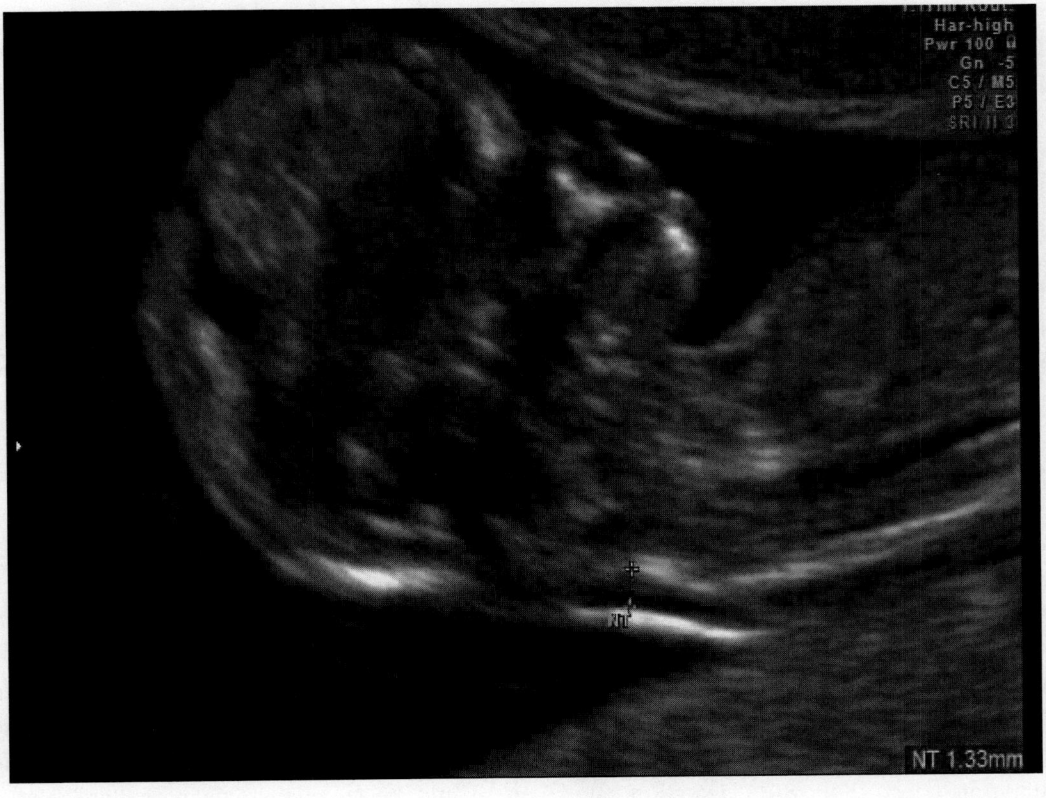

Figure 1: Nuchal translucency (NT).Courtesy of Jean Lea Spitz, MPH, RDMS Program Director, NTQR, Oklahoma City, OK.

Screening Schemes

Several trials have studied ultrasound measurement of nuchal translucency alone and in combination with biochemical markers as a complex first-trimester screening investigation for Down syndrome. A large, National Institutes of Health (NIH)-sponsored, prospective, multi-center study called the Blood, Ultrasound, and Nuchal Translucency (BUN) Trial determined that an algorithm combining NT measurement results in the first trimester (between 11 weeks' and 1 day and 13 weeks' and 6 days' gestation) with the results of maternal serum tests (hCG and PAPP-A) performed in the first trimester detected about 79% of all Down syndrome cases with a false positive rate of 5%.[14] A nested, case-controlled British trial called the Serum, Urine and Ultrasound Screening Study (SURUSS) evaluated both first and second trimester markers for Down syndrome in singleton pregnancies. Results for first trimester screening showed that NT in combination with hCG plus PAPP-A detected 85% of Down syndrome cases with a false positive rate of 5%.[15] The Down syndrome detection rates described in these studies are comparable or better than those for second-trimester "Quad" screening using four maternal serum markers (AFP, hCG, uE3, and inhibin A).

The Society for Maternal Fetal Medicine (SMFM) and the American College of Medical Genetics (ACMG) have provided guidance on the follow-up of normal first trimester pregnancies using combination testing. It is now widely accepted that women should not undergo independent sequential "triple" or "quad" screening in the second trimester of pregnancy to further assess aneuploidy risk if the results of combined NT and serum analyte testing in the first trimester are negative (normal).[16] Independent sequential testing of this sort is associated with an unacceptably high false-positive rate.[17] Instead, women who want a higher detection rate can undergo either an integrated or a stepwise sequential testing, which combines both first- and second-trimester screening results in an efficient way.[7] An integrated approach to screening uses both first-trimester and second-trimester markers to adjust a woman's age-related risk of having a child with Down syndrome. The results are reported only after both first- and second-trimester screening tests are completed. In the FASTER (First- and Second-Trimester Evaluation of Risk) trial, first-trimester screening was performed in 38,167 patients; among them 117 had a fetus with Down syndrome. At a 5% false positive rate, the rates of detection of Down's syndrome were as follows: with first-trimester Combined screening, 87%, 85%, and 82% for measurements performed at 11, 12, and 13 weeks, respectively; with second-trimester Quadruple screening, 81%; with Stepwise Sequential screening, 95%; with Serum Integrated screening, 88%; and with Fully Integrated screening with first-trimester measurements performed at 11 weeks, 96%.[18] For an 85% Down's Syndrome detection rate, the false-positive rate for the Integrated test was 0.9%, the Serum Integrated test (without nuchal translucency) 2.7%, the Combined test 4.3%, the Quadruple test 6.2%, and for nuchal translucency at 11 weeks 15.2%.[19] Using the Integrated test at an 85% detection rate, there would be six diagnostic procedure-related unaffected fetal losses following amniocentesis per 100,000 women screened compared with 35 using the Combined test or 45 with the Quadruple test.[19] Although integrated screening has the highest sensitivity and lowest false-positive rate of noninvasive screening schemes, the main disadvantage of Integrated screening lies in the need to wait 3 to 4 weeks between initiation and completion of the plan. This may result in patient anxiety and the possibility that the patient fails to complete the second-trimester half of the complex screening test after performing the first-trimester half. Another disadvantage is that the patient may miss the opportunity to consider CVS if first-trimester screening indicates a high risk of fetal aneuploidy.

Benefits of first trimester screening include earlier identification of the pregnancy at risk for fetal aneuploidy, in particular, Down syndrome, and the option of earlier confirmation by chorionic villus sampling, if available, which helps the parents decide about the future of the foetus earlier in pregnancy. The Fully Integrated test offers the most effective and safe method of screening for women who attend in the first trimester. The next best test is the Serum Integrated test. First-trimester Combined screening at 11 weeks of gestation is better than second-trimester Quadruple screening but at 13 weeks they are similar (Table1). Both Stepwise Sequential screening and Fully Integrated screening have high rates of detection of Down's syndrome with low false positive rates. There is no justification anymore for retaining the Double or Triple tests, or doing nuchal translucency measurement alone (with or without maternal age) in antenatal screening for Down's Syndrome.

Table 1. Detection rates for a 5% false positive rate for different screening schemes

Test Name	Test Components	DR for a 5% FPR
Stepwise sequential (contingent) test	Same as Integrated test but risk results provided after each step	95%[18]
Fully Integrated test	NT and PAPP-A at 11 completed weeks of pregnancy AFP, uE3, hCG, and inhibin-A at 14-20 completed weeks	96%[18]
Serum integrated test	PAPP-A at 11 completed weeks of pregnancy AFP, uE3, hCG, and inhibin-A in the early second trimester	88%[18]
Combined test	NT, hCG, and PAPP-A at 11 weeks at 12 weeks at 13 weeks	87%[18] 85%[18] 82%[18]
Quadruple test	AFP, uE3, hCG, and inhibin-A at 14-20 completed weeks	81%[18]
Triple test	AFP, uE3, and hCG at 14-20 completed weeks	60%[4]
NT $\geq$ 6 mm, alone	NT at 12-13 completed weeks	38%[10]

In order to make screening more efficient, ACMG have recently introduced the concept of contingent or Stepwise Sequential screening.[20] ACMG guidelines explain that contingent screening, like sequential screening, incorporates components of first and second trimetser screening. However, in contingent screening, the first trimester results are divided into three outcomes: screen positive, screen negative, and intermediate/pending risk. Those patients at intermediate risk will then provide a second trimester sample for testing in order to compute the integrated risk. ACMG guidelines explain that this strategy allows for early diagnosis of Down syndrome among a small, high-risk group (screen positives), early reassurance to a large, low-risk group (screen negatives), and attempts to maintain high performance by having those with intermediate/pending first trimester risk benefit from the integrated test.

Stepwise Sequential screening obviates some of the theoretical disadvantages of Integrated screening. With the sequential approach, the patient is informed of the first-trimester screening result. Those at highest risk might opt for an early diagnostic procedure, and those at lower risk can still take advantage of the higher detection rate achieved with additional second-trimester screening.

First trimester NT testing alone is less sensitive than either first trimester combined screening or second trimester "Quad" screening and, thus, should not be used in isolation for routine fetal aneuploidy screening in singleton pregnancies. In multiple gestations, however, serum analyte testing is unreliable and NT screening alone is sufficiently appropriate. It should be noted that the identification of a cystic hygroma in the first trimester is a very powerful predictor of fetal aneuploidy (Figure 2). In one large, prospective study, a septated cystic hygroma was associated with a 51% likelihood of having a chromosomal abnormality.[21] This finding warrants prompt diagnostic testing with CVS which should not be delayed by serum analyte measurement and further risk calculation. Cystic hygroma has 5-fold, 12-fold, and 6-fold increased risk of aneuploidy, cardiac malformation, and perinatal death, respectively.[21]

Nuchal Translucency Measurement

There are five remarks that the sonographer must consider when performing ultrasound measurement of the fetal NT in the first trimester. First, the absolute measurement of NT thickness significantly decreases with increasing image size which increases the specificity but unfortunately decreases the sensitivity of the NT-derived risk estimation of Down syndrome.[22] Notwithstanding, the feasibility of NT measurement as a screening method requires the standardisation of image magnification criteria so that calipers can detect 0.1 mm differences in measurement. Second, the nuchal translucency measurement must be performed between 10 3/7 weeks and 13 6/7 weeks gestation according to the Nuchal Translucency Quality Review (NTQR) criteria.[23] This is equivalent to a CRL measurement between 38-84 mm. In this window of time CRL accuracy for gestational dating is 3-5 days.

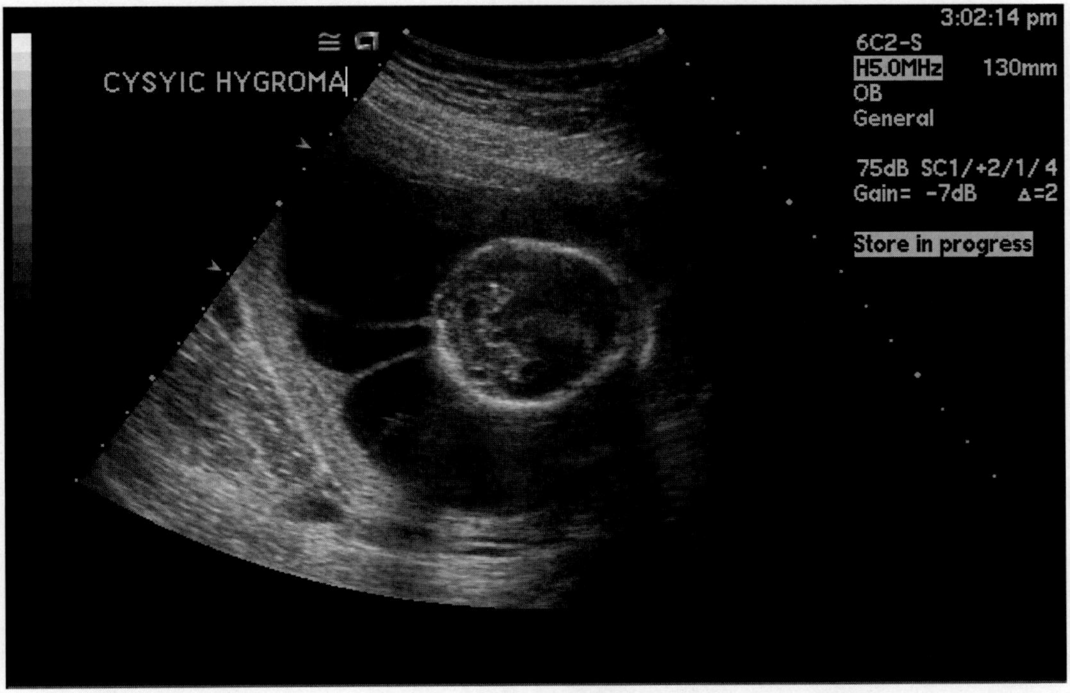

Figure 3. Cystic hygroma.Courtesy of Mark G. Boddy, MD, FACOG Perinatal Center, Macon, GA.

The CRL measurement must be included with NT measurement as the NT measurement is converted into multiples of the median (MOM) for the CRL. The measured CRL is not the actual anatomic CRL but rather the longest straight line measurement of the fetus while its head is maintained in the neutral position. Unlike the NT measurement in which the longest of three good measurements is used, the CRL uses the average from 3 good measurements. Third, a sagittal section of the fetus should be obtained, in a neutral position without hyperflexion or hyperextension. Fourth, the widest part of the translucency should be measured with the amnion seen separate from NT line. Fifth, measurements should be taken with the horizontal lines of the calipers placed on the lines that define the nuchal translucency thickness. Calipers are placed from the outer skull table to the inner skin surface (on-to-on method). The mean difference between the on-to-on and on-to-out nuchal translucency thickness, using transabdominal scanning, is 0.95 +/- 0.14 mm.[24] The differences correlate directly with fetal size and nuchal thickness. Scans performed transvaginally exhibit a smaller difference between the methods (0.90 mm vs. 0.94 mm; $p < 0.05$). Regarding the significance of the smoothness of sonographic contour of NT, a 2001 study showed that a uniformly shaped, increased NT may be more representative of a developmental delay in a normal fetus, whereas a 'notched' nuchal surface may represent abnormal lymphatic or cardiovascular development more commonly seen in DS fetuses.[25]

Poor reproducibility may be a problem with the measurement of NT thickness as reported by a 1995 study. By repeating measurements with a different operator, the same operator using a different still image, and the same operator using the same still image, 18.8%, 17.5%, and 12.4% of NT measurements, respectively, change their classification from normal to abnormal or vice versa.[26] However, a simultaneous study demonstrated that 95% of the time the intraobserver, interobserver and caliper placement repeatability of fetal NT thickness measurment were less than 0.54 mm, 0.62 mm and 0.58 mm, respectively.[27] In addition, the repeatability was unrelated to the NT thickness or image magnification.[28,29] When the NT thickness is measured by well-trained operators, the measurement is highly reproducible. The key word "well-trained" outline the practical problems that could be expected by generalizing ultrasound screening. Thus, the efficacy of the test may seem good in a research environment, however, the effectiveness in everyday use may be less impressive, making its application as a routine screening test in the general population not cost-effective. That is what made some early reports consider the hasty uptake of NT thickness measurement as a screening test in the general population *"imprudent."*[30]

Correct conduction of NT measurement is critical to the accuracy, safety, and effectiveness of various prenatal screening schemes. The NT measurement is highly dependent on the experience of the ultrasonographer. Small differences -- less than one tenth of a millimeter -- in NT measurement can characterize the difference between a negative or "normal" and a positive or "abnormal" result. It is worth reminding that the increased detection rates of chromosomal abnormalities reported with newer non-invasive first and second trimester screening schemes are mostly owing to the contribution of the NT component. However, all published trials that have demonstrated superior detection rates of the new screening strategies incorporating NT thickness have relied on NT measurements performed by highly trained and credentialed ultrasonographers.

Recognizing the potential magnitude of the problem that would result from the performance of NT measurement by untrained sonographers, the Society for Maternal-Fetal Medicine (SMFM) has recommended that first trimester screening not be made widely available until a national program of quality review and oversight is established for the United States. Similarly, the ACOG, the ACMG, the AIUM, and the National Institute of Child Health and Development (NICHD) of the National Institutes of Health (NIH) have cautioned that screening based on NT measurement should only be made available in the setting of quality credentialing and oversight monitoring. Unambiguously, the ACOG stated that *"Specific training, standardization, use of appropriate ultrasound equipment, and ongoing quality assessment are important to achieve optimal nuchal translucency measurement for Down syndrome risk assessment, and this procedure should be limited to centers and individuals meeting these criteria."*[31]

Nuchal Translucency Quality Review (NTQR) initiated by the NT Oversight Committee (NTOC) of the Maternal Fetal Medicine Foundation (MFMF) offers an educational program, credentialing, and an ongoing quality review process for physicians and sonographers (non-physicians) who wish to perform NT measurement as a "credentialed" provider. NTQR is the first US-based national consensus program where physicians and sonographers volunteer to have one of their professional activities epidemiologically reviewed by an independent body that has developed criteria for educational content, proficiency evaluation, and epidemiological monitoring.

NTQR compares the practitioners' measurements to those of a standard referent curve. For review purposes, NT measurements are converted to multiples of the gestational age specific referent median (MOM). The ideal practitioner's median NT should be 1.0 MOM with an expected 90th percentile range from 0.9 to 1.1 MoM. Practitioners with values that are statistically outside the expected range will be considered for improvement.

Soft Markers of Down Syndrome

There are several other findings that can be seen during an ultrasound scan that some researchers feel may have a significant "association" with Down syndrome and increases the efficiency of Down syndrome screening over standard biometry alone (increased nuchal thickness and shortened long bones). These "markers" include intrauterine growth restriction, mild cerebral ventriculomegaly, choroid plexus cysts, echogenic intracardiac foci, congenital heart defects, increased intestinal echogenicity, duodenal atresia (double-bubble sign), renal pelvis dilation, increased iliac wing angle, incurving (clinodactyly) and hypoplasia of the fifth finger, increased space between first and second toes, and two-vessel umbilical cord.

These findings may be present in normal fetuses. "Association" is the key word here; seeing some of these markers on an ultrasound image does not necessarily mean that the fetus has Down syndrome. These markers indicate only that Down syndrome might be present. Scientists are still debating what these markers really mean; parents-to-be should keep in mind that each marker can also be found in a small percentage of normal fetuses. The problem with soft markers is that, even when karyotypic abnormalities are excluded, the mother and her obstetrician will remain in doubt as to their significance–a cause of considerable anxiety. That is why counselling should be provided before parents are told of the presence of ultrasonographic "soft markers" of fetal abnormality.

For the combination of standard biometry (either increased nuchal thickness or short humerus) or gross anatomic defect, Down syndrome detection rate is 53.3%. This increases to 63.2% when subtle anatomic defects (echogenic bowel or clinodactyly) are included in the definition of an abnormal sonogram.[32] Soft markers observed without associated fetal structural malformations individually have low sensitivity (range, 1%-16%), and most fetuses with such markers had normal outcomes. A thickened nuchal fold is the most accurate marker for discriminating between unaffected and affected fetuses and is associated with an approximately 17-fold increased risk of Down syndrome.[33]

Many researchers have attempted to find if any combination of ultrasound markers may be more likely to determine if a fetus has Down syndrome. In a 1992 study, the following scoring system was suggested for the detection of aneuploidy: nuchal fold = 2, major structural defect = 2, and short femur, short humerus, and pyelectasis = 1 each. Selecting fetuses with a score of ≥ 2 would identify 26/32 (81%) of Down syndrome fetuses, and 9/9 (100%) and 2/2 (100%) of fetuses with trisomies 18 and 13, respectively, but only 26/588 (4.4%) of normal fetuses. Using the score of 2 results in a positive predictive value for the 1/250 risk group of 6.87% for Down syndrome and 7.25% for all three trisomies.[1]

Cardiac abnormalities, which are more common in Down syndrome fetuses, are better detected with color doppler ultrasound. It can identify a significantly higher rate of cardiovascular abnormalities in fetuses with Down syndrome, 60% versus 12% for real-time ultrasound.[34] Ultrasound can detect between 60% and 91% of fetuses with Down syndrome depending on the combination of cardiac markers (ventricular septal defect, right-to-left chamber disproportion, tricuspid regurgitation, mitral regurgitation, pericardial effusion, and outflow tract abnormalities) and non-cardiac markers (central nervous system malformations, choroid plexus cysts, abnormal nuchal skin fold, hyperechoic bowel, and pyelectasis) selected in the evaluation.[35] Thus, the use of color Doppler ultrasound to identify fetuses at increased risk for Down syndrome can be an alternative for high-risk patients who decline genetic amniocentesis.

Although congenital heart defects are present in 56% of second trimester fetuses and 44% of newborns with trisomy 21, most studies evaluating second-trimester fetuses at risk for trisomy 21 detect less than 10% of heart malformations. Dr DeVore suggested a 3 level approach that allows the fetal sonographer to incorporate fetal echocardiography, based upon his/her level of skill and experience, when evaluating the fetus at risk for trisomy 21. In Level I examination only noncardiac markers are evaluated with a detection rate of 60% and a false-positive rate of 5.9%. Level II examination incorporates the four-chamber view with non-cardiac markers. If the examiner can identify atrial and/or ventricular chamber disproportion, then the sensitivity is increased to 75%, with a false-positive rate of 6.4%. Level III examination utilizes grayscale and color doppler ultrasound to evaluate the fetal heart. If the examiner can identify ventricular septal defects, atrioventricular septal defects, pericardial effusion, tricuspid regurgitation, and chamber disproportion, then the sensitivity of genetic sonography increases to 91% with a false-positive rate of 14%.[36]

More recently, failure to visualize the fetal nasal bone at around 11-13 weeks was shown to be a very reliable marker for Down syndrome (Figure 3). The absence of the nasal bone could increase the sensitivity of Down syndrome detection to 85% and decrease the false-positive rate to about 1%.[37]

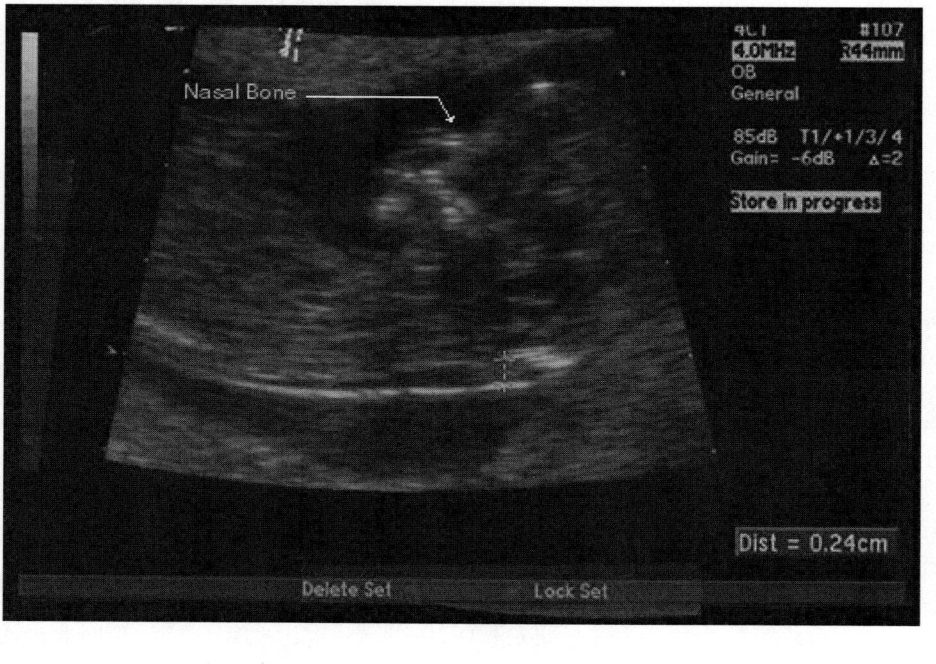

Figure 3. The fetal nasal bone.Courtesy of Jean Lea Spitz, MPH, RDMS Program Director, NTQR, Oklahoma City, OK.

Diagnostic Testing for Down Syndrome

It is important to keep in mind that even the best combination of ultrasound findings and maternal serum variables is only predictive and not diagnostic. Ultrasound is not a substitute for genetic amniocentesis. Physicians need to remind their patients that at least a third of Down syndrome cases can be missed by ultrasound alone. For true diagnosis, the chromosomes of the fetus must be examined.

Even if everything looks normal on a detailed ultrasound, it's still not a guarantee that everything is okay, but it does mean that the baby has a lower risk for chromosomal defects than the general population. This information helps the patient decide whether to go ahead with invasive testing.

There are 2 basic methods for confirming chromosomal abnormalities, such as Down syndrome, in a pregnancy. Amniocentesis involves using a thin needle (generally thinner than what is used to draw blood) to withdraw a small amount of amniotic fluid from the womb for a variety of tests. Although it carries a risk of miscarriage of about 1/250, it remains the safest test available between 15 and 20 weeks of pregnancy to check the fetus for chromosomal abnormalities. Prior to 15 weeks, it is referred to as "early" amniocentesis and carries risks similar to chorionic villus sampling (CVS). CVS is an early test for chromosomal abnormalities, performed between 10 and 14 weeks and is essentially a biopsy of the placenta. While the risk of miscarriage is slightly higher than with amniocentesis (1/150), it carries the advantage of providing early diagnoses for couples at risk.

In deciding whether to have amniocentesis or CVS, the patient will have to weigh her desire to know about her baby's condition against the small risk of miscarriage. Individual parents have different feelings about what risks are acceptable.

Ethical Dispute Regarding Down Syndrome Screening

Routine ultrasound screening was not introduced until recently. ACOG Practice Bulletin # 58 December 2004 of the American College of Obstetricians and Gynecologists (ACOG) reads: "Given the limitations of the evidence, a physician is not obliged to perform ultrasonography in a patient who is at low risk and has no indications."[38] Maternal age 35 years or older at the time of delivery has been used to identify women at highest risk of having a child with Down syndrome. Recently, the practice of using age cutoffs and specific indications to determine whether a woman should be offered screening or invasive diagnostic testing has been challenged by ACOG itself. According to the ACOG Practice Bulletin # 77 January 2007: "Screening and invasive diagnostic testing for aneuploidy should be available to all women who present for prenatal care before 20 weeks of gestation regardless of maternal age."[31] Previously, women were automatically offered genetic counseling and diagnostic testing for Down syndrome by amniocentesis or chorionic villus sampling (CVS) if they were 35 years and older. The new ACOG guidelines recommend that all pregnant women consider less invasive screening options for assessing their risk for Down syndrome before the 20th week of pregnancy. This means that the maternal age of 35 years should no longer be used by itself as a marker to determine who is offered screening versus who is offered invasive diagnostic testing. ACOG advises that all pregnant women, regardless of their age, should have the option of diagnostic testing. The National Down Syndrome Congress, however, did not totally agree with the above recommendations and issued the following: "In formulating the ACOG Guidelines, the mere existence of fetuses, potential persons and living individuals with trisomy 21 is more likely to be considered diminished or devalued, thereby jeopardizing the protections customarily afforded to any fetus, potential person or living individual. Unless specifically requested by a pregnant woman or expectant parents, obstetricians are not justified in rendering any opinion regarding the potential valueî of the life that has been created."[39]

Opinions vary between peoples of different countries. In a 1998 survey in Russia, 33% of respondents indicated that they favoured compulsory termination of pregnancy if testing identified a genetic disorder in the fetus. Compared with the British public, more Russians were in favour of prenatal screening and selective termination.[40] In Denmark, a postal survey identified considerable controversy with respect to abortion for Down's syndrome, indicating that opinions in one country cannot be used to inform decisions in another.[41]

The World Health Organization does not have a formal position on antenatal screening for Down syndrome or other genetic defects since it is the prerogative of individual Member States to decide if and under what circumstances screening procedures are to be applied in the national health care system. The Organization has, however, convened in 1993 a meeting of experts in the field of genetics to discuss the control of hereditary diseases. The report of that meeting devotes a section to the "Ethical, social, and legal aspects of genetic technology in medicine" where they state that "The broadest ethical issue in the area of genetic services is their limited availability. Recent dramatic advances in the development of DNA techniques and their possible medical application make it necessary to update strategies for the control of genetic diseases. Progress in genetic testing techniques, which is much more rapid than progress in treatment, raises social and ethical issues concerned not with the technique itself but with its proper use. In this regard, it is of the utmost importance that scientific, medical and lay organizations should ensure that information and technology are used to preserve the dignity of the individual. The misuse of information can be avoided through discussions at different levels (health care professionals, policy-makers, mass media, schools, etc.) in order to establish a firm understanding of the potential and actual applications of new genetic technology and the achievements of human genome research."[42]

Finally, there are many sound reasons why a woman should have a prenatal ultrasound examination, such as determining the age of the fetus and investigating possible complications or abnormalities. However, ultrasound practices are increasingly facing pressure from their patients to perform entertainment sonograms simply to provide a picture of the fetus or determine fetal gender. The US Food and Drug Administration (FDA) considers the use of ultrasound without a medical indication inappropriate and contradicts the responsible practice of medicine.[43] The FDA has cautioned that persons who promote, sell or lease ultrasound equipment for making keepsake fetal videos should know that the FDA views this as an unapproved use of a medical device. Assuring that prenatal ultrasound scans are done only when medically indicated is important to preserve this valuable technology as a serious medical diagnostic tool.

References

[1] Benacerraf BR, Neuberg D, Bromley B, Frigoletto FD Jr. Sonographic scoring index for prenatal detection of chromosomal abnormalities. *J. Ultrasound. Med.* 1992 Sep;11(9):449-58.

[2] Kuller JA, Laifer SA. Contemporary approaches to prenatal diagnosis. *Am. Fam. Physician* 1995;52: 2277-83,2285-6.

[3] Haddow JE, Palomaki GE, Knight GJ, Williams J, Pulkkinen A, Canick JA, et al. Prenatal screening for Down's syndrome with use of maternal serum markers. *N. Engl. J. Med.* 1992;327:588-93.

[4] Newberger DS. Down syndrome: prenatal risk assessment and diagnosis. *Am. Fam. Physician.* 2000 Aug 15;62(4):825-32, 837-8.

[5] American College of Medical Genetics Clinical Practice Committee. ACMG position statement on multiple marker screening in women 35 and older. American College of Medical Genetics College Newsletter, January 1994;2.

[6] Krantz DA, Larsen JW, Buchanan PD, Macri JN. First-trimester Down syndrome screening: free beta-human chorionic gonadotropin and pregnancy-associated plasma protein A. *Am. J. Obstet. Gynecol.* 1996 Feb;174(2):612-6.

[7] Benn P. A, Kaminsky L. M, Ying J, Borgida A. F, Egan J. F. X. Combined second-trimester biochemical and ultrasound screening for Down syndrome. The American College of Obstetricians and Gynecologists. 2002;100:1168–1176.

[8] Benacerraf BR, Cnann A, Gelman R, Laboda LA, Frigoletto FD Jr. Can sonographers reliably identify anatomic features associated with Down syndrome in fetuses? *Radiology.* 1989 Nov;173(2):377-80.

[9] Benacerraf BR, Fnigoletto FD Jr., Laboda LA. Sonographic diagnosis of Down syndrome in the second trimester. *Am. J. Obstet. Gynecol.* 1985; 153:49-52.

[10] Grandjean H, Sarramon MF. Sonographic measurement of nuchal skinfold thickness for detection of Down syndrome in the second-trimester fetus: a multicenter prospective study. The AFDPHE Study Group. Association Française pour le Dépistage et la Prévention des Handicaps de l'Enfant. *Obstet Gynecol.* 1995 Jan;85(1):103-6.

[11] Souka AP, Von Kaisenberg CS, Hyett JA, Sonek JD, Nicolaides KH. Increased nuchal translucency with normal karyotype. *Am. J. Obstet. Gynecol.* 2005 Apr;192(4):1005-21.

[12] Molina FS, Avgidou K, Kagan KO, Poggi S, Nicolaides KH. Cystic hygromas, nuchal edema, and nuchal translucency at 11-14 weeks of gestation. *Obstet. Gynecol.* 2006 Mar;107(3):678-83.

[13] Pandya PP, Kondylios A, Hilbert L, Snijders RJ, Nicolaides KH. Chromosomal defects and outcome in 1015 fetuses with increased nuchal translucency. *Ultrasound Obstet. Gynecol.* 1995 Jan;5(1):15-9.

[14] Wapner R, Thom E, Simpson JL, Pergament E, Silver R, Filkins K, Platt L, Mahoney M, Johnson A, Hogge WA, Wilson RD, Mohide P, Hershey D, Krantz D, Zachary J, Snijders R, Greene N, Sabbagha R, MacGregor S, Hill L, Gagnon A, Hallahan T, Jackson L; First Trimester Maternal Serum Biochemistry and Fetal Nuchal

Translucency Screening (BUN) Study Group. First-trimester screening for trisomies 21 and 18. *N. Engl. J. Med.* 2003 Oct 9;349(15):1405-13.

[15] Wald NJ, Rodeck C, Hackshaw AK, Walters J, Chitty L, Mackinson AM. First and second trimester antenatal screening for Down's syndrome: the results of the Serum, Urine and Ultrasound Screening Study (SURUSS). *Health Technol. Assess.* 2003;7(11):1-77.

[16] Driscoll DA, Gross SJ. First trimester diagnosis and screening for fetal aneuploidy. *ACMG Practice Guidelines* 2008 January;10(1).

[17] Wapner RJ. First trimester screening: the BUN study. *Semin. Perinatol.* 2005 Aug;29(4):236-9.

[18] Malone FD, Canick JA, Ball RH, Nyberg DA, Comstock CH, Bukowski R, Berkowitz RL, Gross SJ, Dugoff L, Craigo SD, Timor-Tritsch IE, Carr SR, Wolfe HM, Dukes K, Bianchi DW, Rudnicka AR, Hackshaw AK, Lambert-Messerlian G, Wald NJ, D'Alton ME; First- and Second-Trimester Evaluation of Risk (FASTER) Research Consortium. First-trimester or second-trimester screening, or both, for Down's syndrome. *N. Engl. J. Med.* 2005 Nov 10;353(19):2001-11.

[19] Wald NJ, Rodeck C, Hackshaw AK, Rudnicka A. SURUSS in perspective. *BJOG.* 2004 Jun;111(6):521-31.

[20] Wright D, Bradbury I, Benn P, Cuckle H, Ritchie K. Contingent screening for Down syndrome is an efficient alternative to non-disclosure sequential screening. *Prenat. Diagn.* 2004;24:762–766.

[21] Malone FD, Ball RH, Nyberg DA, Comstock CH, Saade GR, Berkowitz RL, et al. First-trimester septated cystic hygroma; prevalence, natural history, and pediatric outcome. *Obstet. Gynecol.* 2005;106:288–94.

[22] Teoh M, Meagher SE, Choong S, Shekleton P, Wallace EM. The effect of image size on screen-positive rates for nuchal translucency screening. *BJOG.* 2006 Apr;113(4):479-81. Epub 2006 Feb 20.

[23] Warsof SL. Criteria for Nuchal Translucency (NT) Measurements. The NT Examiner. Spring 2007. Accessed 10/27/2008. URL: https://ntqr.org/SM /Newsletters/ NTExaminer_3.htm

[24] Herman A, Dreazen E, Samandarov A, Bukovsky Y, Weinraub Z, Maymon R. On-to-on versus on-to-out nuchal translucency measurements. *Ultrasound Obstet Gynecol.* 2000 Feb;15(2):126-30.

[25] Maymon R, Dreazen E, Buckovsky I, Weinraub Z, Herman A. Does a 'notched' nuchal translucency indicate Down syndrome fetuses or other adverse pregnancy outcome? *Prenat. Diagn.* 2001 May;21(5):403–408.

[26] Roberts LJ, Bewley S, Mackinson AM, Rodeck CH. First trimester fetal nuchal translucency: problems with screening the general population. 1. *Br. J. Obstet. Gynaecol.* 1995 May;102(5):381-5.

[27] Pandya PP, Altman DG, Brizot ML, Pettersen H, Nicolaides KH. Repeatability of measurement of fetal nuchal translucency thickness. Ultrasound Obstet Gynecol. 1995 May;5(5):334-7.

[28] Herman A, Maymon R, Dreazen E, Caspi E, Bukovsky I, Weinraub Z. Image magnification does not contribute to the repeatability of caliper placement in measuring nuchal translucency thickness. *Ultrasound Obstet. Gynecol.* 1998 Apr;11(4):266-70.

[29] Stewart Tl and Malone FD. First trimester screening for aneuploidy: nuchal translucency sonography. *Semin. Perinatol.* 23(5): 36-381, 1999.

[30] Kornman LH, Morssink LP, Beekhuis JR, De Wolf BT, Heringa MP, Mantingh A. Nuchal translucency cannot be used as a screening test for chromosomal abnormalities in the first trimester of pregnancy in a routine ultrasound practice. *Prenat. Diagn.* 1996 Sep;16(9):797-805.

[31] Screening for fetal chromosomal abnormalities. ACOG Practice Bulletin No. 77. Washington, DC: ACOG; January 2007.

[32] Deren O, Mahoney MJ, Copel J, Bahdo-Singh RO: Subtle ultrasonographic anomalies: Do they improve the Down syndrome rate? *Am. J. Obstet. Gynecol.* 1998 Mar;178(3):441-5.

[33] Smith-Bindman R, Hosmer W, Feldstein VA, Deeks JJ, Goldberg JD. Second-Trimester Ultrasound to Detect Fetuses With Down Syndrome: A Meta-analysis. *JAMA.* 2001 Feb 28;285(8):1044-55.

[34] DeVore GR, Alfi O. The use of color Doppler ultrasound to identify fetuses at increased risk for trisomy 21: an alternative for high-risk patients who decline genetic amniocentesis. *Obstet. Gynecol.* 1995 Mar;85(3):378-86.

[35] DeVore GR. Trisomy 21: 91% detection rate using second-trimester ultrasound markers. *Ultrasound Obstet Gynecol.* 2000 Aug;16(2):133-41.

[36] DeVore GR. The role of fetal echocardiography in genetic sonography. *Semin Perinatol.* 2003 Apr;27(2):160-72.

[37] Cicero S, Curcio P, Papageorghiou A, Sonek J, Nicolaides K. Absence of nasal bone in fetuses with trisomy 21 at 11-14 weeks of gestation: an observational study. *Lancet.* 2001 Nov 17;358(9294):1665-7.

[38] Ultrasonography in pregnancy. ACOG Practice Bulletin No. 58. Washington, DC: ACOG; December 2004.

[39] Prenatal screening and diagnosis. A Position Statement of the National Down Syndrome Congress. Accessed 10/10/2008. URL: .http://www.ndsccenter.org /resources/position1.php

[40] Gudkov L, Tichtchenko P, Yudin B. Human genetic improvement: a comparison of Russian and British public perceptions. *Bull. Med. Ethics.* 1998;134:20–3.

[41] Norup M. Attitudes towards abortion in the Danish population. *Bioethics* 1997;11:439–49.

[42] Control of hereditary diseases. WHO Technical Report Series No. 865, 1996

[43] Rados C. FDA Cautions Against Ultrasound 'Keepsake' Images. FDA Consumer magazine. January-February 2004;38(1).

In: Handbook of Down Syndrome Research
Editors: Dominicus Jelinek and Gijs Dvorak
ISBN 978-1-60741- 690-6

Chapter 11

Dental Hygiene, Gingival Modified Index (GMI) and Simplified Oral Hygiene Index (OHIS) in the Primary Dentition of Down Syndrome Children

***Marília Fernandes Mathias*[a], *Maria Teresa Botti Rodrigues Santos*[b] *and Renata de Oliveira Guare*[*b]**

[a]School of Dentistry, University of Cruzeiro do Sul,
São Paulo, Brazil

[b]Discipline of Dentistry, Persons with Disabilities Division,
Universidade Cruzeiro do Sul, São Paulo, Brazil

Abstract

Down syndrome (DS) occurs in decorrence of a chromosomic abnormality and is characterized by physical and mental alterations. Individuals with DS are known to have a great predisposition to periodontal disease in early age, due to alterations in their immune system. This study was approved by the Ethics Committee of the Irmandade da Santa Casa de Misericórdia de São Paulo (Brazil). This case-control study aims at evaluating some behavioral characteristics related to dental hygiene, Gingival Modified Index (GMI) and Simplified Oral Hygiene Index (OHIS) in deciduous dentition of DS children. The study group (DS) was composed by 69 DS children, which were compared with 69 children without congenital abnormalities (control group). The oral hygiene habits were obtained by means of a questionnaire, the GMI used was the one proposed by Löe and Silness (1963) and modified by Lobene et al. (1986). The OHI-S was proposed by Greene e Vermillion (1964). Statistical comparisons between the groups were done using Chi-Squared and Fisher's Exact Test or "t" test. The data were analyzed

[*] Address all correspondence to: Renata de Oliveira Guaré DDS, PhD
Discipline of Dentistry, Persons with Disabilities Division Universidade Cruzeiro do Sul Rua Rua Jorge Tibiriçá, 74- apto 113 São Paulo – SP – Brazil, Cep:04126-000, Email: renataguare@uol.com.br, Tel. 55(11) 95770127, Fax.55(11) 25778539.

with the aid of MINITAB® statistical software, 14.2 version. The results demonstrated that the study group (DS) had professional follow-up dental care more frequently (p=0,010) and higher frequency of daily dental brushing (p<0,001). The use of dental floss was, however, rare (p<0,001). A statistically significant difference between the groups related to GMI and OHI-S was observed (p < 0,001). GMI was found to be greater and OHI-S smaller in the study group (DS). Children from the study group (DS) presented better oral hygiene habits and attended regular dental check-ups more often than children from the control group.

Keywords: Pediatric Dentistry, Down Syndrome - Dentistry;Periodontal disease

Introduction

Down syndrome (DS) is known as trisomy 21 or trisomy G[1]. In 1866, John Langdon Down published an article about some of the characteristics of this syndrome, where the patients had aspects similar to those of Asians or Mongolians. The term mongolism prevailed until 1960, when the eponym "Down syndrome" came to be used [2, 3, 4].

In the year 1959, Lejeune, Jacobs, Gautier and Turpin independently confirmed the presence of trisomy in chromosome 21[5] and identified three different genotypes: trisomy-21, translocation and mosaicism. In 1974, Nebuhr suggested that DS could be caused by a duplication of only one part of chromosome 21 in the q22 band [6].

Down syndrome is the most common genetic cause of mental impairment and congenital malformation and it occurs in 25% to 30% of individuals with severe mental impairment, with an intellectual quotient (IQ) lower than 50[5].

In literature, there is a consensus that the prevalence of DS is directly related to maternal age, even though different indices have been used in different studies. According to Pizazzo, Vianna and Lopes [7] (1998), the prevalence of DS in children of Mothers between 18 and 29 years old is of approximately 1.5:1,000 births, increasing up to 29:1,000 in the maternal age group of 40 years old and reaching 92:1,000 in the group of 44 year-old Mothers.

Tannenbaum [8] (1975) reported a DS incidence of 1:2,300 births for children of Mothers under 20 years old and approximately 1:54 for Mothers over 45 years of age.

According to Rogers, Roizen and Capone[5] (1996), the prevalence of DS increases in about 30% for maternal ages over 30 years. Maternal age is also related to the type of chromosomal anomaly, being that 10% of translocations occur in children born to Mothers between 15 and 19 years old.

To Hook, Cross and Schreinemachers[9] (1983) and Johnstone, Barnard and Harrison[10] (1999), the risk of having a child with DS is of 1:1,000 for 30-year-old Mothers and of 9:1,000 for Mothers over 40 years old. The authors Cogulu et al.[11] (2006), Desai and Fayetteville[12] (1997) and Fiske and Shafik[13] (2001) all report that DS is more frequent in the maternal age of above 35 years, having no ethnic, socioeconomic, or gender predilections.

The literature indicates that, in a general manner, the incidence of DS in the population varies between 1:600 and 1:1,000 live births[2,5,12,14,15,16,17,18,19,20].

Fiske and Shafik[13] (2001) reported that the incidence varies from country to country, increasing with maternal age and with consanguineous marriages. According to these authors, the incidence of birth of babies with DS seems to be changing because in 1976 there was 1:700 births; in 1985, there was between 1:1,250 and 1:1,265 births; and recent studies revealed an incidence of 1:854 pregnancies.

From the genetic point of view, this syndrome is caused by an anomaly during cellular division, called non-disjunction. Non-disjunction occurs when an ovule (or sometimes sperm cell) divides itself inappropriately and starts carrying two entire chromosomes. During fertilization, the zygote receives a third copy of chromosome 21, making a total of 47 chromosomes, called trisomy 32 or simple trisomy[12]. This type of anomaly occurs more frequently, constituting 93% to 95% of DS cases. Another mechanism that may cause trisomy 21 is translocation, where an extra fragment originated from chromosome 21 attaches itself to another chromosome (usually chromosome 13, 14, 15, 21 or 22). This type of alteration represents less than 5% of children with DS. Mosaicism, in its turn, is when the individual presents two or more cell lines which are karyotypically or genetically distinct and are originated from a simple zygote. In this case, some cells contain completely normal chromosomes and others present trisomy of chromosome 21. Three percent of cases of DS result from this type of chromosomal alteration[4,5,7,13,19].

Regarding general characteristics, children with DS may have difficulty gaining weight in the initial stages of life. Many factors may contribute to this difficulty, including a low calorie intake associated with inadequate breastfeeding due to weak and slow suction reflexes, as well as an extra need for calories associated to congenital heart disease (CHD). However, after 3 years of age, 30% of these children develop childhood obesity because of excessive caloric intake, a decrease in physical activities, and a low metabolic rate. Concerning neuromotor development, dysfunctions such as hypotonia, hyporeflexia, and reduced primitive reflexes may be present. A delay in the global motor coordination system, involving actions such as sitting without support, walking, and pronouncing the first words, may be observed in the first year of life. Dysgenesis of the cerebral cortex and the cerebellum, such as delayed myelination during the first year of life, probably constitutes the primary neurologic substrate of hypotonia and neural dysfunctions[5,13].

During the first 8 years of life, there is a slow growth rate, reaching the final height around the age of 15 years, which results in a low stature, a large torso, and short arms and legs. Approximately half of the individuals with DS present with a single palmar flexion line in their hands, 30% have a single flexion line in the fifth finger, and 60% present with clinodactyly (Figure 1). Learning difficulties are observed and about 80% of individuals with DS have an IQ between 25 and 50, with rare cases of IQs above 50 [4,13,19]. Nevertheless, in some cases of mosaicism there may be very slight phenotypic alterations and intelligence may be normal or close to normal. Sexual development is also deficient and, while men are sterile, women present with hypogonadism and primary amenorrhea[7].

A detailed description of congenital heart diseases (CHD) in individuals with DS was given by Desai and Fayetteville[12] (1997), Fiske and Shafik[13] (2001), Mustacchi and Rozone[4] (1990) and Rogers, Roizen and Capone[5] (1996), who stated an incidence of 40% to 60% of CHD, basically consisting of: atrioventricular canal defect (51%), ventricular septal defect (28%), atrial septal defect (11%), Tetralogy of Fallot (7%), and patent ductus arteriosus.

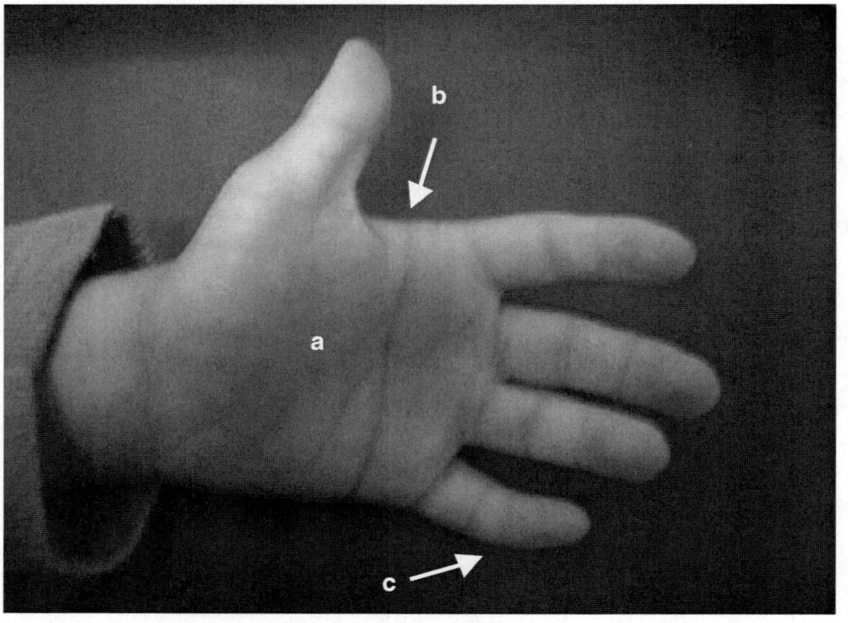

Figure 1. T.A.S., 5 years old, male, with Down syndrome; A) large hand, B) single transverse palmar crease (Simian line), C) short fingers and crooked middle phalanx of the 5th finger.

These authors also mention that children with DS who have CHDs present reduced growth and weight gain rates, increased hypotonia, and delayed motor development, when compared to children with DS without CHD. Adults develop mitral valve prolapse (57%) and 11% develop aortic regurgitation[21].

Pulmonary arterial hypertension with rapid progression of irreversible vascular disease frequently aggravates CHD in individuals with DS. The increase in incidence of pulmonary arterial hypertension is related, in part, to the high incidence of left-to-right shunts and may also be present in chronic upper airway diseases[5].

According to Seagriff-Curtin, Pugliese and Romer[19] (2006), all cardiac alterations described in individuals with DS may be surgically corrected and generally with a good prognosis.

Congenital gastrointestinal malformations are present in 5% of newborns with DS, causing symptoms of intestinal obstruction such as vomiting and abdominal distension. Malformations include frequent duodenal atresia or stenosis (2.4%), non-perforated anus (1%), aganglionic megacolon or Hirschsprung disease (0.5%), tracheoesophageal fistula (0.4%), and pyloric stenosis (0.3%). Although many of these malformations are present in the neonatal period with symptoms of intestinal obstruction, a partial obstruction may occur at a later period in life[5].

Celiac disease, also known as gluten-induced enteropathy, is a disorder of the small intestine consisting of permanent intolerance of gliadin and it affects 6.3% of individuals with DS[22].

Nervous system anomalies are also observed as calcifications of the base ganglions. Massive calcium deposition in the cerebral parenchyma is frequently found in children with DS and it leads to death in the first decade of life. Thirty percent of individuals with DS develop senile plaques and neurofibrillary tangles that are identical to those in Alzheimer disease seen in the general population, with loss of abilities required for daily activities. Also, epilepsy occurs in less than 1% of the general population and affects less than 2% of children with Ds, increasing to 10% at adult ages[4,5,12,13,19].

There is an increased susceptibility to gastrointestinal, urinary, respiratory (otitis media, pneumonia and sinusitis), skin and mucosal infections due to an immune system deficiency, with low counts of T cells. Individuals with DS are 15 to 20 times more likely to develop leukemia, generally acute lymphoblastic leukemia, when compared to individuals without the syndrome[4,5,7].

The reason behind this increased susceptibility to infections is still uncertain, yet, defective neutrophils with shortened life spans are observed. Lymphopenia and eosinopenia are present as well as defective mediator cells and immunoglobulins[13,15]. Individuals with DS who are institutionalized present a seven times greater probability of carrying the surface antigen of the hepatitis B virus than the general population[12,19,23].

Ophthalmologic malformations include almond-shaped palpebral fissures (58%), oblique inclination of the palpebral fissure (62%), Brushfiled spots (50%), and internal epicanthic folds (Figure 2). In the neonatal period, the most important ophthalmologic alteration identified is congenital cataracts, found in 3% of children with DS, which may be associated with absence or distortion of red reflex. Convergent strabismus occurs in 23% to 44% of individuals and refractive errors tend to increase with age, occurring in 30% to 70% of cases[4,5]. As stated by Fiske and Shafik[13] (2001), visual problems such as myopia, hyperopia, astigmatism, and cataracts occur in 50% of children with DS.

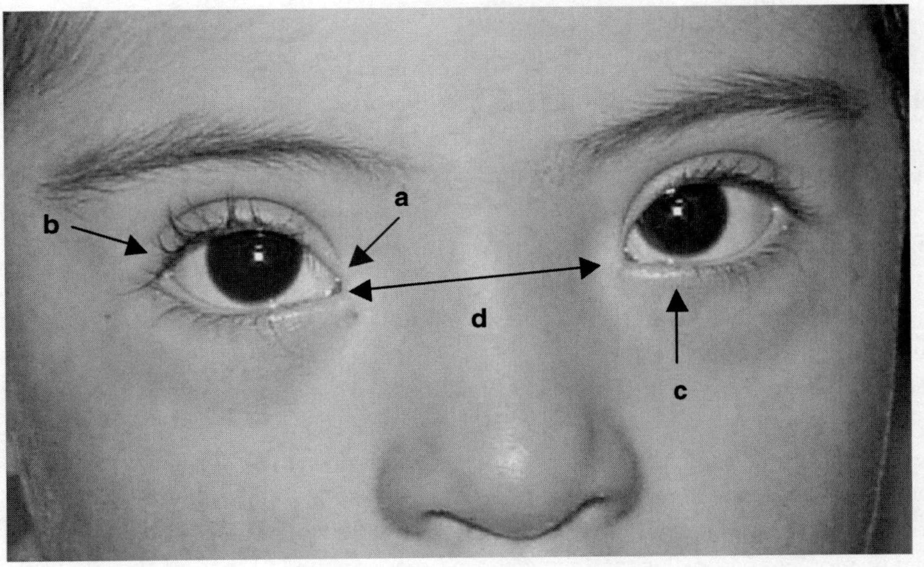

Figure 2. A.D.V., 5 years old, male, with Down syndrome. A) internal epicanthic folds, B) almond-shaped palpebral fissure, C) convergent strabismus, D) telecanthus.

Sixty to eighty percent of children with DS present with hearing loss, which may be conductive, sensorineural or mixed. Conductive hearing loss occurs due to an accumulation of fluids in the middle ear or due to ossicular-chain anomalies and it may result in mild to severe hearing loss, as well as middle ear infections in over 50% of children[5,13].

It is important to emphasize that 12% to 20% of children with DS have transverse ligament laxity between the atlas vertebrae and the odontoid process of the axis vertebrae, as well as in between the atlas vertebrae and the occipital condyle of the base of the cranium. Irreversible damage to the dorsal cord may occur as a result of lesions caused by hyperextension, abrupt flexion, or direct pressure to the neck in cases where the distance between the odontoid process of the axis vertebrae and the anterior arch of the atlas vertebrae exceeds 4.5 to 5 mm, or where there is atlanto-occipital or rotational instability. The taking of a cervical radiograph to verify the presence of atlanto-axial instability is recommended when the child is 3 years old and should be repeated before and at the end puberty[5,7,12].

In regards to the endocrine system of individuals with DS, there is a greater incidence of hypothyroidism as a result of an auto-immune process. This alteration is approximately eight times more common in individuals with DS than in those without the syndrome. Since there is an incidence of 0.7% of congenital hypothyroidism and 0.3% of transient congenital hypothyroidism in DS, the presence of such alterations should be tested in newborn babies[4,5].

Among the craniofacial alterations present in DS, Mustacchi and Rozone[4] (1990) Pinazo, Vianna and Lopes[7] (1998) reported: microcephaly, globular brachycephalic cranium, small suboccipital bregmatic circumference, and a prominent front. There are four fontanelles present, which are large and remain opened for a prolonged period of time. Sphenoid and frontal sinuses are absent and, 90% of the time, the maxillary sinus is hypoplastic. Individuals with DS have a flat facies, skeletal deficiency in the middle third of the face, present with telecanthus, and a flattened nasal bridge (Figure 3).

Underdevelopment of the middle third of the face results in reduction of height, width and depth of the palate. Hypotonia of the orbicular, zygomatic, masseter and temporal muscles may result in severe facial defects. The lips are hypotonic and the lower lip becomes inverted with tongue thrust[7] (Figure 4).

In individuals with Down syndrome, the mouth commonly stays open due to the relatively large tongue in a small oral cavity. This leads to mouth breathing, drooling, angular cheilitis, chronic periodontitis, and infections of the respiratory tract. Occasionally, uvula bifida, cleft lip and/or palate, and enlarged tonsils and adenoids can be seen. Their tongue is hypotonic and may present single, double or multiple fissures in the dorsal surface or on the two anterior thirds[24,25,26].

Thirty-five to fifty-five percent of patients with Down syndrome present with microdontia in both primary and permanent dentitions. The tooth crowns are usually conical, shortened, and smaller than normal and frequently present with enamel hypoplasia and hypocalcification. Congenital absence of teeth is more common in individuals with DS (50%) when compared to the general population (2%), being more frequent in the lower than in the upper jaw, more among males than females, and more on the left than on the right side[24].

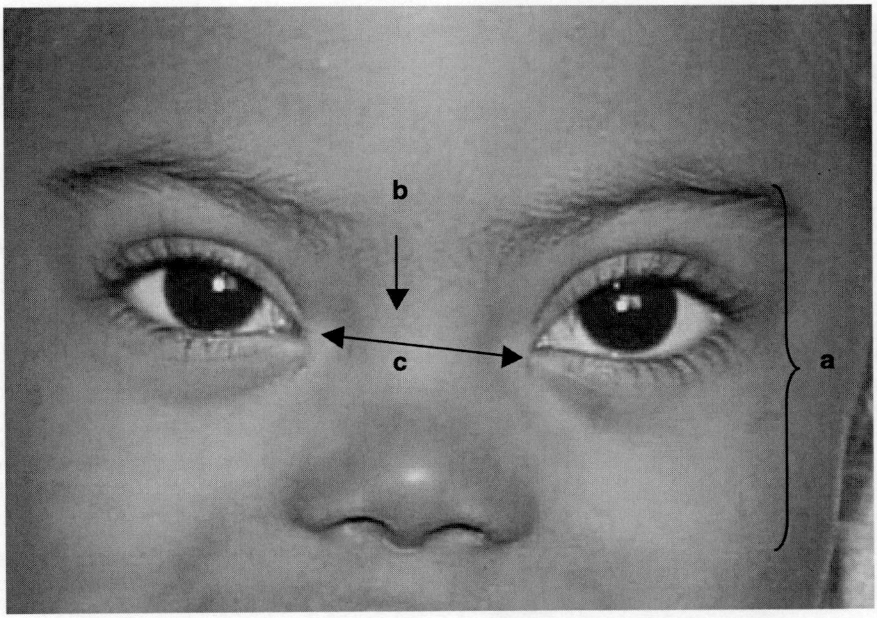

Figure 3. D.B.A., 3 years old, female, with Down syndrome: A) underdevelopment of the middle third of the face; B) flattened nasal bridge; C) telecanthus.

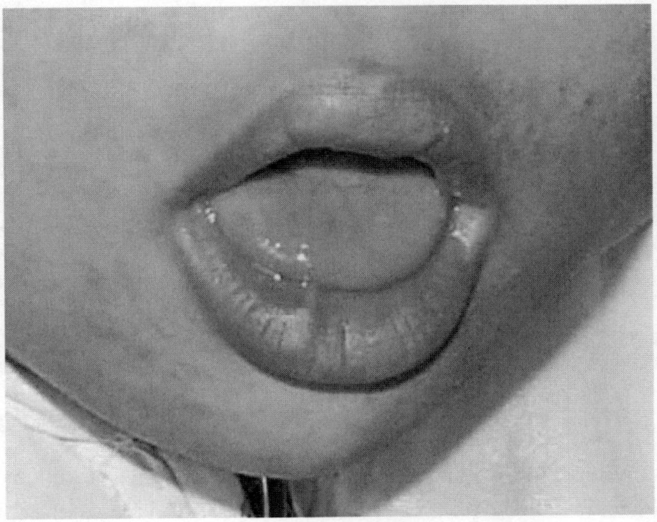

Figura 5. B.M., male, with Down syndrome: lip and tongue hypotonia.

Congenital absence of teeth, or agenesis, occurs mostly on: third molars, second premolars, lateral incisors, and lower incisors, in a decreasing order of frequency. The only teeth not affected by agenesis are the first permanent molars. Taurodontism also occurs more frequently in individuals with DS than in the general population, with a prevalence of 0.54% to 5.6%, where lower second molars are more commonly affected. Furthermore, a delay in eruption of primary teeth can be seen, altering both chronology and sequence of eruption, particularly in the anterior teeth and first molars. In DS, dental eruption generally initiates between 12 to 24 months of age and the primary dentition becomes complete around 4 to 5 years of age. Regarding the permanent dentition, the first molars and lower incisors do not erupt before 8 to 9 years of age[2, 3, 13, 14, 27, 28.]

Individuals with DS usually present malaligned teeth in the primary and permanent dentitions, particularly in the incisor and canine regions. Malocclusion is generally caused by mouth breathing (96%), improper mastication (60%), bruxism (45%), tooth agenesis (12.7%), median line deviation (80%) in the upper arch, anterior open bite (45%), temporomandibular dysfunction (24%), delayed exfoliation and eruption of teeth, tongue thrust, hypotonic TMJ ligaments, and developmental disturbances in the lower and upper jaws. Mandibular-maxillary discrepancies include: mandibular overjet, anterior open bite , posterior crossbite , anterior crossbite, mesial molar relation caused by mandibular protrusion, and sagittal malocclusion. The anterior crossbite is primarily caused by an antero-posterior bone deficiency in the upper arch, as a result of vertical underdevelopment of the maxilla, with evident prognathism (Figures 5 and 6)[2,12,13,24,25,27].

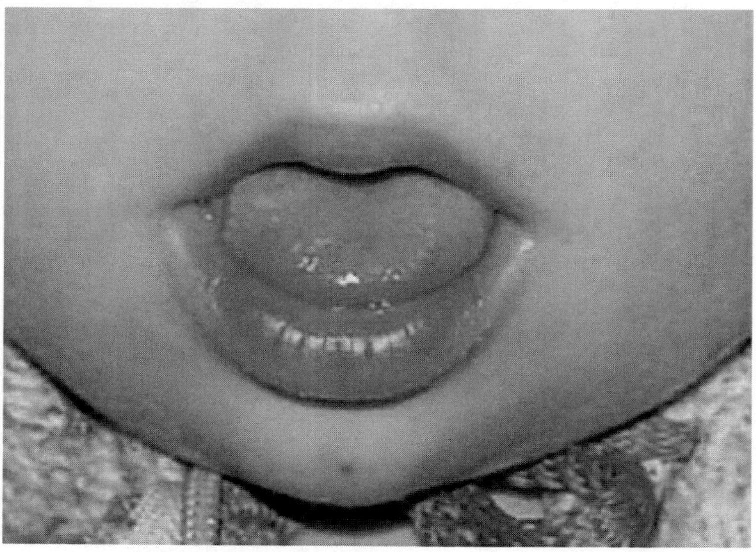

Figure 6. D.A.J., 2 years old, female, with Down syndrome: hypotonic lips and tongue thrust.

There are contradicting views in literature regarding caries experience of individuals with DS. The works of Maclaurin, Shaw and Foster[29] (1985) and Yarat et al.[30] (1999) showed a similar prevalence of dental caries between individuals with DS and the general population. On the other hand, a variety of studies have reported that caries is less prevalent in individuals with DS, due to factors such as: hypodontia, delayed eruption, increased dental spacing, alterations in salivary composition with increased levels of salivary IgA, bruxism, and less cariogenic strands *Streptococcus mutans*[2,7,13,16,30,31,32,33,34,35]. Cutress[1] (1971) and Fung and Alison[36] (2005) reported that when the factors hypodontia and delayed dental eruption are adjusted, dental caries indices are the same among individuals with and without the syndrome.

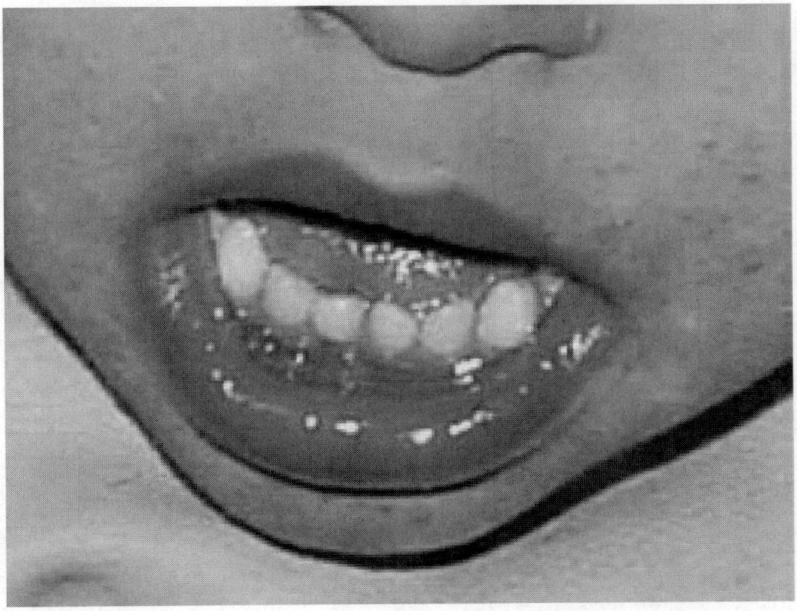

Figure 7. C.B.T.G., 4 years old, male, with Down syndrome: relative mandibular prognathism.

Alterations in the salivary components of individuals with DS were investigated by Siqueira and Nicolau[20] (2002) who compared levels of sialic acid, proteins, salivary flow, pH and amylase and peroxidase activities in 17 individuals with DS and 18 individuals without DS, between 6 and 10 years old. Results showed that individuals with DS had reduced salivary flow in both genders, a lower pH, higher levels of proteins in males, lower concentrations of peroxidase and amylase, and no change in sialic acid when compared to samples of whole saliva from individuals without the syndrome.

There is a consensus in literature that individuals with DS present higher prevalence and susceptibility to periodontal problems. Reuland-Bosma, van Dijk and van der Weele[37] (1986) conducted a study to elucidate some aspects of defense mechanisms using a model of experimental gingivitis and concluded that children with DS present a different leukocytal response associated to more extensive gingival inflammation in relation to children without the syndrome.

Randell, Harth, and Seow[18] (1991) studied 25 non-institutionalized children with DS between 1 and 14 years old, and concluded that children with DS presented worse oral hygiene when compared to the control group. Moreover, a greater number of children with DS had a prolonged habit of using baby bottles after the age of 18 months or consumed drinks using a baby bottle at night, indicating greater risk for the development of dental caries. Children with DS received less help during toothbrushing, had their first dental visit at a later age and presented lower fluoride ingestion. These results indicated that children with DS presented greater disadvantage in relation to oral health practices.

According to Saraiva[38] (1994), the severity of gingivitis found in these patients is associated to immunological alterations. Periodontitis can be observed since childhood, causing loss of primary and permanent teeth. In individuals with DS younger than 30 years old, periodontitis can be observed in 96% of individuals and this disease is more severe in the lower incisors and molars regions.

Shapira and Stablolz[36] (1996) reported that the critical factor responsible for the high incidence of severe periodontal disease in patients with DS is their inability to maintain proper oral hygiene. However, there are some predisposing conditions to the development of early periodontal disease, including occlusal relation alterations, particularly anterior or posterior crossbite, and a high insertion of the anterior mandibular frenum, causing mucogingival defects in the lower incisors. The authors emphasized that severe periodontitis and early loss of lower incisors are common sequelae in these patients.

Desai and Fayetteville[12] (1997) affirmed that individuals with DS develop gingivitis earlier and have manifestations of generalized and acute periodontal disease in adult ages, starting between the ages of 6 and 15 years. The most common problems are: marginal gingivitis, acute and subacute necrotizing gingivitis, advanced periodontitis, gingival recession with formation of gingival pockets, horizontal and vertical bone loss with suppuration, root furcation involvement, and frequent tooth loss, mainly in the lower anterior region.

According to Agholme[23] et al. (1998), the prevalence of periodontal disease in teenagers with DS is of 30% to 40% and reaches values close to 100% at 30 years of age. The authors investigated the periodontal condition and salivary levels of IgA and IgM, all of the subclasses of IgG and albumins in 20 individuals with DS and in 19 individuals of the control group. Gingival inflammation was more extensive ($p<0.05$) in individuals with DS when compared to individuals from the control group and there was more frequent occurrence of periodontal pockets (>4mm) ($p<0.05$). The levels of IgA, IgM, and all subclasses of IgG as well as the concentration of albumins were not significantly different between the groups. However, the proportion of IgG1 expressed as a percentage of the total sum of IgG was significantly higher ($p<0.01$) in individuals with DS when compared to the control group. On the other hand, the proportion of IgG2, IgG3, IgG4 subclasses in saliva was not different between the two groups. The authors concluded that there was an altered distribution of subclasses of IgG in saliva, with a high proportion of IgG1 in individuals with DS compared to the control group.

Agholme, Dahllöf and Modéer[39] (1999); Cichon, Crawford and Grimm[15] (1998), and López-Pérez et al.[17] (2002) stated, despite the deficient oral hygiene in individuals with DS, the presence of biofilm does not seem to be related to the severity of periodontal disease commonly found in these patients. According to the authors, these individuals have an exacerbated immune/inflammatory response as a result of altered mediator and humoral immune cells, chemotaxic alterations and deficient phagocytic system, reduced phagocytic ability of polymorphonuclear leukocytes and of monocytes and defective oxidative response. The number of B lymphocytes in peripheral blood may be reduced in this population and T lymphocytes may be reduced or immature.

In 2000, Amano[40] reported that abnormalities in the defense mechanism, presence of specific periodontopathogenic organisms, susceptibility to infections, altered auto-immune mechanisms, lack of labial seal and tongue thrust are significant factors in the etiology of periodontal disease in individuals with DS. However, the presence of bacterial plaque does not seem to be related to the severity of the disease in these individuals.

Santos et al.[41](2004) reported that patients with DS commonly develop severe periodontal disease at a very early age, being that initial clinical characteristics of this condition in 2 to 5 year-old children resembles Vincent infection.

AIM

This case-control study aims at evaluating some behavioral characteristics related to dental hygiene, Gingival Modified Index (GMI) and Simplified Oral Hygiene Index (OHIS) in the primary dentition of DS children.

Methods

The study group was composed of 69 children with Down syndrome (DS) between 13 and 85 months old. They were examined at the Irmandade da Santa Casa de Misericórdia de São Paulo, Darcy Vargas Children's Hospital, Associação de Pais e Amigos dos Excepcionais (APAE) of the city of Barueri.

The control group consisted of 69 children without congenital anomalies, selected among students of the Marly Teixeira de Almeida kindergarten – Barueri – São Paulo – who were paired to children of the study group according to gender.

Only children with DS in their primary dentition were included in the study and the exclusion criteria was: children with local oral factors (soft or hard tissue tumors, stomatitis, recurrent canker sores or major oral pathologies), and children who had participated in another clinical study 30 days prior to the development of the present study.

The participants' legal guardians read and signed an informed consent form which explained the procedures to be carried out. The participants underwent oral examination, all exams were conducted by a calibrated examiner (Kappa intra-examiner agreement = 89.3%) in a dental office under artificial lighting.

Medical and Dental History

General information regarding the medical and dental history and oral hygiene habits of all children from the study and control groups were obtained from the participants' legal guardians in a questionnaire. Information collected concerning the children's Mothers included age and occupation.

Simplified Oral Hygiene Index – OHI-S

Evaluation of the patient's oral hygiene was done according to the criteria used in the Simplified Oral Hygiene index (OHI-S) proposed by Greene and Vermillion[42] (1964). With the aid of a cotton tip, plaque revealer was applied on the buccal surfaces of the primary upper right central incisor, the lower left central incisor and the upper second molars, bilaterally, as well as on the lingual surfaces of the lower second molars. These surfaces were examined and given a score from zero to three.

Modified Gingival Index (MGI)

For the evaluation of periodontal disease, the index proposed by Löe and Silness (1963) and modified by Lobene et al.[43] (1986) was used, and this technique does not include applying pressure with a probe to determine the presence or absence of gingival bleeding.

The primary teeth evaluated (gingival margins and papillae) in each oral quadrant were: upper right second molar, upper right lateral incisor, upper left primary molar, lower left second molar, lower left lateral incisor, and lower right primary molar. The MGI only consists of visual examination using scores from 0 to 4.

Results

Statistical comparisons between the groups were done using Chi-Squared and Fisher's Exact Test or "t" test. The data were analyzed with the aid of MINITAB® statistical software, 14.2 version.

Table 1. Behavioral Characteristics Of The Study Group and Control Groups: Categorical Variables

Characteristics	Experimental N (%)	Control N (%)	p
Is the child under dental treatment?			0.010*
no	31 (44.9)	46 (66.7)	
yes	38 (55.1)	23 (33.3)	
Oral hygiene orientation?			0.729*
no	29 (42.0)	27 (39.1)	
yes	40 (58.0)	42 (60.9)	
Who brushes the child's teeth?			<0.001*
Does not brush	6 (8.7)	6 (8.7)	
Mother	55 (79.7)	35 (50.7)	
Father	1 (1.5)	1 (1.5)	
Others	1 (1.5)	3 (4.4)	
By him/herself	2 (2.9)	9 (13.0)	
Both parents	4 (5.8)	15 (21.7)	
Daily brushing frequency			0.016*
Does not brush	6 (8.7)	6 (8.7)	
Once	2 (2.9)	14 (20.3)	
Twice	38 (55.1)	31 (44.9)	

Characteristics	Experimental N (%)	Control N (%)	p
Thrice	23 (33.3)	18 (26.1)	
Instrument used for toothbrushing			0.813*
Does not brush	6 (8.7)	6 (8.7)	
Wet cloth	4 (5.8)	3 (4.4)	
Toothbrush	58 (84.1)	59 (85.1)	
Gum massager	1 (1.5)	1 (1.5)	
Use of dental floss			< 0.001*
no	65 (94.2)	48 (69.6)	
yes	4 (5.8)	21 (30.4)	

Table 2. Labor market insertion of mothers: categorical variables

Characteristics	Experimental N (%)	Control N (%)	p
Mother's work (outside household)			0.001*
Does not work	47 (69.1)	29 (42.0)	
Does work	21 (30.9)	40 (58.0)	

Table 3.Summary of statistics regarding characteristics of study and control group: numerical variables

	N	Average	s.d.	minimum	median	maximum
Mother's age (in years): p<0.001						
Experimental	69	34.1	8.5	14	37	47
Control	69	26.1	5.5	16	25	41
MGI: p<0.001						
Experimental	69	2.64	2.45	0	2.00	8.33
Control	69	0.31	0.40	0	0.17	1.50
OHI-S: p=0.017						
Experimental	69	1.11	0.58	0	1.17	2.33
Control	69	1.37	0.66	0	1.50	2.67

Table 4. Ohi-s in the study and control groups: categorical variables

OHI-S	Experimental N (%)	Control N (%)
satisfactory (0 to 1.0)	29 (42.0)	20 (29.0)
regular (1.1 to 2.0)	38 (55.1)	43 (62,3)
deficient (2.1 to 3.0)	2 (2.9)	6 (8.7)
awful (> 3.0)		

Discussion

The association of occurrence of DS with advanced maternal age has long been known[4,7,8,9,10,11,12,13]. According to Rogers, Roizen and Capone[5] (1996), the incidence of this syndrome increases in 30% for Mothers over 30 years old. In the present study, it was observed that the age during pregnancy of Mothers of children with DS varied between 14 and 47 years. The average maternal age was of 34.1 years, while the age of Mothers of children without congenital anomalies varied between 16 and 41 years, with an average of 26.1 years. There was a statistically significant correlation ($p<0.001$) indicating that Mothers of children with DS were older at the time of their pregnancies in comparison to Mothers of the control group.

According to Leujene (1959) apud Rogers, Roizen and Capone[5] (1996), there are three different types of DS: trisomy 21 or simple trisomy, mosaicism, and translocation. Authors agree that 93% to 95% of DS cases are caused by a simple trisomy and that 3% to 5% occurs due to translocation and 1% due to mosaicism[4,5,7,12,13,19]. In this study, the children of the study group were regular patients of the Santa Casa de Misericórdia of São Paulo, Darcy Vargas Hospital and APAE institution of the city of Barueri, that had been diagnosed with DS. Access to the participant's karyotypes was not granted, making it impossible to classify them according to the three genotypes. Since the oral conditions presented by patients of the three different genotypes are similar[6], not having this information did not influence the study.

Fiske and Shafik[13] (2001), Pinazo, Vianna and Lopes[7] (1998), Rogers, Roizen and Capone[5] (1996), Seagriff-Curtin, Pugliese and Romer[19] (2006) reported that approximately 80% of individuals with DS have an IQ between 25 and 50, yet are sweet, imitative, shy and cooperative. The height and weight values were lower at birth and there was a delay in growth and neuromotor development. In the present study, it was observed that many children with DS had trouble articulating words and had a low comprehension level.

From a behavioral point of view, due to their young age and to mental impairment, many of the participants were resistant and difficult to handle during clinical procedures. On the other hand, it was observed that after examination the children displayed signs of affection and acted cordially.

Aside from various systemic health problems, individuals with DS also present craniofacial alterations. In the experimental group, the features observed were: underdevelopment of the middle third of the face, flat nasal bridge and flat facies, hypotonic tongue and orbicular lip muscles, as well as open mouth, tongue thrust, and relative prognathism. Such findings were also observed by Allison, Hannequin and Faulks[27] (2000), Bradley and McAlister[2] (2004), Ciamponi and Guaré[24] (2000), Desai and Fayetteville[12] (1997), Fiske and Shafik[13] (2001) and Rodrigues[26] et al. (1997).

There is a consensus that individuals with DS present a high prevalence and susceptibility to periodontal disease, starting at an early age, associated to immunological alterations[12,17,23,34,36,37,39,40,41].

The Simplified Oral Hygiene index (OHI-S) and the Modified Gingival Index (MGI) were used to verify periodontal conditions in children with SD. Results of the MGI were statistically different ($p<0.001$) between the experimental and control groups, being that children with DS presented higher indices (2.64) than children without the syndrome (0.31). These results are in accordance with those of previously cited authors who reported extensive gingival inflammation of early onset in individuals with DS.

OHI-S results revealed a statistically significant difference ($p=0.017$) between children of the study and control groups, being that children with DS presented a lower index (1.11) than those without the syndrome (1.37). Pinto[44] (2000) classified the OHI-S as satisfactory (0 to 1.0), regular (1.1 to 2.0), deficient (2.1 to 3) and awful (>3.0). Thus, it was observed that the majority of children had regular oral hygiene.

The results found in this study, where the MGI was increased while the OHI-S was regular in children with DS corroborates with the study of Amano (2000). Their observations pointed out that the presence of biofilm was not related to the severity of periodontal disease in individuals with DS, indicating that the main etiological factor would be an abnormality in the defense mechanism of these patients. Agholme, Dahllöf and Modéer[39] (1999), Cichon, Crawford and Grimm[15](1998) emphasized that individuals with DS have an increased immune-inflammatory response due to altered mediator and humoral immune cells, chemotaxic alterations and deficient phagocytic system, reduced phagocytic ability of polymorphonuclear leukocytes and of monocytes and defective oxidative response, leading to severe periodontal disease.

Some information concerning oral hygiene habits were obtained through the use of a questionnaire answered by the participants' legal guardians. The answers showed that 40 children with DS (58%) and 42 children without congenital anomalies (60.9%) had received professional orientation about oral hygiene and there were no statistically significant differences between the two groups ($p=0.729$).

As to the matter of who was responsible for the children's oral hygiene, results showed that, in the study group, toothbrushing was done mostly by the Mothers (79.7%). In control group, toothbrushing was done by the Mothers (50.7%) but also by the children themselves (13%) and by both parents (21.7%), and this difference was statistically significant ($p<0.001$). This difference can be explained by the fact that children with DS were more closely looked after by their Mothers, in part due to their systemic alterations, as well as the children's inability to conduct some chores by themselves. Another fact that may explain this finding is that Mothers of children in the study group did not work outside their households and that was significantly different in relation to Mothers in the control group ($p=0.001$).

In a general manner, children with DS brushed their teeth more frequently (average of 2.13 times) than children in the control group (average of 1.88 times), and this comparison was statistically significant ($p=0.016$). It should be emphasized that 6 children with DS (8.7%) and 6 children without the syndrome (8.7%) did not brush their teeth. There were no differences regarding the instrument used for toothbrushing ($p=0.813$) because the majority of participants from both groups used toothbrushes. Results indicate that the lower OHI-S among participants with DS can be explained by the fact that their Mothers were responsible for their oral hygiene and brushed their teeth more times a day. Furthermore, the higher levels of MGI in the experimental group were not related to dental biofilm but to alterations in the immune system, as mentioned before.

Regarding the use of dental floss, children with DS used it significantly less frequently than children in the control group ($p<0.001$). This result can be explained by the fact that children with DS have difficulty handling floss, which is in agreement with Shapira and Stablolz (1996) who observed that they had a greater inability to maintain good oral hygiene. Nevertheless, independently of having DS or not, the majority of children did not floss their teeth, revealing a lack of motivation and awareness of their legal guardians as to the benefits of this oral hygiene technique.

The investigation of whether the child was under dental treatment revealed that children in the control group attended the dental office significantly more often ($p=0.010$). This result contradicts the study by Allison, Hennequin and Faulks[27] (2000) whose observations pointed out that children with DS in France had difficulty finding dental treatment. In São Paulo city and its suburbs, there are some public hospitals, like the Darcy Vargas Hospital, and charity institutions such as Barueri's APAE, Basic Health Units and dentistry schools, which offer dental treatment and periodical preventive and educational follow-ups for children with DS. However, in many regions of Brazil, especially in more deprived areas, dental treatment for special needs patients is still not accessible.

In general, the children with DS in this study, received more help from their Mothers during toothbrushing, which was performed more frequently during the day, and they attended dental treatment more often than children in the control group. These results are not in accordance with the studies of Shapira and Stablolz[34] (1996), who indicated that children with DS are at an advantage regarding oral health practices.

Considering the results analyzed, it is important to emphasize that the protocol for treatment of children with DS should be based on a detailed medical history taking and should focus on reduction of dental biofilm through mechanical control, use of chemotherapics, and salivary analysis for microbiological examination when possible. Moreover, it is essential to point out that education is still the most effective form of prevention, therefore, parents and legal guardians need to be oriented about oral health care, inserted in a multidisciplinary context, and this orientation should be part of the routine dental treatment.

Conclusion

Children in the study group (DS) presented better oral hygiene habits and attended the dental office more frequently than children in the control group; the OHI-S was lower in the study group; children with DS presented a significantly higher MGI than children without the syndrome.

References

[1] Cutress TW. Dental caries in trisomy 21. *Arch. Oral. Biol.* 1971;16:1329-44

[2] Bradley C, McAlister T. The oral health of children with Down syndrome in Ireland. *Spec. Care Dent.* 2004;24(2):55-60.

[3] Kumasaka S, Miyagi A, Sakai N, Shindo J, Kashima I. Oligodontia: A radiograph comparison of subjects with Down syndrome and normal subjects. *Spec. Care Dent.* 1997;17(4)137-41.

[4] Mustacchi Z, Rozone G. Síndrome de Down: aspectos clínicos e odontológicos. São Paulo: CID; 1990.

[5] Rogers PT, Roizen NJ, Capone GT. Down Syndrome. In: Capute AJ, Accardo PJ. Developmental disabilities in infancy and childhood. 2 ed. Baltimore: Paul H Brookes; 1996. P. 221-43.

[6] Latner LE. The caries experience in three genotypes of Down´s syndrome. *J. Pedod.* 1983;7(2):83-90.

[7] Pinazo JDC, Vianna MIP, Lopes FL. Cárie dentária e placa bacteriana em crianças de 07 a 14 anos portadoras da síndrome de Down, matriculadas em instituições públicas e privadas do município de Salvador – Bahia. *Rev. Fac. Odontol da UFBA*. 1998; 17:15-24.

[8] Tannenbaum KA. The oral aspects of mongolism. *J. Public Health Dent.* 1975;35(2):108.

[9] Hook EB, Cross PK, Schreinemachers DM. Chromosomal abnormality rates at amniocentesis and in live-born infants. *JAMA.* 1983;249(15):2034-8.

[10] Johnstone SC, Barnard KM, Harrison VE. Recognizing and caring for the medically compromised child: 4. Children with other chronic medical conditions. *Dent. Update.* 1999;26:21-6.

[11] Cogulu D, Sabah E, Uzel A, Ozkinay F. Genotyping of *Streptococcus mutans* by using arbitrarily primed polymerase chain reaction in children with Down syndrome. *Arch. Oral Biol.* 2006;51:177-82.

[12] Desai SS, Faytetteville NY. Down syndrome: a review of the literature. *Oral. Surg. Oral Med. Oral Pathol. Oral Radiol. Endond.* 1997;84:279-85.

[13] Fiske J, Shafik HH. Down’s syndrome and oral care. *Dent. Update.* 2001;28:148-156.

[14] Acerbi AG, Freitas C, Magalhães MHCG. Prevalence of numeric anomalies in the permanent dentition of patients with Down syndrome. *Spec. Care Dent.* 2001;21(2):75-8.

[15] Cichon P, Crawford L, Grimm WD. Early-onset periodontitis associated with Down´s syndrome - A clinical interventional study. *Ann. Periodont.* 1998;3(1):370-80.

[16] Cogulu D; Sabah E; Kutukculer N; Ozkinay F. Evaluation of the relationship between caries indices and salivary secretory IgA, salivary pH, buffering capacity and flow rate in children with Down's syndrome. *Arch. Oral Biol.* 2006;51(1):23-8.

[17] López-Pérez R, Borges-Yáñes SA, Jiménez-García G, Maupomé G. Oral hygiene, gingivitis, and periodontitis in persons with Down syndrome. *Spec. Care Dent.* 2002 22(6):214-20.

[18] Randell DM, Harth S, Seow WK. Preventive dental health practices of non-institutionalized Down syndrome children: a controlled study. *J. Clin. Ped. Den*t. 1992;16(3):225-9.

[19] Seagriff-Curtin P, Pugliese S, Romer M. Dental considerations for individuals with Down syndrome. *NYSDJ.* 2006:33-35.

[20] Siqueira Jr WL, Nicolau J. Stimulated whole saliva components in children with Down syndrome. *Spec. Care Dent*. 2002;22(6):226-30.

[21] Barnett ML, Friedman D, Kastner T. The prevalence of mitral valve prolapse in patients with Down's syndrome: implications for dental management. *Oral Surg. Oral Med. Oral Pathol.* 1988;66(4):445-7.

[22] Boyd D, Quick A, Murray C. The Down syndrome patient in dental practice, part II: clinical considerations. *N. Zeland Dent. J.* 2004;100(1):4-9.

[23] Agholme MB, Dahllöf G, Modéer T, Engström PE, Engström GN. Periodontal conditions and salivary immunoglobulins in individuals with Down syndrome. *J. Periodontol.* 1998;69(10):1119-23.

[24] Ciamponi AL, Guaré RO. A criança com trissomia do cromossomo 21 (Síndrome de Down). In: Guedes-Pinto AC. Odontopediatria: resoluções clínicas. Curitiba: *Editora Maio* 2000;(3):301-12.

[25] Ordanza AJL, Blanco R, Valenzuela C. Sequence of eruption of deciduous dentition in a Chilean sample with Down syndrome. *Arch. Oral Bio*l. 1993;42(5):401-6.

[26] Rodrigues MJ, Lima KTF, Carvalho MH, Farias TP. Estudo para avaliar a influência dos hábitos alimentares e de higiene bucal no ceo e cpo-d em pacientes com deficiência mental e síndrome de Down. *Rev. Fac .Odont Pernambuco.* 1997;15(1-2): 25-30.

[27] Allison PJ, Hennequin M, Faulks D. Dental care access among individuals with Down syndrome in France. *Spec. Care Dent.* 2000;20(1):28-34.

[28] Peretz B, Katzenel V, Shapira J. Morphometric variables of the primary second molar in children with Down syndrome. *J. Clin. Ped. Dent.* 1999; 23(4): 333-6.

[29] Maclaurin ET, Shaw L, Foster TD. Dental caries and periodontal disease in children with Down´s Syndrome and other mentally handicapping conditions. *J. Paed. Dent.* 1985;1:15-9.

[30] Yarat A, Akyüz S, Koç L, Erdem H, Emekli N. Salivary sialic acid, protein, salivary flow rate, pH, buffering capacity and caries indices in subjects with Dow's syndrome. *J. Dent. Res.* 1999;22(2):115-8.

[31] Morinushi T, Lopatin DE, Tanaka H. The relationship between dental caries in the primary dentition and anti *S. mutans* serum antibodies in children with Down's syndrome. *J. Clin. Pediat. Dent.* 1995; 19(4): 279-84.

[32] Orner G. Dental caries experience among children with Down´s syndrome and their sibs. *Arch. Oral Biol.* 1975; 20(10):627-34.

[33] Shapira J, Stabholtz A, Schurr D, Sela MN, Mann J. Caries levels, *Streptococcus mutans* counts, salivary pH, and periodontal treatment needs of adult Down syndrome patients. *Spec. Care Dent.* 1991;11(6):248-51.

[34] Shapira J, Stabholz A. A comprehensive 30-month preventive dental health program in a pre-adolescent population with Dows' syndrome: A longitudinal study. *Spec. Care Dent.* 1996;16(1):33-37.

[35] Fung K, Allison PJ. A comparison of caries rates in non-institutionalized individuals with and without Down syndrome. *Spec. Care Dent.* 2005;25(6):302-10.

[36] Stabholz A, Mann J, Sela M, Schurr D, Steinberg D, Dori S, Shapira J. Caries experience, periodontal treatment needs, salivary pH, and *Streptococcus mutans* counts in a preadolescent Down syndrome population. *Spec. Care Dent.* 1991;11(5):203-8.

[37] Reuland-Bosma W, van Dijik LJ, van der Weele L. Experimental gingivitis around deciduous teeth in children with Down´s syndrome. *J. Clin. Periodontol.* 1986;13:294-300.

[38] Saraiva MCP. Ocorrência de doenças periodontais e *actinobacillus actinomycetemcomitans* em pacientes portadores da síndrome de Down. [dissertação]. São Paulo: Faculadade de Odontologia, Universidade de São Paulo; 1994.

[39] Agholme MB, Dahllöf G, Modéer T. Changes of periodontal status in patients with Down syndrome during a 7- year period. Eur J Oral Sci. 1999;107(2):82-8.

[40] Amano A. Kishima T, Akiyama S, Nakagawa I, Hamada S, Morisaki I. Periodontopathic bacteria in children with Down syndrome. *J. Periodontol.* 2000;71(2):249-55.

[41] Santos LM, Moreira EAM, Almeida ICS, Bosco VL. Aspectos bucais da Síndrome de Down: revisão da literatura. *Rev. ABO Nac.* 2004;12(5):278-82.

[42] Greene JC, Vermillion JR. The simplified oral hygiene index. *J. Am. Dent. Assoc.* 1964; 68:7-13.

[43] Lobene RR, Weatherford T, Ross NM, Lamm RA, Menaker L. A modified gingival index for use in clinical trials. *Clin. Prev. Dent.* 1986;8(1):3-6.

[44] Pinto VG. Identificação de problemas. In: Pinto VG. Saúde bucal coletiva. 4a ed. São Paulo: Santos; 2000.p.138-222.

In: Handbook of Down Syndrome Research
Editors: Dominicus Jelinek and Gijs Dvorak ISBN 978-1-60741- 690-6

Chapter 12

Down's Syndrome and Dysphagia

Tracy Lazenby-Paterson
Learning Disabilities Service, NHS Lothian, Edinburgh UK

Abstract

Disorders of eating, drinking and swallowing (also known as 'dysphagia') commonly affect people with Down's syndrome (DS) across the lifespan. This is due to the influence of several factors, including the abnormal oral-facial features that are characteristic of the syndrome, as well as comorbid health conditions that impact on the safety and integrity of the swallowing process. The relevant literature is consulted to explore aspects of the eating, drinking and swallowing process in people with Down's syndrome from birth onwards, and examine how this process differs from that in the general population. Discussion focuses on how the typical eating, drinking and swallowing process in DS individuals is frequently associated with abnormal functioning of the swallowing mechanism at various levels, and how it can very often lead to dysphagia and its potentially life-threatening sequelae. Finally, this paper considers the role of healthcare practitioners in the identification and management of dysphagia in individuals with DS, including implications for treatment planning and health service delivery.

Introduction

Dysphagia (difficulty with eating and drinking and swallowing) is a particular concern for health professionals, as it is commonly considered to be a cause of life-threatening chest illness [1]. Respiratory illness such as aspiration pneumonia is the leading cause of death amongst people with intellectual disabilities (ID), including people with Down's syndrome (DS) [2-7]. Hollins et al. [8] found that out of 2000 individuals with ID, 52% died of respiratory disease, compared with only 17% of females and 15% of males in the general population without ID.

Although the prevalence of dysphagia in people with ID is unknown, dysphagia, nutritional problems, aspiration pneumonia, respiratory illness and asphyxiation are widely considered to be more common in individuals with ID than in the general population [4-6, 9,10].

In studies of stroke patients, dysphagia was found to be an independent predictor of aspiration pneumonia, and is considered to increase risk of aspiration pneumonia by 3 to 7 times [11-14]. It is yet unclear to what extent dysphagia plays a part in the development of aspiration pneumonia in people with ID. Some studies indicate that a sole diagnosis of dysphagia is not a reliable predictor for respiratory illness. Factors such as poor oral health, a history of chest illness, the use of multiple medications, co-existing health conditions and dependency on others for feeding and oral care are also significant predictors for aspiration pneumonia [15-19].

Many of these conditions are more prevalent in people with Down's syndrome and thus increase the risk of respiratory conditions in this population. Bittles et al [20] examined the causes of death in 1332 people with Down's syndrome ranging from 0-73 years. The authors discovered a high mortality rate due to respiratory illnesses and pneumonia across all age groups, with these conditions being the most common cause of premature death in the 19-40 and 40+ age groups.

Dysphagia is commonly considered to be an important risk factor in the development of aspiration pneumonia in people with DS. Dysphagia is also a potential cause of other serious conditions, including malnutrition, obesity, dehydration and upper airway obstruction [8,11,19,21,22]

This chapter examines how the eating, drinking and swallowing process is often impaired in people with DS, and the implications of these difficulties on health service delivery.

Eating, Drinking, Swallowing and Dysphagia

In the general healthy population, the acts of eating, drinking and swallowing are typically categorised into three main events: the *oral phase*, which is subdivided into the *oral preparatory* and *oral transit* stages, the *pharyngeal phase* and the *oesophageal phase*.

Oral phase: Oral preparation begins when food enters the mouth. The lips, tongue, cheeks and jaw act together to control and hold food in the mouth, position it between the teeth, and grind it down. The grinded food mixes with saliva and once sufficiently chewed, it is collected into a cohesive mass referred to as the bolus. It is then positioned and held in a groove formed on the centre of the tongue. Oral transit begins when the anterior portion of the tongue lifts and presses against the hard palate. The mouth closes in order that the jaw can stabilise. The lips close to prevent the bolus from escaping out of the mouth, and buccal musculature ensures that food particles do not escape and collect in the spaces between the jaw and cheek. Increasingly more of the tongue pushes against the hard palate in a front-to-back direction, propelling the bolus towards the pharynx. The soft palate remains lowered and in contact with the posterior portion of the tongue to prevent premature spillage of food into the pharynx. This position of the soft palate also allows for nasal breathing during the oral phase.

The oral phase is under voluntary neural control. Therefore the amount of time taken to complete the oral phase can vary considerably according to an individual's oral motor skills, the rheological properties of food, and the preference of the individual. Upon initiation of the pharyngeal phase, all subsequent processes of the swallow are governed by involuntary reflex actions.

Pharyngeal phase: The pharyngeal swallow reflex initiates due to pressure of the bolus against the anterior faucial arches as it passes into pharynx. A build-up of air pressure is established within the oral cavity due to the closure of the lips and nasopharynx. The soft palate elevates and retracts, sealing off the nasal cavity and preventing material from entering it. Peristaltic movements push the bolus through the pharynx toward the upper oesophageal sphincter (UOS). The aryepiglottic folds, false vocal folds, and true vocal folds close to protect the airway and suspend breathing, also referred to as *swallowing apnoea*. The larynx elevates and moves forward, stretching and increasing the opening of the UOS, which also relaxes to allow the bolus to enter the oesophagus. Additional airway protection is provided by the epiglottis which lowers to cover the larynx when the bolus enters the region of the larynx. The process of coordinating breathing with swallowing is also referred to as the suck-swallow-breathe pattern.

Oesophageal phase: Once the UOS closes on the tail of the bolus, the airway reopens and breathing resumes. Peristaltic waves push the bolus down through the oesophagus towards the lower oesophageal sphincter (LOS), which opens to allow the bolus to enter the stomach [23, 24].

Dysphagia occurs due to impairment of any or all of these phases. As the organs of the swallowing system work in close coordination, if one phase is functionally impaired, the likelihood increases that other phases will also be affected [25-27].

Causes of dysphagia can include illness, injury, tumours, diseases, neurological conditions, structural problems, gastrointestinal disorders, infections and side effects of many medications [21, 28].

Eating, Drinking and Swallowing Problems in Down's Syndrome

People with DS are commonly at risk of dysphagia and its frequently life-threatening consequences. The unique structural and anatomical features typically observed in people with Down's syndrome often impinge on functioning of the eating, drinking and swallowing mechanism. In addition, many illnesses commonly observed in DS, such as congenital heart disease, dental disease, pulmonary conditions and gastroesophageal reflux disease (GORD) can also impact on the swallowing process [4, 10, 20, 29- 34]

From birth, all people with DS have systemic low tone which affects the muscles of the tongue, lips, cheeks, face, jaw, pharynx and larynx. Inadequate strength and range of muscle movement leads to reduced control and coordination of the muscles for eating, drinking and swallowing [35, 36].

Lewis et al. [37] examined the feeding problems of 20 infants with DS reported via parental questionnaire. Many of the problems observed in infants aged from 0-3 months included a weak lip seal, problems with positioning for feeding, a weak, slow and uncoordinated suck-swallow-breathe pattern and severe fatigue, all of which were associated with reduced muscle tone. Potential consequences of these difficulties included coughing, choking, aspiration, vomiting and weight loss.

The typical craniofacial characteristics of individuals with DS include a hypoplastic facial mid-third [38, 39] shortened and narrow palate [43, 44] and apparently large tongue relative to the smallness of the oral cavity [38-43].

The combination of these features and reduced muscle tone lead to tongue protrusion, mouth breathing, upper airway obstruction, malocclusion and poor coordination of breathing and swallowing [36, 37, 44, 45].

Mitchell et al. [36] performed a retrospective review of 29 children with DS ranging from 3 months to 10 years, of which 23 were diagnosed with obstructive sleep apnoea and laryngomalacia (floppy larynx). Airway obstruction and inspiratory stridor characteristic of laryngomalacia were commonly reported in these children, and are likely have a significant impact on the control of breathing and swallowing rhythm.

The large, hypotonic tongue combined with poor oral-motor skills reduces the ability of the tongue to crush food against the palate, collect food within mouth, and form a cohesive bolus. This may lead to the swallowing of inadequately chewed food, loss of food and saliva out of the mouth, and inadequate cleansing of the mouth [22].

Food and saliva loss can also occur as a consequence of malocclusion, tongue thrust, constant open mouth, poor lip control and nasal obstruction. Complications of food and saliva loss include gingivitis, tooth decay, fissuring of the tongue and lips, problems forming a cohesive bolus, and perioral infections such as *Candida albicans* [46].

There exists a very high rate of malocclusion in DS individuals due to the relationship between the underdeveloped maxilla and protruding mandible [38, 47-49]. In their review of the literature, Winter et al. [50] discovered that malocclusion was more prevalent in individuals with DS relative to the general population and other individuals with physical and intellectual disabilities such as cerebral palsy and cleft disorders.

Oral-facial dysmorphology resulting from malocclusion can significantly impair the eating, drinking and swallowing process due to poor contact between the upper and lower arches of the teeth preventing adequate grinding down and chewing of foods.

English et al. [51] examined the implications of malocclusion on chewing performance in the general population. The authors investigated chewing skills in 147 subjects with different types of malocclusion compared to 38 subjects with normal occlusion. The authors found that the subjects with malocclusion had left much larger particle sizes after chewing, and had reported more difficulty chewing harder foods than the subjects with normal occlusion. The subjects with bone class III malocclusion (underbite) experienced the greatest difficulty in both objective and subjective assessments of chewing. Although this study was performed on patients without DS, class III malocclusion is the most common malocclusion reported in people with DS [52]. DS individuals are therefore likely to experience similar difficulties to the Class III test subjects.

Studies in children and young adults with DS suggest that their underlying facial dysmorphology and malocclusion can lock the jaw and prevent adequate lateral movements for chewing [42].

Hennequin et al. [56] examined chewing ability in 11 adults with DS ranging from 17-43 years relative to 12 healthy subjects without DS. The authors discovered that DS subjects inadequately chewed their food, leading them to swallow food whole or inadequately prepared. This may lead to poor digestion, intestinal and oesophageal obstruction, and gastrointestinal problems including gastritis and ulcers [22]. A recent review also suggested that the act of swallowing food whole might lead to less satiety and leading to greater amount of food ingested [57]. This may be a potential cause for the high rates of obesity reported in DS [58-60].

Occlusal instability in DS also commonly leads to orofacial dyskinesias (abnormal and involuntary movements of the jaw and face), bruxism (persistent tooth grinding), an open mouth posture, tongue thrusting, difficulties with lip closure, and a tendency to mouth breathe. Persistent tongue protrusion also occurs as the individual with DS attempts to stabilise the jaw [54]. Difficulties with mouth and lip closure also encourage tongue protrusion in order for the DS individual to create an intraoral seal for swallowing [38, 52-55]. These features can intensify when the person with DS reaches the end of the growth period in early adulthood and can interfere with eating, drinking and swallowing [54].

In addition to malocclusion, poor muscle tone and hypermobility of the temporomandibular joints can also lead to weak and abnormal movements of the jaw and reduce chewing efficiency [61-63]. Other factors that impair chewing function include poor oral hygiene, tooth loss and periodontal disease which are more prevalent in individuals with DS [22, 55, 64-67].

Many studies suggest that DS individuals attempt to compensate for their oral-motor skill deficits by selecting soft foods that place fewer demands on chewing skills [56, 57]. Field et al. [31] examined feeding difficulties reported in the records of 349 children with and without intellectual disability ranging in age from 1 month to 12 years. They discovered a significantly higher prevalence of oral-motor problems, swallowing difficulties and texture selectivity in the 26 children with DS than in the other children without DS.

Suggested implications for texture selectivity include a reduced and restricted diet lacking in important nutrients typically found in harder and textured foods such as raw fruit and vegetables [67]. However current studies have only suggested a correlation between nutritional deficiency and poor masticatory function as opposed to a causal link [22].

Spender et al. [32] also report feeding problems in young DS children who exhibited differences in oral-motor function from typically-developing children. Such oral-motor problems include delayed initiation and poor coordination and sequencing of oral-motor movements, difficulty grading jaw movements for chewing, weak lip closure, and weak and reduced tongue movements. Other studies also find that DS children present with primitive suck patterns, poor coordination of the suck/swallow/breathe pattern, and persistent tongue protrusion [33, 68].

Problems with the pharyngeal phase of swallowing in people with DS have also been reported. Frazier et al. [33] conducted a videofluoroscopic study of oral-motor skills and swallowing function in 19 children with DS. The authors identified a disordered pharyngeal phase including delayed initiation of the pharyngeal swallow reflex in 16 of these children. 10 children aspirated on liquids, with 8 of the 10 having aspirated silently (in the absence of overt signs such as coughing).

Individuals with DS also experience problems at the oesophageal phase of swallowing. The literature reports a higher prevalence of benign oesophageal abnormalities such as atresia and tracheoesophageal fistula in children and adults with DS [69]. Other studies also reveal that oesophageal motor disorders, particularly abnormalities in oesophageal peristalsis and lower oesophageal sphincter function are more common in DS than in the general population [25, 27, 29, 30, 70-72].

In their comparative study of 58 DS adults and 38 adults without DS, Zarate et al. [30] identified a higher prevalence of achalasia in the DS subjects, symptoms of which included dysphagia for solids and liquids, regurgitation, and chest pain.

Oesophageal motor dysfunction can also lead to food loss, food refusal, gagging [31], vomiting, gastro-oesophageal reflux (GOR) [73], choking, weight loss [28], texture selectivity, and respiratory symptoms from aspiration [74-76].

In a clinical audit of 57 adults with Down's syndrome, Wallace [72] discovered that 56 of these patients presented with at least one gastrointestinal problem. Common conditions included celiac disease, achalasia, GOR, unexplained constipation or diarrhoea and over-nutrition. Over half the adults tested positive for Helicobacter Pylori infection. H. Pylori has been reported in various studies to be more prevalent in the learning disabled population, particularly those living in institutionalised settings, and can be responsible for any range of gastrointestinal symptoms such as excessive wind, GOR and vomiting [77-79].

Although the literature reports no clear association between diagnosis of DS and oesophageal carcinoma [80], Moreels et al. [81] report on 2 unusual cases of oesophageal cancer in young DS adults aged 28 and 44. Both individuals had gastro-oesophageal reflux disease, which is commonly reported in DS [31, 32, 34, 36, 82, 83], and which studies have associated with increased risk of oesophageal cancer [84].

Other co-morbid conditions commonly identified in DS children and adults include chronic pulmonary conditions, obstructive sleep apnoea and congenital heart disease. These problems can lead to food loss, food refusal, prolonged feeding times, exhaustion, gagging, vomiting, choking, difficulty progressing to more advanced textures, and increased risk of aspiration [27, 29, 30, 31, 36, 37, 73].

Maladaptive mealtime behaviours can also interfere with the eating and drinking process. Chadwick et al. [85] found that behaviours such as cramming (forcing excessive amounts of food into the mouth at once) and bolting (eating extremely quickly) were common in adults with ID, and were associated with increased risk of asphyxiation.

The literature also suggests an increased prevalence of psychiatric disorders in the DS population [112]. However Nahon et al. [115] referred to four individuals in their study whom had initially been diagnosed with eating disorders of psychogenic cause until it was discovered that they were suffering from disorders of the oesophagus. Gravestock reports several potential causes of eating disorders and abnormal eating behaviours in people with intellectual disability, including physical factors such as oral-motor problems, sensory difficulties and physical health, as well as environmental factors such as sensory deprivation and living in an institutionalised setting [113, 114].

In addition, the natural aging process brings about several changes in the structure, strength, coordination, and sensitivity of the swallowing mechanism that can directly impact on eating, drinking and swallowing function. As the life expectancy of people with DS continues to increase to beyond 60 years at present [86], DS individuals are likely to experience many of the same age-related changes as members of the general elderly population.

Gradual deterioration in muscle mass, reduced flexibility and reduced sensation of the swallowing mechanism, as well as changes in swallow-respiration coordination have been well documented as normal changes associated with aging in adults over 45 [87-93]. These changes reportedly have little functional impact on eating, drinking and swallowing in healthy elderly adults who effectively compensate for any deterioration by increasing functional output. However aging DS individuals are likely to have co-existing eating, drinking and swallowing difficulties as a consequence of their syndrome and therefore will have insufficient functional reserve to compensate for age-related changes to the swallowing mechanism. As a result, the adult with DS is likely to experience increasing difficulties with eating, drinking and swallowing as they get older, due to difficulties compensating for pre-existing swallowing problems as well as coping with any newly emerging problems.

In addition, aging DS adults are also at equal if not greater risk of developing the same illnesses and chronic conditions as the elderly general population, many of which can further impair the swallowing process [94]. These include altered dentition, xerostomia, diabetes, arthritis, stroke, malignant disease, Parkinson's disease, and dementia, all of which have been associated with coughing, choking, regurgitation, and difficulty initiating swallowing [95-97]. Many of the medications prescribed for these conditions can also lead to dysphagia [98, 99]. With several longitudinal studies confirming a premature aging process in DS adults, these conditions might also be observed at a much earlier age in people with DS [100-102].

One clinical condition, dementia of the Alzheimer's type (DAT), merits particular attention because it is well recognized that aging adults with DS are at increased risk of developing DAT than the general population [103]. Dysphagia occurs in virtually all patients with degenerative CNS diseases, including DAT, although the pattern of onset and the progression of oropharyngeal difficulties in adults suffering from DAT are currently not known [104].

In the general population, DAT causes serious impairments in motor function and coordination at both the oral and the pharyngeal phases [105], resulting in difficulties with self-feeding, chewing, initiating swallowing, managing oral secretions, nasal regurgitation, deterioration of the cough reflex, and choking [98, 104, 106]. These problems are well documented in late-stage DAT [98] and often lead to aspiration [104, 107, 108] and aspiration pneumonia [1, 19, 109] which is a major cause of death in people with DAT [110, 111].

Implications for Health Services

While there is a growing awareness that people with DS have the right to the same level of medical care and services as the general population, they are often unable to access these services largely due to a lack of understanding about dysphagia in DS and how it can be best managed [116]. Although many government reports recognise this problem [117, 118] more recent investigations confirm that adults with ID continue to experience health inequalities and discrimination in health services [119-121].

The literature proposes several causes for this. The difficulties of many DS individuals to communicate effectively and self-report symptoms can impede clinical evaluation and delay diagnosis of dysphagia [81]. DS individuals might express symptoms or pain in an atypical manner [123]. For example, Moreels et al. [81] revealed that a feeling of depression was one of the first symptoms of GOR expressed by a subject with DS.

Another cause is in relation to inadequate practitioner knowledge, skills and training about the prevalence of dysphagic conditions in DS, symptoms of dysphagia and communicative behaviours of the individual with DS. As a result, healthcare professionals may misinterpret or ignore early signs and symptoms of dysphagia [119]. If dysphagia is a symptom of an underlying disease or condition such as GORD or H Pylori, delays in evaluation, diagnosis and management can lead to more life-threatening conditions such as oesophageal cancer and potentially shorten life expectancy for people with DS [76, 78].

Several studies highlight that institutional discrimination in the healthcare setting continues to prevent adequate access to services for people with ID [120-122]. Mencap [119] investigated and reported on the premature deaths of 6 individuals with ID of whom one had a diagnosis of DS. All of the patients exhibited problems with eating, drinking or swallowing which were symptomatic of other underlying conditions. The failure to adequately address these symptoms and their underlying causes in the healthcare setting resulted in malnutrition, dehydration, aspiration pneumonia and the eventual death of these patients.

The report stresses that healthcare services fail to account for the diverse medical needs of people with ID. In addition, healthcare practitioners often rely on their own wrongful assumptions about a person's quality of life based on their own mistaken beliefs about ID, rather than taking into account presenting symptoms, patient view or the input of family and caregivers.

Diagnostic overshadowing also denies individuals with ID equity of access to healthcare. Diagnostic overshadowing refers to the failure of health professionals to accurately diagnose health problems in individuals with ID because they wrongly regard them as behavioural features inherent to the intellectual disability, and thus unsuitable for treatment [4, 126-128].

In order to address these healthcare disparities for people with DS, eating, drinking and swallowing skills should be assessed in people with DS as part of their standard health screening, alongside currently recommended screening tests such as those for thyroid conditions, congenital heart problems, and celiac disease. Roizen [129] suggests that individuals with DS would benefit from screening of a particular medical problem if they have a 10% chance of developing it, and if successful interventions exist for that problem. Various techniques are successfully used to support people with DS and eating, drinking and swallowing problems such as orthodontic procedures and specialised dental care [130], occlusal appliances [54, 131] training programmes for medical staff [131] and carers [9], texture modification [133] and environmental manipulation [9]. Regular screening for dysphagia would identify any warning signs early on and address difficulties with appropriate therapeutic techniques and treatments.

Conclusion

Current research in the literature has supported the view that from birth, people with DS suffer from many systemic and structural abnormalities and clinical conditions that impair eating, drinking and swallowing function. However there is an increasing need for further studies examining the prevalence of these problems, given that no prevalence figures of dysphagia in DS are currently available. Most current studies investigate dysphagia in a heterogeneous group of individuals with ID, or focus predominantly on eating, drinking and swallowing difficulties in small groups of children with DS.

Nonetheless it is clear from what is currently available in the literature that people with DS are at significant risk of dysphagia at some point in their lives, and that it is extremely likely that dysphagic problems will change and even worsen with age.

Dysphagia is a serious problem for many people with DS, and it can lead to life-threatening conditions such as respiratory illness, aspiration pneumonia, asphyxiation and death. Improvements in medical care, education and socioeconomic conditions have meant that the population of people with DS is increasing and living longer. However they continue to experience inequalities in access to appropriate healthcare. Difficulties with communication, poor knowledge about DS-specific disorders, and the risk of diagnostic overshadowing impede diagnosis and management of eating, drinking and swallowing problems in this population. It is essential that health care practitioners develop their understanding of the specific dysphagic problems and their signs and symptoms that can occur in this population, with the aim of predicting and identifying symptoms early on, responding proactively with timely and effective treatments, and improving health and quality of life.

References

[1] Martin, B.; Corlew, M.; Wood, H.; Olson, D.; Golopol, L.; Wingo, M.; Kirmani, N. The association of swallowing dysfunction and aspiration pneumonia. *Dysphagia* 1994, *9(1)*, 1–6.

[2] Cooper, S.A.; Melville, C.; Morrison, J. People with intellectual disabilities- Their health needs differ and need to be recognised and met. *BMJ* 2004, *329*, 414-415.

[3] NHS Health Scotland. *Health needs assessment report. People with learning disabilities in Scotland;* NHS: Edinburgh, 2004.

[4] National Patient Safety Agency. *Understanding the patient safety issues for people with learning disabilities*. NPSA: London, 2004

[5] Stewart, L. Development of the Nutrition and Swallowing Checklist, a screening tool for nutrition and swallowing risk in people with intellectual disability. *J Intell Dev Disabil* 2003, *28*, 171-187.

[6] Carter, G.; Jancar, J. Mortality in the mentally handicapped: a 50 year survey at the Stoke Park group of hospitals (1930-1980). *J Ment Def Res* 1983, *27*, 143-156

[7] Day, S.; Strauss, D.J.; Shavelle, R.M.; Reynolds, R.J. Mortality and causes o fdeath in persons with Down syndrome in California. *Dev Med Child Neurol* 2005, *47*, 171-176.

[8] Hollins, S.; Attard, M. T.; von Fraunhofer, N.; McGuigan, S.; Sedgwick, P. Mortality in people with learning disability: risks, causes, and death certification findings in London. *Dev Med Child Neurol* 1998, *40(1)*, 50-56.

[9] Chadwick, D.; Joliffe, J.; Goldbart, J. Adherence to eating and drinking guidelines for adults with intellectual disabilities and dysphagia. *Am J Ment Retard* 2003, *108(3)*, 202-211.

[10] Chadwick, D.D.; Joliffe, J. A descriptive investigation of dysphagia in adults with intellectual disabilities. *J Intell Disabil Res* 2009, *53(1)*, 29-43.

[11] Singh, S.; Hamdy, S.Dysphagia in stroke patients. *Postgrad Med J* 2006, *82*, 383-391.

[12] Holas, M.A.; DePippo, K.L.; Reding, M.J. Aspiration and relative risk of medical complications following stroke. *Arch Neurol* 1994, *51*, 1051–1053.

[13] Kidd, D.; Lawson, J.; Nesbitt, R.; MacMahon J. The natural history and clinical consequences of aspiration in acute stroke. *QJM* 1995, *88*, 409–413.

[14] Mann, G.; Hankey, G.J.; Cameron, D. Swallowing function after stroke: prognosis and prognostic factors at 6 months. *Stroke* 1999, *30*, 744–8.

[15] Langmore, S.E.; Terpenning, M.S.; Schork, A.; Chen, Y.; Murray, J.T.; Lopatin, D.; Loesche, W.J. Predictors of aspiration pneumonia: how important is dysphagia? *Dysphagia* 1998, *13*, 69-81.

[16] Masiero, S.; Pierobon, R.; Previato, C.; Gomiero, E. Pneumonia in stroke patients with oropharyngeal dysphagia: a six-month follow-up study. *Neuro Sci* 2008, *29(3)*, 139-45.

[17] Weir, K.; McMahon, S.; Barry, L.; Ware, R.; Masters, I.B.; Chang, A.B. Oropharyngeal aspiration and pneumonia in children. *Pediatr Pulmonol* 2007, *42*, 1024-1031.

[18] Terpenning, M. Geriatric oral health and Pneumonia Risk. *CID* 2005, 40, 1807-1810.

[19] Kikawada, M.; Iwamoto, T.; Takasaki, M. Aspiration and infection in the elderly. Epidemiology, diagnosis and management. *Drugs Aging* 2005, *22(2),* 115-130.

[20] Bittles, A.H.; Bower, C.; Hussain, R.; Glasson, E.J. The four ages of Down syndrome. *Eur J Public Health* 2006, *17(2)*, 221–225.

[21] Samuels, R.; Chadwick, D.D. Predictors of asphyxiation risk in adults with intellectual disability and dysphagia. *J Intell Disabil Res* 2006, *50(5)*, 362-370.

[22] N'Gom, P.I.; Woda, A. Influence of impaired mastication on nutrition. *J Prosthet Dent* 2002, *87*, 667-673.

[23] Rogers B, Arvedson J (2005) Assessment of infant oral sensorimotor and swallowing function. *Ment Retard Dev Disabil Res Rev* 11: 74-82.

[24] Logemann, J.A. *Evaluation and Treatment of Swallowing Disorders*, 2nd edition. Pro-ed: Austin, TE, 1998, pp. 24-35.

[25] Dekel, R.; Pearson, T.; Wendel, C.; De Garmo, P.; Fennerty, M.B.; Fass, R. Assessment of oesophageal motor function in patients with dysphagia or chest pain - the Clinical Outcomes Research Initiative experience. *Aliment Pharmacol Ther* 2003, *18*, 1083-1089.

[26] Logemann, J.A. *Evaluation and Treatment of Swallowing Disorders*, 2nd edition. Pro-ed: Austin, TE, 1998, p 110.

[27] Triadafilopoulos, G.; Hallstone, A.; Nelson-Abbott, H.; Bedinger, K. Oropharyngeal and esophageal interrelationships in patients with nonobstructive dysphagia. *Dig Dis Sci* 1992, *37(4)*, 551-557.

[28] Mittal, R.; Bhalla, V. Oesophageal motor functions and its disorders. *Gut* 2004, *53(10)*, 1536-1542.

[29] Zárate, N.; Mearin, F. ; Gil-Vernet.; J.M. ; Camarasa, F.; Malagelada, J.R. Achalasia and Down's syndrome: coincidental association or something else? *Am J Gastroenterol* 1999, *94(6)*, 1674-1677.

[30] Zárate, N.; Mearin, F.; Hidalgo, A.; Malagelada, J.R. Prospective evaluation of esophageal motor dysfunction in Down's syndrome. *Am J Gastroenterol* 2001, *96 (6)*, 1718-1724.

[31] Field, D.; Garland, M.; Williams, K. Correlates of specific childhood feeding problems. *J Paediatr Child Health* 2003, *39*, 299–304.

[32] Spender, Q.; Stein, A.; Dennis, J.; Reilly, S.; Percy, E.; Cave, D. An exploration of feeding difficulties in children with Down syndrome. *Dev Med Child Neurol* 1996, *38*, 681–694.

[33] Frazier, J.; Friedman, B. Swallow function in children with Down syndrome: a retrospective study. *Dev Med Child Neurol* 1996, *38*, 695-703.

[34] Kerins, G.; Petrovic, K.; Bruder, M.B.; Gruman, C. Medical conditions and medication use in adults with Down syndrome: A descriptive analysis. *Downs Syndr Res Pract* 2007, *12(2)*, 1-7.

[35] Desai, S.S. Down syndrome: a review of the literature. *Oral Surg Oral Med Oral Pathol Oral Radiol Endod* 1997, *84*, 279-285.

[36] Mitchell, R.B.; Call, M.S.; Kelly, J. Ear, nose and throat disorders in children with Down Syndrome. *Laryngoscope* 2003, *113*, 259-263.

[37] Lewis, E.; Kritzinger, A. Parental experiences of feeding problems in their infants with Down syndrome. *Downs Syndr Res Pract* 2004, *9(2)*, 45-52.

[38] Fisher-Brandies, H. Cephalometric comparison between children with and without Down syndrome. *Eur J Orthodont* 1988, *10(1)*, 255-263.

[39] Dagklis, T.; Borenstein, M.; Peralta, C.F.A.; Faro, C.; Nicolaide, K.H. Three-dimensional evaluation of mid-facial hypoplasia in fetuses with trisomy 21 at 11 + 0 to 13 + 6 weeks of gestation. *Ultrasound Obstet Gynecol* 2006, *28(3)*, 261 – 265.

[40] Austin, J.; Preger, L.; Siris, E.; Taybi, H. Short hard palate in newborn: roentgen sign of mongolism. *Radiology* 1969, *92*, 775-776.

[41] Bhagyalakshmi, G.; Renukarya, A.J.; Rajangam, S. Metric analysis of the hard palate in children with Down syndrome - a comparative study. *Downs Syndr Res Pract* 2007, *12(1)*, 55-59.

[42] Hennequin, M.; Faulks, D.; Veyrune, J.L.; Bourdiol, P. Significance of oral health in persons with Down syndrome: a literature review. *Dev Med Child Neurol* 1999, *41*, 271-283.

[43] Guimaraes, C.V.; Donnelly, L.F.; Shott, S.R.; Amin, R.S.; Kalra, M. Relative rather than absolute macroglossia in patients with Down syndrome: implications for treatment of obstructive sleep apnea. *Pediatr Radiol* 2008, *38(10)*, 1062-1067.

[44] Nargozian, C. The airway in patients with craniofacial abnormalities. *Pediatr Anesth* 2004, *14*, 53-59.

[45] Boston, M.; Rutter, M. Current airway management in craniofacial anomalies. *Curr Opi Otolaryngol Head Neck Surg* 2003, *11*, 428-432.

[46] Meningaud, J.P.; Poramate, R.A.; Chikhani, L.; Bertrand, J.C. Drooling of saliva: A review of the etiology and management options. *Oral Surg Oral Med Oral Pathol Oral Radiol Endod* 2006, *101(1),* 48-57.

[47] Cohen, M.M.; Winer, R.A. Dental and facial characteristics in Down´s syndrome (Mongolism). *J Dent Res* 1965, *44*, 197-208.

[48] Kisling, K. Craneal morphology in Down's syndrome. A comparative roentencephalometric study in adults males. *Munksgaard* 1960, *107*, 90-98.
[49] Oliveira, A.C.; Paiva, S.M.; Campos, M.R.; Czeresnia, D. () Factors associated with malocclusions in children and adolescents with Down syndrome. (Online only) *Am J Orthod Dentofacial Orthop* 2008, *489*, e1-e8.
[50] Winter, K.; Baccaglini, L.; Tomar, S. A review of malocclusion among individuals with mental and physical disabilities. *Spec Care Dentist* 2008, *28(1)*, 19-26.
[51] English, J.D.: Buschang, P.H.; Throckmorton, G.S. Does malocclusion affect masticatory performance? *Angle Orthod* 2002, *72(1)*, 21-27.
[52] Alió-Sanz, J.J. A new cephalometric diagnostic method for Down's Syndrome patients with open bite. *Med Oral Patol Oral Cir Bucal* 2008, *1,13(3)*, E171-5
[53] Haw, C.; Barnes, T.; Clark, K.; Crichton, P.; Kohen, D. Movement disorder in Down's syndrome: a possible marker of the severity of mental handicap. *Mov Dis* 1996, *11(4)*, 395–403.
[54] Faulks, D.; Veyrune, J.L.; Hennequin, M. Consequences of oral rehabilitation on dyskinesia in adults with Down's syndrome: a clinical report. *J Oral Rehabil* 2002, *29*, 209-218.
[55] Hennequin, M; Allison, P.J.; Veyrune, J.L. Prevalence of oral health problems in a group of individuals with Down syndrome in France. *Dev Med Child Neurol* 2000, *42*, 691-698.
[56] Hennequin, M.; Allison, P.J.; Faulks, D.; Orliaguet, T.; Feine, J. Chewing indicators between adults with Down syndrome and controls. *J Dent Res* 2005, *84(11)*, 1057-1061.
[57] Faulks, D.; Collado, V.; Mazille, M.N.; Veyrune, J.L.; Hennequin, M. Masticatory dysfunction in persons with Down's syndrome. Part 1: aetiology and incidence. *J Oral Rehabil* 2008, *35(11)*, 854-862.
[58] Delrue, M.A.; Michaud, J.L. Fat chance: genetic syndromes with obesity. *Clin Genet* 2004, *66*, 83-93.
[59] Prasher, V.P. Overweight and obesity amongst Down's syndrome adults. *J Intell Disabil Res* 1995, *39*, 437-441.
[60] Braunschweig, C.L.; Gomez, S.; Sheean, P.; Tomey, K.M.; Rimmer, J.; Heller, T. Nutritional status and risk factors for chronic disease in urban-dwelling adults with Down syndrome. *Am J Ment Retard* 2004, *109*, 186-193.
[61] Sato, S.; Ohta, M.; Goto, S.; Kawamura, H.; Motegi, K. Electromyography during chewing movement in patients with anterior disc displacement of the temporomandibular joint. *Int J Oral Maxillofac Surg* 1998, *27*, 274-277.
[62] Bhowate, R.; Dubey, A. Dentofacial changes and oral health status in mentally challenged children. *J Indian Soc Pedod Prev Dent* 2005, *23(2)*, 71-73.
[63] Woda A.; Mishellany, A.; Peyron, M.A. The regulation of masticatory function and food bolus formation. *J Oral Rehabil* 2006, *33*, 840-849.
[64] Helm, S.; Petersen, P.E. Causal relation between malocclusion and periodontal health. *Acta Odontol Scand* 1989, *47*, 223-228.
[65] Oredugba, F. Oral health condition and treatment needs of a group of Nigerian individuals with Down syndrome. *Downs Syndr Res Pract* 2007, *12(1)*, 72-77.
[66] Gabre, P.; Martinsson, T.; Gahnberg, L. Longitudinal study of dental caries, tooth mortality and interproximal bone loss in adults with intellectual disability. *Eur J Oral Sci* 2001, *109*, 20-26.

[67] Waldman, H.B.; Perlman, S.P.; Swerdloff, M. Orthodontics and the population with special needs. *Am J Orthod Dentofacial Orthop* 2000, *118*, 14-17.

[68] Glatz-Noll, E.; Berg, R. Oral dysfunction in children with Down syndrome: an evaluation of treatment effects by means of videoregistration. *Eur J Orthod* 1991, *31*, 446–451.

[69] Bianca, S.; Bianca, M,; Ettore, G. Oesophageal atresia and Down syndrome. *Downs Syndr Res Pract* 2002, *8(1)*, 29-30.

[70] Boeckxstaens, G.; Jonge, W.; van den Wijngaard, R.; Benninga, M. Achalasia: From new insights in pathophysiology to treatment. *J Pediatr Gastroenterol Nutr* 2005, *41(1)*, S36-S37.

[71] Okawada, M.; Okazaki, T.; Yamataka, A.; Lane, G.J.; Miyano, T. Down's syndrome and esophageal achalasia: a rare but important clinical entity. *Pediatr Surg Int* 2005, *21*, 997-1000.

[72] Wallace, R.A. Clinical audit of gastrointestinal conditions occurring among adults with Down syndrome attending a specialist clinic. *J Intell Dev Disabil* 2007, *32*, 45-50.

[73] Marder, E.; Dennis, J. Medical management of children with Down's syndrome. *Curr Paediatr* 2001, *11*, 57–63.

[74] Roizen, N.; Patterson, D. Down's syndrome. *Lancet* 2003, *361*,1281–1289.

[75] Seddon, P.C.; Khan, Y. Respiratory problems in children with neurological impairment. *Arch Dis Child* 2003, *88(1)*, 75–78.

[76] Prakash, C.; Clouse, R.E. Esophageal motor disorders. *Curr Opin Gastroenterol* 2002, *18*, 454-463.

[77] Beange, H.; Lennox, N. Physical aspects of health in the learning disabled. *Curr Opin Psychiatry* 1998, *11*, 531–534.

[78] Duff, M.; Scheepers, M.; Cooper, M.; Hoghton, M.; Baddeley, P. Helicobacter pylori: Has the killer escaped from the institution? A possible cause of increased stomach cancer in a population with intellectual disability. *J Intell Disabil Res* 2001, *45(3)*, 219-225.

[79] Morad, M.; Merrick, J.; Nasri, Y. Prevalence of Helicobacter pylori in people with intellectual disability in a residential care centre in Israel. *J Intell Disabil Res* 2002, *46(2)*, 141-143.

[80] Hill, D.A.; Gridley, G.; Cnattingius, S.; Mellemkjaer, L.; Linet, M.; Adami, H.O.; Olsen, J.H.; Nyren, O.; Fraumeni, J.F. Jr. Mortality and cancer incidence among individuals with Down syndrome. *Arch Intern Med* 2003, *163*, 705-711.

[81] Moreels, T.G.; van Vliet, E.P.M.; Tilanus, H.W.; Tran, T.C.K.; Kuipers, E.J.; Siersema, P.D. Down syndrome and esophageal cancer. *Dis Esophagus* 2007, *20*, 183-186.

[82] Bohmer, C.J.; Klinkenberg-Knol, E.C.; Niezen-de Boer, M.C.; Meuwissen, S.G. Gastroesophageal reflux disease in intellectually disabled individuals: how often, how serious, how manageable? *Am J Gastroenterol* 2000, *95*, 1868-1872.

[83] Carr, M.; Nguyen, A.; Nagy, M.; Poje, C.; Pizzuto, M.; Brodsky, L. Clinical presentation as a guide to the identification of GERD in children. *Int J Pediatr Otorhinolaryngol* 2000, *54*, 27-32.

[84] Lagergren, J. Adenocarcinoma of oesophagus: what exactly is the size of the problem and who is at risk? *Gut* 2005, *54*, (Suppl I) il-5.

[85] Chadwick, D.D.; Samuels, R. Predictors of asphyxiation risk in adults with intellectual disabilities and dysphagia. *J Intell Disabil Res* 2006, *50(5)*, 362-370.

[86] Glasson, E.J.; Sullivan, S.G.; Hussain, R.; Petterson, B.A.; Montgomery, P.D.; Bittles A.H. The changing survival profile of people with Down's syndrome: implications for genetic counselling. *Clin Genet* 2002, *62*, 390–393.

[87] Jaradeh, S. Neurophysiology of swallowing in the aged. *Dysphagia* 1994, *9(4)*, 218–220.

[88] Fucile, S.; Wright, P.M.; Chan, I.; Yee, S.; Langlais, M.E.; Gisel, EG. Functional oral-motor skills: do they change with age? *Dysphagia* 1998, *13*, 195–201.

[89] Volpi, E.; Nazemi, R.; Fujita, S.; Muscle tissue changes with aging. *Curr Opin Clin Nutr Metab Care* 2004, *7*, 405–410.

[90] Nicosia, M.; Hind, J.; Roecker, E.; Carnesm M.; Doylem J.; Dengelm G.; Robbinsm J. Age effects on the temporal evolution of isometric and swallowing pressure. *J Gerontol* 2000, *55A(11)*, M634–M640.

[91] Peyron, M.A.; Blanc, O.; Lund, J.P.; Woda, A. Influence of age on adaptability of human mastication. *J Neurophysiol* 2004, 92, 773–779.

[92] Barczi, S.; Sullivan, P.; Robbins, J. How should dysphagia care of older adults differ? Establishing optimal practice patterns. *Semin Speech Lang* 2000, *21(4)*, 347–363.

[93] Robbins, J.; Gangnon, R.; Theis, S.; Kays, S.; Hewitt, A.; Hind, J. The effects of lingual exercise on swallowing in older adults. *J Am Geriatr Soc* 2005, *53*, 1483–1489.

[94] Kawashima, K.; Motohashi, Y.; Fujishima, I. Prevalence of dysphagia among community-dwelling elderly individuals as estimated using a questionnaire for dysphagia screening. *Dysphagia* 2004, *19*, 266–271.

[95] Martin-Harris, B.; Brodsky, M.B.; Michel, Y.; Ford, C.; Walters, B.; Heffner, J. Breathing and swallowing dynamics across the adult lifespan. *Arch Otolaryngol Head Neck Surg* 2005, *131(9)*, 762–770.

[96] Hirst,L.; Ford, G.; Gibson, G.; Wilson, J. Swallow-induced alterations in breathing in normal older people. *Dysphagia* 2002,17, 152–161.

[97] Achem, S.; DeVault, K. Dysphagia in aging. *J Clin Gastroenterol* 2005, *39(5)*, 357–371.

[98] Priefer, B.; Robbins, J. Eating changes in mild-stage Alzheimer's disease: a pilot study. *Dysphagia* 1997, 12(4), 212–221.

[99] Morris, H. Dysphagia in the elderly - a management challenge for nurses. *Br J Nurs* 2006, *15(10)*, 558–562.

[100] Holland, A.J. Down's Syndrome. In *Dementia, Aging, and Intellectual Disabilities: A Handbook;* Janicki, M.; Dalton, A.; Eds; Brunner/Mazel: New York, NY, 1998, pp 184–185.

[101] Carmeli, E.; Kessel, S.; Bar-Chad, S.; Merrick, J. A comparison between older persons with Down syndrome and a control group: Clinical characteristics, functional status and sensorimotor function. *Downs Syndr Res Pract* 2004, *9(1)*, 17–24.

[102] Burt, D.; Primeaux-Hart, K.; Loveland, K.; Cleveland, L.; Lewis, K.; Lesser, J.; Pearson, P. Aging in adults with intellectual disabilities. *Am J Ment Retard* 2005, *110(4)*, 268–284.

[103] Bush, A.; Beail, N. Risk factors for dementia in people with Down syndrome: issues in assessment and diagnosis. *Am J Ment Retard* 2004, *109(2)*, 83–97.

[104] Wada, H.; Nakajoh, K.; Satoh-Nakagawa, T.; Suzuki, T.; Ohrui, T.; Arai, H.; Sasaki, H. Risk factors of aspiration pneumonia in Alzheimer's disease patients. *Gerontology* 2001, *47*, 271–276.

[105] Silverman, W.; Zigman, W.; Huykang, K.; Krinsky-McHale, S.; Wisniewski, H. Aging and dementia among adults with mental retardation and Down Syndrome. *Top Geriatr Rehabil* 1998, *13(3)*, 49–64.
[106] Buchholz, D.; Robbins, J. Neurologic diseases affecting oropharyngeal swallowing. In *Deglutition and Its Disorders- Anatomy, Physiology, Clinical Diagnosis and Management;* Perlman, A.; Schulze-Delrieu, K.; Eds.; Singular: San Diego, CA, 1997; pp 326–327.
[107] Horner, J.; Alberts, M.; Dawson, D.; Cook, G. Swallowing in Alzheimer's disease. *Alzheimer Dis Assoc Disord* 1994, *8(3)*, 177–189.
[108] Kalia, M. Dysphagia and aspiration pneumonia in patients with Alzheimer's disease. *Metabolism* 2003, *52(10)*, 36–38.
[109] Loeb, M.; McGeer, A.; McArthur, M.; Walter, S.; Simor, A. Risk factors for pneumonia and other lower respiratory tract infections in elderly residents of long-term care facilities. *Arch Intern Med* 1999, *159(17)*, 2058–2064.
[110] Marik, P.; Kaplan, D. Aspiration pneumonia and dysphagia in the elderly. *Chest* 2003, *124(1)*, 328–336.
[111] Ganguli, M.; Dodge, H.; Shen, C.; Pandav, R.; DeKosky, S. Alzheimer disease and mortality: a 15-year epidemiological study. *Arch Neurol* 2005, *62(5)*, 779–784.
[112] Myers, B.; Pueschel, S. Psychiatric disorders in persons with Down syndrome. *Journal Nerv Men Dis* 1991, *179(10)*, 609-613.
[113] Gravestock, S. Eating disorders in adults with intellectual disability. *J Intell Disabil Res* 2000, *44(6)*, 625-637.
[114] Gravestock, S. Diagnosis and classification of eating disorders in adults with intellectual disability: the Diagnostic Criteria for Psychiatric Disorders for Use with Adults with Learning Disabilities/Mental Retardation (DC-LD) approach. *J Intell Disabil Res* 2003, *47(1)*, 72-83.
[115] Nahon, S.; Boudet, MJ.; Godeberge, P.; Mal, F.; Lévy, P.; Perniceni. T.; Gayet, B. Achalasie mimant des troubles du comportement alimentaire. *Gastroenterol Clin Biol* 2001, *25*, 313-315.
[116] Disability Rights Commission (DRC). *Equal treatment: Closing the gap. A formal investigation into the physical health inequalities experienced by people with learning disabilities and/or mental health problems;* Disability Rights Commission: London, 2006.
[117] Department of Health. *Valuing people: A new strategy for learning disabilities for the 21st Century*; Department of Health: London, 2001
[118] Scottish Executive. *The same as you? A review of services for people with learning disabilities*; Scottish Government: Edinburgh, 2000.
[119] Mencap. *Death by Indifference, Following up the Treat me right! Report.* Mencap: London, 2007.
[120] Michael, Sir J, *Healthcare for all: Report of the independent inquiry into access to healthcare for people with learning disabilities.* London, July 2008.
[121] House of Lords, House of Commons Joint Committee on Human Rights. *A Life Like Any Other? Human Rights of Adults with Learning Disabilities,* Seventh Report of Session 2007–08, Vol 1.
[122] Healthcare Commission. *A life like no other: a national audit of specialist inpatient healthcare services for people with learning difficulties in England;* December 2007.
[123] Hennequin, M. ; Morin, C. ; Feine, J.S. Pain expression and stimulus localization in individuals with Down's syndrome. *Lancet* 2000, *356*, 1882-1887.

[124] Puri, B.K.; Lekh, S.K.; Langa, A.; Zaman, R.; Singh, I. Mortality in a hospitalized mentally handicapped population: a 10-year survey. *J Intell Disabil Res*, 1995, *39*, 442-446.
[125] Kmietowicz, Z. Down's children received "less favourable" hospital treatment. *BMJ* 2001, *322*, 815.
[126] Reiss, S.; Levitan, G.W.; Szysko, J. Emotional disturbance and mental retardation: diagnostic overshadowing. *Am J Ment Def* 1982, *86*, 567-574.
[127] Mason, J.; Scior, K. 'Diagnostic overshadowing' amongst clinicians working with people with intellectual disabilities in the UK. *J App Res Intell Disabil* 2004, *17*, 85-90.
[128] Leslie, P.; Crawford, H.; Wilkinson, H. People with a Learning Disability and Dysphagia: A Cinderella Population? *Dysphagia* 2008, in press.
[129] Roizen, N. The early interventionist and the medical problems of the child with Down syndrome. *Inf Young Child* 2003, *16(1)*, 88-95.
[130] Musich, D.R. Orthodontic intervention and patients with Down syndrome. The role of inclusion, technology and leadership. *Angle Orthod* 2006, *76(4)*, 734-735.
[131] Mazille, M.N.; Woda, A.; Nicolas, E.; Peyron, M.A.; Hennequin, M. Effect of occlusal appliance wear on chewing in persons with Down syndrome. *Physiology Behavior* 2008, *93*, 919-929.
[132] Rosenvinge, S.; Starke, I. Improving care for patients with dysphagia. *Age Ageing* 2005, *34(6)*, 587-593.
[133] Logemann, J.A. *Evaluation and Treatment of Swallowing Disorders*, 2nd edition. Pro-ed: Austin, TE, 1998, pp 202-203.

In: Handbook of Down Syndrome Research
Editors: Dominicus Jelinek and Gijs Dvorak
ISBN 978-1-60741- 690-6

Chapter 13

Advances in Prenatal Screening for Down Syndrome

***Aggeliki Kolialexi*[1]*, Georgia Tounta*[1]*, Nikolas Papantoniou*[2]*, George Th. Tsangaris*[3] *and Ariadni Mavrou*[1]**

[1] Department of Medical Genetics, Athens University School of Medicine, Athens, Greece

[2] 1st Department of Obstetrics and Gynecology, Athens University School of Medicine, Athens, Greece

[3] Proteomics Research Unit, Centre of Basic Research II, Biomedical Research Foundation, Academy of Athens, Athens, Greece

Abstract

Prenatal screening is based on maternal serum biochemistry and ultrasound examination which are non invasive and are used as a first line for investigation. In the 2nd trimester of gestation, the multiple marker combination with the highest screening performance currently available is alpha-fetoprotein (AFP), unconjugated estriol (uE3), human chorionic gonadotropin (hCG), and inhibin A, in combination with maternal age. With this combination, a detection rate of 80% at a 5% false positive rate is achieved. First trimester screening tests combining maternal age, fetal nuchal translucency (NT) thickness and maternal serum free beta-hCG and PAPP-A are at least as accurate as traditional 2nd trimester testing and provide results earlier in pregnancy.

In this chapter, the various options for prenatal screening for DS are outlined. Current research efforts made to improve non invasive prenatal diagnosis based on fetal cells, cell free fetal DNA and proteins present in maternal circulation are also discussed.

Introduction

Down Syndrome (DS) is the most common genetic cause of mental retardation and one of the few aneuploidies compatible with post-natal survival [1]. It occurs in 1 out of 700 live births and has the same incidence in all ethnic groups [2]. DS is caused by the presence of an additional copy of chromosome 21 [1] which is usually the result of a maternal meiotic nondisjunction. Approximately 4% of cases are due to an unbalanced segregation of a Robertsonian translocation. Besides mental retardation, present in all individuals with DS, trisomy 21 is associated with characteristic facial appearance and with more than 80 phenotypic features including congenital heart disease, duodenal stenosis or atresia, imperforate anus, Hirschprung disease, muscle hypotonia, immune system deficiencies, increased risk of leukemia and early onset Alzheimer's disease [3]. In about 1% of the patients, mosaicism is present and these individuals may have a milder phenotype.

Prenatal diagnosis of DS is desirable for many patients and is based on a) diagnostic tests following amniocentesis or chorionic villus sampling (CVS) which allow for the definite assessment and are most often used as a second line of study, due to their invasiveness and relative risk for fetal loss and b) screening tests based on maternal serum biochemistry and ultrasound examination which are non invasive and are used as the first line for investigation.

Currently, many maternal serum schemes and ultrasonographic options are availables but these tests can only estimate the risk of the pregnant woman to carry a fetus with DS. Patients who screen positive are generally offered genetic counselling and definitive diagnosis through cytogenetic analysis of either CVS in the 1st trimester or amniotic fluid cells in the 2nd trimester. Women with a DS affected fetus frequently choose to terminate their pregnancy [4].

The aim of this review is to summarize the various screening tests that have been developed in recent years in order to identify women at increased risk for DS.

Second Trimester Biochemical Screening

The relationship between advanced maternal age and the risk of having a fetus with DS has been well recognized for the last 40 years. For this reason the original screening test for DS was based on maternal age with women >=35 years old being at the highest risk [5]. Until 1970s advanced maternal age was the only risk factor considered to identify women advised to undergo amniocentesis and fetal karyotyping. Maternal age alone however, is a poor risk assessment criterion for DS as the majority of children with DS are born to women who are less than 35 years old.

With the advent of maternal serum AFP screening for open neural tube defects Merkatz et al. [6] noted that fetal trisomy 21 was associated with lower levels of maternal serum AFP suggesting that a combination of AFP levels with maternal age could improve prenatal detection of pregnancies at high risk for DS [7,8].

Knowledge that maternal serum markers can provide information about fetal chromosome aneuploidies and especially DS prompted the search for additional screening markers. Bogart et al [9] reported that 2nd trimester maternal serum human chorionic gonadotropin (hCG) levels are on average elevated when the fetus has DS. Measurment of hCG appeared to be superior to AFP in detecting fetal chromosome abnormalities and due to the widespread availability of hCG assays for pregnancy detection and monitoring this marker was rapidly incorporated into DS screening.

In 1988, a reduction of unconjugated estriol (uE3) in 2nd trimester maternal serum was noted in cases with DS fetuses implying that this marker could also be used for DS screening [10,11]. Although there has been some controversy as to the value of this marker [12], data from multiple studies indicated that uE3 is nearly as useful as hCG and is more powerful than AFP in distinguishing between affected and unaffected pregnancies.

In 1992, van Lith et al [13], using an immunoassay that measured all forms of inhibin and its A subunit, reported that 2nd trimester maternal serum total inhibin levels were found to be elevated in DS pregnancies. Subsequently, with the advent of a specific immunoassay that measured only inhibin A, levels of inhibin A, were reported to be more elevated in DS pregnancies than the levels of total inhibin [14-20]. Inhibin A is the newest addition to 2nd second trimester serum screening and is measured using a monoclonal two-site ELISA test validated for use in prenatal screening.

The serum markers described above have been combined using mathematical methods based on a multivariate Gaussian model to produce double (usually AFP and hCG) [21], triple (AFP, uE3, and hCG) [22], or quadruple (AFP, uE3, hCG, and INH-A) tests [23]. The triple test is the most popular one. Clinical studies demonstrated that triple marker testing results in a detection rate of approximately 70% of fetal DS cases with a false-positive rate of 5% [24]. At the same false-positive rate, addition of inhibin A can result in a detection rate of approximately 80%.

Optimal 2nd trimester screening requires accurate estimation of gestational age and efficacy is maximized when results are based on an ultrasound determination of gestational age [25,26]. Additionally, since known factors independently affect analyte concentrations appropriate adjustments are made. These include maternal weight, ethnicity, diabetic status, cigarette smoking,, parity, *in vitro* fertilization and analyte concentrations in a previous pregnancy. Other factors that affect serum marker levels include maternal rhesus blood type, twin pregnancy and maternal systemic lupus erythematosus. Thus, marker screening for fetal DS in the 2nd trimester allows the detection of the majority of cases with fetal DS, with an acceptably low false-positive rate.

Second Trimester Sonographic Markers

Second trimester ultrasound screening may identify either major fetal structural abnormalities or other less-defined features associated with DS, known as «soft markers». Approximately one-third of fetuses with DS have one or more sonographically detectable major structural malformations in the following systems: cardiovascular, central nervous system, gastrointestinal system, and craniofacial abnormalities. Nicolaides et al [27] observed that the risk for aneuploidy is directly related to the number of defects identified, with an increasing risk when several sonographically-detected defects are present.

«Soft markers» include increased nuchal fold thickness, short femur and humerus, echogenic cardiac foci, renal pyelectasis, echogenic bowel and presence of choroid plexus cysts [28, 29]. Use of these soft markers in the development of a standardized risk-assessment system has been termed «genetic sonogram». Although not pathologic themselves, these markers have been used to screen for, or adjust the risk for DS. A normal ultrasound is associated with a reduction in DS risk from approximately 60% to 83% compared with the age-related empiric risk [30]. In a low-risk patient, however, detection of an isolated marker (eg, a short femur or pyelectasis) changes only minimally from the *a priori* risk and is probably not clinically relevant. Approximately 50% of DS fetuses will not have any abnormal findings on ultrasound.

Because nuchal fold thickness and proximal long bone measurements can be treated as continuous variables, it is possible to combine these markers into a multivariate Gaussian marker model that can include maternal serum analytes. A protocol therefore that combines the quadruple test with nuchal thickness and long bone measurements was developed which can achieve a 90% detection rate at the 5% false-positive standard [31]

First Trimester Markers for Down Syndrome Screening

Screening in the 1st trimester can provide women with an earlier reassurance and if termination of pregnancy is required, it can often be completed before fetal movements are evident.

Two 1st trimester maternal serum screening markers, pregnancy-associated plasma protein-A (PAPP-A) and free β-human chorionic gonadotropin (β-hCG), are useful for identifying women at increased risk for carrying a fetus with DS. When these markers are used to modify maternal individual age related risk, they can detect 42% and 29% of DS fetuses respectively, at a false positive rate of 5% [32]. When these two are combined, the detection rate for trisomy 21 is 60% at a false positive rate of 5% in an unselected low risk population of women <35 years old [33, 34]. In women > 35 years, the detection rate is approximately 75-80% at a similar false positive rate.

As in the case for 2nd trimester serum markers, it is appropriate to adjust the observed concentrations of the 1st trimester analytes to reflect patient race/ethnicity [35] and weight [36]. Twin pregnancies show an approximately two-fold concentration of β-hCG and PAPP-A, allowing the computation of a pseudo-risk for an affected pregnancy [37]. Other factors influencing the concentrations include maternal smoking, gravidity, parity, fetal gender, gestational diabetes, and assisted reproduction [36, 38, 39].

Measurement of an enlarged thickness of the subcutaneous fluid-filled space at the back of the neck of the developing fetus, known as nuchal translucency (NT) has been demonstrated to be an indicator for fetal trisomy 21 (figure 1) [40].

Fluid accumulation causing NT enlargement or nuchal cystic hygroma has been attributed to aortic isthmus narrowing or other cardiovascular defects which cause overperfusion of the head and neck. Other explanations for NT enlargement include abnormal or delayed development of the lymphatic system. Numerous studies have confirmed this association [41-45]. Nicolaides et al [46] reviewed fetal NT measurements present in predominantly high-risk women undergoing chorionic villi biopsy because of advanced maternal age or family history of chromosome abnormality. Using a fixed cut-off for the NT measurement of 3 mm, 18 of 28 (64%) of chromosomally abnormal cases could be identified, while only 33 of the 799 (4.1%) fetuses with normal karyotypes showed similar NT enlargement. Subsequently a Gaussian model for the NT variable was developed. This model allows for this test to be combined with other markers [47]. Using NT measurements and maternal age alone, it was estimated that 73% of DS affected pregnancies would be identified if the false-positive rate was set at 5% [48]. Subsequent studies demonstrated that NT increases with gestational age [49, 50] and that the sensitivity of NT measurement depends on inter-observer variability. It is highly recommended, therefore, that measurement of NT must be performed according to standardized protocol after appropriate training and accreditation [34].

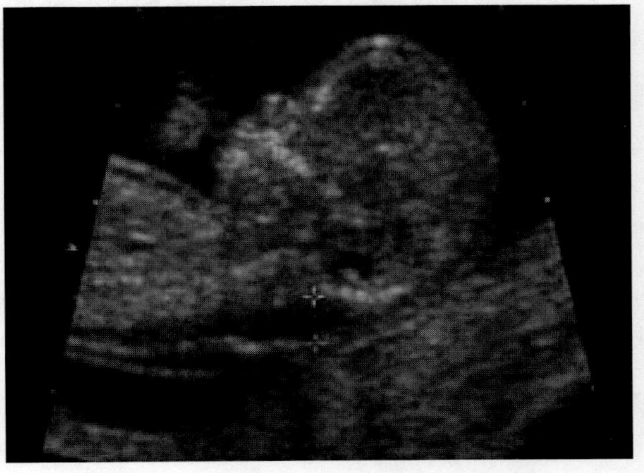

Figure 1. Representative ultrasonographic picture of a fetus with Down syndrome diagnosed in the 1st trimester of gestation by increased nuchal translucency measurement.

There is also increasing evidence that an enlarged NT measurement is indicative of a high risk for spontaneous abortion and for fetal abnormalities that are not detectable by cytogenetic analysis. Women whose fetuses show enlarged NT, therefore, need first trimester counseling regarding their risk for carrying a DS fetus and the possibility of other adverse pregnancy outcomes.

Absence of nasal bone (NB) has also been proposed as another marker for 1st trimester ultrasound screening for DS. Cicero et al [50] investigated this marker in pregnancies which screen positive by NT plus maternal age and noted that 43 of 59 (73%) DS fetuses showed absence of the NB, while only 3 of 603 (0.5%) unaffected fetuses had this marker. This observation was further confirmed by Nikolaides et al [51], but other recent studies have questioned its value. The 1st and 2nd trimester evaluation of risk (FASTER) multi-centre trial performed in the United States found that an acceptable nasal image was obtained in only 76% of over 6000 patients undergoing evaluation in the 1st trimester [52]. In addition to this, none of the cases of trisomy 21 in the group were detected using this method.

Abnormal Doppler flow patterns of the ductus venosus have been also associated with an increased risk for trisomy 21. However, like the NB, difficulty in measuring ductus venosus flow limits the use of this marker clinically [53].

First Trimester Combined Screening Strategies

A combination of NT measurement with β-hCG and PAPP-A in the 1st trimester comprises the «combined test» [54] that is estimated to achieve 80% detection at a 5% false-positive rate, which is better than that obtained with maternal age and serum markers or maternal age with NT. Orlandi et al [55] evaluated the performance of «combined testing» and reported an overall detection rate of 87% at a 5% false-positive rate. In a prospective study of 1467 patients who underwent combined first trimester screening, De Baisio et al reported a trisomy 21 detection rate of 85% at a false-positive rate of 3.3% [56]. The SURUSS study among 47.053 singleton pregnancies reported an 85% detection rate at a false-positive rate of 6.1% for the «combined test» [57], while more recently in the FASTER trial among women from the general population, the detection rates for trisomy 21 were 87%, 85% and 82% at a 5% false-positive rate 11, 12, and 13 weeks' of gestation, respectively [58]. «Combined testing» with NT and serum markers has been shown to be more effective than either one alone and is even better than the quadruple test in the 2nd trimester. The main advantage of the «combined test» is the availability of the results late in the 1st trimester, which allows karyotyping by chorionic villus sampling and early surgical termination of pregnancy when this is indicated.

First trimester testing could also be combined with 2nd trimester maternal serum screening tests to obtain even higher levels of efficacy [59]. This is the concept of «stepwise sequential screening» and «contingent sequential screening». In the first one, results are provided to patients after both the 1st and 2nd trimester tests are available and only patients who screen negative for the 1st trimester are screened again in the 2nd. In this case 2nd trimester screening analyses take into account the results of the earlier first-trimester screen for any given individual.

Contingent sequential screening also begins with combined 1st trimester screening using both nuchal translucency and 1st trimester serum screening. However, based on these results, there are three options: 1) high risk women who are offered invasive prenatal diagnostic testing, 2) women at moderate risk who go on to 2nd trimester serum screening and 3) pregnancies at low risk who require no further testing.

There are, however, several practical limitations to «stepwise sequential screening» and «Contingent Sequential screening». These include scheduling of testing within relatively narrow gestational age intervals, availability of appropriately trained ultrasonographers for NT measurement, risks associated with chorionic villus biopsy and cost.

Recent Progress in Non-Invasive Prenatal Diagnosis for Down Syndrome

Prenatal DS screening has evolved over the last few decades through the sequential addition of maternal serum analytes and ultrasound-based procedures in order to reduce the need for invasive, but definitive, tests such as amniocentesis. However, current screening procedures still report high numbers of false-positive cases relative to true-positive ones in order to gain high detection rates [57]. Among women who screen positive for fetal DS, follow-up amniocentesis causes fetal loss in 1 out of every 1600 cases [60], a rate significantly lower than previous estimates [61] but one which still represents a serious concern. Consequently, the need for further development of noninvasive prenatal DS screening still exists.

Application of Proteomics for the Identification of Biomarkers for Down Syndrome in Maternal Plasma

Use of global approaches, such as proteomics for biomarker discovery, is hoped to reveal a greater panel of markers which will improve screening and perhaps diagnosis of DS [62]. Such a panel might allow for the absence/presence of a protein in DS that would otherwise characterize a healthy fetus.

Proteomic analytic procedures applied for the analysis of reproductive fluids could be divided in two major groups, namely techniques used for profiling and techniques used for differential protein detection. The most common and widely accepted approach for the analysis of reproduction-related biological fluids relies upon a coordinated use of two-dimensional gel electrophoresis (2-DE), image analysis, mass spectrometry (MS) protein identification and bioinformatics/database construction [63-66]. In addition, the advance of fluorescence two-dimensional differential in-gel electrophoresis (DIGE) and multidimensional protein identification technology (MudPIT) coupled with MS allowed the quantitative comparison of related samples, such as AF obtained at different times during pregnancy and maternal serum obtained from women carrying chromosomally normal and DS fetuses [67]. Emerging proteomic techniques, however, such as top-down/bottom-up and peptidomics, have not as yet been applied in reproduction related research.

Application of these high throughput methodologies in pregnancy-related pathology can contribute to the comprehension of the underlying pathophysiologies and the successful identification of relevant protein biomarkers that can potentially change early diagnosis and treatment of several medical conditions related to human pregnancy. Tsangaris et al. [68] applied MS-based proteomics to identify proteins differentially expressed in amniotic fluid samples from pregnancies with DS fetuses and chromosomally normal ones. This comparison revealed seven proteins differentially expressed in samples obtained from pregnancies with DS fetuses as compared to the control group. Alpha -1-microglobulin, collagen alpha 1(I) chain, collagen alpha 1(III) chain, collagen alpha 1(V) chain d, and basement membrane-specific heparin sulfate proteoglycan core protein were increased in cases with DS, whereas insulin-like growth factor-binding protein was decreased by 40% as compared to chromosomally normal fetuses. In the same study, splicing factor arginine/serine-rich protein was identified as present only in amniotic fluid samples from cases with DS fetuses, and was completely absent in the chromosomally normal ones.

Nagalla's study in 2007 [67] was the first attempt to use MS technology in order to identify biomarkers for non-invasive prenatal diagnosis of Down syndrome. Nagalla et al. analyzed 1st and 2nd -trimester maternal serum samples of DS and gestational age-matched controls, using multiple complementary proteomic approaches, DIGE, 2-dimensional liquid chromatography-chromatofocusing, MudPIT, LC/LC-MS/MS and MALDI-TOF-MS peptide profiling. They found 28 and 26 proteins differentially present in first- and second-trimester samples, respectively. Of those, 19 were specific for the first and 16 for the 2nd trimester and 10 were differentially present in both trimesters. They reported that analysis of MALDI-TOF-MS peptide profiles with pattern-recognition software also discriminated between DS and controls in both trimesters, with an average recognition capability that approached 96%.

Kolialexi et al [69], analysed plasma from 8 women carrying a DS fetus and 12 with non-DS fetuses matched for gestational age, maternal age and ethnicity, in the 2nd trimester of pregnancy, using 2-DE coupled with MALDI-TOF-MS. Gel comparison revealed nine proteins differentially expressed in maternal plasma in women with DS fetuses. Eight proteins, Transthyretin (TTHY), Ceruloplasmin (CERU), Afamin (AFAM), Alpha-1-microglobulin (AMBP), Apolipoprotein E (APOE), Serum amyloid P-component (SAMP), Histidine-rich glycoprotein (HRG) and Alpha-1-antitrypsin (A1AT) were up-regulated and one, Clusterin (CLUS), down- regulated. All nine proteins detected in this study are known to be involved in fetal growth and development, while APOE, SAMP, AFAM and CLUS are associated with the DS phenotype. All differentially expressed proteins are candidate biomarkers for DS, providing opportunities for the development of non invasive prenatal diagnosis. Before any meaningful application of these proteomic biomarkers, however, extensive validation in the form of well-designed, statistically significant human clinical trials must be performed.

Fetal Cells and Nucleic Acids in Maternal Blood

Another alternative to the use of invasive procedures is the analysis of fetal cells or nucleic acids, including DNA and RNA, in maternal circulation. While these approaches hold some promise, their utility is presently limited by a number of factors, including the sporadic presence and/or nonproliferative nature of fetal cell types in maternal serum, the difficulty in distinguishing maternal and female fetal material, and the small amounts of fetal nucleic acids present in maternal serum.

During the last few years, extensive research has been conducted towards the development of non-invasive methods for prenatal diagnosis of chromosomal abnormalities such as DS on the basis of the enrichment and analysis of intact fetal cells entering maternal circulation. Although this method has been successfully used for the detection of many aneuploidies [70,71,72], complete distinction of fetal from maternal cells is not yet possible, because, according to several reports, maternal cells may constitute up to 50% of the isolated nucleated red blood cells (NRBCs) [73,74]. It is well known that NRBCs are absent from the peripheral blood of healthy adults, but pregnancy *per se* induces their appearance in maternal circulation. We have previously demonstrated that the number of NRBCs in maternal blood depends on the anemic status of the mother [75]. FISH analysis of the isolated cell population can facilitate distinction between fetal and maternal NRBCs in cases with male embryos, but hybridization efficiency is very low due to enrichment procedures and the apoptotic status of the isolated fetal cells [76, 77]. It has also been proposed that determination of the number of NRBCs in maternal circulation, alone or in combination with biochemical or ultrasonographic tests in both trimesters of pregnancy, could indicate fetal DS, since an increase of NRBCs is noted in maternal peripheral blood when the fetus has trisomy 21. Bianchi *et al*. [70, 71] estimated a six-fold increase in the number of fetal cells identified in the peripheral blood of women carrying fetuses with DS and similar results were also reported by other investigators [78,79,80,81]. In a previous study Mavrou et al [82] determined that NRBC count had a 100% detection rate for DS and therefore the number of fetal cells in maternal blood during pregnancy is likely to be applied as a non-invasive method for the assessment of pregnancies at risk for DS in order to reduce the number of amniocenteses among the positive screened women .

Use of cell free fetal-DNA (cff-DNA) for non invasive prenatal detection of fetal trisomy 21 is severely hampered by the fact that fetal material represents only 3–5% of the total circulatory DNA in maternal plasma during pregnancy [83]. This makes the determination of fetal STRs or SNPs that could be used to determine fetal aneuploidies very difficult.

One alternative now seems to be provided by the presence of placentally derived cell-free fetal messenger RNA (cff-RNA) in maternal plasma [84]. The main advantage of cff-RNA over cff-DNA is that it is possible to select for placenta-specific mRNA sequences not expressed by any maternal tissues. Analysis of cff-RNA represents fetal genes completely absent from the maternal genome and therefore can be considered in the same way. The Hong Kong group focused it attention on the *PLAC4* gene, which is known to be expressed only in the placenta. Since this gene is located on chromosome 21, quantitative analysis of its expression can be useful in determining the number of copies of this chromosome. In another study, the same group, enumerated chromosome 21 levels using SNPs located in the *PLAC4* gene by mass spectrometry with a sensitivity of 90% and a specificity of 96%. In cases where the fetus was heterozygous for a SNP locus, the *PLAC4* mRNA transcripts would, in cases of normal ploidy, contain equal ratios of each allele (1:1 ratio). If, however, an aneuploidy was present, then the ratio would shift to 2:1.

Recently, Fan et al [85] directly sequenced cell-free DNA from the plasma of pregnant women using high-throughput shotgun sequencing technology and obtained, on average, 5 million sequence tags per sample. This enabled them to measure the over- and under-representation of chromosomes from an aneuploid fetus. This sequencing approach is polymorphism independent and therefore universally applicable for the non-invasive detection of fetal aneuploidy. Using this method, they successfully identified nine cases of trisomy 21 at the 14th week of gestation. Although this approach, appears to be very promising, follow-up experiments are needed in order to evaluate the relevance of these findings.

References

[1] Lejeune, J; Gauthier, M; Turpin, R. Les chromosomes humains en culture des tissues. *C. R. Acad. Sci.,* 1959 248, 602–603.

[2] Egan, JF; Benn, P; Borgida, AF; Rodis, JF; Campbell, WA; Vintzileos AM. Efficacy of screening for fetal Down syndrome in the United States from 1974 to 1997. *Obstet. Gynecol.,* 2000 96, 979-85.

[3] Torfs, CP; Christianson, RE. Anomalies in Down syndrome individuals in a large population-based registry. *Am. J. Med. Genet.*, 1998 77, 431-8.

[4] Verp, MS; Heckerling, PS. Use of decision analysis to evaluate patients' choices of diagnostic prenatal test. *Am. J. Med. Genet.*, 1995 58, 337-44.

[5] Akesson, HO; Forssman, H. A study of maternal age in Down's syndrome. *Ann Hum Genet*, 1966 29, 271-6.

[6] Merkatz, IR; Nitowsky, HM; Macri, JN; Johnson, WE. An association between low maternal serum alpha-fetoprotein and fetal chromosomal abnormalities. *Am J Obstet Gynecol,* 1984 148, 886-94.

[7] Cuckle, HS; Wald, NJ; Lindbaum, RH. Maternal serum alpha-fetoprotein measurement: a screening test for Down syndrome. *Lancet,* 1984 1, 926–929.

[8] Fuhrmann, W; Went, P; Weitzel, HK. Maternal serum AFP as screening test for Down syndrome. *Lancet,* 1984 2, 413.

[9] Bogart, MH; Pandian, MR; Jones, OW. Abnormal maternal serum chorionic gonadotropin levels in pregnancies with fetal chromosome abnormalities. *Prenat. Diagn.*, 1987 7, 623-30.

[10] Canick, JA; Knight, GJ; Palomaki, GE; Haddow, JE; Cuckle, HS; Wald; NJ. Low second trimester maternal serum unconjugated oestriol in pregnancies with Down's syndrome. *Br. J. Obstet. Gynaecol.*, 1988 95, 330-3.

[11] Wald, NJ; Cuckle, HS; Densem, JW; Nanchahal, K; Royston, P; Chard, T; Haddow, JE; Knight, GJ; Palomaki, GE; Canick, JA. Maternal serum screening for Down's syndrome in early pregnancy. *BMJ,*1988 297, 883-7.

[12] Macri, JN; Kasturi, RV; Krantz, DA; Cook, EJ; Sunderji, SG; Larsen, JW. Maternal serum Down syndrome screening: unconjugated estriol is not useful. *Am. J. Obstet. Gynecol.*, 1990 162, 672-3.

[13] Van Lith, JM; Pratt, JJ; Beekhuis, JR; Mantingh, A; Second-trimester maternal serum immunoreactive inhibin as a marker for fetal Down's syndrome. *Prenat. Diagn.*, 1992 12, 801-6.

[14] Canick, JA; Lambert-Messerlian, GM; Palomaki, GE. Maternal serum dimeric inhibin is elevated in Down syndrome pregnancy. *Am. J. Hum. Genet.*, 1994 55, p. A9.

[15] Lambert-Messerlian, GM; Canick, JA; Palomaki, GE; Schneyer, AL. Second trimester levels of maternal serum inhibin-A, total inhibin, α inhibin precursor and activin in Down's syndrome pregnancies. *J. Med. Screen.* 1996 3, 58–62.

[16] Wald, N; Densem, J; George, L; Muttukrishna, S; Knight, PG. Prenatal screening for Down's syndrome using inhibin-A as a serum marker. *Prenat. Diagn.*, 1996 16, 143–153.

[17] Aitken DA; Wallace, EM; Crossley, JA; Swanston, IA; van Pareren, Y; van Maarle, M; Groome, NP; Macri, JN; Connor, JM. Dimeric inhibin-A as a marker for Down's syndrome in early pregnancy. *N. Engl. J. Med.*, 1996 334, 1231–1236.

[18] Cuckle, HS; Holding, S; Jones, R; Groome, NP; Wallace, EM. Combining inhibin A with existing second-trimester markers in maternal serum screening for Down's syndrome. *Prenat. Diagn.*, 1996 16, 1095–1100.

[19] Spencer, K; Wallace, EM; Ritoe, S. Second trimester dimeric inhibin-A in Down's syndrome screening. *Prenat. Diagn.*, 1996 16, 1101–1110.

[20] Wallace, EM; Swanston, IA; McNeilly, AS; Ashby, JP; Blundell, G; Calder, AA; Groome, NP. Second trimester screening for Down's syndrome using serum dimeric inhibin-A. *Clin. Endocrinol.*, 1996 44, 17–21.

[21] Mooney, RA; Peterson, CJ; French, CA; Saller, DN Jr; Arvan, DA. Effectiveness of combining maternal serum alpha-fetoprotein and hCG in a second-trimester screening program for Down syndrome. *Obstet Gynecol*, 1994 84, 298-303.

[22] Wald, NJ; Cuckle, HS; Densem, JW; Nanchahal, K; Royston, P; Chard, T; Haddow, JE; Knight, GJ; Palomaki, GE; Canick, JA. Maternal serum screening for Down's syndrome in early pregnancy. *BMJ*, 1988 297, 883–887.

[23] Wald, NJ; Densem, JW; George, L; Muttukrishna, S; Knight, PG. Prenatal screening for Down's syndrome using inhibin-A as a serum marker. *Prenat. Diagn.*, 1996 16, 143-53.

[24] Wald, NJ; Hackshaw, A. Tests using multiple markers. In *Antenatal and Neonatal Screening* (2nd edn), Wald, N; Leck, I (eds). Oxford University Press: New York, 2000, 23–57.

[25] Wald, NJ; Cuckle, HS; Densem, JW; Kennard, A; Smith, D. Maternal serum screening for Down's syndrome: the effect of routine ultrasound scan determination of gestational age and adjustment for maternal weight. *Br. J. Obstet. Gynaecol.*, 1992 99, 144–149.

[26] Benn, PA; Borgida, A; Horne, D; Briganti, S; Collins, R; Rodis, JF. Down syndrome and neural tube defect screening: the value of using gestational age by ultrasonography. *Am. J. Obstet. Gynecol.*, 1997 176, 1056–1061.

[27] Nicolaides, KH; Snijders, RJ; Gosden, CM; Berry, C; Campbell, S. Ultrasonographically detectable markers of fetal chromosomal abnormalities. *Lancet*, 1992 340, 704–707.

[28] Drugan, MP Johnson; Evans, MI. Ultrasound screening for fetal chromosome anomalies. *Am. J. Med. Genet.*, 2000 90, 98–107.

[29] Smith-Bindman, R; Hosmer, W; Feldstein, VA; Deeks, JJ; Goldberg, JD. Second-trimester ultrasound to detect fetuses with Down syndrome: a meta-analysis. *JAMA*, 2001 285, 1044–1055.

[30] Nyberg, DA; Souter, VL; El-Bastawissi, A; Young, S; Luthardt, F; Luthy, DA. Isolated sonographic markers for detection of fetal Down syndrome in the second trimester of pregnancy. *J .Ultrasound Med.*, 2001 20, 1053–1063.

[31] Kaminsky, L; Egan, J; Ying, J; Borgida, A; DeRoche, M; Benn, P. Combined second trimester biochemical and ultrasound screening for Down syndrome is highly effective. *Am J Obstet Gynecol*, 2001 185, S78.

[32] Haddow, JE; Palomaki, GE; Knight, GJ; Williams, J; Miller, WA; Johnson, A. Screening of maternal serum for fetal Down's syndrome in the first trimester. *N. Engl. J. Med*,. 1998 338, 955-61.

[33] Wapner, R; Thom, E; Simpson, JL; Pergament, E; Silver, R; Filkins, K; Platt, L; Mahoney, M; Johnson, A; Hogge, WA; Wilson, RD; Mohide, P; Hershey, D; Krantz, D; Zachary, J; Snijders, R; Greene, N; Sabbagha, R; MacGregor, S; Hill, L; Gagnon, A; Hallahan, T; Jackson, L. First Trimester Maternal Serum Biochemistry and Fetal Nuchal Translucency Screening (BUN) Study Group. First-trimester screening for trisomies 21 and 18. *N .Engl. J. Med.*, 2003 349, 1405-13.

[34] Malone, FD; Canick, JA; Ball RH; Nyberg, DA; Comstock, CH; Bukowski, R; Berkowitz, RL; Gross, SJ; Dugoff, L; Craigo, SD; Timor-Tritsch, IE; Carr, SR; Wolfe, HM; Dukes, K; Bianchi, DW; Rudnicka, AR; Hackshaw, AK; Lambert-Messerlian, G; Wald, NJ; D'Alton, ME. First- and Second-Trimester Evaluation of Risk (FASTER) Research Consortium. First-trimester or second-trimester screening, or both, for Down's syndrome. *N. Engl. J. Med.*, 2005 353, 2001-11.

[35] Spencer, K; Ong, CYT; Liao, AWJ; Nicolaides, KH. The influence of ethnic origin on first trimester biochemical markers of chromosomal abnormalities. *Prenat. Diagn.*, 2000 20, 491–494.

[36] de Graaf, IM; Cuckle, HS; Pajkrt, E; Leschot, NJ; Bleker, OP; van Lith, JM. Co-variables in first trimester maternal serum screening. *Prenat Diagn*, 2000 20, 186–189.

[37] Spencer, K; Nicolaides, KH. First trimester prenatal diagnosis of trisomy 21 in discordant twins using fetal nuchal translucency thickness and maternal serum free beta-hCG and PAPP-A. *Prenat. Diag.*, 2000 20, 683–684.

[38] Ong, CY; Liao, AW; Spencer, K; Munim, S; Nicolaides, KH. First trimester maternal serum free beta human chorionic gonadotrophin and pregnancy associated plasma protein A as predictors of pregnancy complications. *BJOG*, 2000 107, 1265–1270.

[39] Liao, AW; Heath, V; Kametas, N; Spencer, K; Nicolaides, KH. First-trimester screening for trisomy 21 in singleton pregnancies achieved by assisted reproduction. *Hum. Reprod.*, 2001 16, 1501–1504.

[40] Szabó, J; Gellén, J. Nuchal fluid accumulation in trisomy-21 detected by vaginosonography in first trimester. *Lancet*, 1990 336, 1133.

[41] Cullen, MT; Gabrielli, S; Green, JJ; Rizzo, N; Mahoney, MJ; Salafia, C; Bovicelli, L; Hobbins, JC. Diagnosis and significance of cystic hygroma in the first trimester. *Prenat. Diagn.*, 1990 10, 643–651.

[42] Ville, Y; Lalondrelle, C; Doumerc, S; Daffos, F; Frydman, R; Oury, JF; Dumez, Y. First trimester diagnosis of nuchal anomalies: significance and fetal outcome. *Ultrasound Obstet. Gynecol.*, 1992 2, 314–316.

[43] Shulman, LP; Emerson, DS; Felker, RE; Phillips, OP; Simpson, JL; Elias, S. High frequency of cytogenetic abnormalities in fetuses with cystic hygroma diagnosed in the first trimester. *Obstet Gynecol.*, 1992 80, 80–82.

[44] Van Zalen-Sprock, RM; Van Vugt, JMG; Van Geijn, HP. First trimester diagnosis of cystic hygroma-Course and outcome. *Am. J. Obstet. Gynecol.*, 1992 167, 94–98.

[45] Savoldelli, G; Binkert, F; Achermann, J; Schmid W. Ultrasound screening for chromosomal abnormalities in the first trimester of pregnancy. *Prenat Diagn*, 1993 13, 513–518.

[46] Nicolaides, KH; Brizot, ML; Snijders, RJM. Fetal nuchal translucency; ultrasound screening for fetal trisomy in the first trimester of pregnancy. *Br. J. Obstet. Gynaecol.*, 1994 101, 782–786.

[47] Pandya, PP; Snijders, RJ; Johnson, SP; De Lourdes Brizot M; Nicolaides KH. Screening for fetal trisomies by maternal age and fetal nuchal translucency thickness at 10 to 14 weeks of gestation. *Br. J. Obstet. Gynaecol.*, 1995 102, 957–962.

[48] Malone, FD; D'Alton, ME. Society for Maternal-Fetal Medicine.First-trimester sonographic screening for Down syndrome. *Obstet. Gynecol.*, 2003 102, 1066-79.

[49] Roberts, LJ; Bewley, S; Mackinson, AM; Rodeck, CH. First trimester fetal nuchal translucency: problems with screening the general population. *Br. J. Obstet. Gynaecol.*, 1995 102, 381–385.

[50] Cicero, S; Curcio, P; Papageorghiou, A; Sonek, J; Nikolaides KH. Absence of nasal bone in fetuses with trisomy 21 at 11–14 weeks of gestation: an observational study. *Lancet*, 2001 358, 1665–1667

[51] Nicolaides, KH; Spencer, K; Avgidou, K; Faiola, S; Falcon, O. Multicentre study of first-trimester screening for trisomy 21 in 75821 pregnancies: results and estimation of the potential impact of individual risk orientated two-stage first-trimester screening Ultrasound. *Obstet. Gynecol.*, 2005 25, 221–226.

[52] Malone, FD; Ball, RH; Nyberg, DA; Comstock, CH; Saade, G; Berkowitz, RL; Dugoff, L; Craigo, SD; Carr, SR; Wolfe, HM; Tripp, T; D'Alton, ME. FASTER Research Consortium. First-trimester nasal bone evaluation for aneuploidy in the general population. *Obstet. Gynecol*,. 2004 104, 1222-8.

[53] Matias, A; Montenegro, N; Areias, JC; Brandão, O. Anomalous fetal venous return associated with major chromosomopathies in the late first trimester of pregnancy. *Ultrasound Obstet. Gynecol.*, 1998 11, 209-13.

[54] Wald, NJ; Hackshaw, AK. Combining ultrasound and biochemistry in first-trimester screening for Down's syndrome. *Prenat. Diagn.*, 1997 17, 821–829.

[55] Orlandi, F; Damiani, G; Hallahan, TW; Krantz, DA; Macri, JN. First-trimester screening for fetal aneuploidy: biochemistry and nuchal translucency. *Ultrasound Obstet. Gynecol.*, 1997 10, 381–386.

[56] De Biasio, P; Siccardi, M; Volpe, G; Famularo, L; Santi, F; Canini, S. First-trimester screening for Down syndrome using nuchal translucency measurement with free beta-hCG and PAPP-A between 10 and 13 weeks of pregnancy-the combined test. *Prenat. Diagn*,. 1999 19, 360–363.

[57] Wald, NJ; Rodeck, C; Hackshaw, AK; Walters, J; Chitty, L; Mackinson, AM. SURUSS Research Group. First and second trimester antenatal screening for Down's syndrome: the results of the Serum, Urine and Ultrasound Screening study (SURUSS). *Health Technol. Assess*, 2003 7, 1–77.

[58] Malone, FD; Canick, JA; Ball, RH; Nyberg, DA; Comstock, CH; Bukowski, R; Berkowitz, RL; Gross, SJ;, Dugoff, L; Craigo, SD; Timor-Tritsch, IE; Carr, SR; Wolfe, HM; Dukes, K; Bianchi, DW; Rudnicka, AR; Hackshaw, AK; Lambert-Messerlian, G; Wald, NJ; D'Alton, ME. First- and Second-Trimester Evaluation of Risk (FASTER) Research Consortium. *N. Engl. J. Med.*, 2005 353, 2001–2011.

[59] Ndumbe, FM; Navti, O; Chilaka, VN; Konje, JC. Prenatal diagnosis in the first trimester of pregnancy. *Obstet. Gynecol. Surv.*, 2008 63, 317-28.

[60] Eddleman, KA; Malone, FD; Sullivan, L; Dukes, K; Berkowitz, RL; Kharbutli, Y; Porter, TF; Luthy, DA; Comstock, CH; Saade, GR; Klugman, S; Dugoff, L; Craigo, SD, Timor-Tritsch, IE; Carr, SR; Wolfe, HM; D'Alton, ME. Pregnancy loss rates after midtrimester amniocentesis. *Obstet. Gynecol.*, 2006 108, 1067-72.

[61] Caughey, AB; Hopkins, LM; Norton, ME. Chorionic villus sampling compared with amniocentesis and the difference in the rate of pregnancy loss. *Obstet. Gynecol*,. 2006 108, 612-6

[62] Avent, ND; Plummer, ZE; Madgett, TE; Maddocks, DG; Soothill, PW. Post-genomics studies and their application to non-invasive prenatal diagnosis. *Semin. Fetal. Neonatal. Med.*, 2008 13, 91-8.

[63] Liberatori, S; Bini, L; De Felice, C; Magi, B; Marzocchi, B; Raggiaschi, R; Frutiger, S; Sanchez, JC; Wilkins, MR; Hughes, G; Hochstrasser, DF; Bracci, R; Pallini, V. A two-dimensional protein map of human amniotic fluid at 17 weeks' gestation. *Electrophoresis*, 1997 18, 2816-22.

[64] Fountoulakis, M; Langen, H. Ligand-independent dimerization of the extracellular domain of the leptin receptor and determination of the stoichiometry of leptin binding. *Anal. Biochem.*, 1997 250, 153-156.

[65] Park, SJ; Yoon, WG; Song, JS; Jung, HS; Kim, CJ; Oh, SY; Yoon, BH; Jung, G; Kim, HJ; Nirasawa, T. Proteome analysis of human amnion and amniotic fluid by two-dimensional electrophoresis and matrix-assisted laser desorption/ionization time-of-flight mass spectrometry. *Proteomics*, 2006 6, 349-363.

[66] Tsangaris, GT; Kolialexi, A; Karamessinis, PM; Anagnostopoulos, AK; Antsaklis, A; Fountoulakis, M; Mavrou, A. The normal human amniotic fluid supernatant proteome. *In Vivo*, 2006a 20, 479-490.

[67] Nagalla, SR; Canick, JA; Jacob, T; Schneider, KA; Reddy, AP; Thomas, A; Dasari, S; Lu, X; Lapidus, JA; Lambert-Messerlian, GM; Gravett, MG; Roberts, CT Jr; Luthy, D; Malone, FD; D'Alton, ME. Proteomic analysis of maternal serum in down syndrome: identification of novel protein biomarkers. *J. Proteome Res.*, 2007 6, 1245-57.

[68] Tsangaris, GT; Karamessinis, P; Kolialexi, A; Garbis, SD; Antsaklis, A; Mavrou, A; Fountoulakis, M. Proteomic analysis of amniotic fluid in pregnancies with Down syndrome. *Proteomics*, 2006b 6, 4410-4419.

[69] Kolialexi, A; Tsangaris, GT; Papantoniou, N; Anagnostopoulos, AK; Vougas, K; Bagiokos, V; Antsaklis, A; Mavrou, A. Application of proteomics for the identification of differentially expressed protein markers for Down syndrome in maternal plasma. *Prenat. Diagn.*, 2008 28, 691-8.

[70] Bianchi, DW; Williams, JM; Sullivan, LM; Hanson, FW; Klinger, KW; Shuber, AP. PCR quantitation of fetal cells in maternal blood in normal and aneuploid pregnancies. *Am. J .Hum. Genet.*, 1997 61, 822–829.

[71] Bianchi, DW; Simpson, JL; Jackson, LG; Elias, S; Holzgreve, W; Evans, MI; Dukes, KA; Sullivan, LM; Klinger, KW; Bischoff, FZ; Hahn, S; Johnson, KL; Lewis, D; Wapner, RJ; de la Cruz, F. Fetal gender and aneuploidy detection using fetal cells in maternal blood: analysis of NIFTY I data. National Institute of Child Health and Development Fetal Cell Isolation Study. *Prenat. Diagn.*, 2002 22, 609-15

[72] Al-Mufti, R; Hambley, H; Farzaneh, F; Nicolaides, KH. Investigation of maternal blood enriched for fetal cells: role in screening and diagnosis of fetal trisomies. *Am. J. Med. Genet*,. 1999 85, 66-75.

[73] Troeger, C; Zhong, XY; Burgemeister, R; Minderer, S; Tercanli, S; Holzgreve, W; Hahn, S. Approximately half of the erythroblasts in maternal blood are of fetal origin. *Mol. Hum. Reprod.*, 1999 5, 1162-5.

[74] Kolialexi, A; Vrettou, C; Traeger-Synodinos, J; Burgemeister, R; Papantoniou, N; Kanavakis, E; Antsaklis, A; Mavrou, A. Noninvasive prenatal diagnosis of beta-

thalassaemia using individual fetal erythroblasts isolated from maternal blood after enrichment. *Prenat. Diagn.*, 2007 27, 1228-32

[75] Mavrou, A; Kolialexi, A; Antsaklis, A; Krikos, X; Koratzis, A; Metaxotou, C. Detection of fetal NRBCs in maternal blood of pregnant carriers of beta-thalassemia using anti-gamma and anti-epsilon monoclonal antibodies. *Ann. N Y Acad. Sci.*, 2001 945, 151-2.

[76] Sekizawa, A; Samura, O; Zhen, DK; Falco, V; Farina, A; Bianchi, DW. Apoptosis in fetal nucleated erythrocytes circulating in maternal blood. *Prenat. Diagn.*, 2000 20, 886-9.

[77] Kolialexi, A; Tsangaris, GT; Antsaklis, A; Tzortzatou, F; Amentas, C; Koratzis, A; Mavrou, A. Apoptosis in maternal peripheral blood during pregnancy. *Fetal. Diagn. Ther.*, 2001 16, 32-7

[78] Farina, A; Bianchi, DW. Fetal cells in maternal blood as a secondnon-invasive step for fetal Down syndrome screening. *Prenat. Diagn.*, 1998 18, 983–984.

[79] Parano, E; Falcidia, E; Grillo, A; Takabayashi, H; Trifiletti, RR; Pavone, P. Fetal nucleated red blood cell counts in peripheral bloodof mothers bearing Down syndrome fetus. *Neuropediatrics*, 2001 32, 147–149.

[80] Falcidia, E; Parano, E; Grillo, A, Pavone, P; Takabayashi, H; Trifiletti, RR; Scollo, P; Dallapiccola, B; Grammatico, P; Novelli, A; Paladini, D; Monni, G; Gulisano, A; Scassellati G. Fetal cells in maternalblood: a six-fold increase in women who have undergoneamniocentesis and carry a fetus with Down syndrome: a multicenterstudy. *Neuropediatrics*, 2004 35, 321–324.

[81] Krabchi, K; Gros-Louis, F; Yan, J; Bronsard, M; Massé, J; Forest, JC; Drouin, R. Quantification of all fetalnucleated cells in maternal blood between the 18th and 22nd weeksof pregnancy using molecular cytogenetic techniques. *Clin. Genet.*, 2001 60, 145–150.

[82] Mavrou, A; Kouvidi, E; Antsaklis, A; Souka, A; Kitsiou Tzeli, S; Kolialexi, A. Identification of nucleated red blood cells in maternal circulation: a second step in screening for fetal aneuploidies and pregnancy complications. *Prenat. Diagn.*, 2007 27, 150-3

[83] Lo, YM; Chiu, RW. Prenatal diagnosis: progress through plasma nucleic acids, *Nat. Rev. Genet.*, 2007 8, 71–77.

[84] Lo YM; Tsui, NB; Chiu, RW; Lau, TK; Leung, TN; Heung, MM; Gerovassili, A; Jin, Y; Nicolaides, KH; Cantor, CR; Ding, C. Plasma placental RNA allelic ratio permits noninvasive prenatal chromosomal aneuploidy detection. *Nat. Med.*, 2007 13, 218-23.

[85] Fan, HC; Blumenfeld, YJ; Chitkara, U; Hudgins, L; Quake, SR. Noninvasive diagnosis of fetal aneuploidy by shotgun sequencing DNA from maternal blood. *Proc. Natl. Acad. Sci. U S A*, 2008 105, 16266-71.

In: Handbook of Down Syndrome Research
Editors: Dominicus Jelinek and Gijs Dvorak
ISBN 978-1-60741- 690-6

Chapter 14

Machine Learning Applied to Second-Trimester Down's Syndrome Screening

***Vicenç Soler**[*1,2]* ***and Marta Prim**[†2]*
[1]Biomonitorization Group of the CIBER-BBN Center
(Biomedical Research Center on Network in Bioengineering,
Biomaterials and Nanomedicine)
[2]Dept. Microelectrònica i Sistemes Electrònics, Universitat Autònoma de Barcelona,
Bellaterra, Spain

Abstract

This chapter presents a new methodology to detect Down's syndrome during the second-trimester of gestation. We propose a Fuzzy Logic based classification method that is able of both improving the classification accuracy of the existing screening methods and extracting a set of intelligible rules that explain the system found. The accuracy is improved by reducing the False Positive rate up to 3%-4%, with a 60% of True Positive rate. Never before a screening method could reduce the FP rate below 5%, with a 60% of TP. The intelligibility is obtained by getting a reduced set of rules, expressed in a fuzzy way, which helps to explain the knowledge contained in the classification system found. Finally, conclude that the medical staff was able to understand the system expressed in the Fuzzy rules found, where its number of rules is just 10.

Introduction

The work presented in this chapter consists in developing a new method to solve the problem of early detection of Down syndrome in human fetuses, from numerical data

* vicenc.soler@uab.es.
† Edifici Q, Campus UAB,08193 Bellaterra, Spain, Tel. +34 93 581 3555, marta.prim@uab.es.

obtained from the mother. The approach to find such a method is carried out in the field of Machine Learning (Artificial Intelligence), as it allows a wide versatility in terms of number of today's techniques.

The Down syndrome's biochemical screening [[5]][[6]] is the method used today by most of hospitals in the world as a non-invasive method. It consists of a combination of statistical and mathematical operations, such as the calculation of medium and application of experimental regression formulas, from data obtained from the mother. It can be applied to the first or second trimester of pregnancy and has a reliability of 80-90% for the first trimester and 60-70% for the second, with an upper bound of 5% of false positive for the latter, although normally they are between 7% and 8%. In next section will be exposed the method age/LR, the most usual method applied in the second trimester of pregnancy for calculating the risk of having a fetus with Down syndrome.

Regarding the type of data set to analyze, it is needed to recall that it is an imbalanced data set. Imbalanced data sets [[1]] have the especial characteristic that one of the classes has a much higher number of cases than the other one, and it is a strong feature that restricts the type of Machine Learning method to be used. Regarding to the number of cases, from now on we will refer to the negative class as the *major-class* and the positive class as the *minor-class*, since in this application we have many more cases of babies born who do not have Down syndrome than those who do.

The goal of the work presented in this chapter is to expose a new methodology for the detection of Down syndrome, able to improve the performance of existing non-invasive methods applied to the second trimester of pregnancy. We want to emphasize that this work aims to improve numerical methods, reducing the number of applications of invasive methods, which have 1% probability of causing an irreversible damage on the fetus.

Another issue presented in this chapter is that the final system to be found should extract intelligible information able to help medical staff, based on the knowledge acquired by the final system found. Following this idea, a system that fits these constraints is a Fuzzy System, especially adapted to work with imbalanced datasets. The main problem arisen from working with imbalanced datasets come from the fact that, as one class has much more cases than the other one, the system either classifies all the results on the major-class or the system produces a lot of rules for the minor-class. The latter case has to be avoided, since the final system should provide a generalized solution for both classes.

The analysis of the medical results presented in this chapter has been supervised by a medical staff.

This chapter is structured in 5 sections. The first section is this introduction, which describes the topic which is dealt with in this chapter. In the second section related work is reviewed. The third section details the development and the characteristics of our new method (FLAGID). In the following section, we present the results obtained by applying the FLAGID method to the dataset corresponding to the Down's syndrome. Finally, the conclusions of the work presented in this chapter are presented.

Related Work

This section is divided into two parts. The first one summarizes the current non invasive method used in most of countries to detect Down syndrome in the second trimester. The second one shows the related work in terms of Machine Learning methods applied to solve this problem.

The most popular screening method currently used to detect Down syndrome in the second trimester of pregnancy is defined by the combination of two statistical methods: Maternal age risk and Likelihood ratio. This method is statistically based and is explained in the following paragraphs.

The *risk of maternal age* is the risk that a pregnant woman has, to give birth to a fetus affected by trisomy. Cuckle [[3]] found that cases of trisomy 21 increases with maternal age, and provides specific risk for trisomy 21 by maternal age at the probable date of birth, between 18 and 50 years, by the formula expressed in Equation 1.

$$p = 0.000627 + e^{-16.2395+[0.286\cdot(age-0.458)]} \quad \text{Eq. 1.}$$

where $age \in \mathfrak{R}$ is the mother's age.

The *Likelihood Ratio (LR)* is one way to describe the behavior of a diagnostic test and contains the same information as the sensitivity / specificity. The LR value, for a concrete screening value, is the probability of the test result in diseased individuals, divided by the probability of that result in healthy individuals.

The LR for a specific biochemical marker or ultrasound, with a normal distribution, is calculated based on prior knowledge of the Gaussian distribution for an affected population group and other not affected by trisomy 21 (Down syndrome). The basis for calculating the likelihood ratio (LR) is the relationship between the distances representing the height of the Gauss curve of the concentration of the marker, in relation to the fetuses affected and not affected of trisomy 21.

Screening methods for the second trimester need to work with all the markers standardized and having a Gaussian distribution shape, since the concentration of various markers in maternal serum varies with the time of pregnancy. This implies the need to find a method that makes independent the value of the marker during the pregnancy. To do it, the markers have to be transformed into multiples of the median (MoM), where a value of 1 indicates that the value has the same value that the median of the sample. A MoM, for a marker, includes all the rest of non-markers variables (gestational age of the fetus, alcohol consumption, etc.) except mother's age, since the information provided by the age is too important to be dissolved with the rest of variables.

Therefore, for each marker we must know the mean and standard deviation of normal distribution of the MoM of the population affected and not affected by trisomy 21, in this case. It is also useful to know the correlation coefficients between each pair of markers, since the fact of using combinations of markers whose correlation is very low or absent would cancel their capacity to detect the disease.

The final risk, combined from the Risk of maternal age (odds expressed) and LR methods, is shown in the formula expressed in Equation 2.

$$R = odds\_age \cdot LR(x) \qquad \text{Eq 2.}$$

This method achieves a 60-70% of detection, with a 7-8% of false positives. From now on, this method will be called *age/LR.*

Regarding the related work concerning the use of Machine Learning methods applied to Down syndrome detection, Sordo [[10]] compared the performance of different architectures of neural networks and learning algorithms in the diagnosis of Down syndrome in fetuses. The data used were 8 variables (maternal age, gestational age and hormonal markers) of 459 patients (410 negative and 49 with Down syndrome). To solve the problem, a 3-50-1 RBF network was used. The test results were 84% of cases correctly classified, that improves the 60-70% of the above method. However, there were a 35% of false positives, compared to the 7-8% of the above method. This suggests that the use of these networks is not acceptable for this type of problem, as well as for the type of network used. The greater benefit of the classification contrasts with the cost of the number of false positives.

Flagid: The Machine Learning Method

The method proposed in this chapter has the goal of achieving an accurate Fuzzy Classification System from an imbalanced dataset. A Fuzzy System is composed, mainly, by two parts: the Fuzzy Variables and the Fuzzy Rules. The fuzzy method mentioned above is called FLAGID (Fuzzy Logic and Genetic Algorithms applied to Imbalanced Datasets) and it uses a Fuzzy Clustering method to obtain the Fuzzy Variables and a Genetic Algorithm to obtain the Fuzzy Rules.

The FLAGID method consists of several steps:

1) A clustering method (DDA/RecBF algorithm) is used to get a first set of membership functions from the dataset. This method needs that the user defines previously the Fuzzy Output Variable.
2) The membership functions found by the DDA/RecBF algorithm are recombined (method ReRecBF) in order to obtain a new set of membership functions adapted to imbalanced datasets.
3) Finally, a genetic algorithm is applied to find a set of fuzzy rules that uses the membership functions obtained in step 2.

Figure 1 shows a schema of the FLAGID method.

In this chapter, the FLAGID method is presented as a new method to obtain good accuracy from Down syndrome data. As mentioned above, this method is based on the combination of other methods: DDA/RecBF, ReRecBF and Genetic Algorithms. In the following lines will be summarized the existing DDA/RecBF and Genetic Algorithms methods, and later explained in detail the ReRecBF method, a method created by the authors specifically for managing Fuzzy Variables in Imbalanced Datasets, and to be integrated into FLAGID.

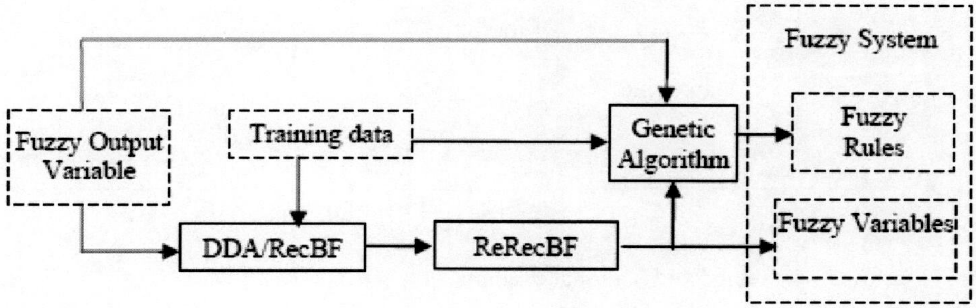

Figure 1. FLAGID method's schema. Solid line rectangles represent algorithms (DDA/RecBF, ReRecBF and Genetic Algorithm) and dashed ones represent sets (dataset, fuzzy rules set and fuzzy variables set).

Fuzzy Logic is a mathematical theory developed by Lotfi A. Zadeh in 1965 at the University of Berkeley (California) [[11]]. It is a different logic from classical logic since not everything is true or false, but there are degrees of certainty. This feature makes it a logical, being closer to human reasoning, since in the concept of Fuzzy Set introduced by Zadeh, lies the idea that the elements on which the human mind is built are not numbers but linguistic labels. Therefore, the fuzzy logic can represent the qualitative common knowledge in a mathematical (quantitative) way through this theory, also called Fuzzy Sets Theory.

In order to understand later some arguments referred to Fuzzy Logic, we will explain some concepts about the Fuzzy Logic processing. Fuzzy Logic processing follows the schema shown in Figure 2.

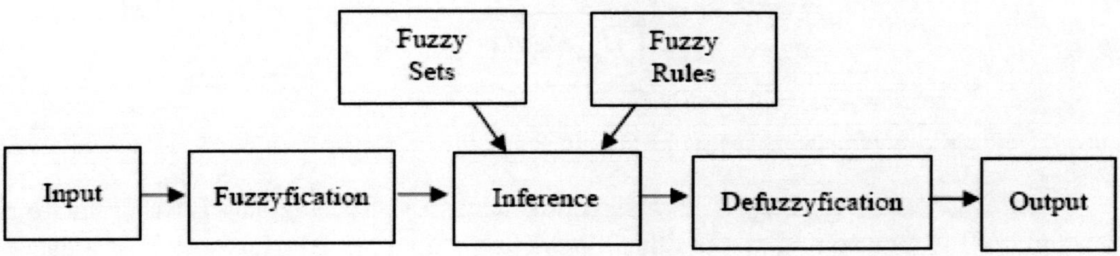

Figure 2. Fuzzy system processing schema.

During the fuzzyfication process, the input data is applied to every rule. The following example shows a rule and the fuzzyfication process applied. First, the corresponding Fuzzy Sets that appear in the rule are chosen from every Fuzzy Variable. Then, the input data (V1=60 and V2=178) is applied in the X-axis, giving a value in the Y-axis. The Y value is called α-cut, since it "cuts" the function in this value. The minimum of both values is the final α-cut applied to the output variable (see Figure 3).

Rule: IF V1 is low and V2 is medium THEN Output is NO

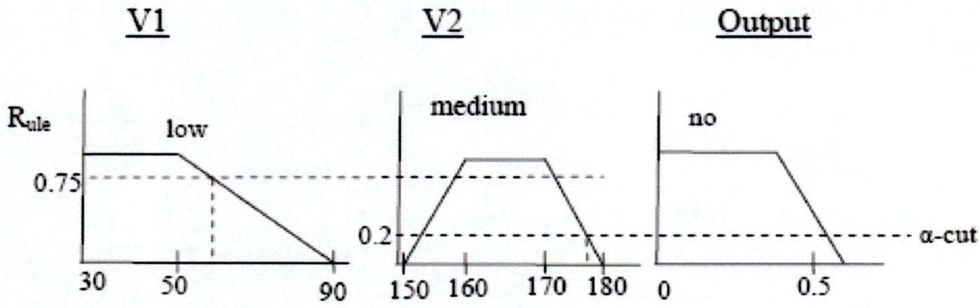

Figure 3. Fuzzification method with an α-cut example.

In this case, the system has 5 rules (the above one is R_3, one of them). Once all the 5 rules are applied to the output fuzzy sets (in this case 2 fuzzy sets of the output variable), a shape is obtained (see Figure 4, at right) and a defuzzyfication method is applied to extract the output value (in this case the Centroid formula).

Result:

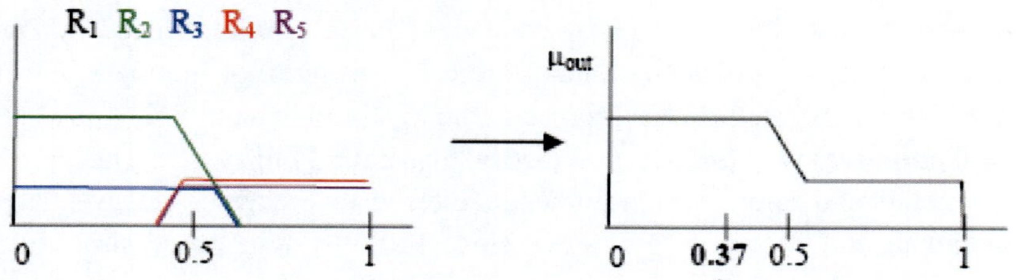

$$centroid = \frac{\int x\mu_{out}(x)dx}{\int \mu_{out}(x)dx}$$

Figure 4. Defuzzification method. The figure at right shows the final shape.

The *DDA/RecBF* (Dynamic Decay Adjustment for Rectangular Basis Functions) algorithm [[2]] is a clustering method that allows to obtain a RecBF Network from a dataset and a definition of the clusters (classes) of the output variable in a set of fuzzy membership functions. RecBF Networks [[2]] are a variation of RBF networks, in which the representation is a set of hyper-rectangles belonging to the different classes of the system. Every dimension of the hyper-rectangles represents a membership function of every variable (one variable per dimension). Figure 5 shows an example of a 2-dimension hyper-rectangle (or also called Fuzzy Point) corresponding to a system with 2 input variables, where the Support Region and Core Regions are clearly defined.

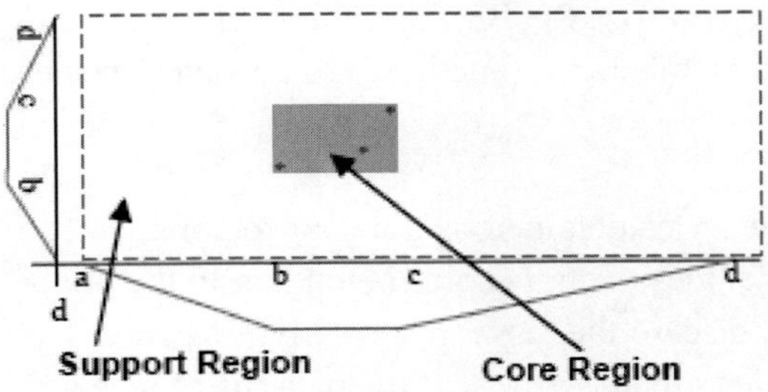

Figure 5. Example of a 2 dimensions Fuzzy Pointy, its associated membership functions defined by its 2 regions. The a, b, c and d points are different for every dimension.

The algorithm which produces the RecBFN from the dataset and from the definition of the classes of the system is called DDA/RecBF. The set of membership functions defined by this method are usually well suited for classification, although usually produces overlapping Fuzzy Points producing overlapping Fuzzy Sets in every variable.

These membership functions will be used to obtain a set of rules by means of a Genetic Algorithm. Although first, a previous step to transform the set of membership functions (output of the DDA/RecBF) has to be done since they need to be adapted for working with imbalanced data. This task is done through the *ReRecBF* algorithm by recombining the set of membership functions.

Genetic Algorithms [[4]] are used to derive fuzzy rules from the set of recombined membership functions. Genetic algorithms are methods based on principles of natural selection and evolution for global searches. Given a problem, a genetic algorithm runs repeatedly by using the three fundamental operators: reproduction, crossover and mutation. These operators, combined randomly, are based on a fitness function evolution to find a better solution in the searching space. Chromosomes represent the individuals of the genetic algorithms and a chromosome is composed of several genes. Genetic algorithms are used to find solutions to problems with a large set of possible solutions and they have the advantage of only requiring information concerning the quality of the solution. This fact makes genetic algorithms a very good method to solve complex problems.

The following subsections will explain both the developed ReRecBF algorithm and the application of the Genetic Algorithm.

Rerecbf Algorithm: Recombining Rectangular Basis Functions (RECBFS).

After obtaining the Fuzzy Variables from the DDA/RecBF algorithm, the ReRecBF algorithm performs the shape of the Fuzzy Variables in order to be adapted to work with imbalanced datasets.

Since overlapping membership functions are given as result of the RecBF algorithm, due to we are working with a dataset with overlapped classes (boundary not well defined), these membership functions are not adequate to obtain an accurate set of fuzzy rules from an imbalanced dataset. The tests on different datasets demonstrated that the membership functions obtained from the DDA/RecBF algorithm were not discriminant enough and some transformations of these membership functions are needed. On these grounds we propose to (argued in [[8]]):

1) Take only the intervals obtained by the core-regions.
2) Transform to triangles the trapezoids belonging to the minor-class.
3) If it is possible, discard the less representative RecBFs. That is, RecBFs whose core-region includes less than the 10% of the patterns of its class.

The core-regions delimit the areas where the training patterns are, and the support-regions (without taking into account the core ones) are the undefined areas between the core ones. In these undefined regions, the algorithm does not know how to classify the possible patterns included there. Then, we can affirm that the only place where we are sure that a pattern belongs to a class is into the core-regions of that class.

Out of them, the RecBF represents a grading of the level in which the instance belongs to the class. In this way, the nearer the value is to the core area, the higher the possibilities to belong to the class. So, in this case, the set of overlapped membership functions belonging to a variable and a class will be split into new ones, selecting only the areas defined by the core-regions. Thanks to this operation, we will have the membership function areas divided into sectors, and this fact will improve the quantity of patterns matched by the rules found.

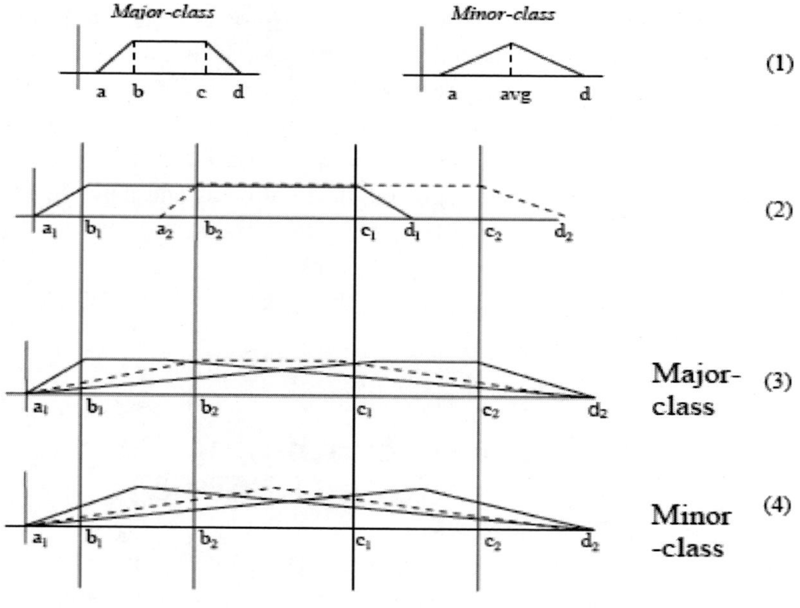

Figure 6. (1) Trapezoids for major-class membership functions and triangles for minor-class membership functions. (2) Example of 2 overlapped trapezoids. (3) Three trapezoids will be obtained from above if the membership functions would belong to the major-class and (4) Three triangles if would belong to the minor-class. Both (3) and (4) have membership functions with the minimum and the maximum in the limits of the variable.

Finally, the recombination procedure shown in Figure 6 consists in creating new membership function by splitting the existing ones by its core-region (points b and c) and eliminating the old ones. For every new membership function created, the support-area will be defined from the minimum to the maximum values of that variable. The membership functions created from examples belonging to the minor-class are transformed into triangles (having its maximum in the average point of its original trapezoid) and the major-class ones as trapezoids.

We can obtain the following conclusions about the proposed transformation:

1) More uncertainty is introduced in the definition of the membership function because we do not discard that a membership function can be evaluated in the whole variable space.
2) Every value for a membership function is always greater than 0, so always the α-cut will be greater than 0.
3) As the value of a rule will be determined by the minimum of the α-cuts, and as the importance of a class is determined by the maximum of the α-cuts of all its rules, we can affirm that the final importance of a class in a pattern can be determined by only one rule, and that rule has to have all membership function as near as possible the values of the example treated.
4) The minor-class membership functions introduce more uncertainty because they are treated as triangles. If we do not have much information about how that class is (the case for highly imbalanced datasets), we can consider an area centered in the average of the membership function's core-region and its belonging value decreasing as far away it is.

Thanks to these characteristics, the membership functions are not so rigid and they have many more possibilities to participate in every rule. Thus, we give to the system more feasible tools to adapt itself to the given dataset.

The following subsection explains how the rule set will be extracted by a genetic algorithm, once the membership functions have been calculated by the previously specified procedure.

Genetic Algorithm: Obtaining the Rule Set

The codification of one chromosome of our genetic algorithm is expressed in the following line: $(x_{1,1},...,x_{1,n},x_{2,1},....,x_{2,n},x_{m,1},...,x_{m,n})$ where n is the number of variables (input variables plus output variables) and m is the number of rules. $x_{i,j}$ is the value that a gene can take, which is an integer value compressed in the interval $[0,n\_fuzzysets_j]$ and $n\_fuzzysets_j$ is the number of membership functions of the jth variable. If a $x_{i,j}$ has value 0 it expresses that this variable is not present in the rule. If the 0 value is assigned to the output fuzzy set, the rule is not taken into account to evaluate the rules. So, the system is able to find a set of rules less than m, just putting 0 in the output fuzzy set of the rule. Every $x_{i,1}$,..., $x_{i,n}$ corresponds to a rule of the system.

The initial population is either taken randomly or by an initial set of rules. Every gene of a chromosome is generated randomly in the interval [0,n_fuzzysets$_j$], but some rules can be fixed for the entire simulation or just given as an initial set of rules, if needed. If a fuzzy set is 0, it means that the variable is not taken into account in the rule.

In the case of this chapter, the initial rules have been generated randomly and no restriction has applied on them.

The classification of the data, in a Fuzzy Logic System, depends on the shape of the membership functions of the input and output variables and the rules. The membership functions of the input variables are obtained by the ReRecBF method, the rules by means of this genetic algorithm and the output variable has to be defined from the beginning. So, another important fact in the matching of the examples by the rule set is the shape of the output trapezoids. We can choose between symmetric (they have the same area and shape) or non-symmetric (they have different shapes and areas, see Figure 7), that is, both classes will have either the same importance or not.

In this chapter, 4 different types of asymmetry were tested. They have been chosen in order to represent different degrees of asymmetry to provide one degree more of freedom in the learning process. Figure 7 (1) represents a high degree of asymmetry, and Figure 7 (2) is symmetric.

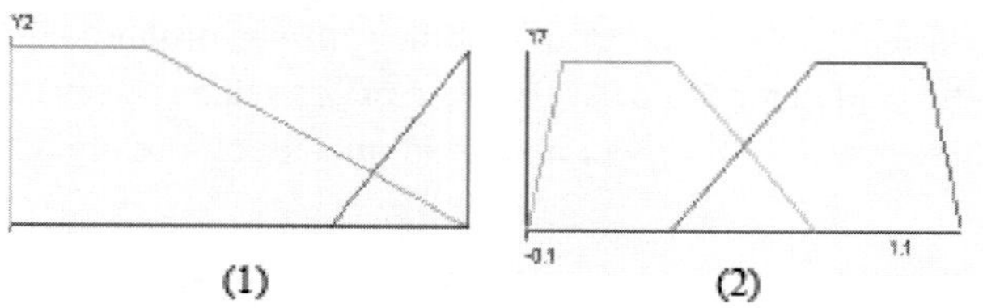

Figure 7. Example of (1) non-symmetric and (2) symmetric 2-class output.

The symmetric one is much better, because the fuzzy rules will be much easier intelligible.

Regarding the stopping criteria, it is difficult to apply an early-stopping method based on the test of a small quantity of data, since usually the minor-class is provided with a reduce number of patterns. In this case, the genetic algorithm will stop when a determinate threshold value in its fitness function is reached.

Flagid Results on Down Syndrome Data

This section will present the results obtained by the FLAGID method. To perform the tests, the method needs to adjust some parameters. These parameters are:

1) Respecting to the DDA / RecBF algorithm:

- Order of patterns: ordered or disordered classes.

- • Scope: the algorithm works with a restricted area defined by either the scope of the training patterns or ∞ area or another.

2) Respecting to the ReRecBF method:

- Discard or not the less representative Fuzzy Points of a class, that is, the ones that have been created with less than 10% of its class patterns.

3) Respecting to the Genetic Algorithm (GA):

- The number of rules to be found.
- The definition of the fuzzy membership functions of the output variable.

All these parameters are important, and were taking into account during the learning process. This section will explain below how these parameters were considered.

Since the problem to be solve is a 2-class problems, the only issue that affects the definition of the fuzzy output variable is if it is symmetric or asymmetric, in order to provide more weight to one class. For a 2-class system, it is not decisive for the DDA/RecBF algorithm and it is to the GA. The variable must have two functions belonging to the values found in both classes, and the shape of these functions does not influence on the DDA/RecBF algorithm, but yes on the GA. For this reason it was not mentioned in point 1).

The aim of the tests, primarily, is to find a Fuzzy System that tries to improve the performance of the method used today for the detection of Down syndrome in the second trimester of pregnancy, the combined age/LR method explained above.

In this type of data, the negative patterns are the one that do not have Down syndrome and compose the largest class (major-class). The positive ones are the ones that have Down syndrome and compose the smallest class (minor-class).

This section will examine first the Down syndrome data set and then the results are compared between the current method (age/LR) and the proposed in this paper (FLAGID). It will be verified that the solution found has better results than any other of the methods, lowering the rate of false positives (FP), without improving the true positives (TP), which will remain in the same values as the age/LR method.

Furthermore, as one of the objectives proposed in this paper is to extract information from the solution found, we will see that the information provided by the solution found can be interpretable by the medical staff.

Down Syndrome Data

The Down syndrome data available contains only physical parameters (age, race, hormone markers, etc.). The data contains many variables, and only a few quantity of them will be used for the work presented in this chapter (advised by the medical group): the race of the mother, the number of fetuses during gestation, the mother's age and weight, gestational age of the fetus, the presence of diabetes, the level of consumption of alcohol and cigarettes, the Alpha-Fetoprotein (AFP) and the human Chorionic Gonadotropin (hCG) hormone markers, and their MoM.

Based on these variables, the problem was focused only on white women and single fetus, since changing the race or the number of fetuses, the value of hormone markers varies.

Therefore, the input variables will be the mother's age and weight, gestational age of the fetus, the presence of diabetes, the level of consumption of alcohol and cigarettes, and the hormonal markers AFP, hCG, and their MoM. Since almost all MoM include input variables, the input variables are divided into two groups:

1) One composed by the age of the mother and the two MoM markers (MoM-AFP and MoM-hCG).
2) Other group consisting in 8 variables that are not expressed in MoM: the mother's age and weight, gestational age of the fetus, the presence of diabetes, the level of consumption of alcohol and cigarettes, and the hormonal markers AFP and hCG.

The data provided is divided into three groups: one with 3109 cases (3096 positive and 13 negative), another of 818 cases (816 negative and 2 positive) and another of 4995 cases (4980 negative and 15 positive), in chronological order. The first two groups correspond chronologically and their difference lies in the method used to measure the gestational age of the fetus. The last set, called Down_total in Table 1, is the sum of the previous three. Table 1 shows the characteristics of the three data sets and the total one.

Table 1. Features of the 3 datasets and the total one

Set name	#cases	#neg	#pos	%neg	%pos
Down_3109	3109	3096	13	99.60%	0.40%
Down_818	818	816	2	99.75%	0.25%
Down_4995	4995	4980	15	99.70%	0.30%
Down_total	8922	8892	30	99.66%	0.34%

The chronological split is important, since a deterioration has been observed in the collection of data. This is due to the fact that at the beginning of the study the medical staff tries to write the data carefully, and just a reduced quantity of them is in charge of this work. It was observed that this accuracy was not followed during posterior years, mainly because of the moving of medical staff.

In the age/LR method, the data is truncated by the upper and lower limits of the MoM variables, due to an adjustment of the function, which needs to have Gaussian shape. To meet the Gaussian, the limits are set at approximately 3 times the variance. So, looking at Table 2, the upper limits should be set at 1.1 +3 x 0.2 and 1.3 +3 x 0.8.

Table 2. Average and variance of both MoM markers

	averag e	variance
MoM (AFP)	1.1	0.2
MoM (hCG)	1.3	0.8

In the case of the work presented in this chapter, the truncation will only affect the upper bound of the two markers hCG and AFP, with the aim of grouping all the cases that exceed this threshold. It was decided, observing the data, to increase the limit from 3 to 5 times the variance. This will expand the scope of the variable without removing the desired effect. For the markers AFP and hCG not expressed in MoM, the same upper limit is applied, proportional to the value of 5MoM. Table 3 shows these limits.

Table 3. Upper limits of both hormonal markers

	MoM	No MoM
AFP	5	115
hC G	5	85

If this truncation were not be done, the DDA/RecBF would have some troubles in creating the Fuzzy Sets from variables with too large scope, having 95% of the cases concentrated in 10% of its space.

Results from the Age/LR Method

This section will examine the results of the data sets of Down syndrome with the age/LR method. Table 4 shows the results for Down_4995 data set from Table 1. The cutting level is the threshold that considers a case risky or not risky. The values with odds under this threshold are risky considered.

Table 4. Sensibility, specificity, rates of true positives (TP) and false positives (FP) for different cutting levels of the datatset Down_4995. The measures were obtained by means of the *SsdwLab* software [[7]]

Cutting level	%Sensibility	%Specificity	%TP	%FP
1:850	60.0	80.1	60.0	19.9
1:400	53.3	89.3	53.3	10.7
1:350	46.6	90.3	46.6	9.65
1:270	40.0	92.3	40.0	7.71

The normal cutting level is 1:270 (risk of 1 possibility among 270). For this cutting level, results in Table 4 are very poor, since the success rate in cases of Down syndrome is only 40%. To achieve a rate of 60%, a cutting level of 1:850 is needed, which does increase excessively the rate false positives (20%).

Therefore, the data set Down_4995 is a set that not complies with the standard cutting level of 1:270. Maybe this is due to noise (measurement errors, mistakes introducing the data, etc.). However, these formulations will not be ruled out of the data set, as the final system should operate if there is or not noise in the data set.

Results with FLAGID

As discussed previously, the main objective of this work is to find a Fuzzy System able to improve the today results to detect Down syndrome (trisomy 21) in a fetus during the second trimester of pregnancy.

The fitness function chosen for the genetic algorithm is described in Equation 3.

$$fitness() = \begin{cases} \dfrac{\%TP}{\%FP} & if \quad \%VP \geq threshold \\ \\ 0 & otherwise \end{cases} \qquad \text{Eq. 3}$$

Regarding the variables used, 4 types of different data sets have been created:

1) MoM: comprises three variables: age of the mother, and AFP MoM and hCG MoM markers.
2) 4var: Includes 4 variables: maternal age, weight of the mother, and the markers AFP and hCG.
3) 5var: comprises 5 variables: age of the mother, mother's weight, gestational age of the fetus, and the markers AFP and hCG.
4) 8var: Includes 8 variables: age of the mother, mother's weight, gestational age of the fetus, degree of alcohol and cigarettes usually consumed, presence of diabetes in the mother, and the markers AFP and hCG.

The best results obtained by using the FLAGID method are shown in Table 5. The data used corresponds to the datasets Down_3109 and Down_818, since they have a cutting level of 1:250 (remember what was mentioned above: the first datasets have less noise than the second one, Down_4995 in this case, and for better comparing the age/LR standard results with the FLAGID results, it is better to use the first datasets). The training data is the 70% of the Down_3109 dataset, and the test data is the remaining 30% plus the Down_818 dataset.

The resulting dataset has a total of 1750 patterns, with 1744 positives and 6 negatives. Thus, Table 5 shows that the results are very good, generally improving the age/LR method, especially for the *5var* dataset.

Once good results were obtained by using a dataset without noise, it was also necessary to use the Down_4995 (noisy) dataset. To do these tests, FLAGID worked with all three datasets, using them as training datasets in several executions.

Table 5. Summary of the test results training with 70% of Down_3109 dataset, and taking its 30% of cases and the Down_818 dataset to perform the test

Dataset	TP	TN	FP	FN	%TP	%FP	Fitness (%TP/%FP)
MoM	5	1669	75	1	83.33%	4.30%	19.38
4var	3	1699	45	3	50.00%	2.58%	19.38
5var	6	1679	66	0	100.00%	3.78%	26.44
8var	4	1696	49	2	66.67%	2.81%	23.74

The Fuzzy System solution must have a successful test and must be stable. That is, should not have high variations in the results of a test to another, to simulate as closely as possible how it will behave with future data.

Taking the best result shown in Table 5, the test with Down_4995 gives a result of TP=60% and FP=3.98%, making a total of TP and FP = 60% = 3.93%. Similar results are obtained by joining all the data, shuffle it, and perform the train/test several times, as cross-validation does. In this case, cross-validation train/test method was not performed due to the small quantity of case of the minor-class.

In conclusion, this result does not improve the FN rate, but yes the FP one.

Finally, the Fuzzy System solution found is a 10 rules Fuzzy System (8 belonging to the major-class and 2 belonging to the minor-class), taking the 5 input variables: age and weight of the mother, gestational age of the fetus, and the markers AFP and hCG.

Conclusion

In this chapter has been presented a new method that finds a better solution, in terms of false positives, than the existing one, for the early detection of Down syndrome for the second trimester of pregnancy. The method, called FLAGID (Fuzzy Logic and Genetic Algorithms for Imbalanced Datasets) is a Fuzzy System built from a dataset of two classes and has the characteristic of being imbalanced, meaning that one class has many more cases than the other one.

The FLAGID method is based on taking profit of the good results provided by the clustering algorithm DDA/RecBF, to obtain a first set of the membership functions of the Fuzzy Variables, which are then transformed by another algorithm presented in this paper, called ReRecBF. Once the Fuzzy Variables are defined, only is needed to find the Fuzzy Rules. A Genetic Algorithm (GA) is in charge of this task, by using the Fuzzy Variables found by ReRecBF and the dataset.

This chapter contributes to the field of medicine in the fact that it has found a new set of variables, different from those used so far (were age of the mother and 2 MoM). The package is composed of 5 variables: the mother's age and weight, gestational age of the fetus and the two markers hormone hCG and AFP, without applying any MoM processing. This is the first time that the False Positives rate lowered the threshold of 5%, in this case between 1%-2%, maintaining a minimum of 60%-70% of True Positives detection. The only change applied was to truncate over the values of hCG and AFP to facilitate the learning. So, the FLAGID method does not improve the success of TP rate, but reduced the rate of FP.

In addition, the medical staff confirmed that the rules were understood, confirming that the FLAGID method extracts intelligible information from the dataset, expressed in a Fuzzy System. This information is expressed in a small number of rules (10 rules: 8 positives and 2 negatives). This fact means that the rules are not specialized in cases of the minor-class, but they are distributed among both classes. This was one of the goals to be achieved by the method.

References

[1] Japkowicz N.; S. Stephen. (2002). The Class Imbalance Problem: A Systematic Study, *Intelligent Data Analysis*, Volume 6, Number 5, pp. 429-450.

[2] Berthold M.; K.P. Huber. (1999). "Constructing Fuzzy Graphs from Examples", *Intelligent Data Analysis*, 3, pp. 37-53.

[3] Cuckle HS; Wald NJ; Thompson SG. (1987). Estimating a woman's risk of having a pregnancy associated with Down's syndrome using her age and serum alpha fetoprotein level. *Br J Obstet Gynaecol*;94:387-2.

[4] Goldberg, D.E. (1989). *Genetic Algorithms in Search, Optimization, and Machine Learning*. Addison-Wesley.

[5] Norgaard-Pedersen, L. et al. (1990). *Maternal serum markers in screening for Down syndrome*.

[6] Sabrià, J. (1998). Screening bioquímico del segundo trimestre. Nuestra experiencia, *Progresos en Diagnóstico Prenatal*, vol. 10, nº 4, pag.147-153.

[7] SsdwLab: Software from SbpSoftware. Available from: http://www.sbpsoftware.com/

[8] Soler, V.; Roig, J.; Prim, M. (2006). Adapting Fuzzy Points for Very-Imbalanced Datasets. *NAFIPS*. Conference.

[9] Soler, V.; Roig, J.; Prim, M. (2002). Finding Exceptions to Rules in Fuzzy Rule Extraction. *KES, Knowledge-based Intelligent Information Engineering Systems*, Part 2, pp.1115-1119.

[10] Sordo M. (1995). *Neural Nets for Detection of Down's Syndrome*. MSc Thesis, Department of Artificial Intelligence, University of Edinburgh, UK.

[11] Zadeh L.A. (1965). *Fuzzy Sets. Information Control*, p. 338-353.

In: Handbook of Down Syndrome Research
Editors: Dominicus Jelinek and Gijs Dvorak

ISBN 978-1-60741- 690-6

Chapter 15

The Influence of Oromotor Functions and Diet Consistency on Caries Experience and Growth Rate in Cerebral Palsied Individuals

Maria Teresa Botti Rodrigues Santos[a], Maria Cristina Duarte Ferreira[b], Paula Celiberti[c], and Renata Oliveira Guare[a]

[a]Discipline of Dentistry, Persons with Disabilities Division, Post Graduation Professor, Universidade Cruzeiro do Sul, São Paulo, Brazil.
[b]Universidade Paulista (UNIP), São Paulo, Brazil
[C]Department of Orthodontics and Pediatric Dentistry, School of Dentistry, University of São Paulo (USP), São Paulo, Brazil

Introduction

Cerebral palsy (CP) describes a group of movement and posture development disorders attributed to non-progressive disturbances in the developing fetal or infant brain, causing activity limitations and being the most common cause of severe physical disability in childhood. The motor disorders of CP are often accompanied by disturbances of sensation, cognition, communication, perception, behavior, and seizure disorders.[1]

Oromotor dysfunction and oral-ingestive problems, as uncoordinated control mechanisms of orofacial and palatolingual musculatures [2], are often observed in CP individuals, and varies from mild to severe.[3] These disabilities are expressed by drooling, coughing, choking, rejection of solid food, food loss, and spillage during eating. Difficulties in spoon-feeding, biting, chewing, cup drinking, straw drinking, swallowing and clearing are also observed.[2]

Another nutritional issue to be considered is the common inability of severely oromotor impaired CP individuals to ingest solid food, which often leads to an exclusively liquid or semi-solid diet. In spite of contributing to some degree to growth and nutritional disturbances, especially at an early age, food consistency may also cause a significant impact on oral health. Therefore, a timely nutritional rehabilitation and preventive measures in oral health may significantly improve the quality of life of these individuals,[4-6] as well as prevent deleterious and noxious habits such as bottle feeding. Performing an adequate oral hygiene on CP individuals however, can be a very difficult task for the caregivers, due to the patient's persistent pathological biting reflex[7]

Food consistency, sugared beverages, and long term oral medicines [4,8], associated with oromotor dysfunction and oral hygiene difficulties, may explain the high incidence of caries and periodontal diseases exhibited by the CP population.[9-13]

The influence of oromotor impairment in CP individuals as a risk factor in caries experience was not studied yet. Therefore, this study aimed at evaluating the influence of oral motricity and diet consistency on caries experience and growth rate in CP individuals.

Material and Methods

Subject's Selection

A group of 78 non-institutionalized CP individuals of both genders, aged 4 to 14 years old (9.5±2.3), living in Sao Paulo - Brazil (0.7 mg/L F- in water supply), and attending the Special Children's Elementary School of Lar Escola São Francisco – Rehabilitation Center (Federal University of Sao Paulo, Brazil) were enrolled in this study. The main inclusion criterion was the CP medical diagnosis.

This study was approved by the Ethics in Human Research Committee of the Federal University of Sao Paulo School of Medicine, Brazil. After receiving detailed explanations about the study and agreeing to participate, a written consent for participation and publication of data was obtained from the adult responsible for each CP individual.

Patient medical records were reviewed for demographic and clinical data, including gender, age, type of movement disorder (spastic, dystonic, with athetosis or with ataxia, or a mixture of these disorders), clinical patterns of involvement (quadriplegia, diplegia, hemiplegia or double hemiplegia), and severity of CP. By means of Gross Motor Function Classification System (GMFCS), CP severity was measured and allocated in levels (I-V14), where each level indicates:

- level I: walking without restrictions, but with limitations in more advanced gross motor skills;
- level II: walking without assistive devices, but with limitations walking outdoors and in the community;
- level III: walking with assistive mobility devices, and with limitations walking outdoors and in the community;
- level IV: self-mobility with limitations. The patient is transported or uses a power mobility outdoors and in the community;
- level V: severely limited self-mobility, even with assistive technology.

Orofacial Motor Function Assessment

The assessment of individuals' orofacial motor functions was carried out by one examiner according to the Orofacial Motor Function Assessment Scale (OFMFAS).15 For OFMFAS assessment, individuals were positioned in the best sitting position, in a ventilated room, with trunk and pelvis aligned and without hip hyperextension. The shoulder girdle was kept forward, with abduction of the scapulae and the cervical spine elongated.

Guidelines of the Orofacial Motor Function Assessment Scale

The oral motor evaluation involves assessment of oral posture and movements. The guidelines of the OFMFAS are consisted of 13 items considered important criteria for the assessment of oral-facial motor function in CP individuals. Each sub-item can be rated using a Likert scale ranging from 0 (unable to perform or determine, inconsistent) to 2 (adequately performed).

Items 1 to 12 assess voluntary movements, i.e., response to a verbal command. Item 13 involves the assessment of oral reflexes, such as suckle, tonic bite, gag, and rooting, which are stimulated by the examiner's forefinger. These items are presented in Table 1.

During the assessment of all voluntary tasks, the examiner stimulated the individuals by performing all movements and showing the individuals how they should be performed. The examiner must be positioned opposite to the patient and should perform each movement at least three times, consecutively.

Table 1. Items of the OFMFAS

1. Jaw mobility Subtotal:
a) voluntary jaw opening ☐ yes = 2 ☐ no = 0 ☐ unable to determine = 0 b) jaw opening ☐ midline = 2 ☐ right / left deviation = 1 ☐ inconsistent = 0 c) open against resistance ☐ normal / adequate = 2 ☐ weak = 1 ☐ unable to determine = 0 d) close against resistance ☐ normal / adequate = 2 ☐ weak = 1 ☐ unable to determine = 0
2. Voluntary jaw protrusion Subtotal:
a) ☐ yes = 2 ☐ no = 0 ☐ unable to determine = 0 b) ☐ midline = 2 ☐ right / left deviation = 1 ☐ inconsistent = 0

3. Voluntary lateral jaw movements Subtotal:

a) right
☐ yes = 2 ☐ no = 0 ☐ unable to determine = 0
b) left
☐ yes = 2 ☐ no = 0 ☐ unable to determine = 0
c) presence involuntary jaw movements during jaw lateral movements
☐ yes = 0 ☐ no = 2

4. Rapid coordinated jaw movements Subtotal:

a) tooth tap
☐ present = 2 ☐ slow/ slows with time/ irregular/ erratic = 1 ☐ unable P/D = 0
b) excursion jaw lateral
☐ present = 2 ☐ slow/ slows with time/ irregular/ erratic = 1 ☐ unable P/D = 0

5. Voluntary facial movements Subtotal:

a) show teeth
☐ symmetrical = 2 ☐ right/ left weakness = 1 ☐ unable P/D = 0
b) pucker lips
☐ symmetrical = 2 ☐ right/ left weakness = 1 ☐ unable P/D = 0

6. Lip muscle strength: puff-out cheeks/maintain pressure Subtotal:

☐ present and strong = 2 ☐ present and weak = 1 ☐ unable P/D = 0

7. Rapid coordinated lip movements Subtotal:

a) protrusion/retraction of lips
☐ present = 2 ☐ slow/ slows with time/ irregular/ erratic = 1 ☐ unable P/D = 0
b) pa-pa-pa-pa-pa-pa
☐ present = 2 ☐ slow/ slows with time/ irregular/ erratic = 1 ☐ unable P/D = 0

8. Glossopharyngeal and vagal motor activity Subtotal:

ah!
☐ symmetrical = 2 ☐ right/ left weakness = 1 ☐ unable P/D= 0

9. Rapid coordinated palatal movements Subtotal:

mm-bah, mm-bah
☐ adequate = 2 ☐ poor = 1 ☐ unable P/D= 0

10. Hypoglossal motor: voluntary tongue movements Subtotal:

tongue protrusion
a) ☐ yes = 2 ☐ no = 0 ☐ unable to determine = 0
b) ☐ midline = 2 ☐ right/left deviation = 1 ☐ inconsistent = 0

11. Voluntary elevation and lateralization of tongue Subtotal:
a) back incisors = ttt ☐ yes = 2 ☐ no = 0 ☐ unable to determine = 0 b) back soft palate = ing ☐ yes = 2 ☐ no = 0 ☐ unable to determine = 0 c) right corner mouth ☐ yes = 2 ☐ no = 0 ☐ unable to determine = 0 d) left corner mouth ☐ yes = 2 ☐ no = 0 ☐ unable to determine = 0
12. Rapid coordinated movements of tongue Subtotal:
a) t-t-t-t-t ☐ present = 2 ☐ rhythm slows with time/ erratic = 1 ☐ unable P/D = 0 b) k-k-k-k-k ☐ present = 2 ☐ rhythm slows with time/ erratic = 1 ☐ unable P/D = 0
13. Oral abnormal reflexes Subtotal:
a) suckle ☐ present = 0 ☐ absent = 2 a) tonic bite ☐ present = 0 ☐ absent = 2 a) gag ☐ present = 0 ☐ absent = 2 a) rooting ☐ present = 0 ☐ absent = 2
TOTAL:
* P/D = perform or determine

Item 1: Jaw Mobility Evaluation

In order to evaluate individuals' ability to coordinate the movements of their jaw, individuals are asked to voluntarily open their mouth (sub-item a). When the movement is performed adequately, score 2 is given to this sub-item (Figure 1). When individuals are unable to perform the task, or when the examiner is unable to determine whether individuals do not understand the oral command (concerning a cognitive deficiency *or* mental retardation), the sub-item is marked with score 0. During jaw opening (sub-item b), the examiner must observe whether it is performed in the midline (score 2) or with right/left deviation (score 1).

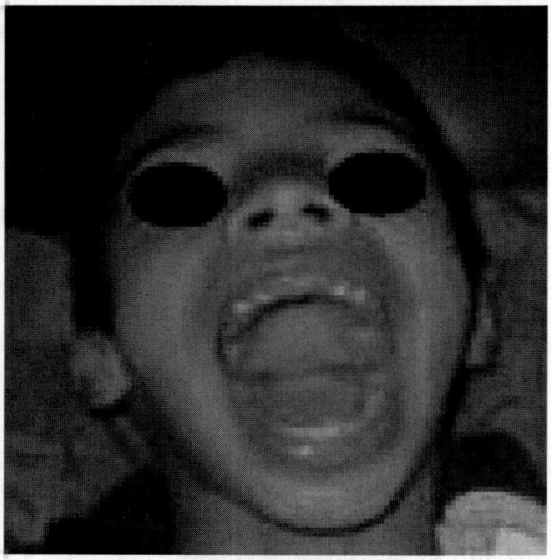

Figure 1. Evaluation of jaw mobility during opening movement.

The score is recorded as inconsistent when lateral movements are made in an uncoordinated form during mouth opening, or when individuals are unable to perform the task.

In order to test the ability to open (sub-item c) and close (sub-item d) the mouth against resistance, the examiner position one hand on the top of the individual's head and the other hand is positioned with the thumb under the chin (open movement) or with the forefinger between the dental arches (close movement), creating a light resistance against the movement tested (Figure 2). According to the individuals' ability to open and close the mouth, Score 2 is given when the movements against resistance is performed adequately, score 1 when it is performed weakly, and score 0 when it is difficult to know whether individuals do not understand the oral command or are unable to perform the task.

Item 2: Jaw Protrusion

Individuals are asked to make a protrusive jaw movement, (Figure 3) (sub-item a). A light forefinger stimulus can be applied to the chin to encourage the individual to accomplish the movement. If the lower dental arch protrudes beyond upper dental arch, score 2 is given. When individuals cannot perform the protrusion, or when the examiner cannot determine whether individuals do not want to or do not know how to do perform the task (unable to determine), the score is recorded as 0. During the movement (sub-item b), it must be observed if the task is performed in the midline (score 2) or with right/left deviation (score 1). The task is recorded as inconsistent when individuals alternate midline and deviated jaw protrusive movements or are unable to perform them.

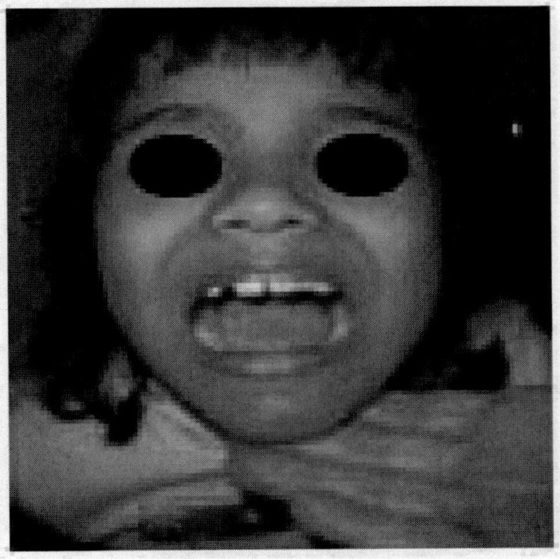

Figure 2. Evaluation of jaw mobility during opening against resistance.

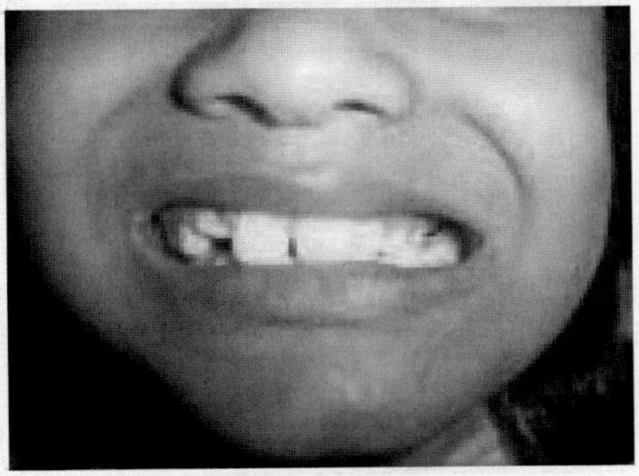

Figure 3. Evaluation of jaw mobility during protrusive movement.

Item 3: Lateral Jaw Movements

Individuals are asked to move the jaw from the midline to the right (sub-item a) and back, and from the midline to the left and back (sub-item b) (Figure 4). In order to encourage individuals, a light forefinger stimulus can be applied to the cheek, on the opposite side of the movement tested. Score 2 is registered when lower midline is deviated to the right (right jaw lateral movement) or the left (left jaw lateral movement). When individuals cannot perform lateral movements, or when the examiner cannot determine whether the patient does not want to or does not know how to do the task, score 0 is given. The observation of involuntary movements (sub-item c) during jaw lateral movements is scored as 0 (yes) or 2 (no).

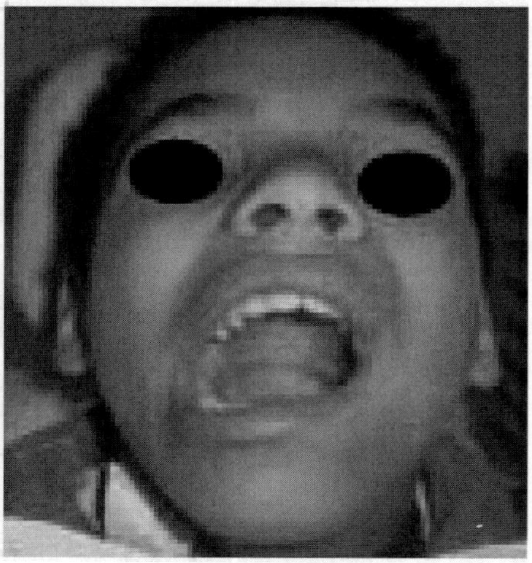

Figure 4. Evaluation of jaw mobility during lateral movements.

Item 4: Rapid Coordinated Jaw Movements

To evaluate individuals ability to perform rapid and coordinated movements (sub-item a), the examiner must ask them to tap their teeth in rhythmic and coordinated movements for at least five seconds. When individuals are able to perform the movement, maintaining the rhythm, the score is recorded as 2. When, individuals are able to do only a few slow rhythmic taps before stopping, present a rhythm that slows with time, or if the taps are irregular, erratic, and without rhythm, the score is recorded as 1. The inability to determine whether individuals do not want to or do not know how to perform the task is scored as 0.

To evaluate the ability to perform excursion jaw lateral movements (item b), individuals are asked to perform side-to-side movements in a continuous way. The item is scored as 2 when the movements are adequately performed. When individuals are able to perform only a few slow rhythmic movements before stopping, with a rhythm that slows with time, or if the movements are irregular, erratic, or without rhythm, the item is scored as 1. The inability to determine whether individuals do not want to or do not know how to perform the task is scored as 0.

Item 5: Voluntary facial movements

The voluntary facial movements are tested by asking individuals to smile (Figure 5), show the teeth as in a grin (sub item a), and pucker the lips as in sending kisses (sub item b) (Figure 6). For both conditions, score 2 is registered when facial movements are symmetrical and score 1 when the movements observed present lateral deviation or have a weak result. The inability to determine whether individuals do not want to or do not know how to perform the task is scored as 0.

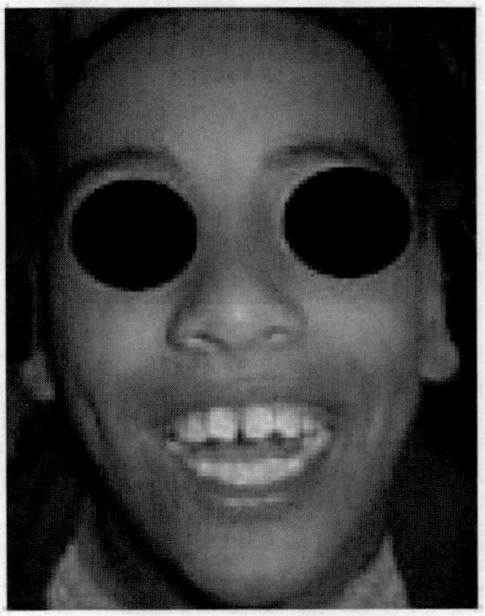

Figure 5. Evaluation of voluntary facial movements (showing the teeth).

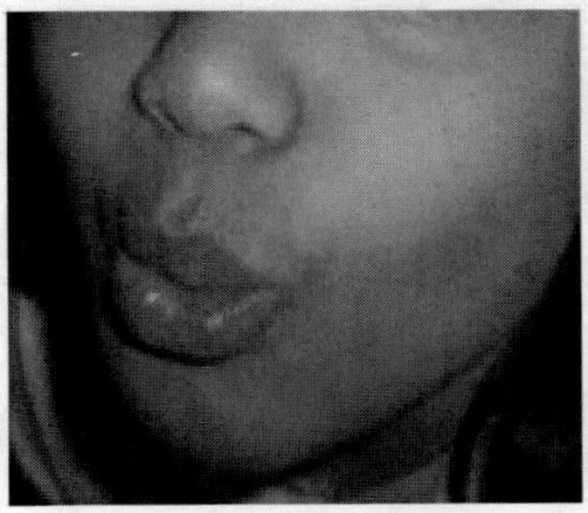

Figure 6. Evaluation during puckering the lips, as in sending kisses.

Item 6: Lip Muscle Strength

In order to test lip muscle strength, individuals are asked to inflate the cheeks and keep the air inside the mouth with sealed lips for a few seconds (Figure 7). The score is recorded as 2 when individuals are able to maintain cheeks inflated strongly, 1 when the task is performed weakly, and 0 when the examiner does not know whether individuals do not want to or do not know how to perform the task.

Item 7: Rapid Coordinated Lip Movements

In this sub-item, individuals are asked to perform rapid coordinated lip movements, with a protrusion/retraction of lips, i.e. from smile to pucker, consecutively. Afterwards (sub-item b) individuals are asked to say "pa-pa-pa-pa". For both sub-items the scores are the same as described in item 4.

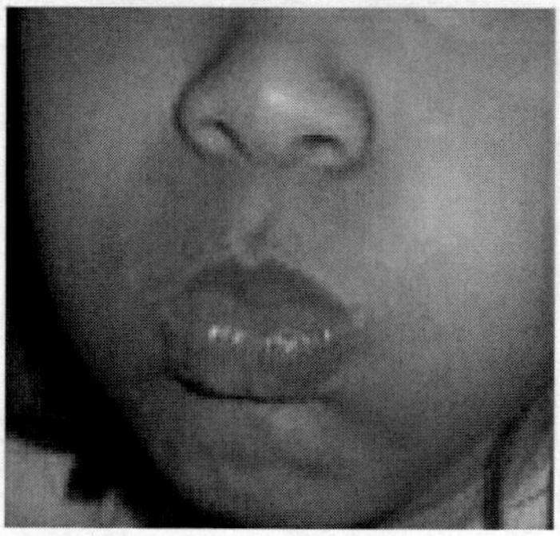

Figure 7. Evaluation of lip muscle strength by inflating cheeks and keeping the air inside the mouth with sealed lips.

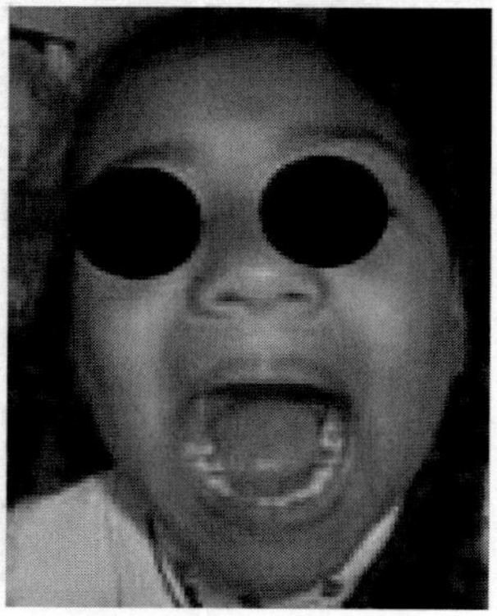

Figure 8. Evaluation of glossopharyngeal and vagal motor movements saying "ah".

Item 8: Glossopharyngeal And Vagal Motor

Individuals are asked to say "ah" in order to verify glossopharyngeal and vagal motor movements (Figure 8). Score 2 is registered when the examiner observes the soft palate elevation in a symmetrical way, score 1 when the elevation occurs in an asymmetrical or weak way, and 0 when the examiner is unable to know whether individuals do not want to or do not know how to perform the task.

Item 9: Rapid Coordinated Palatal Movements

Individuals are asked to repeat the sounds "mm-bah" in a continuously way, in order to verify the ability to perform rapid coordinated palatal movements. Score 2 is registered when individuals are able to perform the task adequately, 1 when individuals are able to perform in a poor way (when it is not possible to distinguish the sounds clearly), and 0 when the examiner is unable to know whether individuals do not want to or do not know how to perform the task.

Item 10: Hypoglossal Motor: Voluntary Tongue Movements

In order to test the ability to perform voluntary tongue movements, (sub-item a), individuals are asked to protrude the tongue (Figure 9). If they are able to perform the movement adequately, score 2 is registered. The protrusion in the midline (sub-item b) receives score 2, when movement is performed with right/left deviation, score 1 is given. On both sub-items, score 0 is registered when the examiner is unable to know whether individuals do not want to or do not know how to perform the task

Item 11: Voluntary Elevation and Lateralization of Tongue

Individuals' ability to voluntarily elevate and lateralize the tongue is evaluated by asking them to lift the tongue apex towards the palatal face of upper incisors (Figure 10) saying "t-t-t-t" (sub-item a), to lift the tongue apex and position it rewards in the direction of the soft palate saying "ing" (sub-item b), to position the tongue apex on right corner of the mouth (Figure 11a) (sub-item c) and finally to the left corner of the mouth (Figure 11 b) (sub-item d). For all tasks in this item, score 2 is registered for able to perform, and 0 for not performed or unable to determine.

Item 12: Rapid Coordinated Movements of Tongue

Individuals are asked to perform rapid and coordinated tongue movements performing the sounds "t-t-t-t" (sub-item a) and "k-k-k-k" (sub-item b) in a continuously and rhythmic way. Scores are the same as described for item 4.

Item 13: Abnormal Oral Reflexes

The evaluation of the presence or absence of oral reflexes is achieved by observing the individuals' reaction to stimuli. The rooting reflex is evaluated after a touch stimulus made by the examiner's forefinger above the upper lip, below the lower lip, and on labial comissura. The presence of this reflex is observed when the patient rotates the head towards the stimulus direction (Figure 12). For the suckle-swallow reflex, the forefinger is gently placed on the tongue apex. Its presence is confirmed when backward-forward tongue movements, such as suction movements, are observed (Figure 13). Biting is assessed by touching the buccal gum, near lower molars. An upward jaw movement into a strongly clenched posture is observed when the reflex is present, making it difficult for the patient to open the mouth (Figure 14).

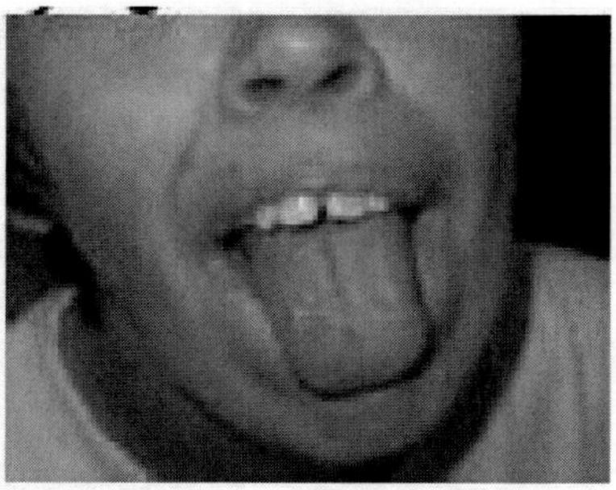

Figure 9. Evaluation of Hypoglossal motor voluntary tongue protrusive movements.

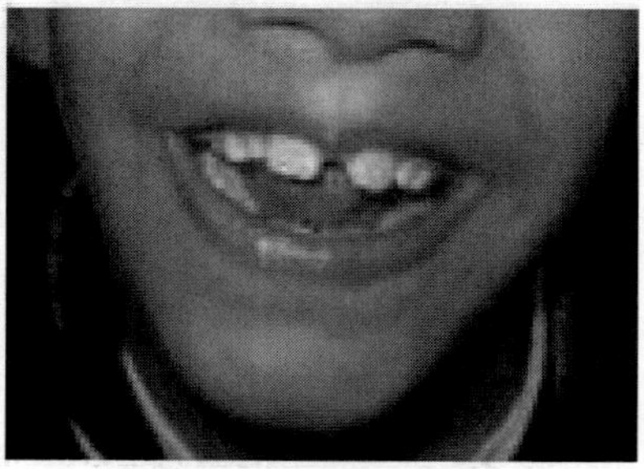

Figure 10. Evaluation of voluntary elevation of tongue.

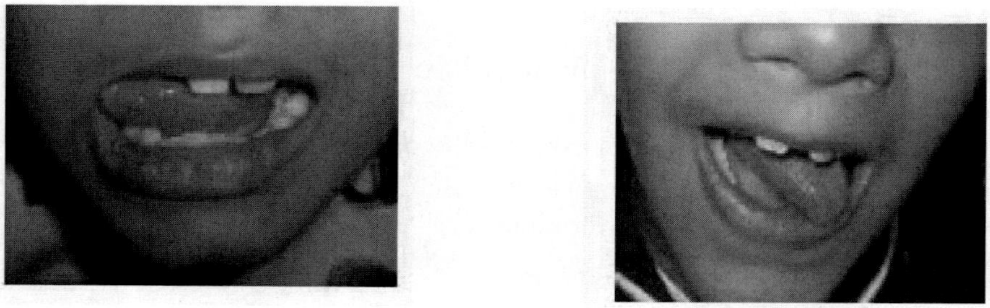

Figure11. Evaluation of voluntary lateralization of tongue to the right (11a) and left (11b).

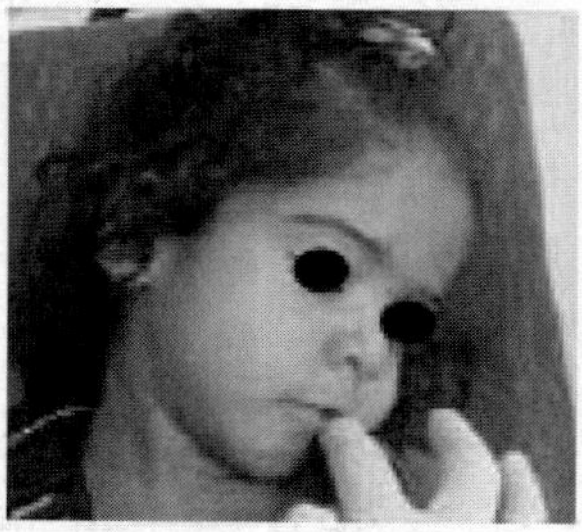

Figure 12. Evaluation of the rooting reflex.

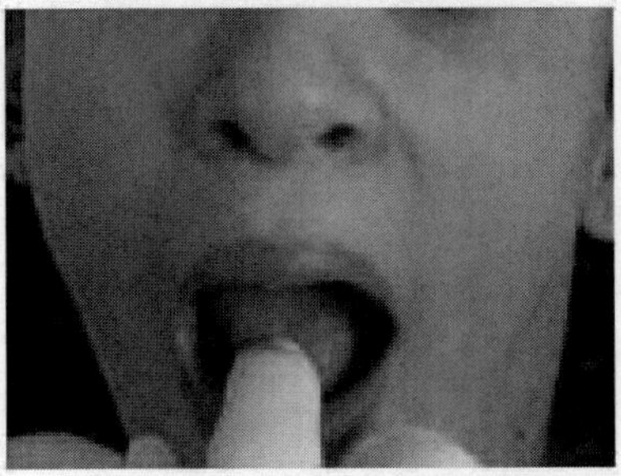

Figure 13. Evaluation of the suckle-swallow reflex.

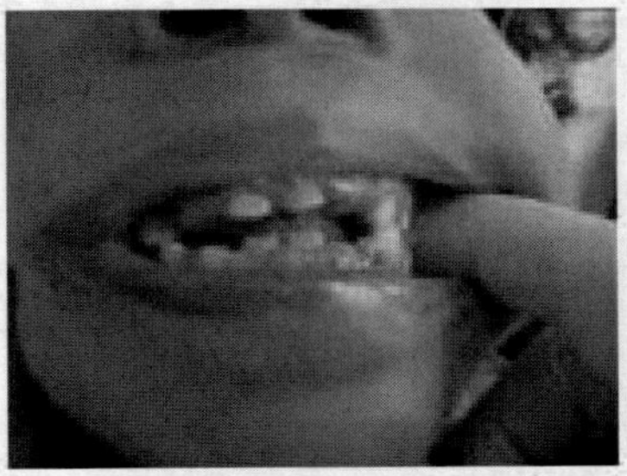

Figure 14. Evaluation of the biting reflex.

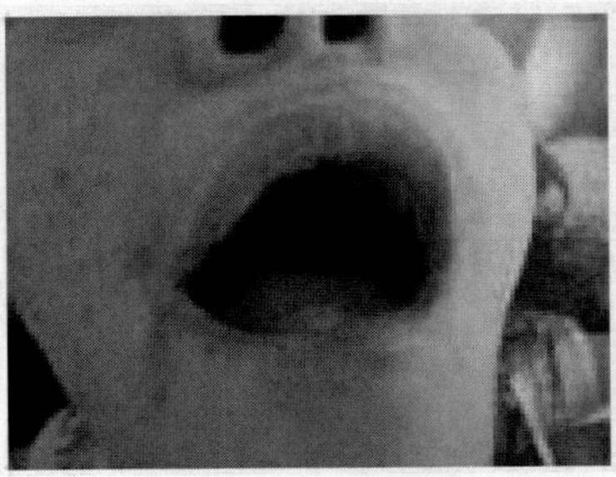

Figure 15. Evaluation of the gagging reflex.

The gagging reflex is tested through a touch that begins on the tongue apex moving rearward up to the tongue anterior 2/3. This reflex is present when the contraction of the oropharyngeal muscles is observed (Figure 15).

The individual's OFMFAS final score was obtained by adding all sub-item values. Individuals were then classified as severely impaired (1st quartile: score ≤19), moderately impaired (2nd quartile: score between 20 and 31), slightly impaired (3rd quartile: score between 32 and 41) or very slightly impaired (4th quartile: score ≥ 42).

Oral Health and Caries Experience Assessment

After receiving a new tooth brush and dentifrice, the caregivers were instructed how to perform oral hygiene correctly. Then, under supervision, each CP individual had their teeth brushed by the respective caregiver.

Afterwards, the air-dried teeth were submitted to visual and tactile examinations on a dental unit, under artificial illumination, with the use of a plane intra-oral mirror and a round-ended dental probe.

Oral health status assessment was performed by a trained and calibrated single examiner, according to standard procedures.[16] Caries experience was assessed using the DMFT/dmft index, for permanent and primary dentition, respectively (Figure 16). For children with mixed dentition, dmft and DMFT were recorded. Decayed teeth were assessed only at cavity threshold. Teeth exhibiting white spot lesions were, therefore, considered sound.

In order to evaluate the intra-examiner reproducibility, 10 random children were submitted to two subsequent examinations with a 7 day interval between them, and with no assess or knowledge of the CP individuals previous oral health status (Kappa=0.89). No radiographic examination was carried out.

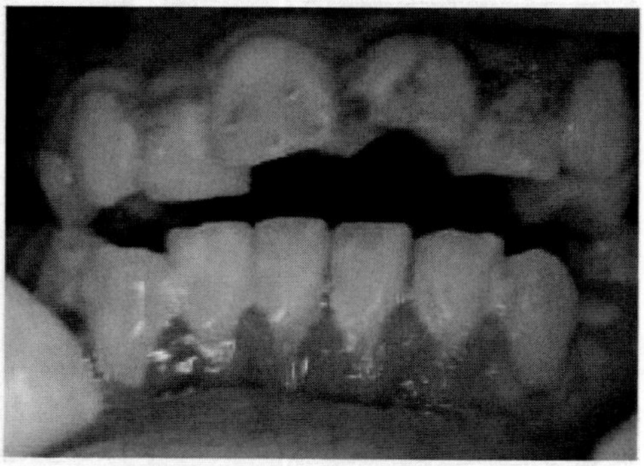

Figure 16. Intra-oral aspects of an individual with cerebral palsy.

Diet Consistency Assessment

CP individuals enrolled in this study were periodically controlled by speech therapists (Lar Escola São Francisco). These professionals, beyond other orientations to the caregivers, also prescribed the adequate diet consistency for each individual, based on their feeding difficulties, with the objective to avoid choking and food aspiration. Diet consistency was divided in 3 groups, as follows:

- Solid food: This food consistency is one normally offered to individuals with no severe oromotor dysfunction, and consisted of food in pieces, which needed to be chewed (Figure 17).

- Semi-solid food: Food with a paste-like consistency, but still presenting pieces of the smashed, kneaded or triturated foods. Cereals, vegetables, cookies or bread smashed with milk and triturated or finely pulled meat are examples of semi-solid food. (Figure 18).
- Liquid food: Food has to be homogeneous, smooth and without pieces. This consistency is obtained through mixing, beating, or blending food with the use of a mixer. Fruits, soups, and cooked vegetables and meat can be prepared like this, but afterwards, they have to be strained. Custards and yogurts are also indicated (Figure 19).

In order to assess the consistency of the CP individuals diet, the caregivers were asked which of the 3 consistencies were prescribed by the speech therapist and if they were in accordance to the real dietary habits of these individuals.

Growth Rate

Growth rate was assessed through the measurement of weight and height. Individuals were weighted on a digital scale in a thin layer of clothing and dry diaper or underwear (Figure 20).

Due to CP individuals' difficulties on standing straight, height was measured through the knee segment length *KH* (Figure 21) and the estimation of stature (S) were determined from segmental measures in the equation:

Knee height (KH in cm): $S = 2.69 \times (KH) + 24.2cm$ [17]

The results were compared to CP growth curves[18] on the P10, P25, P50, P75, and P90 percentiles for height and weight, according to age and gender (Figures 22, 23, 24 and 25).

For statistical analyses Chi square, Fisher exact, Kruskall-Wallis and Dunn tests were used. The significance level was set at $p<0.05$.

Results

Regarding the Gross Motor Function Classification System, from the 78 CP individuals enrolled in this study, 4 (5.1%) presented GMFCS level I, 2 (2.6%) presented level II, 6 (7.7%) presented level III, 44 (56.4%) presented level IV, and 22 (28.2%) level V of GMFCS.

Concerning the type of movement disorder, 64 individuals (82.1%) presented spastic CP, 13 (16.6%) presented dystonic CP with athetosis and 1 (1.3%) presented ataxia. About the clinical patterns of involvement, quadriplegic CP was present in 36 (46.2%) of the patients, diplegia was found in 25 (32.1%) of the patients and hemiplegia in 3 (3.8%) of them.

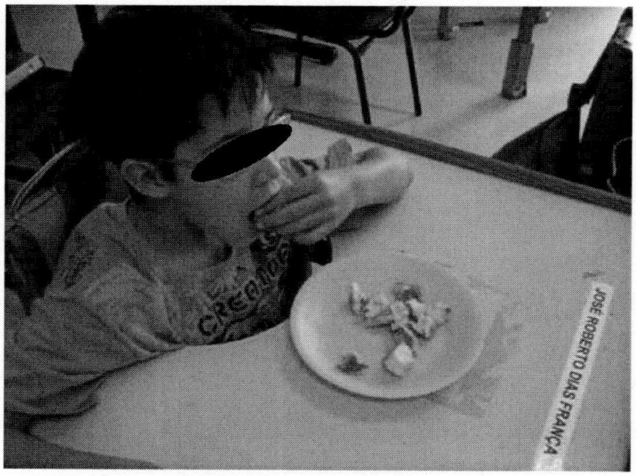

Figure 17. Solid food.

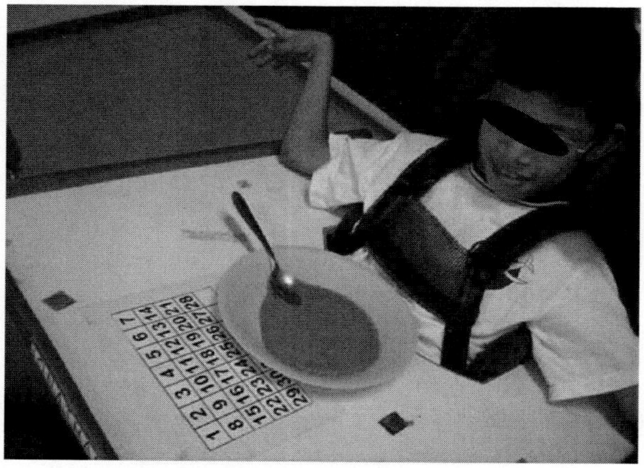

Figure 18. Semi-solid food

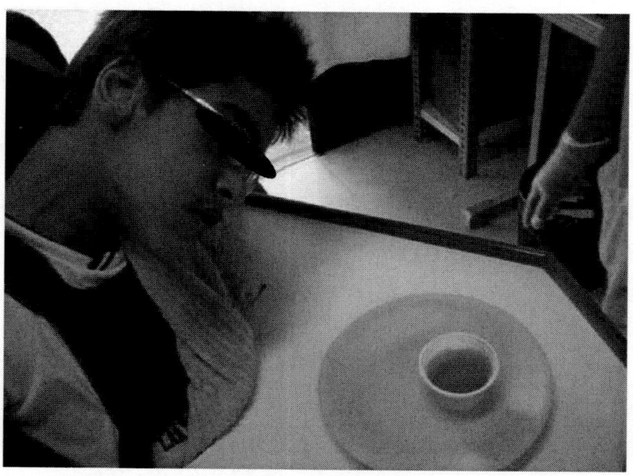

Figure 19. Liquid food

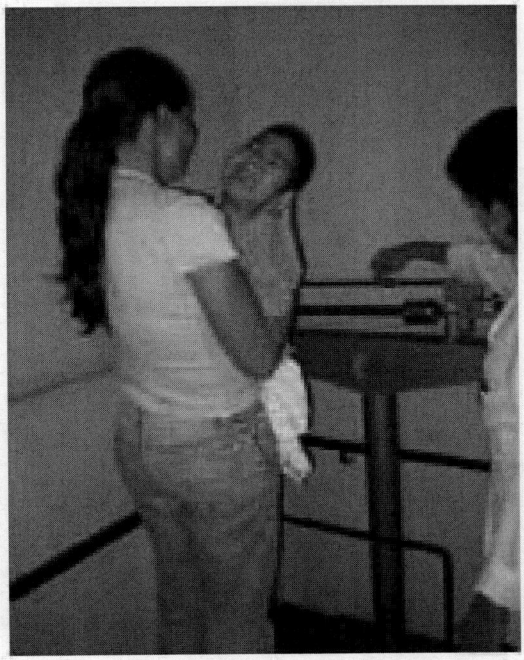

Figure 20. Weight measured with the CP individual being carried by the caregiver.

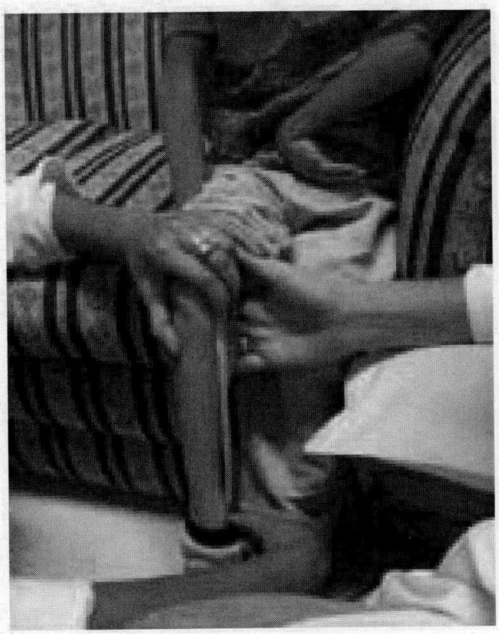

Figure 21. Height measured using the knee segment length.

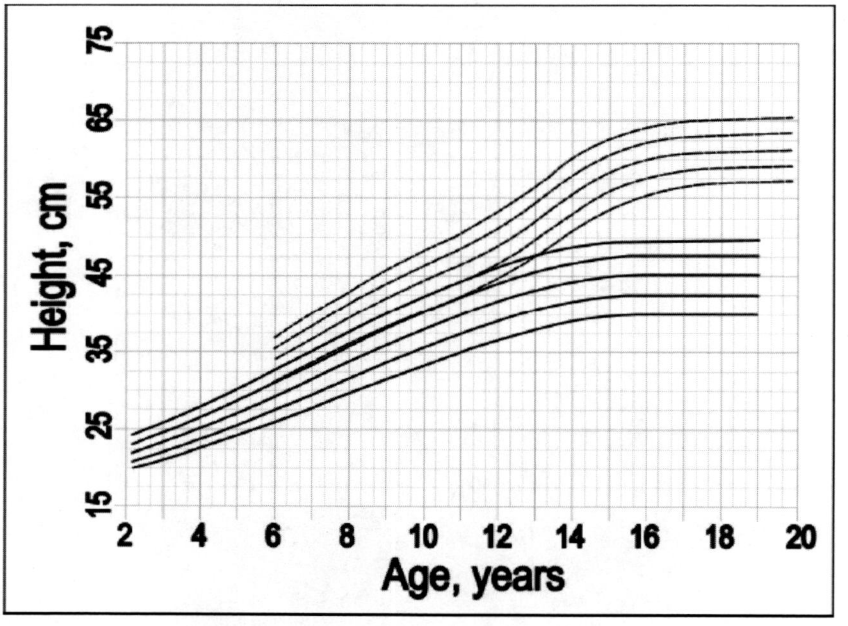

Figure 22. Height for CP girls ( ) and healthy girls (-------), according to Stevenson et al. [17]

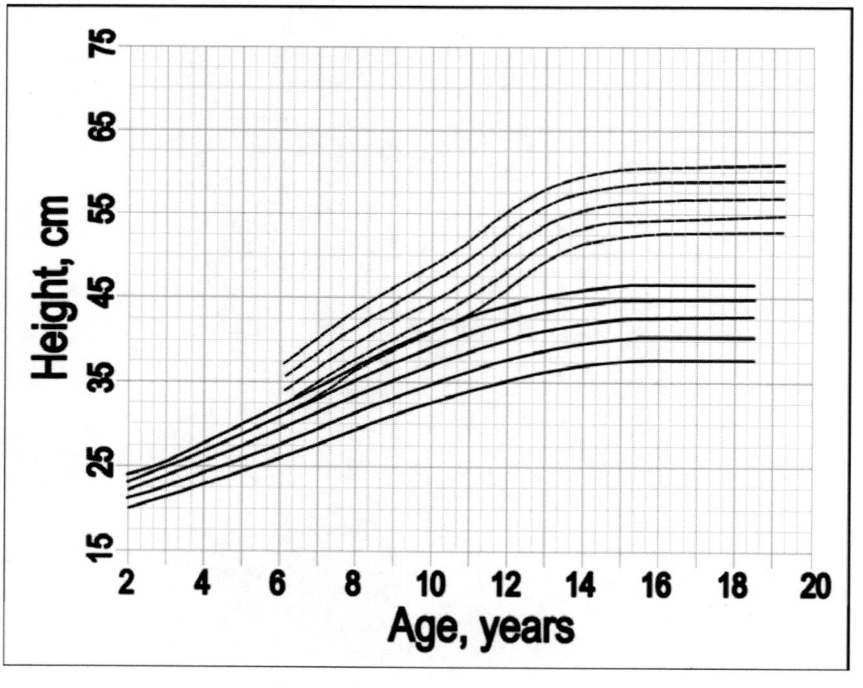

Figure 23. Height for CP boys ( ) and healthy boys (-------), according to Stevenson et al. [17]

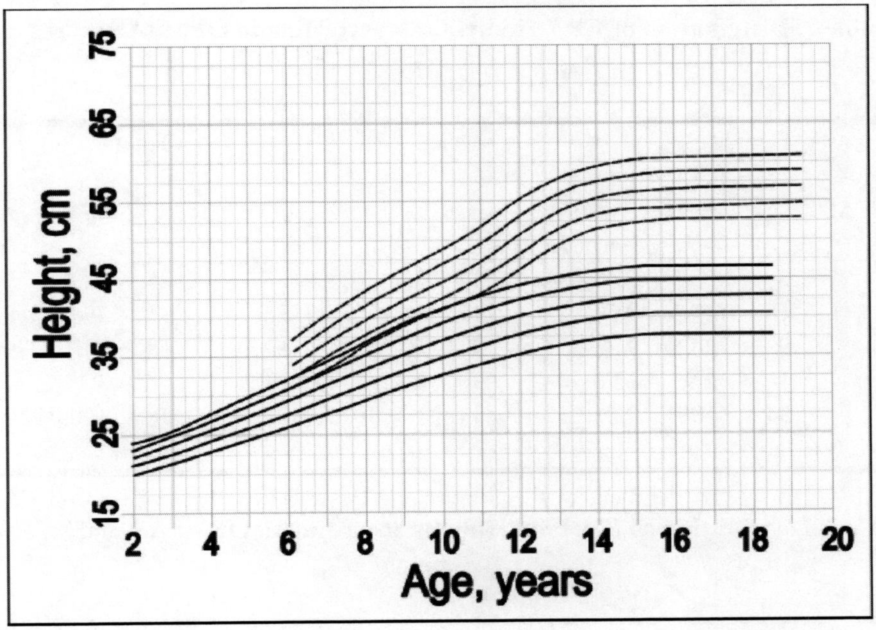

Figure 24. Weight for CP girls ( ) and healthy girls (-------), according to Stevenson et al. [17]

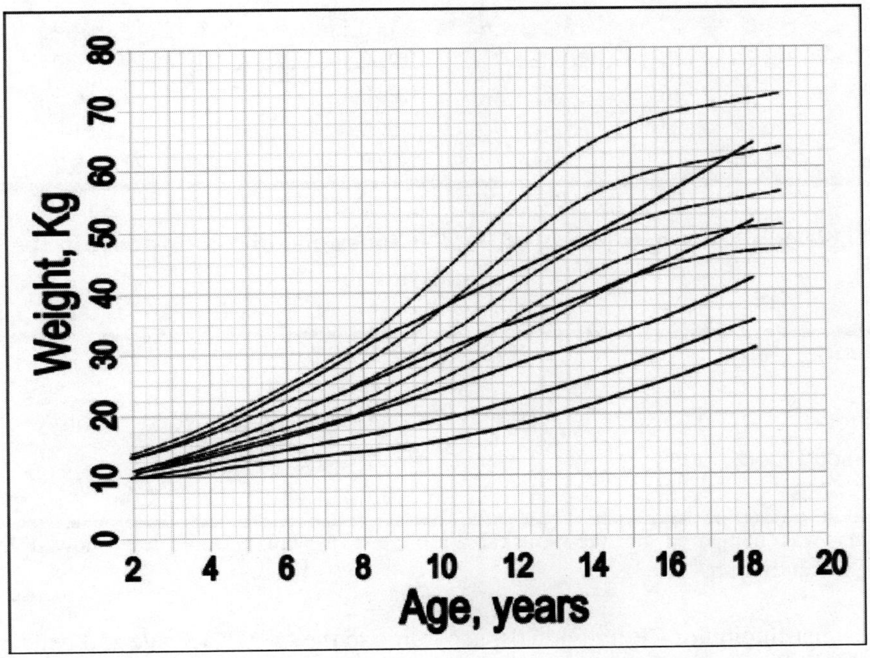

Figure 25. Weight for CP boys ( ) and healthy boys (-------), according to Stevenson et al. [17]

Table 2. Distribution of CP 78 individuals according to OFMFAS scores, age and gender

	Female			Male			Total		
OFMFAS	n	%	Age (mean±SD)	n	%	Age (mean ±SD)	n	%	Age (mean±SD)
I	8	23.5	9.4±2.3	17	38.6	9.6±2.7	25	32.1	9.5±2.5
II	16	47.1	9.5±2.2	15	34.1	8.3±2.0	31	39.7	8.9±2.1
III	9	26.5	9.3±2.1	9	20.5	10.1±2.4	18	23.1	9.7±2.2
IV	1	2.9	12.0±.0	3	6.8	12.0±1.7	4	5.1	12.0 ±1.4
Total	34	100.0	9.5±2.1	44	100.0	9.4±2.5	78	100.0	9.5±2.3

Table 3. Distribution of 78 CP individuals according to OFMFAS scores, weight and height

	Female				Male			
OFMFAS	n	%	Weight	Height	n	%	Weight	Height
I	8	23.5	18.4 ± 4.6	1.1±0.1	17	38.6	17.0±4.4	1.1±0.1
II	16	47.1	20.0±5.7	1.2±0.1	15	34.1	19.8±6.9	1.1±0.1
III	9	26.5	25.7±4.8	1.2±0.1	9	20.5	25.6±6.1	1.2±0.1
IV	1	2.9	35.6±0.0	1.5±0.0	3	6.8	36.9±14.5	1.3±0.1
Total	34	100.0	21.6±6.2	1.2±0.1	44	100.0	21.1±8.2	1.1±0.1

Table 4. Mean scores [± SD] of DMF-T index and diet consistence of the 78 CP individuals

Diet consistency	n	DMFT (mean ±SD	P
Solid food	21	1.5±1.9 [a]	0.0053*
Semi-solid food	23	2.9±2.4 [b]	
Liquid food	34	3.6±2.2 [c]	

The data was compared by the Kruskal-Wallis test *$P<0.05$. Dunn test showed that [a] differs significantly from [b] and [c].

The distribution of CP individuals, according to the OFMFAS, age and gender are shown in Table 2. The sample was shown to be homogenous regarding gender ($p=0.701$).

Considering oromotor function and gender, 23.5% of female (F) individuals and 38.6% of male (M) were found to be severely impaired, 47.1%F and 34.1%M moderately impaired, 26.5%F and 20.5%M slightly impaired, and 2.9%F and 6.8%M very slightly impaired.

The distribution of CP individuals, according to the OFMFAS scores, weight and height are shown in Table 3.

Oromotor function was found to be a statistically significant factor on CP individuals' weight and height ($p<0.05$) when compared to CP growth curves18 on the P10, P25, P50, P75, and P90 percentiles. Severely and moderately impaired individuals exhibited the P10 and P25 percentiles more frequently than slightly and very slightly impaired ones.

The distribution of the CP individuals according to diet consistency and DMFT index is shown in Table 4.

The Kruskal-Wallis test demonstrated a statistically significant difference on total DMFT values ($p=0.0053$) and diet consistency (Table 4). The Dunn test verified that individuals on solid food diet intake presented statistically significantly the lowest DMFT ($p<0.05$) compared to the ones on a semi-solid and a liquid food diet intake.

Oral motricity was shown to be significantly associated with weight and stature in both genders ($p<0.05$), presenting the severely and moderately impaired groups a greater number of cases on the P10 and P25 percentiles, when compared with the CP growth curves[18] on the P10, P25, P50, P75 and P90 percentiles for height and weight, according to age and gender.

Discussion

Understanding the impact of oromotor dysfunction, and its consequences, on oral health status, may be helpful in identifying individuals at high risk of developing dental caries and for planning preventive strategies and dental treatment for these individuals.

The sample of this study included CP individuals of both genders, attending the Special Children's Elementary School of Lar Escola São Francisco – Rehabilitation Center, and aged 4 to 14 years old (9.5±2.3). The eligibility criterion for students was that they should not have a cognitive deficit higher than 3 years of their chronological age, independently of global motor deficit. According to chronological limits established by the school, the students up to 4 years old were not evaluated.

In relation to gender, the male/female ratio found was of 1.3:1. Similar results were observed by Kiely et al.[19], in which the ratio found was of 1.4:1. Despite the greater prevalence of male gender observed in this study, when OFMFAS was considered, severely and moderately impaired individuals (I and II) were found similarly in both genders (72.7% e 70.6%).

It was observed for both genders that individuals with OFMFAS I and II presented the lower corporal weight values. This data suggests that the severity observed in OFMFAS evaluation may be helpful in reflecting the low weight in relation to age. This information can be of great value when patients need to be medicated according to their corporal weight, as when local anesthesia, antibiotics, analgesics and anti-inflammatories are needed. In severely compromised CP children, this must be respected in order to achieve an adequate dosage in these patients.

The direct measures of the stature are not possible in the majority of CP individuals due to the presence of contractions, articular deformities, scoliosis and involuntary movements.[20] The use of the shinbone (tibia) length may result in overestimated values with greater standard error of estimation (1.4 cm), when compared with a knee height of 1.1cm. [17]

Generally, the corporal mass rate is not an adequate screening for malnutrition, being a better indicator of acute malnutrition than for the chronic.[21] The CP child generally experiences long periods of malnutrition, being considered chronic cases.

The knee height was used as an alternative stature measure in individuals with impaired mobility, as an accurate, reliable and affordable substitute for assessing length in this type of individual.[17]

In relation to the height, it was observed that the female gender presented lightly superior values when compared with male gender, what is similar to that observed in no neurological impaired children.[22]

Oromotor dysfunctions at an early age disturb both growth and nutritional status and, therefore, CP children must receive early rehabilitation interventions.[4-5]

This study observed that CP individuals who were fed with a liquid diet presented total-DMF significantly higher than those who were fed semi-solid and solid diets. The individuals with severe oromotor impairment were unable to ingest solid food and the harmful role of a liquid diet consumed at an early age should be taken into account.[4,8,23] Probably these factors must be considered in relation to growth and development of CP individuals that presented minor weight/height rates in both genders as well.

High caries prevalence in CP individuals has been reported in the literature[.9-13] Food consistency, the number of carbohydrate exposures per day [4,8,23], the difficulty found in mastication due to the biting reflex [7], reduced salivary flow[24], long-term liquid oral medication[25] extremely high dental treatment needs[26] and problems related to dental management[27] are some of the points described in the literature. However, none of the studies took into account oromotor impairment in CP individuals as a risk factor.

Severely orofacial motor impaired individuals (score range ≤19 – OFMFAS I) were those fed on a liquid diet and presented the highest total-DMF. In view of the fact that the presence of caries in deciduous teeth exposes the individuals to high risk in permanent teeth[28], it is a fundamental requirement that these individuals begin to receive early preventive measures and, as part of this program, their caregivers should receive proper instruction, training and motivation regarding the realization of adequate oral hygiene, plaque control, dental floss use and fluoride therapy, as well as promoting adequate diet consistency; thus preventing deleterious and noxious habits such as bottle feeding.

The severity of the neurological damage is reflected, in a direct way, in the oral cavity through the oral motricity impairment, being directly associated with growth patterns in those individuals.

Conclusion

Oromotor dysfunction in children with CP is associated with poor growth and increased caries experience

Acknowledgments

This study was approved by the Ethics Committee of the Federal University of Sao Paulo School of Medicine, Brazil, under the protocol number 0425/03.

References

[1] Bax M, Goldstein M, Rosenbaum P, Leviton A, Paneth N, Dan B, Jacobsson B, Damiano D; Executive Committee for the Definition of Cerebral Palsy. Proposed definition and classification of cerebral palsy. *Dev. Med. Child Neurol.* 2005; 47:571-6.

[2] Meningaud JP, Pitak-Arnnop P, Chikhani L, Bertrand JC. Drooling of saliva: a review of the etiology and management options. *Oral Surg. Oral Med. Oral Pathol. Oral Radiol. Endod.* 2006; 101:48-57.

[3] Yilmaz S, Basar P, Gisel EG. Assessment of feeding performance in patients with cerebral palsy. *Int. J. Rehabil. Res.* 2004; 27:325-9.

[4] Gangil A, Patwari AK, Aneja S, Ahuja B, Anand VK. Feeding problems in children with cerebral palsy. *Indian Pediatr.* 2001; 38:839-46.

[5] Sonis A, Castle J, Duggan C. Infant nutrition: implication for somatic growth, adult onset diseases, and oral health. *Curr. Opin. Pediatr*. 1997; 9:289-97.

[6] Sullivan PB, Lambert B, Rose M, Ford-Adams M, Johnson A, Griffiths P. Prevalence and severity of feeding and nutritional problems in children with neurological impairment: Oxford Feeding Study. *Dev. Med. Child Neurol.* 2000; 42:674-80.

[7] Dos Santos MT, Nogueira ML. Infantile reflexes and their effects on dental caries and oral hygiene in cerebral palsy individuals. *J. Oral. Rehabil.* 2005; 32:880-5.

[8] Hou M, Fu P, Zhao JH, Lan K, Zhang H. Oral motor dysfunction, feeding problems and nutritional status in children with cerebral palsy. *Zhonghua Er. Ke Za Zhi.* 2004; 42:765-8.

[9] Gupta DP, Chowdhury R, Sarkar S. Prevalence of dental caries in handicapped children of Calcutta. *J. Indian Soc. Pedod. Prev. Dent.* 1993;11:23-7.

[10] Bhavsar JP, Damle SG. Dental caries and oral hygiene amongst 12-14 years old handicapped children of Bombay, India. *J. Indian Soc. Pedod. Prev. Dent. 1*995; 13:1-3.

[11] dos Santos MT, Masiero D, Simionato MRL. Risk factors for dental caries in children with cerebral palsy. *Spec. Care Dentist* 2002; 22:103-7.

[12] Rodríguez Vázquez C, Garcillan R, Rioboo R, Bratos E. Prevalence of dental caries in an adult population with mental disabilities in Spain. *Spec. Care Dentist* 2002; 22:65-9.

[13] Guare R. de O, Ciamponi AL. Dental caries prevalence in the primary dentition of cerebral palsied children. *J. Clin. Pediatr. Dent.* 2003; 27:287-92.

[14] Wood E, Rosenbaum P. The gross motor function classification system for cerebral palsy: a study of reliability and stability over time. *Dev. Med. Child. Neurol.* 2000;42:292-6.

[15] Santos MT, Manzano FS, Ferreira MC, Masiero D. Development of a novel orofacial motor function assessment scale for children with cerebral palsy. *J. Dent. Child (Chic)* 2005; 72:113-8.

[16] World Health Organization. Oral health surveys: basic methods, 4th edn. Geneva: WHO; 1997.

[17] Stevenson RD. Use of segmental measures to estimate stature in children with cerebral palsy. *Archives of Pediatric and Adolescent Medicine* 1995; 149: 658-62.

[18] Stevenson RD, Conaway M,Chumlia WC, Rosembaum P, Fung EB, Henderson RC, Worley G. Growth and health in children with moderate-to-severe cerebral palsy. Pediatrics 2006; 118: 1010-8.

[19] Kiely M, Lubin R, Kiely J. Descriptive epidemiology of cerebral palsy. Public Health Review 1984; 12: 79-101.

[20] Patrick J, Boland M, Stolski D, Murray GE. Rapid correction of wasting in children with cerebral palsy. *Dev. Med. Child Neurol.* 1986; 28:734-9.

[21] Radheshyam B. A comparison of five anthropometric indices for identifying factors of malnutrition. *American Journal of Epidemiology* 1987; 126:258-67.

[22] Day SM, Strauss DJ, Vachon PJ, Rosenbloom L, Shavelle RM, Wu YW. Growth patterns in a population of children and adolescents with cerebral palsy. *Dev. Med. Child Neurol.* 2007; 49:167-71.

[23] Haschke F. The nutrition commission of the Austrian Society of Pediatrics and Adolescent Medicine. Prevention of caries. *Padiatr. Padol.* 1992; 27:109-11.

[24] Santos MT, Siqueira WL, Nicolau J. Flow rate, pH and buffer capacity in saliva of adolescents with cerebral palsy. *J. Disabil. Oral Health* 2006; 7:185-8.

[25] Sahgal J, Sood PB, Raju OS. A comparison of oral hygiene status and dental caries in children on long term liquid oral medications to those not administered with such medications. *J .Indian Soc. Pedod .Prev. Dent* .2002; 20:144-51.

[26] Mitsea AG, Karidis AG, Donta-Bakoyianni C, Spyropoulos ND. Oral health status in Greek children and teenagers, with disabilities. *J. Clin. Pediatr. Dent*. 2001; 26:111-8

[27] Dicks JL. Outpatient dental services for individuals with mental illness: a program description. *Spec. Care Dentist.* 1995; 15:239-42.

[28] Skeie MS, Raadal M, Strand GV, Espelid I. The relationship between caries in the primary dentition at 5 years of age and permanent dentition at 10 years of age - a longitudinal study. *Int. J. Paediatr. Dent.* 2006; 16:152-60.

In: Handbook of Down Syndrome Research
Editors: Dominicus Jelinek and Gijs Dvorak

ISBN 978-1-60741- 690-6

Chapter 16

Craniofacial Growth in Patients with Down Syndrome

***José Lorenzo*[1], *Carmen Iglesias*[2] *and Juan J. Alió*[1]**
[1]Odonthopediatrics and Orthodontics Department, Universidad Complutense de Madrid, Madrid, Spain
[2]Private practice, Ourense, Spain

The set of clinical manifestations known as Down syndrome (DS) was formally described for the first time by John Langdon Down in 1886 in an article published in *London Hospital Reports*. He described the typical physical characteristics of this syndrome, which he called "idiocia mongoliana" with the intention of combining the idea that the appearance of these children is similar to that of the Mongol people with the idea of a certain degree of mental retardation. [1]

Almost an entire century would have to pass from the description made by Down before Jerome Lejeune, in 1959, would identify a chromosome 21 trisomy as the fundamental cause of the syndrome. And it has been just in the past few years that geneticists have succeeded in identifying the specific region of the 21st chromosome where the genes responsible for the characteristic phenotype lie. [2]

Down syndrome is the most common chromosome abnormality in humans. It is estimated that Down syndrome is present in 1 of every 1000 conceptions, but that between 50% and 70% of these embryos are spontaneously aborted in the first trimester of pregnancy. This rate is much higher than for other chromosomal abnormalities and trisomic syndromes. About 8% of all human embryos conceived suffer from some kind of chromosomal abnormality, but natural selection only allows 0.5% to be born, and of these, approximately 30% have Down syndrome, that is, 0.15% of all births. Of all the chromosomal abnormalities, Down syndrome is the most frequent viable aneuploidy among live births. Put another way, it is the alteration in the number of chromosomes of the human karyotype that best outwits the natural "quality control" mechanisms of embryonic development.[2,3]

Today, Down syndrome is found in approximately 1 per 1,250 births, falling from the rate from 20 years ago estimated at 1 of every 700 births. Although the specific reasons for this decrease are not clear, modern prenatal diagnostic techniques (maternal serum analyte screening, fetal ultrasonography, amniocentesis, etc.) and voluntary abortions may have played an important role [4]

There is a high survival rate among people suffering from Down syndrome, especially since 1960, when modern treatment methods started correcting congenital heart defects at an early age and antibiotics became widespread, thereby greatly reducing the mortality rate. Today, the average lifespan for Down syndrome patients is around 57 years, while in 1963 it was 26 and in 1929 it was only 9. About 80% of people with Down syndrome live past their 30th birthday and around 14% are still alive at the age of 68. It is thought that life expectancy will continue to increase over the next few decades as it has done throughout the 20th century and in the year 2020 it is estimated that today's figures will have increased by 50%. Medical advances, along with improvements in the education system and the tireless work that has been done by a number of foundations and associations of families affected by Down syndrome, have brought about notable improvements in longevity as well as functional results. People with DS are gradually finding their place in society and becoming much more integrated.[1,5,6]

The most common kind of Down syndrome is the trisomy of the 21st chromosome due to the nondisjunction of this chromosome in one of the parents, usually the mother. As with any other cellular mechanism, errors can occur in chromosomal disjunction and at times produce aneuploid gametes. The odds of these errors in cellular division occurring depends on the age of the mother. Older mothers, especially over 35, have a very high risk of conceiving children with DS (1:2300 at 20 years old, 1:290 at 35 years old, 1:50 at 45 years old). The age of the father has also been shown to have an effect when he is over the age of 50, although to a much lesser extent. Overall, it is estimated that 95% of all DS cases are due to a chromosomal error in the mother, and only 5% are ascribed to a chromosomal error in the father.[3,5]

Down syndrome can be identified by a large number of stigmas or clinical manifestations in practically all of the systems that make up the human body: upward slanting eyes, flat bridge of the nose, sensorial deficiencies, congenital gastrointestinal and heart defects, atlantoaxial instability, muscular hypotonia, slow development of motor skills, poor bone development in general, as well as immunological, endocrine and metabolic disorders. However, none of these clinical signs can be considered pathognomonic of the syndrome and preliminary diagnoses must always be confirmed through a karyotypic study.[6] The most significant symptom of Down syndrome is the mental retardation that is invariably present. The intelligence quotient of these patients usually ranges between 20 and 75, with the average being 50.[7]

Every type of Down syndrome (trisomy 21, translocations and mosaicisms) has in common an "overdose" of genetic information. It is thought that this excess of genes causes disorders in the normal processes that regulate embryogenesis, but the ultimate mechanism remains unknown. The excess of genetic material breaks the balance and harmony necessary build the organism correctly and makes possible the excessive production of substances that in the long run are harmful to the normal workings of the body. This excess of genetic material also produces a large number of structural and functional anomalies in Down syndrome patients, and the severity of these anomalies (from brain abnormalities to heart defects) depends on how the chromosome 21 genes interrelate with the genes in the rest of the organism. After all, one of the basic functions of genes is to regulate the functioning of other genes.[5] Consequently, the differing degrees of physical and mental limitations is enormous when dealing with Down syndrome, and a wide range of grey areas exist between the most and least severe cases.

It is known that the malformations associated with Down syndrome are due to an "incomplete", rather than "abnormal", embryogenesis, as can be seen in the atrioventricular communication, tracheoesophageal fistulas, anal atresia, syndactyly and neuronal and synaptic immaturity. This suggests that the products synthesized by the additional genes can suspend the development of organs or anatomical structures.[2] This reasoning carried to the field of craniofacial growth might explain the shortening of the anterior cranial base and maxillary hypoplasty described in Down syndrome by several authors.[8-11]

Many authors have studied different aspects of craniofacial growth in Down syndrome patients, but they have not always arrived at the same conclusions and there is a certain amount of controversy. People with Down syndrome are often described as having maxillary hypoplasty,[8,12] a short, flat cranial base,[10,11,13,14] and a smaller palate in its three dimensions: width, length and height.[15] Some studies point out that all craniofacial measurements in Down syndrome are smaller than normal, thereby describing a kind of generalized microcephaly.[16,17] Other authors, however, have pointed out that the palatal height is not different from that found in the general population, despite being shorter and narrower.[18,19] The mandible often protrudes notably in the facial profile of these individuals with respect to their cranial base and upper maxilla, which is usually considerably smaller than the mandible.[12]

Almost all of the authors agree on the prevalence of malocclusions found in Down syndrome patients.[20-24] More specifically, there is a higher frequency of anterior and posterior crossbites, Angle's Class III and anterior open bites in these individuals than in other mentally disabled people or in the general population.

In any case, despite the numerous longitudinal studies carried out on craniofacial growth in the general population, nothing comparable has been done for people with Down syndrome. Cephalometric analyses of Down syndrome patients are extremely scarce and are done over transversal samples, often on subjects with great differences in age. Moreover, most of the studies are limited to the study of some isolated craniofacial structure (cranial base, hard palate, etc.). Others merely describe the craniofacial morphology in Down syndrome using cephalometric norms established for genetically normal individuals,[25,26] but in no case do they offer a dynamic, global vision of craniofacial growth as a whole.

The purpose of this paper is to analyze the changes brought about by growth in the craniofacial area in individuals with Down syndrome and compare them to the growth that occurs in the general population. In order to do so, we have carried out a longitudinal study on a sample of genetically diagnosed subjects with Down syndrome, recording craniofacial growth taken from cephalometric radiographs at yearly intervals. We will discuss all of the morphological aspects related to craniofacial growth found in our study, contrasting our findings with those published by other authors. By way of clarity, we will divide the discussion section into three main parts: cranial base growth, maxillary growth and mandibular growth in Down syndrome.

Material and Method

The experimental group included 47 subjects (25 boys and 22 girls), all having been diagnosed with Down syndrome. The average age of the group in the initial x-ray was 11 years, 8 months, with a range of 7 years, 7 months, to 16 years, 4 months. The average age in the last x-ray was 14 years, 1 month, with a range of 8 years, 7 months, to 18 years, 6 months. To draw comparisons between the different stages of growth, the sample was divided into 3 age groups: prepubescent (ages 8-11), pubescent (ages 12-14), and postpubescent (ages 15-18). This classification was made according to other authors who concur that the pubescent period in Down syndrome occurs similarly to that in the general population, although with a lower rate of growth.[27-30]

The control group included 38 subjects, 16 girls and 22 boys. Subjects in the control group satisfied the following criteria: between the ages of 8 and 16 at the time of the first x-ray, no apparent craniofacial deformities, no history of craniofacial trauma or congenital anomalies, occlusal stability with clear intercuspation, no extractions of permanent teeth, no dental anomalies, and no maxillofacial surgery or surgical treatment. The average ages at the first x-ray were 10 years, 4 months, for the girls and 10 years, 1 month, for the boys. At the time of the last x-ray, the ages were 13 years, 6 months, for the girls and 13 years, 8 months, for the boys.

At least one lateral cranium x-ray was taken of each patient annually for as long as they participated in the study. All the x-rays were done using the same machine, with a magnification index of 1:1.10 (10%).

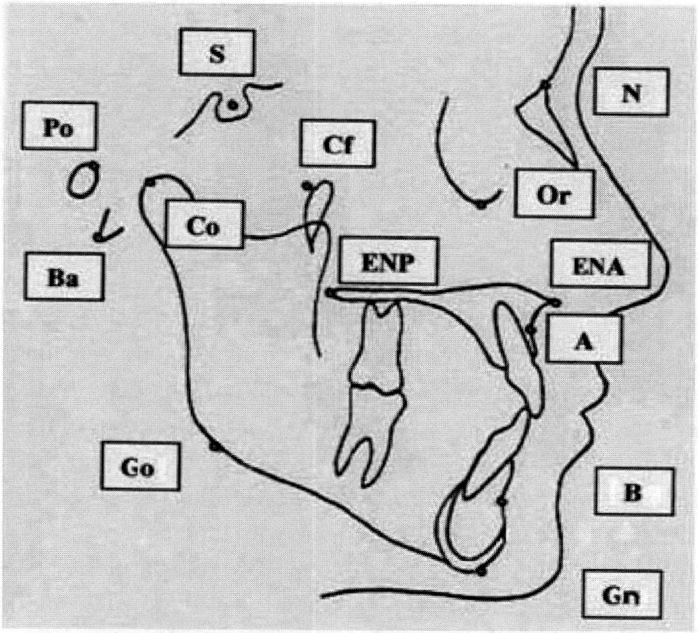

Figure 1. Cephalometric landmarks used in the study.

Table I. Cephalometric parameters used in the study

CEPHALOMETRIC PARAMETERS	DEFINITION	ANATOMICAL REGION
Anterior Cranial Base Length	Sella-Nasion (SN) Distance	CRANIAL BASE
Posterior Cranial Base Length	Sella-Basion (SBa) Distance	
Cranial Base Angle	Basion-Sella-Nasion (Ba-S-N) Angle	
Height of the midfacial area	Nasion-ANS Distance	MAXILLA
Palatal Plane Length	ANS-PNS Distance	
Effective Mandibular Length	Condylion-Gnathion (Co-Gn) Distance	MANDIBLE
Mandibular Plane	Angle between (Go-Gn) and Frankfort (FH)	

Table II. Superimposition method according to anatomical region studied

ANATOMICAL REGION	PLANE OF SUPERIM POSITION	HORIZONTAL CHANGES (FH)	VERTICAL CHANGES (Vp)	ROTATIONAL CHANGES
Cranial Base	SN at S	N and Ba	N and Ba	BaSN Angle
Maxilla	BaN at N	A	ANS and PNS	Palatal Plane
Mandible	BaN at CC	B	Go and Gn	Mandibular Plane

In all the lateral cranium x-rays, a cephalometry was traced with a computerized analysis (Nemotec Studio®, Nemoceph Dental System©) by marking the following cephalometric landmarks (Figure 1): S (sella), N (nasion), Ba (basion), ANS (anterior nasal spine), PNS (posterior nasal spine), point A, Po (porion), Or (suborbital), Co (condylion), point B, Gn (gnathion), Go (gonion) and Me (menton). The following cephalometric parameters were then traced using those landmarks (Table 1): S-N length, S-Ba length, Ba-S-N angle (cranial base angle), ANS- PNS (palatal plane length), N-ANS (height of the midfacial area), Co-Gn (effective mandibular length) and Go-Gn (mandibular plane).

In order to gather as much information as possible from the cephalometric x-rays, in addition to studying the variation over time of the cephalometric measurements that we have just defined, we also carried out superimpositions of the cranial base, maxilla and mandible with all of the tracings of each patient. We were then able to quantify the changes in the sagittal plane of the following cephalometric landmarks and planes (Table II):

- In the cranial base: N, Ba and base angle (Ba-S-N).
- In the maxilla: point A, ANS, PNS and palatal plane (ANS-PNS).
- In the mandible: point B, Go, Gn and mandibular plane (Go-Gn).

The computer program we used allowed us to superimpose the cephalometric tracings making the basicranial plane (Ba-N) coincide with the nasion, or with the pterygomaxillary (CC), as described by Ricketts[31] to study maxillary and mandibular changes, respectively; and to study the cranial base we used the SN line anchored at S, as recommended by Björk due to its being a stable reference throughout adolescence.[32]In all three situations, two main axes of reference were traced:

- Frankfort Plane (FH): the plane the passes through the porion and suborbital.
- Vertical Pterygoid (Vp): perpendicular line to Frankfort from the most posterior point of the pterygomaxillary fossa.

Over the first axis we measured the horizontal changes of N, Ba, point A and point B. Over the second we measured the vertical changes of N, Ba, ANS, PNS, Go and Gn.

A positive value was given to horizontal changes when the displacement of the point in the superimposition was forward. Likewise, a positive value was given to the vertical changes when the displacement of the point in question was downward.

We also recorded the rotational changes of the maxilla and mandible using the palatal plane (ANS-PNS) and the mandibular plane (Go-Gn). The rotation was considered positive when the final position of the palatal plane had undergone a counterclockwise turn with respect to the initial position (Figure 3). For the mandible we gave the rotation a positive value when it rotated clockwise (Figure 4). We also recorded the changes that took place in the Ba-S-N angle, giving a positive value to increases in the angle (Figure 2).

All cephalometric analyses were made by two researchers. These researchers calibrate their instruments annually to prevent errors in the cephalometric measurements. Once having done the tracings, they compared their findings and obtained these possibilities:

- Concordance Type I: absolute coincidence of the two tracings.
- Concordance Type II: differences were considered valid until 1 mm for linear measurements and 2° for angular measurements.
- Concordance Type III: a greater difference than in Type II.

In concordance type II, the arithmetic mean between the 2 values is established for the parameter that does not coincide. When the difference is greater (Concordance Type III), the tracings are re-drawn, and the measurements are made again, bearing in mind the 3 types of concordance.

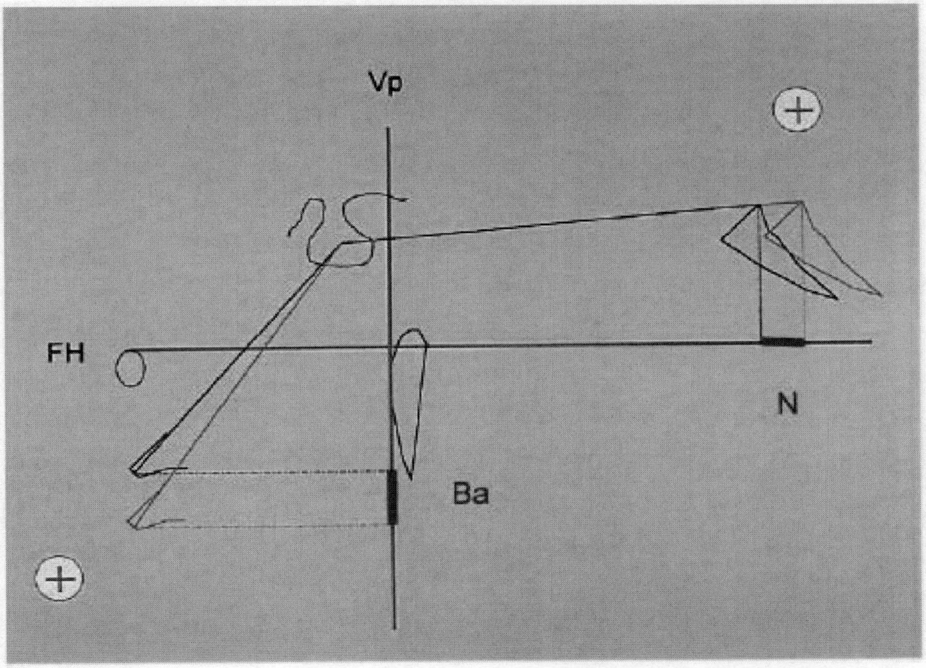

Figure 2. Method used for the superimposition of the cranial base. SN tracing in S.

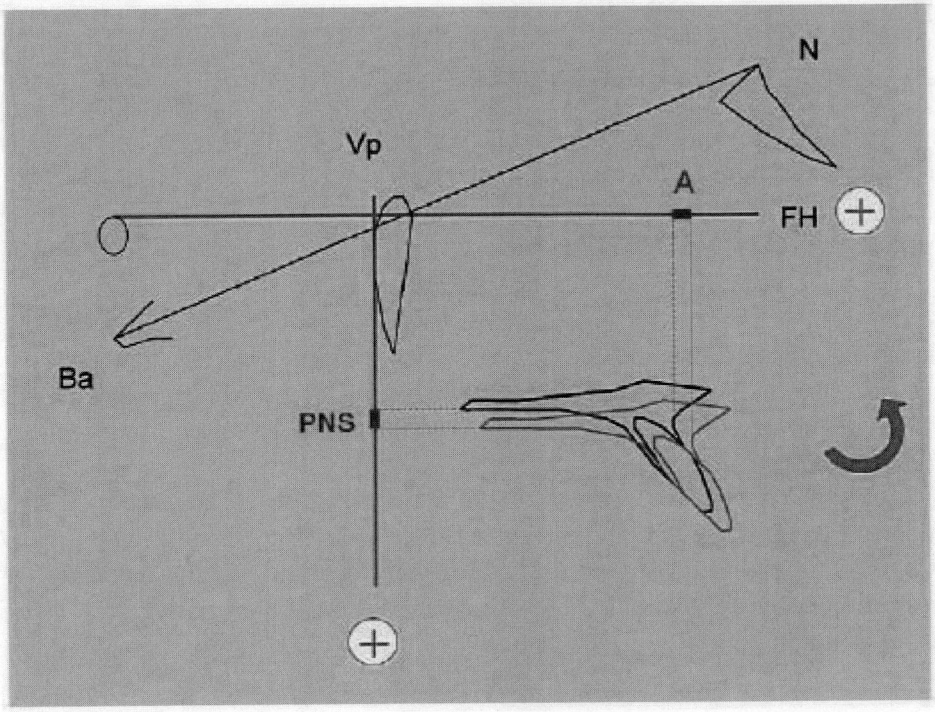

Figure 3. Method used for superimposition of the maxilla. BaN at N.

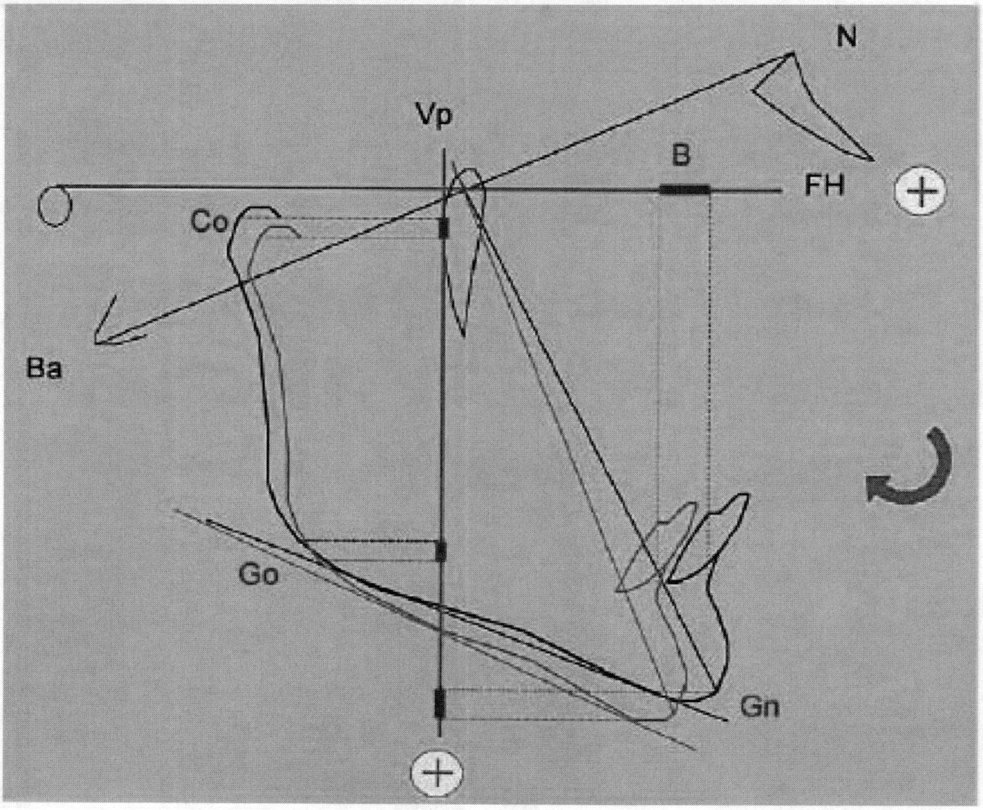

Figure 4. Mandibular superimposition. BaN at CC.

We carried out a statistical analysis of the data applying the Student *t* test, analysis of variance (ANOVA) and the Duncan multiple range test.

Results

Table III contains the results obtained (average, standard deviation and statistical significance) with the cephalometric parameters studied for the whole sample and for each age group. Similarly, Table IV shows the results obtained from the cephalometric superimpositions.

In two other tables we present the differences between the sexes found in the cephalometric parameters (Table V) and in the cephalometric superimpositions (Table VI).

We have also included charts of the variables studied to help the reader achieve a better understanding of the results which are presented here in a more visual way than in the numerical tables.

Table III. Results for the whole sample and each age group

	Variable		Group	TOTAL (8-18 years)			Prepubescent (8-11 years)			Pubescent (12-14 years)			Post-pubescent (15-18 years)		
				Average	S.D.	Sig.	Average	S.D.	Sig.	Average	S.D.	Sig.	Average	S.D.	Sig.
Cranial base	SN	(mm)	D	63.77	4.04	$p < 0.001$	61.85	3.68	$p < 0.001$	63.99	3.91	$p < 0.001$	64.81	3.98	$p < 0.001$
			C	72.26	2.84		71.15	2.68		73.02	2.80		73.83	2.00	
	SBa	(mm)	D	42.33	3.22	$p < 0.001$	39.94	2.91	$p < 0.001$	43.04	3.00	$p < 0.001$	43.31	2.81	$p < 0.001$
			C	46.30	3.03		45.53	2.78		46.78	3.13		47.52	3.02	
	Ba-S-N	(°)	D	14.40	4.76	$p < 0.001$	143.30	5.37	$p < 0.001$	142.60	4.06	$p < 0.001$	144.00	4.83	$p < 0.001$
			C	13.90	4.12		133.90	3.95		133.50	4.19		135.60	4.31	
Maxilla	PP length	(mm)	D	4.33	3.37	$p < 0.001$	40.91	2.81	$p < 0.001$	43.61	3.56	$p < 0.001$	44.65	2.69	$p < 0.001$
			C	5.23	3.46		51.48	2.88		54.42	3.15		55.71	3.42	
	N-ANS	(mm)	D	46.52	3.90	$p < 0.001$	44.13	4.29	$p < 0.001$	46.28	3.18	$p < 0.001$	48.23	3.27	$p < 0.001$
			C	54.30	3.53		52.52	3.33		55.50	3.04		56.86	2.52	
Mandible	Eff. Mand. length	(mm)	D	107.00	9.70	$p < 0.001$	97.36	7.38	$p < 0.001$	107.70	7.26	$p < 0.001$	112.50	7.93	$p < 0.001$
			C	112.20	6.07		108.70	4.92		113.90	4.59		119.80	5.36	
	Stein. MP	(°)	D	33.54	5.68	n.s.	35.32	3.50	n.s.	32.99	5.22	n.s.	32.82	6.76	n.s.
			C	34.48	5.30		34.78	5.36		34.45	5.30		33.45	5.25	

D. - down syndrome group; C. - control group; Sig. - statistical significance; NS. - not significant

Table IV. Cephalometric superimposition

	Variable		Group	TOTAL (8-18 years)			Prepubescent (8-11 years)			Pubescent (12-14 years)			Post-pubescent (15-18 years)		
				Average	S.D.	Sig.	Average	S.D.	Sig.	Average	S.D.	Sig.	Average	S.D.	Sig.
Cranial base	N Horiz.	(mm/year)	D	0.47	0.49	–	0.49	0.37	$p < 0.01$	0,69	0.60	n.s.	0.25	0.33	$p < 0.01$
			C	0.75	0.41		0.77	0.42		0,73	0.42		0.76	0.29	
	N Vert.	(mm/year)	D	0.13	0.15	–	0.18	0.18	n.s.	0,17	0.14	n.s.	0.05	0.11	$p < 0.05$
			C	0.14	0.07		0.14	0.06		0,14	0.08		0.15	0.06	
	Ba Horiz.	(mm/year)	D	0.48	0.53	–	0.77	0.62	$p < 0.01$	0,55	0.50	n.s.	0.21	0.33	$p < 0.05$
			C	0.40	0.45		0.32	0.40		0,48	0.52		0.49	0.24	
	Ba Vert.	(mm/year)	D	0.36	0.45	n.s.	0.60	0.56	n.s.	0,41	0.46	n.s.	0.16	0.23	n.s.
			C	0.40	0.47		0.47	0.46		0,32	0.50		0.25	0.22	
Maxilla	A	(mm/year)	D	0.12	0.24	n.s.	0.14	0.20	n.s.	0,12	0.14	n.s.	0.11	0.32	n.s.
			C	0.20	0.29		0.22	0.31		0,19	0.28		0.11	0.21	
	ANS	(mm/year)	D	0.62	0.76	n.s.	1.15	0.93	n.s.	0,72	0.65	n.s.	0.15	0.37	$p < 0.05$
			C	0.98	0.65		1.05	0.47		0,97	0.85		0.48	0.25	
	PNS	(mm/year)	D	0.70	0.77	n.s.	1.05	0.78	n.s.	0,92	0.85	n.s.	0.25	0.38	n.s.
			C	1.02	0.58		1.09	0.49		1,03	0.68		0.49	0.27	
Mandible	B	(mm/year)	D	1.21	1.44	n.s.	1.63	1.24	$p < 0.05$	1,33	1.51	n.s.	0.88	1.45	n.s
			C	1.10	0.75		1.02	0.63		1,23	0.93		0.98	0.28	
	Co	(mm/year)	D	0.31	0.42	n.s.	0.26	0.36	n.s.	0,57	0.53	n.s.	0.14	0.20	n.s
			C	0.25	0.40		0.11	0.17		0,44	0.55		0.29	0.25	
	Gn	(mm/year)	D	1.04	1.23	$p < 0.05$	1.32	1.18	n.s.	1,45	1.34	n.s.	0.56	0.99	n.s
			C	1.54	0.76		1.57	0.60		1,55	0.97		1.24	0.59	

D. -Down syndrome group; C. - control group; Sig. - statistical significance; NS. - not significan

Table V. Cephalometric variables. Differences between sexes in the DS group and the control group. (Student's t)

	Variable	Group	FEMALES Average	FEMALES S.D.	MALES Average	MALES S.D.	STAT. SIG.
Cranial base	SN (mm)	D	61.15	2.32	65.84	3.92	$p < 0.001$
		C	71.29	2.73	73.03	2.71	$p < 0.001$
	S-Ba (mm)	D	40.37	2.68	43.88	2.75	$p < 0.001$
		C	45.36	2.45	47.04	3.26	$p < 0.001$
	SN-Ba (°)	D	144.14	4.75	142.76	4.71	n.s.
		C	135.65	4.15	132.55	3.55	$p < 0.001$
Maxilla	PP length (mm)	D	41.17	2.03	45.05	3.23	$p < 0.001$
		C	52.53	2.66	53.79	3.91	$p < 0.05$
	N-ANS (mm)	D	44.90	2.83	47.81	4.15	$p < 0.001$
		C	54.69	3.41	53.98	3.61	n.s.
Mandible	Eff. Mand length (mm)	D	100.68	6.83	111.95	8.71	$p < 0.001$
		C	110.83	5.73	113.26	6.15	$p < 0.05$
	Mand. plane (°)	D	34.77	4.91	32.48	6.10	$p < 0.05$
		C	34.94	5.01	34.12	5.52	n.s.

Table VI. Cephalometric variables of superimposition. Differences between sexes in the DS group and the control group. (Student's t)

	Variable	Group	FEMALES Average	FEMALES S.D.	MALES Average	MALES S.D.	STAT. SIG.
Cranial base	Horiz. N (mm / year)	D	0.48	0.56	0.46	0.43	n.s.
		C	0.68	0.40	0.81	0.41	n.s.
	Vert. N (mm / year)	D	0.13	0.15	0.12	0.15	n.s.
		C	0.15	0.08	0.13	0.06	n.s.
	Horiz. Ba (mm / year)	D	0.45	0.48	0.50	0.56	n.s.
		C	0.27	0.33	0.50	0.50	$p < 0.01$
	Vert. Ba (mm / year)	D	0.46	0.48	0.29	0.42	n.s.
		C	0.18	0.25	0.58	0.53	$p < 0.01$
Maxilla	A (mm/ year)	D	0.10	0.18	0.14	0.28	n.s.
		C	0.29	0.37	0.13	0.18	$p < 0.01$
	ANS (mm/ year)	D	0.64	0.79	0.60	0.75	n.s.
		C	0.71	0.47	1.21	0.69	$p < 0.001$
	PNS (mm/ year)	D	0.73	0.75	0.68	0.79	n.s.
		C	0.84	0.61	1.18	0.51	$p < 0.01$

Table VI. (Continued)

			FEMALES		MALES		STAT. SIG.
Mandible	B	D	1.07	1.34	1.33	1.53	n.s.
		C	1.08	0.65	1.11	0.82	n.s.
	Co	D	0.31	0.40	0.31	0.43	n.s.
		C	0.30	0.49	0.21	0.30	n.s.
	Gn	D	0.95	1.39	1.11	1.08	n.s.
		C	1.26	0.72	1.76	0.72	$p < 0.001$

Discussion

In this section we discuss our findings by looking at each of the three anatomical structures studied (cranial base, maxilla and mandible) while we contrast our results with those previously published in medical literature.

A) Cranial Base Growth

The cephalometric variables used to assess the cranial base (SN and SBa) showed a shorter anterior cranial base and posterior cranial base ($P<0.001$) in individuals with Down syndrome (DS). The shortening of the cranial base has been described by several authors [3,9,11,33-35] and in other studies[16,17,36] we find references of general microcephaly in Down syndrome. This lack of growth compared to normal subjects remains the same throughout the study, with a constant rate of growth. That is, the cranial base grows in the same way in both populations between the ages of 8 and 18, so we can conclude that there is a difference in cranial base size at earlier ages than the ones considered in our study.[37] Some studies[38,39] report that cranial length and perimeter are similar in Down syndrome babies and normal babies at birth, but in the first four years of life the growth rate in children with DS decreases and thereby gives rise to these differences. Other authors [9] find a smaller anterior cranial base by as much as 4 mm at birth, coming to the conclusion that these differences already exist during the pregnancy.

The shortening of the cranial base has been related to the lack of pneumatization of the frontal sinus[17,40,41] and to the lack of development of the nasal bone that often appears in DS.[42] However, neither reason seems to be enough to explain the shortening of the cranial base.[41] In any case, when we analyzed the cephalometric superimposition variables (Table IV) we observed that the horizontal growth of the nasion point is considerably less in the DS group than in the control group, and after the age of 15 years nasion and basion growth seems to stop in both the horizontal and vertical planes. This is completely consistent with the stabilization of the SN and SBa distances observed in the pubescent and post-pubescent groups with DS42 and agrees with our results which indicate the end of nasal bone growth in

DS subjects around the age of 16. These differ from what happens in the general population where cranial base growth continues until the individual is 18-20 years old.[32, 37 y 43]

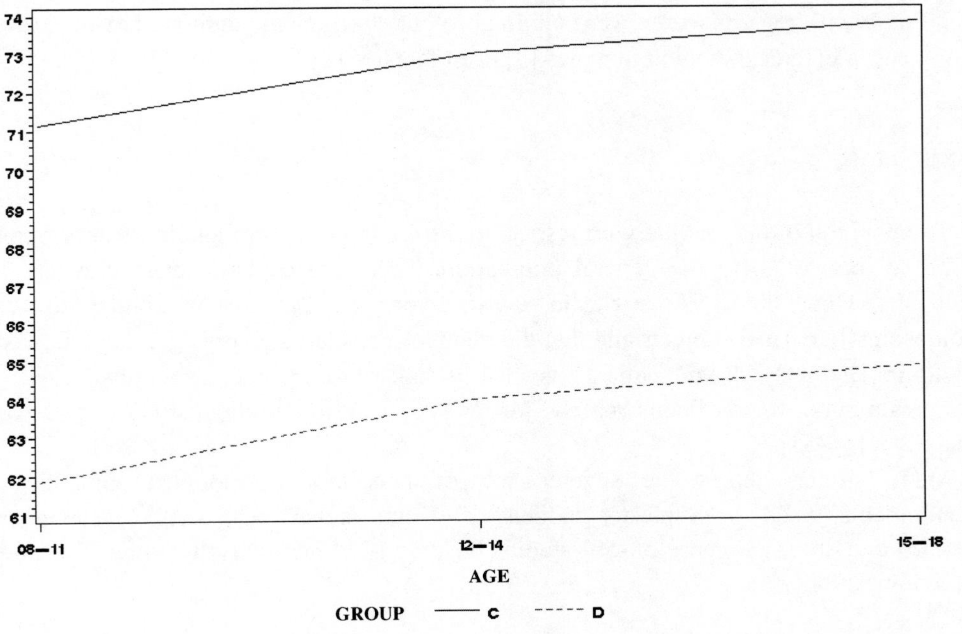

Figure 5: Anterior cranial base. SN (mm)

However, the floor area of the middle cranial fossa and the glenoid fossa of the temporal bone reveal completely normal size and development in DS patients.[26,37]

Several different studies report the flattening of the cranial base in DS.[8,14,15,46] The angulation of the cranial base was analyzed with the Ba-S-N angle. This measurement shows us a flatter cranial base in the DS group ($P<0.001$), that is, a wider in the Ba-S-N angle in the DS group with respect to the control group. The flattening of the cranial base can be understood as a vertical hypoplasty of the central part of the cranium accompanied by a lowering of the sella turcica, due to a lesser degree of cerebral development. [25] This agrees with observations which describe a hypoplastic sphenoid bone and poor general pneumatization of the cranial base, including the sphenoidal sinus, in Down syndrome.[17,47]

On the other hand, the mediosphenoidal or intersphenoidal synchondrosis does not close until the seventh year in DS, while in the general population it usually ossifies by the time of birth or in the first months of life.[48,49] There would seem to be a relation between the degree of flattening of the base and the closing of the synchondrosis, leading some authors to attribute the cause of a flat cranial base in Down syndrome to the late ossification of the intersphenoidal synchondrosis.[46] Once the intersphenoidal synchondrosis closes, the angle of the cranial base remains constant in Down syndrome,[14,37] just as it does in the general population.[49]

A certain degree of sexual dimorphism has been described in that males have a bigger cranial base than females.[3,23,37] In the general population, the differences in cranial base size with respect to sex appears at the age of 5.[44,45 In Down syndrome sexual dimorphism of the cranial base also seems to be present at a very early age and both sexes share the same annual growth rate in the following years.[3,42] The differences in the angulation of the cranial base with regards to sex were minimal in our study. Some authors, however, did find differences: a greater flattening in males,[3] or in females.[8]

B) Maxillary Growth

The position of the maxilla with respect to the cranial base throughout its development is similar to that found in the general population. There are cephalometric studies[8,25,35] which note that the SNA angle in Down syndrome patients is similar to that of chromosomally normal subjects and that this remains constant at every age. Sagittal maxillary growth in Down syndrome patients is clearly linked to cranial base growth, with both structures moving forward coordinately, just as is seen in longitudinal studies of the general population. [50-53]

Many studies report the severe lack of maxillary development in DS. Using measurements taken from plaster models of dental arches [15,18,19,54] cephalometric [8,25,35] and anthropometric[55-58] studies have verified maxillary hypoplasty in the three spatial dimensions.

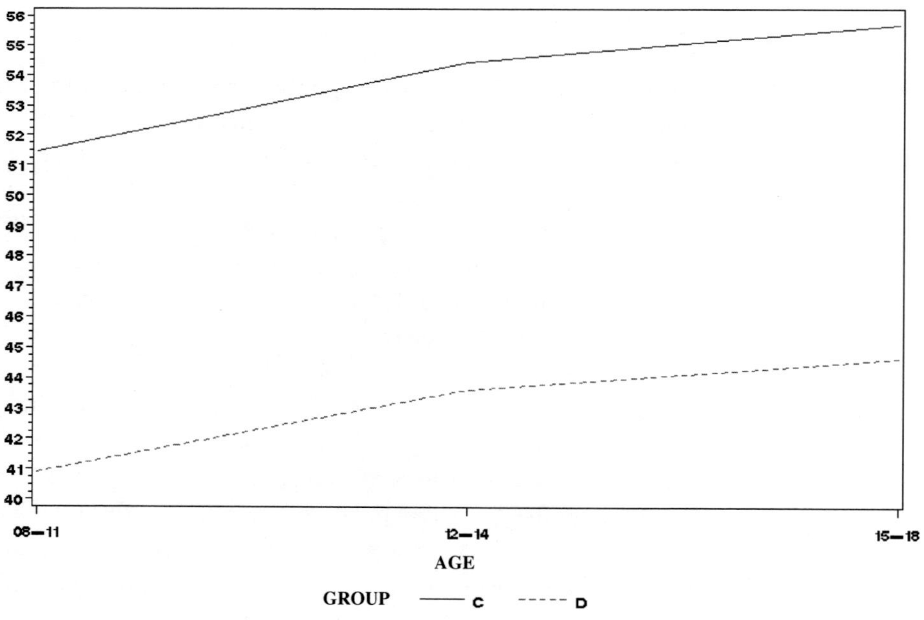

Figure 6: Palatal plane length. PNS-ANS (mm)

If the maxilla grows in accordance with the cranial base, and hypoplasty is present in both structures, logically the cephalometric variables that relate the maxilla to the cranial base, such as the SNA angle, remain unchanged within the cephalometric norm.[35]

In our study, cephalometric superimpositions were done assessing the evolution of the projection of point A over the Frankfort plane, and of the ANS and PNS over the vertical pterygoid, in order to monitor sagittal maxillary growth independently of the anterior cranial base (Figure2). We find that the annual maxillary growth rates are always less in the DS group compared to the control group, whether it be from point A, ANS or PNS, despite not reaching statistical significance. The average measurement recorded for each one of these points was 0.12 mm/year, 0.62 mm/year and 0.70 mm/year, respectively (Table IV). The ANS and PNS descend at practically the same speed, which means the maxilla in individuals with DS does not undergo any rotation in its vertical descent during facial development.[8,9]

Palatal plane length (ANS-PNS) is significantly diminished over the course of our study. Maxillary size increases proportionally as it does in the control group while differing by about 10 mm in the amount of growth. Vertically, the height of the midfacial area (N-ANS) also showed a significant shortening of about 8 mm (Table III).

However, despite the hypoplasty, palatal plane length development over time was very similar to that of the control group, with the both groups having parallel tracings, which indicates that Down syndrome subjects have a smaller maxilla to begin with but its development is quite stable over time. In other words, these individuals present, as we have seen, a vertically and especially sagittally hypoplastic maxilla, but it grows at the same rate as in the general population. So, the smaller maxillary size of Down syndrome subjects must already be present at earlier ages than those considered in our study.

In the analysis according to sex, independently of hypoplasty, males with DS had bigger maxillas than women (Table V), indicating that sexual dimorphism is present in maxillary size. This is also true in the general population.[59]

C) Mandibular Growth

Several authors report DS patients having a hypoplastic mandible to a greater or lesser degree, whether it be in its total size[21,23,25] or in one of its parts.[33] But there have also been studies that consider both the ramus as well as the mandibular body similar in size to those in the general population.[26]

However, a simple facial exploration is usually enough to see that the mandible of DS subjects sticks out with respect to other elements of the facial profile. In cephalometric[25,35] as well as in anthropometric[33] studies and intraoral clinical explorations done on these patients, an intermaxillary relation of skeletal Class III is usually found. That is, the mandible is in a more forward position than the maxilla. This is because mandibular hypoplasty in DS is less severe than maxillary hypoplasty,[12,35] which is highly influenced by the lack of anterior cranial base development. That is, even though hypoplasty or a smaller size can be present in both the maxillary and mandibular structures, it is much greater in the maxilla. Therefore, the resulting intermaxillary (maxillomandibular) relation is Class III, but this is essentially due to the maxilla.

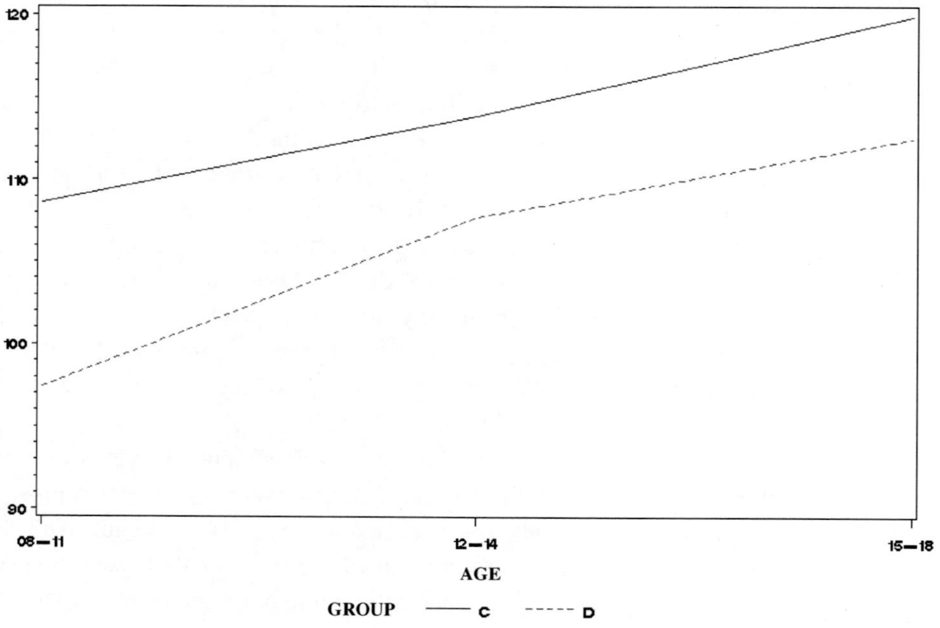

Figure 7: Effective mandibular length. Co-Gn (mm)

Furthermore, as some authors have pointed out,[25,35 we should rule out the possibility of postural advance of the mandible due to the relative macroglossia described in the syndrome[60] and pay attention to the anatomical characteristics of the structural elements of the craniofacial area of these subjects. We must focus on the flattening of the cranial base,[9,37] (that is, basal morphology which does not tend towards mandibular prognathism,) hypoplasty with a totally normal placement of the glenoid cavity[26,37] where the mandible articulates with the cranial base, and a hypoplastic maxilla.[8,25,35,55-58] Bearing these points in mind, one must conclude that the supposed mandibular prognathism initially attributed to Down syndrome should be put into context and understood as a deficit in the other two facial thirds (cranial base and maxilla). Consequently, measures taken to place the mandible in front of the cranial base can be misled by the shortening of the cranial base, especially by a position behind the nasion, and what is really reflected here is the smaller size of the anterior cranial base.[25]

In our study, we have basically verified everything that has been put forth so far in this paper. We have observed significantly hypoplastic mandibular length (Co-Gn) in DS patients (Table III) with an average deficit of 5 mm. That is, the mandible is affected to a lesser degree than the maxilla, where, as has been stated above, the sagittal development is some 10 mm less. The mandible in DS, even though it is slightly hypoplastic, has a growth potential comparable to that in the general population,[12] and greater than that of the maxilla (Table IV). Additionally, we have seen a horizontal growth pattern in DS with a mandible that undergoes a slight antero-rotation (counterclockwise) in the mandibular plane throughout the duration of the study (Table III). This might explain the greater horizontal growth recorded in the superimpositions at point B, especially from 8-11 years ($p<0.05$) since a mandibular antero-rotation supposes a greater forward projection of point B (Table IV). Regarding the direction of facial growth, the published studies do not all coincide: some studies[25 find, as we do, a horizontal pattern in DS, while others report a vertical pattern with a counterclockwise mandibular rotation which progressively makes facial growth more horizontal, and there are still other studies that identify a mesofacial growth pattern[26,61]. We should point out here that the vertical hypoplasty described in the maxilla would bring about a mandibular antero-rotation and horizontal growth pattern in DS.

In the mandibular superimpositions we observe that the two points studied in the vertical plane (Go and Gn) (Table IV) generally showed lower values in the DS group, but behave similarly in both the DS group and in the control group, with high peaks of growth in the pubescent stage (12-14 years), which coincides in time with the greatest increase in mandibular length (Co-Gn).

With respect to sexual dimorphism, we found greater mandibular length in males, reaching statistical significance (Table V), but not in the annual growth rates obtained from the mandibular superimpositions (Table VI). This means the growth rate in similar in both sexes and that the size difference in established at an earlier age than those considered in our study.

References

[1] Smith GF, Berg JM. Síndrome de Down. Edición española. Editorial Médica y Técnica, s.a. Barcelona 1978

[2] Hayes A, Batshaw ML. Síndrome de Down. Clínicas Pediátricas de Norteamérica. 1993; 3: 555-569

[3] Griffiths AJF, Miller JH, Suzuki DT. Genética. McGraw-Hill Interamericana

[4] Hoekelman RA, Adam HM. Atención primaria en pediatría. Vol II. Ediciones Harcourt 2002

[5] Asociación para el síndrome de Down de Madrid. El síndrome de Down hoy: perspectivas de futuro. 1991

[6] Pueschel SM, Pueschel JK. Síndrome de Down. Problemática biomédica. Ediciones Científicas y Técnicas, s.a. Masson-Salvat 1994

[7] Forfar JO, Arneil GC. Tratado de Pediatría. Tomo I. Salvat Editores 1986

[8] Fischer-Brandies H, Schmid RG, Fischer-Brandies E. Craniofacial development in patients with Down's syndrome from birth to 14 years of age. *Eur. J. Orhod.* 1986; 8(1): 35-42

[9] Fischer-Brandies H. Cephalometric comparison between children with and without Down's syndrome. *Eur. J. Orthod.* 1988; 10(3): 255-63

[10] Roche AF, Roche PJ, Lewis AB. The cranial base in trisomy 21. *J. Ment. Defic. Res.* 1972;16(1): 7-20

[11] Seward FS, Roche AF, Sunderland S. The lateral cranial silhouette in mongolism. *Am. J. Roentgenol.* 1961; 85: 653-8

[12] Fink GB, Madaus WK, Walker GF. A quantitative study of the face in Down's syndrome. *Am. J. Orthod.* 1975; 67(5): 540-53

[13] Alonso-Tosso A, Naval-Gias L, Hernandez-Vallejo G, Lucas-Tomas M. Etude céphalometrique de la base crânienne dans 133 cas de syndrome de Down. *Rev. Stomatol. Chir. Maxillofac.* 1985; 86(4): 234-40

[14] Burwood RJ, Gordon IRS, Taft RD. The skull in mongolism. *Clin. Radiol.* 1973 ; 24(4): 475-80

[15] Westerman GH, Johnson R, Cohen MM Variations of palatal dimensions in patients with Down's syndrome. *J. Dent .Res.* 1975; 54(4): 767-71

[16] Austin JHM. Short hard palate in new born: roetgen sign of mongolism. Radiology 1969; 92: 775-7

[17] Spitzer R. Observations on congenital dentofacial disorders in Mongolism and microcephaly. *Oral Surg. Oral Med. Oral Pathol.* 1967; 24(3): 325-32

[18] Redman RS, Shapiro BL, Gorlin RJ. Measurement of normal and reportedly malformed palatal vaults. III Down's syndrome. *J. Pediatr.* 1965; 67(2): 162-5

[19] Shapiro BL, Gorlin RJ, Redman RS, Brulh HH The palate and Down's syndrome. N *Engl. J. Med.* 1967; 276(26): 1460-3

[20] Alió JJ, Soto MT, Moreno JP. Prevalencia de maloclusiones en pacientes con síndrome de Down. *Rev. Ibero. Am. Ortod.* 1992; 11(2): 48-53

[21] Cohen MM, Arvystas MG, Baum BJ. Occlusal disharmonies in trisomy G. *Am. J. Orthod.* 1970; 58: 367-72

[22] Gullikson JS. Oral findings in children with Down's syndrome. *J. Dent. Child* 1973; 40: 293-7

[23] Jensen GM, Cleall JF. Dentoalveolar morphology and developmental changes in Down's syndrome. *Am. J. Orthod.* 1973 ;64: 607-18

[24] Vigild M. Prevalence of malocclusion in mentally retarded young adults. Community *Dent. Oral Epidemiol.* 1985; 13(3): 183-4

[25] Menéndez M, Alarcón JA, González E. Estudio de la morfología craneofacial en el síndrome de Down. Ortodoncia Española 1992; 33: 223-32

[26] Suarez Quintanilla J, Biedma BM, Rodriguez MQ, Mora MT, Cunqueiro MM, Pazos MA. Cephalometrics in children with Down's syndrome. *Pediatr. Radiol.* 2002; 32(9): 635-43

[27] Klain U. Pubertá e mongolismo (Studio auxologico di 10 casi). *Minerva Pediatr.* 1965; 17 (23): 1248-9

[28] Rarick GL, Wainer H, Thissen D, Seefeldt V. A double logistic comparison of growth pattern of normal children and children with Down's syndrome. *Ann. Hum. Biol.* 1975; 2: 339-46

[29] Arnell H, Gustafsson J, Ivarsson SA, Anneren G. Growth and pubertal development in Down syndrome. *Acta Paediatr. Scand.* 1996; 85(9): 1102-06

[30] Toledo C, Alembik Y, Aguirre JA, Stoll C. Growth curves of children with Down syndrome. *Ann. Genet.* 1999; 42(2): 81-90

[31] Ricketts RM. Cephalometric analysis and synthesis. *Angle Orthod.* 1961; 31: 141-56

[32] Björk A. Cranial base development. *Am. J. Orthod.* 1955; 41:198-225

[33] Gosman SD, Vimeland NJ. Facial development in mongolism. *Am. J. Orthod.* 1951; 37: 332-49

[34] Baer MJ, Gavan JA. Symposium on bone growth as revealed by in vivo markers. *Am. J. Phys. Antropol.* 1968; 29(2): 157-6

[35] Naval Gías L. Análisis telerradiográfico del desarrollo craneofacial en pacientes mongólicos. Tésis Doctoral. Zaragoza 1983.

[36] Benda CE. Growth disorder of the skull in Mongolism. Am J Pathol 1940;16: 71-86

[37] Alió JJ, Lorenzo J, Iglesias C Cranial base growth in patients with Down syndrome: A longitudinal study *Am. J. Orthod. Dentofac. Orthoped.* 2008;133(5):729-37

[38] Roche AF, Seward FS, Sunderland S. Growth changes in the mongoloid head. *Acta Paediatr. Scand.* 1961; 50: 133-140

[39] Roche AF, Seward FS, Sunderland S. Non-metrical observations on cranial roentgenograms in mongolism. *Am. J. Roentgenol.* 1961; 85: 659-62

[40] Spitzer R. Developmental anomalies in teeth and skull in mental defectives. *Int. Dent. J.* 1963; 3(4): 678-83

[41] Roche AF. The cranium in mongolism.*Acta Neurolica Scandinavica* 1966;42:62-78

[42] Frostad WA, Cleall JF, Melosky LC. Craniofacial complex in the tisomy 21 syndrome (Down's syndrome). *Arch. Oral Biol.* 1971;16(7):707-22

[43] Brodie AG. On the growth pattern of the human head from the third month to the eigth year of life. *Am. J. Anat.* 1941; 68: 209-62

[44] Baughan B, Demirjian A. Sexual dismorphism in the growth of the cranium. *Am. J. Phys. Anthropol.* 1978; 49: 383-90

[45] Roche AF, Lewis AB. Sex differences in the elongation of the cranial base during pubescence. *Angle Orthod.* 1974; 44: 279-94

[46] Michejda M, Menolascino FJ. Skull base abnormalities in Down's syndrome. *Ment. Retard.* 1975; 13(1): 24-6

[47] James AE Jr, Merz T, Janower ML. Radiological features of the most common autosomal disorders:trisomy 21-22 (mongolism or Down's syndrome), trisomy 13-15, and the cri du chat syndrome. *Clin. Radiol.* 1971; 22(4): 417-33

[48] Michejda M. The role of basiocranial synchondroses in flexure process and ontogenic development of skull base. *Am. J. Phys. Anthropol*.1972;37: 143-150

[49] Lewis AB, Roche AF. The saddle angle: constancy or change? *Angle Orthod.* 1977; 47(1):46-54

[50] Walker GF, Kowalski CJ. On the use of the SNA and SNB angles in cephalometric analyses. *Am. J. Orthod*.1973;64:517-23

[51] Kerr WJ. A longitudinal cephalometric study of dento-facial growth from 5 to 15 years. *Br .J. Orthod.* 1979;6(3):115-21

[52] Bishara SE. Longitudinal cephalometric standards from 5 years of age to adulthood. *Am. J. Orthod.* 1981;79(1):35-44

[53] Bishara SE, Jakobsen JR. Longitudinal changes in three normal facial types. *Am. J. Orthod.* 1985;88(6):466-502

[54] Dellavia C, Sforza C, Orlando F, Ottolina P, Pregliasco F, Ferrario VF. Three-dimensional hard tissue palatal siza and shape in Down sindrome subjects. *Eur. J. Orthod.* 2007;29:417-22

[55] Farkas LG, Munro IR, Kolar JC. Abnormal measurements and disproportions in the face of Down's syndrome patients: preliminary report of an anthropometric study. *Plast. Reconstr .Surg* .1985;75(2):159-69
[56] Farkas LG, Posnik JC, Hreczko T Anthropometry of the head and face in 95 Down syndrome patients. *Prog. Clin. Biol. Res.* 1991;373:53-97
[57] Farkas LG, Katic MJ, Forrest CR. Surface anatomy of the face in Down's syndrome: age-related changes of anthropometric proportion indices in the craniofacial regions. *J. Craniofac. Surg* .2002;13(3):368-74
[58] Allanson JE, O'hara P, Farkas LG, Nair RC. Anthropometric craniofacial pattern profiles in Down syndrome. *Am. J. Med. Genet.* 1993 1; 47(5): 748-52
[59] Ursi WJ, Trotman CA, McNamara JA Jr, Behrents RG. Sexual dimorphism in normal craniofacial growth. *Angle Orthod.* 1993;63(1):47-56
[60] Ardran GM, Harker P, Kemp FH. Tongue size in Down's syndrome. *J. Ment. Defic. Res.* 1972;16:160-66
[61] Soto MT, Alió JJ, Barbería E. Morfologia y alteraciones dentarias en el Síndrome de Down. *Rev. Ibero. Am. Ortod.* 1992;11(2):43-7

In: Handbook of Down Syndrome Research
Editors: Dominicus Jelinek and Gijs Dvorak
ISBN 978-1-60741- 690-6

Chapter 17

Hearing Loss and Middle Ear Disorders in Children with Down Syndrome: The Need for Screening and Surveillance Systems

***Iris Hoi-Yee Ng* [1] *and Carlie Driscoll* [2]**
[1]Institute of Human Communicative Research, and
Department of Otorhinolaryngology, Head and Neck Surgery
The Chinese University of Hong Kong
Hong Kong, China
[2]School of Health and Rehabilitation Sciences, University of Queensland
Queensland, Australia

Abstract

Evidence has been well-documented that persons with Down syndrome are particularly susceptible to hearing loss and middle ear pathology. Hearing loss associated with Down syndrome is usually late-onset and progressive in nature, deeming the regular practices of universal newborn hearing screening insufficient. The authors have carried out hearing screening and diagnostic assessment on schoolchildren with Down syndrome, in both special schools and mainstream schools, in two different nations in the past few years. The prevalence of hearing loss in these school-age populations, as well as the common degree, nature and underlying pathology of hearing loss/middle ear disorders, were investigated. This chapter presents discussion of the developmental implications of such hearing impairment for schoolchildren with Down syndrome, in addition to its influence on learning. Technological options for hearing and middle ear screening are explored, culminating in feasible and practical screening and surveillance protocols for this population. Finally, the authors discuss medical and audiological treatment options and outline recommendations for meeting the audiological rehabilitation needs of children with Down syndrome.

Introduction

When providing services for children with Down syndrome, medical professionals are often aware of the associated intellectual impairment, as well as the craniofacial anomalies evident in many. Yet, this population is also particularly susceptible to otological and audiological disorders. Congenital abnormalities predispose them to hearing loss, often of a type that cannot be detected by universal neonatal hearing screening programs. Furthermore, hearing loss is sometimes not viewed as the primary concern in caring for this population and, thus, audiological monitoring and rehabilitation provided to children with Down syndrome can be relatively limited. By adopting an objective, reliable and time-efficient hearing screening protocol, the feasibility and practicality of hearing surveillance among children with Down syndrome are asserted. As an increasingly wide array of rehabilitative technologies become available, timely otological treatment and audiological (re)habilitation for this population shall no longer be inaccessible.

Prevalence and Underlying Pathology of Hearing Loss Associated with Down Syndrome

For decades, it has been established that the prevalence of hearing loss in those with Down syndrome is higher in comparison with the general population, and that the prevalence disproportionately increases with age [1-5]. Estimates of the incidence of hearing loss in pediatric populations with Down syndrome vary from 38% to as high as 78% [6]. The authors' previous findings in two different school-aged populations revealed a 40% to an astonishing 90% point prevalence using a transient evoked otoacoustic emissions (TEOAE) screening protocol [2,7]. The hearing loss reported in these studies was usually mild to moderate in degree. Such prevalence rates compare unfavorably with the 1 to 3 in 500 rates, inclusive of late-onset permanent childhood hearing impairment, typically cited for the general population [8].

Hearing loss among children with Down syndrome can be both congenital and acquired later in life. Inner ear abnormalities (including a tendency for smaller cochleas, Mondini deformity, shortened organ of Corti, endolymphatic hydrops, remnant tissue in the round windows, as well as fewer fibres in the ventral cochlear nuclei), as reviewed in histological research, predispose this population to a loss of sound sensitivity at their cochlear sensory cells or neural pathways beyond the inner ear, known as sensorineural hearing loss [9]. Early onset presbycusis, probably contributed to by age-related bone apposition in the fundus of the internal auditory meatus, was also noted by different researchers [10-13]. "Early onset" refers to the condition being acquired in advance of the normal age period. "Presbycusis" refers to hearing loss that is associated with the degenerative processes of aging. Typically, the loss is slowly progressive and affects the basal area of the cochlea, the region responsible for high frequency hearing, first. Relatively young persons with Down syndrome, even in their second decade of life, are already exhibiting this high frequency sensorineural hearing loss [14]. This is a condition that the general population does not usually encounter until their sixth decade of life.

Besides deformity and degeneration of the cochlea, leading to sensory hearing loss, craniofacial anomalies including Eustachian tube problems, remnant tissue in the middle ear cavity, stenosis of the external auditory canal, defects of the external pinna, adenoidal hypertrophy, constriction of the nasopharynx and mastoid hyperplasia are not uncommon among those with Down syndrome [1,4,11,15-20]. Middle ear dysfunction clearly affects a greater proportion of this population than persons without the condition, where prevalence rates for Caucasian children are usually in the vicinity of 13% [21]. The middle ear anomalies and dysfunction are believed to cause a high incidence of recurrent episodes of otitis media and other middle ear pathologies, with rates varying from 48% to 89% depending on the particulars of the participant sample and criterion selected. A conductive hearing loss results [2,17]. Such hearing loss may either be a consequence of the destructed sound conduction pathway (before the signal reaches the inner ear), and, thus, permanent, or fluctuating in accordance with the status of middle ear infection and effusion.

Malformed or stenotic external auditory canals can also create a transient conductive hearing loss. This anatomical difference prevents cerumen/earwax from migrating outwards and, hence, promotes its accumulation and occlusion of the external auditory canal. One of the authors' previous studies indicated that 13.9% of ears in children with Down syndrome, examined on one occasion, had an occlusive degree of cerumen and needed cleaning by physicians [7]. Another report on otological monitoring of children with Down syndrome mentioned that over 90% of children required cerumen cleaning under microscope in the otolaryngologist's office before audiological evaluations could be performed [6].

Effects of Hearing Loss on Development

Despite all the known etiology of rapidly deteriorating or fluctuating hearing loss, the precise hearing status of children with Down syndrome is often unknown to caregivers and medical practitioners. One of the authors' studies, conducted in special schools in Queensland, Australia, indicated that a startling 70.4% of the participants with Down syndrome were suspected by their caregivers as having an undiagnosed hearing loss at the time of testing. No participating children were identified by caregivers or school staff as having a previously diagnosed hearing loss, while 85.2% of students were reported to have had hearing assessments in the past [2]. Hearing evaluation for children with Down syndrome, especially those who are intellectually challenged and exhibiting developmental skills inconsistent with their chronological age, is often easier said than done. Regular hearing screening provided to this population, at general out-patient or special education settings such as special schools, special units or developmental centers, usually comprises a standard behavioral battery of audiological tests (e.g., pure tone audiometric screening and immittance audiometry). Though audiologists are usually well-trained to observe various developmentally appropriate behaviors, ranging from hand-raising, play task performing (such as dropping a toy block in a bucket), head-turning, to even eye-widening and quieting, in response to sound stimuli, behavioral hearing screening is sometimes simply impossible. Voluntary behavioral responses are often limited by attentional constraints, poor psychomotor skills, lack of cooperative behavior, atypical and unreliable response characteristics, and deficient interest in non-meaningful sound stimuli. As a consequence, the time required to complete the screening, if possible at all, is grossly increased and electrophysiological diagnostic tests are often deemed necessary in estimating the hearing status of these children.

A study has suggested that as few as 50% of students with significant developmental delay could be assessed behaviorally, while, for many others, results had to be supplemented by diagnostic auditory brainstem responses (ABR) [22]. This diagnostic, electrophysiological tool is, however, a much more costly option if applied in regular screening and monitoring, as a very quiet, preferably sound-treated and electrically-shielded environment is needed for a good ABR recording. The person being tested has to be quiet, inactive and not vocalizing as well, to prevent interference by physiological noise and, therefore, sedation and sometimes general anesthesia would be necessary to obtain recordings among those with developmental delay. The average test duration varies between different protocols, yet a fair estimation would be that well over 30 minutes to an hour is required for frequency-specific, threshold estimation measurements. Such could explain the lack of hearing screening, particularly using ABR measurement, that is directed to this population. In view of all the constraints and limitations of screening, any deficit, change or fluctuation in hearing status may be overlooked.

The intricacy in diagnosis of hearing status in children with Down syndrome, who are almost universally facing intellectual challenge and global development delay, may lead to a delay in identification of hearing loss and subsequent (re)habilitation and this may substantially hinder their progress. A study of over a thousand school-aged children with no other disability revealed that even a minimal sensorineural hearing loss of above 20 dB HL at the major speech frequencies, or a mere mild high-frequency loss, did impact upon the children's educational and functional test performances, and over 30% of such children failed at least one grade of schooling [23]. Other research has clearly indicated that a mild degree of untreated hearing loss may impede children's speech, language, literacy, educational, psychosocial and emotional development [24-33].

Given the developmental delay and intellectual challenge inclining children with Down syndrome towards speech and language delay, as well as an expected lack of repair strategies as are used by hearing-impaired adults when understanding speech in context, any level of hearing difficulty does complicate daily understanding of verbal conversations and instructions. Timely identification of hearing loss in this population is, thus, necessary for optimal habilitation.

Technological Options for Screening

Several researchers and academics have proposed the use of otoacoustic emissions (OAEs) in the hearing evaluation of populations with special needs [7,9,34,35]. OAE screening involves a simple and non-invasive technique, with no behavioral response and minimal cooperation required, providing an objective and reliable overview of cochlear outer hair cell function. It can robustly be administered in non-sound treated testing environments and takes no more than a couple of minutes to perform [36]. OAEs may be defined as low-intensity acoustic energy produced by the cochlea and recorded in the ear canal, and are believed to reflect energy leakage that is radiated out by the cochlea, as a result of the active processing and amplification of low-intensity sound input by the outer hair cells [37]. Transient evoked otoacoustic emissions (TEOAEs) and distortion-product otoacoustic emissions (DPOAEs) are elicited and measured as a result of deliberate acoustic stimulation, forming part of the "evoked" class of OAEs. The testing procedure essentially involves placing a soft, disposable plastic probe tip into the entrance of the external auditory canal, as the equipment presents a series of soft acoustic stimuli, either clicks or tones, and measures the energy radiated out of the ear in response. The presence of a recordable evoked emission essentially indicates normal functioning of the cochlea, a fundamental part of the sensorineural hearing apparatus, along with normal middle ear function, a vital part of the conductive hearing apparatus. The TEOAEs, obtained with click stimulus in particular, are present in almost all normal ears, and are reduced in amplitude when pure tone hearing thresholds between the frequency range of 1 and 4 kHz exceed 20 dB HL, while basically absent when thresholds are worse than 30 dB HL [38,39]. Although not a test of hearing levels, evoked OAEs are frequently used in the screening context to identify ears with hearing levels worse than 25 dB HL, in accordance with the conventional definition of hearing loss.

Apart from this, immittance audiometry, a test of middle ear function, should also be an integral part in the battery of hearing monitoring for children with Down syndrome, in view of a high prevalence of otitis media and middle ear effusion. With a soft, flexible probe tip inserted into the entrance to create an airtight seal in the external auditory canal, the acoustic admittance can be measured in seconds and interpreted according to Jerger's classification of tympanometric shapes [40]. Such enhances identification of middle ear problems.

To date, however, few publications detailing the results of such an integrated testing protocol in special populations have appeared. One study has reported on the outcomes of immittance and DPOAE testing of children with Down syndrome [17]. Along with frequently pathological immittance findings, these researchers reported lower mean DPOAE amplitudes in children with Down syndrome than was observed in their control counterparts. In addition, DPOAE results for the target group were suggestive of early age-related inner ear impairment (early onset presbycusis). This particular study was, however, an investigation conducted within a clinical context and with a strong diagnostic focus. The utilization and results of other types of OAE testing, such as TEOAEs, within school hearing screening programs for children with Down syndrome, have not been widely discussed thus far.

The current authors conducted OAE and immittance testing in school-based settings, on two different populations of children with Down syndrome and other special needs [2,7,41]. No sound-treated test room was employed and no sedation or anesthesia was necessary, while the tests were conducted by an audiologist and assisted by nursing personnel. It was demonstrated that the vast majority (74%) of our total sample of 581 schoolchildren with intellectual impairment (age range 1.9–20.3 years) were able to be tested successfully and swiftly using the TEOAE and immittance test protocol, whereas 75% of our sample of 119 schoolchildren with Down syndrome (age range 2.7–20.3 years) could comply with the hearing screening [2,7,41]. The remaining results were unobtainable because of behavioral or medical reasons, including absence from school. Such a protocol was found to be more than feasible as an effective screening tool in our two samples of schoolchildren with Down syndrome in two different nations. Overall, findings suggested that a combined protocol of OAE and immittance measurements may be a more practicable option than behavioral screening and a less costly alternative to electrophysiological measurements for hearing screening among children with Down syndrome.

It is worth noting that OAE measurement is not an assessment of hearing status, in the sense that it does not provide precise hearing threshold levels at specific frequencies, but evaluates the integrity of the peripheral auditory system up to the outer hair cells in the cochlea. Nonetheless, it still serves as a beneficial part of a hearing screening and surveillance battery. With age and gender specific normative data for the particular population established, and results supplemented by immittance measurements, the presence of significant sensory and/or conductive hearing loss in children with Down syndrome can be reliably screened and monitored with a quick protocol.

The Need for Continued Surveillance of Hearing Status

In spite of the availability of technological options for objective hearing screening, some parents/caregivers, healthcare professionals and educators may misguidedly feel that the need for a hearing screening and monitoring program is fading, as universal neonatal hearing screening programs develop rapidly around the world. Though the goals of early identification of hearing loss and early intervention were partly attained by this multitude of well-organized neonatal screening programs, a large cohort from the pre-screen era, including most of the school-agers and teenagers to date, still need to be followed by school-based or community-based programs. In addition to this, other medical concerns or contraindications among the population with Down syndrome during the neonatal period may preclude them from some of the screening programs designed for well-infants. That is, these high-risk children may be intentionally or otherwise excluded from newborn screening. A recent US study has confirmed the strong association between poor health at birth, high risk of hearing loss and missed neonatal hearing screens [42]. Furthermore, the fluctuating nature of the conductive hearing loss often experienced by this group, along with the real possibility of early-onset presbycusis (which is progressive and not evident in the newborn stage), also dictate the need for vigilant monitoring of those with Down syndrome throughout childhood and early adulthood.

Therefore, hearing screening for children with Down syndrome beyond the neonatal period can be considered a current necessity, yet it is a necessity that has not been fulfilled. Hearing screening in special schools, special units or developmental centers, where young people with Down syndrome are likely receiving at least part-time education, is usually not routinely conducted. This is despite the existence of multiple international consensus statements and guidelines on universal neonatal hearing screening, which stipulate that the hearing of all children must be regularly monitored throughout childhood, and that monitoring and surveillance systems are crucial [43].

Some clinicians have proposed a protocol of close monitoring, as well as aggressive medical and surgical management of otological and audiological problems in this population [6]. Children with Down syndrome were suggested to be enrolled into a surveillance system before the age of two years and provided with full otolaryngological and audiological check-up at least every six months. Phone follow-up was also recommended bi-weekly to monitor for any episode of otitis media diagnosed and treated by primary care physicians. Hearing assessment with behavioral techniques was attempted at six months of age or older, and the children would undergo electrophysiological hearing assessment whenever they were unable to cooperate or respond to a behavioral test [6]. The preliminary results of this management protocol were very promising, in that 98% of children, all below the age of 4 years, had hearing levels within normal limits after the program was run for less than 2 years. This suggests that the hearing status of those with Down syndrome could possibly be better than previously observed [6].

Apart from meticulous surveillance commencing shortly after birth, another potential opportunity for hearing and middle ear status screening for children with Down syndrome beyond the newborn period arises upon commencement of schooling, e.g., entry into special education facilities. Once schooling has started, a regular hearing surveillance program could be conducted within school-based settings, where those with developmental and intellectual challenges may be screened with the aforementioned OAE and immittance technologies.

In addition to a hearing screening and surveillance system, a clear referral pathway and a total team management approach would be necessary in allowing children with Down syndrome to achieve their highest potentials. The team approach may enhance collaborations among pediatricians or primary care physicians (who can attend to a high prevalence of cerumen occlusion and otitis media), otolaryngologists (who can regularly clean ears and examine tympanic membranes), audiologists (who can perform appropriate hearing screening, assessment and auditory rehabilitation), and many other (re)habilitation specialists, so that an effective management program could be tailor-made for this population.

Treatment Options – Medical and Audiological

Two of the major causes of transient conductive hearing loss among children with Down syndrome (namely the recurrent middle ear effusion and the cerumen occlusion in their stenotic external auditory canals) may potentially be remedied by timely monitoring. Regular visits to an otolaryngologist for microscopic examination may not only clear the cerumen occlusion and cure the associated transient conductive hearing loss, but also reveal any signs of otitis media or middle ear effusion, which probably cannot be visualized adequately under conventional otoscopic check because of the canal anatomy. Shott and her colleagues' investigation found that 83% of their study population had pressure equalization (PE) tubes placed at least once because of middle ear effusion over a study period of less than two years, while one of our studies revealed that 19.1% of ears in the study population screened on one occasion were suspected to have middle ear effusion [6,7]. Aggressive medical treatment, involving antibiotics and PE tubes, commencing as early as possible after birth, can substantially improve hearing levels in this population, so that audiological intervention, aside from monitoring, may then be unnecessary [6]. However, it was noted that chronic otitis media with effusion in this population usually does not resolve but returns after the PE tubes have been extruded, so that multiple sets of tubes are required [6]. Whilst hearing may be improved, optimal hearing levels may still not always be maintained.

Among those with Down syndrome for whom the middle ear pathology cannot be medically ameliorated, the associated conductive hearing loss may be persistent. Additionally, for those with disordered sensorineural hearing apparatus, the loss is nearly always permanent and untreatable. One of the authors' studies on schoolchildren with Down syndrome, conducted in special schools in Hong Kong, China, suggested that the children's classroom audibility, calculated according to their average hearing levels, could be as low as less than 20% of words correctly understood [7,44]. Thus, for them, audiological rehabilitation is essential, in which standard hearing aid amplification is often recommended to maximize their reception of auditory and speech signals. Hearing aid technologies have advanced enormously over the past couple of decades. Hearing aids nowadays are small and light-weight enough to fit on pediatric ears, or malformed pinna in some of the children with Down syndrome. Their digital-based programmable settings and adjustments allow fitting for almost any configuration of hearing loss, while such flexibility, along with frequent audiological consultations and close monitoring, accommodate the changing amplification needs of fluctuating or progressive hearing loss common among these children as well. Recent developments also permit specific fitting prescriptions, and objective processes of verification and validation, even with limited cooperation from the children. Personalized hearing aid fitting for children with Down syndrome, or other special needs including intellectual challenge, should be attainable once a hearing loss is diagnosed and the degree is estimated. With a large variety of hearing aid accessories available in the market to assist in children's adaptation, in addition to specific hardware and software designs in the hearing aids, safe and proper use by young children or those with developmental delay is also ensured. Hearing aid fitting for young children with Down syndrome and associated hearing loss, thus, should not be precluded. As a matter of fact, if the hearing loss is congenital or developed shortly after birth, amplification should be provided by the age of 6 months to achieve optimal language development [33].

For those attending school or developmental centers, however, the listening environment is usually less than optimal compared to the home environment, in terms of background noise, signal-to-noise ratio, reverberation and distance from communication partners [45]. According to the guidelines published by the American National Standards Institute, the background noise level of a classroom is recommended not to exceed 35 dB A, yet the background noise levels of the typical quiet special school classrooms where the authors conducted their hearing screening of schoolchildren with Down syndrome ranged from 31 to 61 dB A, with an average of about 40 dB A [7,41,46]. In this relatively high level of noise, hearing aids are sometimes commented to be amplifying both the speech signals and the background noise, providing insufficient improvement in terms of signal-to-noise ratio (which is how much the speech signal is standing out from the background noise as a difference in intensity).

Sound-field amplification is an alternative to standard hearing aids in school environments, for enhancing speech reception and improving access to auditory information, especially when students have difficulties in self-caring and manipulation of the hearing aids, as well as difficulties in the reporting of any fluctuation of hearing status. Well-designed installation of a sound-field amplification system has been reported as cost-effective and beneficial in improving classroom acoustics. These systems can selectively increase instructors' speech level, and drastically improve and stabilize the signal-to-noise ratio throughout the whole classroom [45,47-49]. Investigation has been performed on a small group of schoolchildren with Down syndrome using sound-field amplification in their classrooms, where significantly superior speech perception was revealed [50]. Sound-field amplification is, in particular, advantageous to those with fluctuating hearing loss in classrooms, such as children with recurrent otitis media associated with Down syndrome [51]. Apart from these, prescription of personal listening systems and implantation of bone-anchored hearing aids are also potential options. Study has revealed that the quality of life of children with Down syndrome, including social and physical function, has been improved with bone-anchored hearing aids, while both the children and their parents/caregivers were motivated to maintain such a device [52]. The exact choice of rehabilitation is dependant upon individual case-related factors and, although none could be considered as without possible complication or limitation, all options have been shown to be successful under specified circumstances. If classroom acoustic modifications are employed in addition, such as low-noise air-conditioning systems, double-paned windows, sound-absorbing materials for floor and hard surfaces, and rearrangement of classroom furniture, reception of speech and auditory signals by schoolchildren with Down syndrome can be further enhanced [53].

Conclusion

The authors' studies on schoolchildren with Down syndrome, echoing many other researchers over past decades, clearly indicate a high prevalence of hearing loss, with a large proportion most probably attributed to middle ear pathologies. Considering the intellectual challenge and developmental delay faced by many children with Down syndrome, this population is usually viewed as "difficult to test" in audiological evaluation. Yet any undiagnosed or untreated hearing loss, or fluctuation in their hearing status, does hinder (re)habilitation progress and restricts these children from achieving their highest potential. Thus, a more feasible, time-efficient and objective hearing surveillance battery, such as a combination of immittance and OAE measurements, has been proposed by the authors. It is hoped that by identifying any hearing loss among children with Down syndrome, close monitoring of their hearing status over time, and referring for full medical and/or audiological consultations, appropriate (re)habilitations can be provided. Communication needs in the home, school, institution and work environment can then be fulfilled and, hence, higher achievements can be realized.

References

[1] Balkany TJ, Downs MP, Jafek BW, Krajicek MJ. Hearing loss in Down's syndrome. *Clin Pediatr* 1979;18:116-118.

[2] Driscoll C, Kei J, Bates D, McPherson B. Tympanometry and TEOAE testing of children with Down syndrome in special schools. *Aust NZ J Audiol* 2003;25:85-93.

[3] Kattan HA, Jarrar RF, Mahasin ZZ. A pilot study of the relationship between Down's syndrome and hearing loss. *Saudi Med J* 2000;21:931-933.

[4] Mazzoni DS, Ackley RS, Nash DJ. Abnormal pinna type and hearing loss correlations in Down's syndrome. *J Intellect Disabil Res* 1994;38:549-560.

[5] Roizen NJ, Wolters C, Nicol T, Blondis TA. Hearing loss in children with Down syndrome. *J Pediatr* 1993;123:S9-S12.

[6] Shott SR, Joseph A, Heithaus D. Hearing loss in children with Down syndrome. *Int J Pediatr Otorhinolaryngol* 2001;61:199-205.

[7] McPherson B, Lai SPS, Leung KKK, Ng IHY. Hearing loss in Chinese school children with Down syndrome. *Int J Pediatr Otorhinolaryngol* 2007;71:1905-1915.

[8] Mehl AL, Thomson V. Newborn hearing screening: The great omission. *Pediatrics* 1998;101(1):e4.

[9] Kile JE. Audiologic assessment of children with Down syndrome. *Am J Audiol* 1996;5:44-52.

[10] Brooks DN, Wooley H, Kanjilal GC. Hearing loss and middle ear disorders in patients with Down syndrome (Mongolism). *J Ment Defic Res* 1972;16:21-29.

[11] Kanamori G, Witter M, Brown J, Williams-Smith L. Otolaryngologic manifestations of Down syndrome. *Otolaryngol Clin North Am* 2000;33:1285-1292.

[12] Keiser H, Montague J, Wold D, Maune S, Pattison D. Hearing loss of Down's syndrome adults. *Am J Ment Defic* 1981;85:467-472.

[13] Krmpotic-Nemanic J. Down syndrome and presbyacusis. *Lancet* 1970;2(7674):670-671.

[14] Buchanan LH. Early onset of presbyacusis in Down syndrome. *Scand Audiol* 1990;19:103-110.

[15] Brown PM, Lewis GTR, Parker AJ, Mau AR. The skull base and nasopharynx in Down's syndrome in relation to hearing impairment. *Clin Otolaryngol* 1989;14:241-246.

[16] Glass RB, Yousefzadeh DK, Roizen NJ. Mastoid abnormalities in Down syndrome. *Pediatr Radiol* 1989;19:311-312.

[17] Hassmann E, Skotnicka B, Midro AT, Musiatowicz M. Distortion products otoacoustic emissions in diagnosis of hearing loss in Down syndrome. *Int J Pediatr Otorhinolaryngol* 1998;45:199-206.

[18] Jacobs IN, Gray RF, Todd NW. Upper airway obstruction in children with Down syndrome. *Arch Otolaryngol Head Neck Surg* 1996;122:945-950.

[19] Shibahara Y, Sando I. Congenital anomalies of the Eustachian tube in Down syndrome. *Ann Otol Rhinol Laryngol* 1989;98:543-547.

[20] Strome M. Down's syndrome: A modern otorhinolaryngological perspective. *Laryngoscope* 1981;91:1581-1594.

[21] Nozza RJ, Sabo DL, Mandel EM. A role for otoacoustic emissions in screening for hearing impairment and middle ear disorders in school-age children. *Ear Hear* 1997;18(3):227-239.

[22] Rupa V. Dilemmas in auditory assessment of developmentally retarded children using behavioural observation audiometry and brain stem evoked response audiometry. *J Laryngol Otol* 1995;109:605-609.

[23] Bess F, Dodd-Murphy J, Parker R. Children with minimal sensorineural hearing loss: Prevalence, educational performance, and functional status. *Ear Hear* 1998;19(5):339-354.

[24] Blamey PJ, Sarant JZ, Paatsch LE, Barry JG, Bow CP, Wales RJ, et al. Relationships among speech perception, production, language, hearing loss and age in children with impaired hearing. *J Speech Lang Hear Res* 2001;44:264-285.

[25] Jerger S. Current state of knowledge: Perceptual processing by children with hearing impairment. *Ear Hear* 2007;28(6):754-765.

[26] Levitt H. Interrelationships among the speech and language measures. In: Levitt H, McGarr NS, Geffner D, editors. *Development of language and communication skills in hearing-impaired children* (ASHA monographs no. 26). Rockville, MD: American Speech-Language-Hearing Association; 1987. p. 123-139.

[27] Meadow K. Studies of behaviour problems of deaf children. In: Stein LK, Mindel ED, Jabaley T, editors. *Deafness and Mental Health.* New York: Grune and Stratton; 1981. p. 3-22.

[28] Moeller MP. Early intervention and language development in children who are deaf and hard of hearing. *Pediatrics* 2000;106:e43.

[29] Moeller MP. Current state of knowledge: Psychosocial development in children with hearing impairment. *Ear Hear* 2007;28(6):729-739.

[30] Moeller MP, Tomblin JB, Yoshinaga-Itano C, McDonald Connor C, Jerger S. Current state of knowledge: Language and literacy of children with hearing impairment. *Ear Hear* 2007;28(6):740-753.

[31] Prior MR, Glazner EA, Sanson A, Debelle G. Temperament and behavioural adjustment in hearing impaired children. *J Child Psychol Psychiatr* 1988;29:206-216.

[32] Yoshinaga-Itano C. Development of audition and speech: Implications for early intervention with infants who are deaf or hard of hearing. *Volta Rev* 1998;100(5):213-236.

[33] Yoshinaga-Itano C, Sedey AL, Coulter DK, Mehl AL. Language of early- and later-identified children with hearing loss. *Pediatrics* 1998;102(5):1161-1171.

[34] Grewe TSC, Danhauer JL, Danhauer KJ, Thornton ARD. Clinical use of otoacoustic emissions in children with autism. *Int J Pediatr Otorhinolaryngol* 1994;30:123-132.

[35] Hall JW. *Handbook of otoacoustic emissions*. San Diego: Singular; 2000.

[36] Kemp DT. Developments in cochlear mechanics and techniques for non invasive evaluation. *Advance for Audiologists* 1988;5:27-45.

[37] Probst R, Lonsbury-Martin BL, Martin GK. A review of otoacoustic emissions. *J Acoust Soc Am* 1991;89(5):2027-2067.

[38] Prieve BA, Gorga MP, Schmidt A, Neely S, Peters J, Schultes L, et al. Analysis of transient-evoked otoacoustic emissions in normal-hearing and hearing-impaired ears. *J Acoust Soc Am* 1993;93:3308-3319.

[39] Taylor CL, Brooks RP. Screening for hearing loss and middle-ear disorders in children using TEOAEs. *Am J Audiol* 2000;9:50-55.

[40] Jerger JF. Clinical experience with impedance audiometry. *Arch Otolaryngol* 1970;92:311-324.

[41] Driscoll C, Kei J, Bates D, McPherson B. Transient evoked otoacoustic emissions in children studying in special schools. *Int J Pediatr Otorhinolaryngol* 2002;64:51.

[42] Christensen M, Thomson V, Letson GW. Evaluating the reach of universal newborn hearing screening in Colorado. *Am J Prev Med* 2008;35(6):594-597.

[43] Joint Committee on Infant Hearing. Year 2007 Position Statement: Principles and guidelines for early hearing detection and intervention programs. *Pediatrics* 2007;120(4):898-921.

[44] Pavlovic CV. Speech recognition and five articulation indexes. *Hear Instrum* 1991;42(9):20-23.

[45] McSporran E. Towards better listening and learning in the classroom. *Educ Rev* 1997;49:102-111.

[46] American National Standards Institute. *Acoustical performance criteria, design requirements, and guidelines for schools*. 2002;ANSI S12.60-2002.

[47] Berg FS, Blair JC, Benson PV. Classroom acoustics: The problem, impact, and solution. *Lang Speech Hear Serv Sch* 1996;27:16-20.

[48] Flexer C, Millin J, Brown L. Children with developmental disabilities: The effects of sound field amplification on word identification. *Lang Speech Hear Serv Sch* 1990;21:177-182.

[49] Flexer C, Crandell C, Smaldino J. Considerations and strategies for amplifying the classroom. In: Crandell C, Smaldino J, Flexer C, editors. *Sound-field FM Amplification: Theory and Practical Applications.* San Diego: Singular; 1995. p. 125-147.

[50] Bennetts LK, Flynn MC. Improving the classroom listening skills of children with Down syndrome by using sound-field amplification. *Downs Syndr Res Pract* 2002;8:19-24.

[51] Flexer C. Individual and sound-field FM systems: Rationale, description, and use. *Volta Rev* 1997;99:133-162.

[52] McDermott A-, Williams J, Kuo MJ, Reid AP, Proops D. The role of bone anchored hearing aids in children with Down syndrome. *Int J Pediatr Otorhinolaryngol* 2008;72(6):751-757.

[53] Siebein GW, Gold MA, Siebein GW, Ermann MG. Ten ways to provide a high-quality acoustical environment in schools. *Lang Speech Hear Serv Sch* 2000;31:376-384.

In: Handbook of Down Syndrome Research
Editors: Dominicus Jelinek and Gijs Dvorak
ISBN 978-1-60741- 690-6

Chapter 18

The Dental Evidence for Prenatal and Early Postnatal Growth Insults in Down Syndrome

***Uri Zilberman*[1,2] *David Keinan*[1] *and Patricia Smith*[1]**
[1]Laboratory of Bioanthropology and Ancient DNA, Faculty of Dental Medicine, Hebrew University, Jerusalem, Israel
[2]Pediatric Dental Clinic, Barzilai Medical Center, Ashkelon, Israel

Abstract

Down Syndrome (DS) (Trisomy 21) is a relatively common anomaly occurring in one in every 600-700 live births and characterized by impaired growth and development and early senescence. Signs of abnormal development have been observed on ultrasound as early as the first trimester. They include abnormal flow velocity patterns in the ductus venosus and hypoplasia of the nasal bone in addition to increased fetal nuchal translucency. By the second trimester additional signs are evident on ultrasound, affecting skeletal growth as well as other organ systems. Dental anomalies include reduced tooth size and number, thin enamel and abnormal crown form as well as taurodont roots and a high frequency of missing teeth. The severity of the dental defects varies along the tooth row with later developing teeth most severely affected. Recent studies carried out on exfoliated (shed) deciduous teeth using a combination of serial microCT scans and SEM have enabled us to reconstruct the chronology and extent of intrauterine and infant growth insults in DS infants, expressed in growth and differentiation of the developing teeth. Our results for the deciduous teeth show that in DS, there is accelerated dental development in the first trimester followed by progressive growth retardation associated with impaired differentiation of the dental tissues. These changes appear to primarily affect cells derived from ectoderm and affect cell division and differentiation. This results in a smaller modified tooth germ with impaired enamel matrix formation and bio-mineralization. The resulting enamel is thin and hypomineralized and this may contribute to the severe abrasion seen in the teeth of DS children despite the associated lack of muscle tone.

Introduction

Down syndrome (DS) is a relatively common anomaly and is the best known example of impaired growth and development associated with chromosomal anaploidy. It is primarily associated with cognitive impairment and craniofacial dysmorphia. Phenotypic variants include congenital heart defects, gastrointestinal tract abnormalities, acute megakaryoblastic leukemia, immunological defects and endocrine abnormalities, neuropathology leading to dementia, and dysmorphic body proportions (Moore and Roper 2007). Leukocyte expression patterns in DS differ from those of the general population, with key regulators of growth and proliferation affected (Malago *et al.* 2005). Individuals with DS have a higher risk of leukemia and testicular cancer when compared to the general population (Patja *et al.* 2006).

First trimester ultrasound screening of DS fetuses shows abnormal flow velocity patterns in the *ductus venosus* in addition to increased fetal nuchal translucency (Prefumo *et al.* 2005). Impaired growth of the nasal bone, maxilla and humerus has been shown in ultrasound images taken in the second semester (Benacerraf *et al.* 1986) and autopsies carried out on DS fetuses have shown an increase in the hypertrophic portion of rib cartilage with a concomitant decrease in the proliferating and resting zone (Garcia-Ramirez *et al.* 1998). Mean birth weight for DS boys and girls recently reported by Weijerman *et al.* (2008) in the Netherlands was 3.119 kg and 2.901kg respectively, averaging 300-400 gm less than that of the general population, while mean duration of gestation at 38 weeks was one week less than that of the general population. Bone mineral density in DS is also reduced compared to that of controls (Angelopoulou *et al.* 1999, 2000, Sepulveda *et al.* 1995, Baptista *et al.* 2005), and has been related to muscular hypotonia (Angelopoulou *et al.* 1999, 2000).

Oral and dental characteristics associated with DS include high and antero-posterior shortened palate (Shapiro *et al.* 1967, Skrinjaric *et al.* 2004) (Figure 1), macroglossia and scrotal tongue and microdontia of permanent teeth (Figure 2), although some primary teeth are larger (Cohen 1970, Townsend 1983, 1987, Peretz *et al.* 1999) with altered crown shape (Brown and Townsend 1984,(Peretz *et al.* 1998). Enamel hypoplasia (Figure 3), taurodontism (Jasper 1981) and hypodontia are common (McMillan and Kashgarian 1961) (Figure 4), with third molar agenesis four times more frequent than in controls (Lomholt *et al.* 2002). Caries prevalence in DS is lower than in controls and related to elevated salivary *S. mutans* specific IgA concentrations and different profiles of *S. mutans* based on AP-PCR typing (Lee *et al.* 2004, Cogulu *et al.* 2006). The roots of DS teeth have thin cementum similar to that observed in leukocyte adhesion deficiency and aggressive periodontitis (Bimstein *et al.* 2008).

Deciduous teeth offer an excellent model with which to reconstruct the timing and progress of growth insults such as those associated with DS. Their development is a strictly ordered hierarchical process that is highly correlated with chronological age and begins in the 6th to 8th week *in utero* (Kraus and Jordan 1965, Ten Cate 1998). Developmental insults leave a permanent imprint whose onset and severity can be identified in fully formed teeth.

Both oral ectoderm and neural crest ecto-mesenchyme are involved in tooth formation. Initiation and morphogenesis appear to be primarily determined by the ectodermally derived enamel organ, which also gives rise to the ameloblasts that form the enamel matrix.

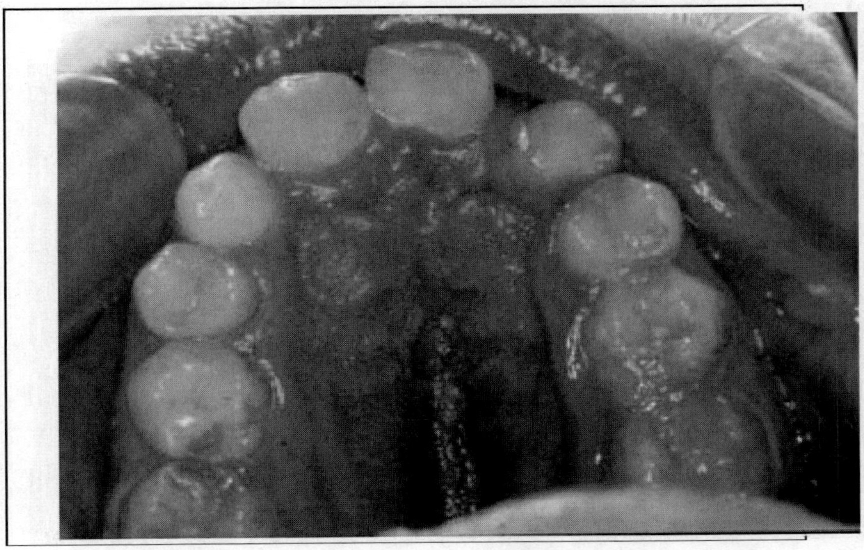

Figure 1. The palate in DS -very high and short antero-posterior.

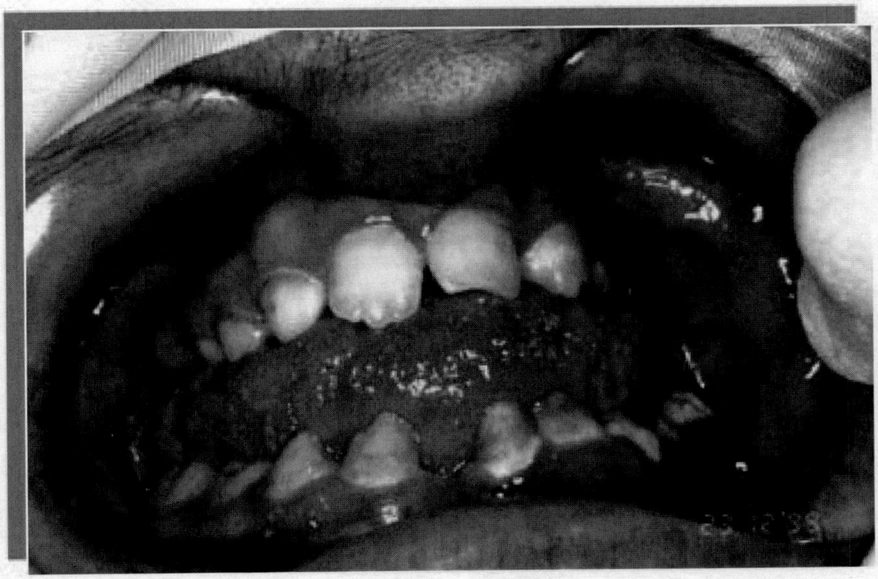

Figure 2. Macroglossia, scrotal tongue, and malformed permanent teeth in DS.

The ecto-mesenchyme forms the dental sac and dentin-pulp complex.

Crown size is determined by two phases:

The early stage is defined by the dentin-enamel junction (DEJ) that denotes the extent and pattern of cell proliferation and differentiation. The final stage is defined by the thickness of the enamel shell overlying the DEJ and represents the activity of the ameloblasts that secrete the enamel matrix. The thickness of enamel varies in different locations, modifying the outline presented at the DEJ (Ten Cate 1998).

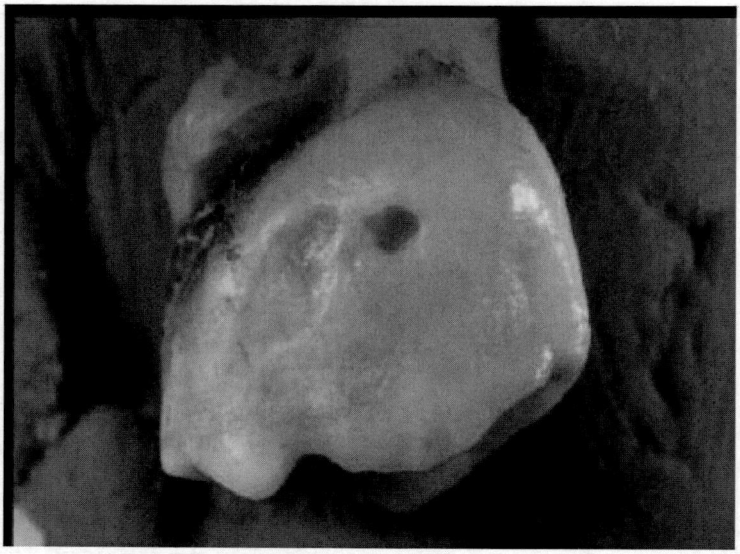

Figure 3. Abnormal cusp number and enamel hypoplasia on an upper DS deciduous first molar.

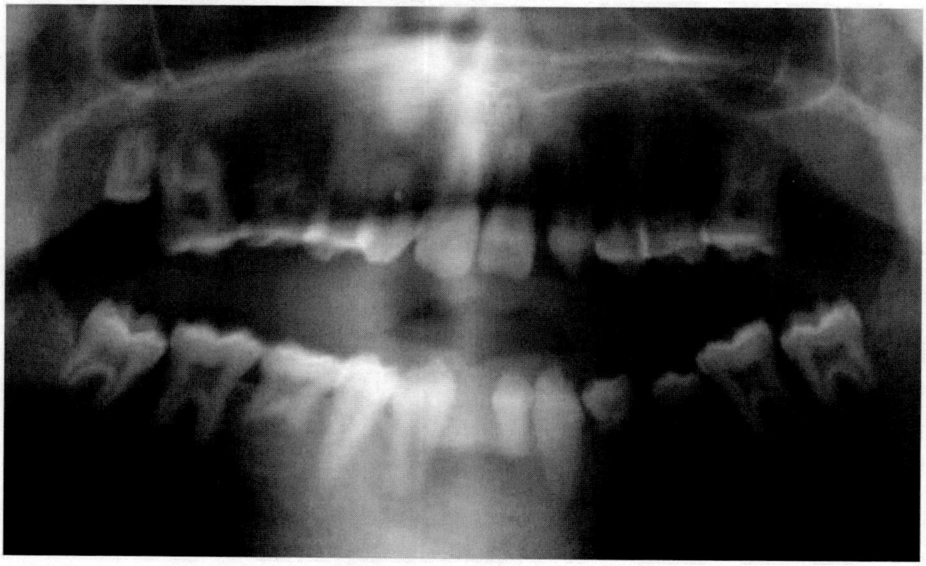

Figure 4. Hypodontia in DS (16 permanent teeth missing).

Deciduous Tooth Size in Down Syndrome

Brabant (1975), Barden (1980), Townsend (1983) and Brown and Townsend (1984) all reported that deciduous incisors, canines and first molars in DS children were larger than those of controls, but the second deciduous molars tended to be smaller than controls. Barden (1983) attributed these size differences to age related effects of growth factors on the developing teeth in DS embryos. He proposed that the large size of the first deciduous teeth initiated, namely the incisors, canines and first molars, was due to a transient acceleration of growth in the first trimester of DS embryos while the later developing second deciduous molars showed the effects of the declining growth rates typical of the condition that are more pronounced in the permanent teeth. More specific information as to the extent to which cell proliferation versus the amount of enamel matrix formed contributes to the size differences exhibited in these teeth has been obtained through the use of clinical radiographs and ground sections.

Stereomicroscopic Studies of Down Syndrome Incisors

Bell *et al.* (2001) examined mid-sagittal sections of exfoliated mandibular deciduous and extracted permanent incisors of individuals with DS using a stereomicroscope. They found that DS permanent incisors were smaller than those of controls with both enamel and dentin affected. They also exhibited a flattened labio-lingual profile as opposed to the more convex outline shown by controls. Bell *et al.* (2001) attributed this to the progressive slowing down of proliferation during the development of the crown from tip to neck. They reported that there were no major differences between DS and control deciduous incisors, although mean values for DS central incisors were larger than in controls and enamel thickness in deciduous lateral incisors of the DS sample was reduced.

Radiographic Studies of Tooth Components in Down Syndrome Molars

Dental radiographs that are routinely taken in the course of dental treatment provide clear differentiation between the outer enamel shell of the teeth, dentin-pulp complex and roots, so that they constitute a primary source of information on the extent to which successive phases of tooth formation are affected. In order to examine this issue in DS molars, Zilberman *et al.* (2004) examined routine diagnostic bitewing radiographs of 45 patients with cytogenetically determined DS and a control group comprising 250 individuals. The teeth measured were lower deciduous second molars and first permanent molars.

Six measurements were taken on each tooth crown (Figure 5). Enamel height (EH), dentin height (DH) and pulp height (PH) were measured along a line drawn parallel to the long axis of the tooth, one millimeter mesial to the central fossa. Maximal pulp width (PW), mesial enamel width (EW) and maximal crown width (CW) were all measured perpendicular to the long axis of the tooth. All measurements were also expressed as a ratio of mesio-distal CW, in order to assess the effect of variation in CW or magnification on tooth proportions.

The results showed that the mesio-distal crown diameter (CW) of second primary molars in children with DS was smaller than that of the control group, with thinner dentin and increased pulp height (Table 1).

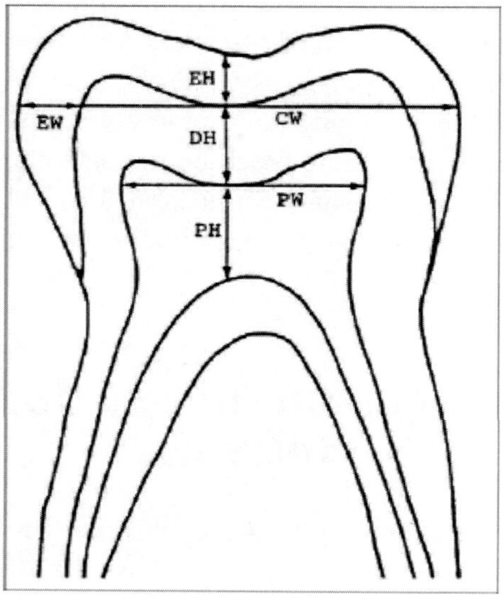

Figure 5. Components measurements obtained from bite-wing radiographs for each molar.

Table 1. Tooth components dimensions in DS and control molars measured from bite-wing radiographs

		Dm2		M1	
		CONTROLS	DS	CONTROLS	DS
	Mean	0.96	0.92	1.66	1.42*
	N.	175	28	160	41
EH	S.D.	0.15	0.16	0.40	0.18
	Min	0.64	0.73	0.64	0.87
	Max	1.64	1.53	2.78	1.72
	Mean	2.83	2.27*	3.30	2.85*
	N.	175	28	160	39
DH	S.D.	0.38	0.46	0.52	0.33
	Min	2.08	1.33	2.03	2.36
	Max	3.92	2.91	4.92	3.57
	Mean	1.10	1.52*	1.69	1.81
	N.	175	28	160	39
PH	S.D.	0.40	0.59	0.60	0.87
	Min	0.33	0.69	0.47	0.64
	Max	2.28	2.55	3.55	3.89
	Mean	0.83	0.88	1.32	1.22
	N.	175	26	160	41
EW	S.D.	0.10	0.13	0.29	0.18
	Min	0.59	0.75	0.62	0.76
	Max	1.16	1.37	2.12	1.53

		Dm2		M1	
		CONTROLS	DS	CONTROLS	DS
	Mean	5.00	4.54	4.57	4.38
	N.	175	28	160	39
PW	S.D.	0.41	0.35	0.49	0.51
	Min	3.93	4.03	3.35	3.39
	Max	5.87	5.42	6.02	5.32
	Mean	10.25	9.77*	11.39	11.11*
	N.	175	28	160	41
CW	S.D.	0.49	0.37	0.73	0.74
	Min	9.07	8.79	9.61	9.70
	Max	11.44	10.60	12.96	12.27
	Mean	0.09	0.09	0.14	0.13
EH1	N.	175	28	160	41
	S.D.	0.01	0.02	0.03	0.01
	Mean	0.28	0.23*	0.29	0.26
DH1	N.	175	28	160	39
	S.D.	0.04	0.05	0.04	0.03
	Mean	0.11	0.15*	0.15	0.16
PH1	N.	175	28	160	39
	S.D.	0.04	0.06	0.05	0.08
	Mean	0.08	0.09	0.12	0.11
EW1	N.	175	26	160	41
	S.D.	0.01	0.02	0.02	0.02
	Mean	0.49	0.46	0.40	0.39
PW1	N.	175	28	160	39
	S.D.	0.03	0.03	0.05	0.04

Note: Dm2= Deciduous second molar
M1= Permanent first molar
EH= Enamel Height
DH= Dentin Height
PH= Pulp Height
EW= Enamel Width
PW= Pulp Width
CW= Crown Width
EH1= EH/CW
DH1= DH/CW
PH1= PH/CW
EW1= EW/CW
PW1= PW/CW
*= P<0.05

One way analysis of variance (ANOVA, REGWR procedure. Post-hoc, α=5%) for each tooth component, showed significant differences between DS and control groups in the deciduous second molars. The main variables contributing to these differences were dentin and pulp height and crown width. The differences were statistically significant and indicative of reduced mitotic activity as well as dentin-matrix formation by the odontoblasts. Moreover, the roots were taurodont, probably as a result of a delay in the apically growing root sheath to produce the horizontal flaps that unite to form the root bifurcation.

The DS, permanent first molars, like the deciduous second molars, were characterized by smaller crown width than controls, with thinner dentin and taurodont roots (Table 1). They also had thinner enamel, as shown by enamel height/crown width ratios. This may reflect the increased severity of the growth insult in the later developing permanent molars. On the other hand, since samples sizes were small, the error of measurement may have obscured differences in enamel thickness between teeth.

The findings of Bell *et al.* (2001) for incisors agree with those of Zilberman *et al.* (2004) for the molars, in showing that both cell proliferation and matrix formation are more severely affected in permanent teeth than in deciduous teeth of the same tooth type. The normal appearance of the DS deciduous incisors probably reflects their early intra-uterine development, since their crowns are nearly complete at birth (Deutsch *et al.* 1985). In contrast crown formation in the second deciduous molars is only finalized between 10 month and 1 year (Coughlin and Christensen 1966).. Thus the significant differences they reported between DS and controls for this tooth, is in keeping with the known progressive effect of DS on growth and development.

Histological Evidence of Prenatal Growth and Development in Down Syndrome Tooth Enamel

Examination of the ultrastructure of the enamel of exfoliated deciduous teeth has provided more detailed information on the extent of qualitative and quantitative changes in DS.

Biomineralization of tooth enamel begins at the future cusp tip and spreads apically as adjacent cells along the inner enamel epithelium overlying the dental sac progressively differentiate into matrix producing ameloblasts (Ten Cate 1998). The enamel matrix is laid down in daily increments, rather like growth rings in a tree, and like them can be related to chronological age (Ten Cate 1998). Once formed this matrix undergoes maturation, a process in which the organic content decreases from some 30% to less than 4% (Deutsch and Gedalia 1980, Deutsch and Pe'er 1982, Deutsch and Shapira 1987). Impaired ameloblast function modifies the quantity and integrity of the organic matrix and so affects the orientation and growth of the apatite crystals and subsequent degradation and removal of the organic matrix, as observed in fluorosis (Robinson *et al.* 2004).

Biomineralization of the crown of the upper primary canine starts later than the incisors, between 17-20 weeks *in utero* and is completed at 9 months after birth, while that of the second primary molar begins around 20 weeks *in utero* and is completed between 10 months and 1 year after birth. In the case of the canine the three regions that develop successively (incisal third, middle third and cervical third) provide a means of comparing early and late stages of growth. In the case of the deciduous incisor, comparison of the mesial and distal cusps serves the same purpose. Comparison of these two deciduous teeth that show a similar developmental age.different regions of the jaw enables us to differentiate between regional effects and chronological effects on growth

To this end, Keinan *et al.* (2006, 2007) examined thin sections of exfoliated deciduous teeth; 20 upper deciduous canines and 12 lower second deciduous molars from a control population and 12 upper deciduous canines and 7 lower second deciduous molars from children with DS. The neonatal line, a layer of hypomineralized enamel formed immediately after birth, was used to distinguish between crown formation before and after birth (Skinner and Dupras 1993). For the canines the thin sections were cut bucco-lingually through the cusp tip. For the molars one section was cut to bisect mesio-buccal and mesio-lingual cusps and the second section bisected the disto-buccal and disto-lingual cusps. Each section was viewed with a light microscope at low magnification.

Measurements taken are shown in Figure 6a and 6b. They included: (1) the thickness of the prenatal and postnatal enamel on outer and inner surfaces of all cusps taken 1mm below the dentine cusp tip, and (2) the distance between the cervical-enamel junction (CEJ) and the location of the neo-natal line at the DEJ; and (3) the distance between the CEJ and dentin cusp tip.

Significantly more enamel was formed prenatally in DS upper primary canines (56%) than in controls (36%), although total enamel width was similar (Table 2). Furthermore, comparison of the distance between the CEJ and location of the neonatal line at the DEJ showed that relatively more of the crown was present in DS canines than in controls at birth.

The lower second deciduous molars exhibited an opposite trend (Table 2). The DS molars had significantly less enamel laid down prenatally in mesial cusps than controls (24% and 33% respectively). However, total enamel width in DS was similar to that of controls with more enamel formed after birth. These results suggest that prenatal growth rates of the deciduous canines in DS children were faster than those of controls, with crown formation more advanced at birth. The reverse applies to the second deciduous molars. Crown formation in these teeth was less advanced than that of controls at birth suggesting that the differences observed in radiographic studies (Zilberman *et al.* 2004) have an early developmental origin.

Chemical Composition of Down Syndrome Teeth

In order to determine the association between the amount of enamel matrix formed *in utero* and its degree of mineralization, Keinan *et al.* (2007) estimated the Ca/P ratio of enamel in a sub-sample of the DS and control upper deciduous canines and second deciduous molars described above.

The hardest mineral component of mature tooth enamel is hydroxyapatite with a Ca/P ratio of 1.67. Primary teeth have a higher Ca/P ratio than permanent teeth as a result of calcium bonded to other elements than phosphate (Deutsch and Shapira 1987), making them softer and less resistant to acid attack. The chemical composition of enamel and dentin was evaluated for the teeth using an energy dispersive X-ray spectrometer (EDS) in order to identify and quantify the main elements in the enamel and dentin tip of each cusp in the deciduous canines and second molars, and in the labial and lingual cervical region in the canines.

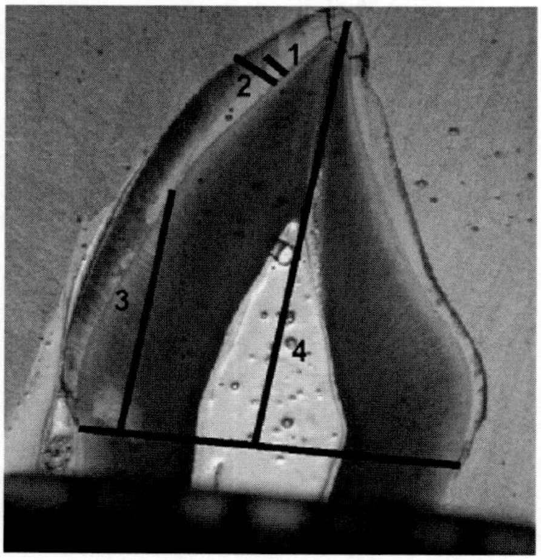

Note: 1- Prenatal enamel width
2- Total enamel width
3- Apical position of neonatal line
4- Dentin cusp height

Figure 6a. Measurements on histology slices in canines.

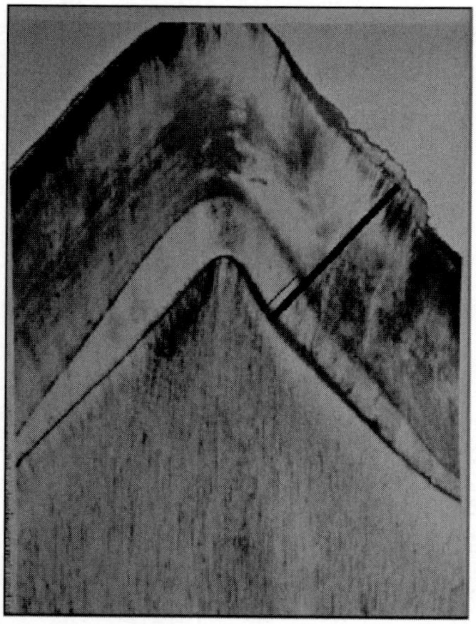

Note: Thick line- total enamel thickness.
Thin line- prenatal enamel thickness.

Figure 6b. Measurements on histology slices in second primary molars cusps.

Table 2. Total enamel thickness and the prenatal enamel ratio in DS deciduous teeth

Tooth/Dev	Cusps	Aspect		Control (11)		DS(8)	
				Mean	Range	**Mean**	Range
U canine 17wiu-9m		Outer	**Total**	**0.70**	0.58-0.78	**0.72**	0.63-0.92
			Ratio	**0.36**	0.29-0.45	**0.56***	0.44-0.56
L dm2 22wiu-12m	MB+ML	Outer	**Total**	**0.94**	0.64-1.46	**0.79**	0.65-1.20
			Ratio	**0.33**	0.17-1.15	**0.24***	0.13-0.31
L dm2 26wiu-12m	DB+DL	Outer	**Total**	**0.95**	0.77-1.15	**0.85**	0.69-1.20
			Ratio	**0.26**	0.14-0.38	**0.29**	0.15-0.41

wiu= weeks in utero

*= P value<0.05 compared to control group

Table 3. Ca/P ratio in DS deciduous teeth compared to control group

		Upper c		**Lower dm2**		**Lower dm2**	
	Cusps			MB+ML		DB+DL	
		Mean	Range	**Mean**	Range	**Mean**	Range
Control	Enamel	**2.10**	2.00-2.38	**2.09**	1.74-2.24	**2.22**	2.12-2.51
	Dentin			**2.13**	1.70-2.37	**2.29**	1.98-2.54
DS	Enamel	**2.04**	1.99-2.12	**2.19**	2.07-2.32	**2.18**	2.01-2.31
	Dentin			**2.13**	2.03-2.24	**2.12**	2.05-2.27

The most prevalent elements that were found were: Calcium, Phosphate, Oxygen and Carbon. Traces of Aluminium, Fluoride, Magnesium and Sodium were also present (less than 3%). The Ca/P ratio of enamel for each tooth was calculated for each location on the tooth and differences between control and DS teeth were analyzed using non-parametric statistical tests (Table 3).

In the canines, no significant differences were found between the cervical and cusp tip. Values were accordingly averaged for subsequent comparisons. No significant differences were found between the DS and control canines with the Ca/P ratios low in both groups. In the DS molars, Ca/P ratios were high in both cusps. This may be related to a reduction in the amount of prenatal enamel formation in these teeth.

To further investigate the differences in enamel structure of DS lower second deciduous molars, Keinan *et al.* (2008) used Atomic Force Microscopy (AMF) to analyze the structure of the organic matrix of the dental enamel after exposure to acid treatment. This was carried out on eight teeth treated for 10 seconds with 0.1 mol% citric acid. Measurements were performed on three points in the enamel close to the outer surface, post natal enamel, and three points in the enamel close to the dentin, pre natal enamel (Figure 7).

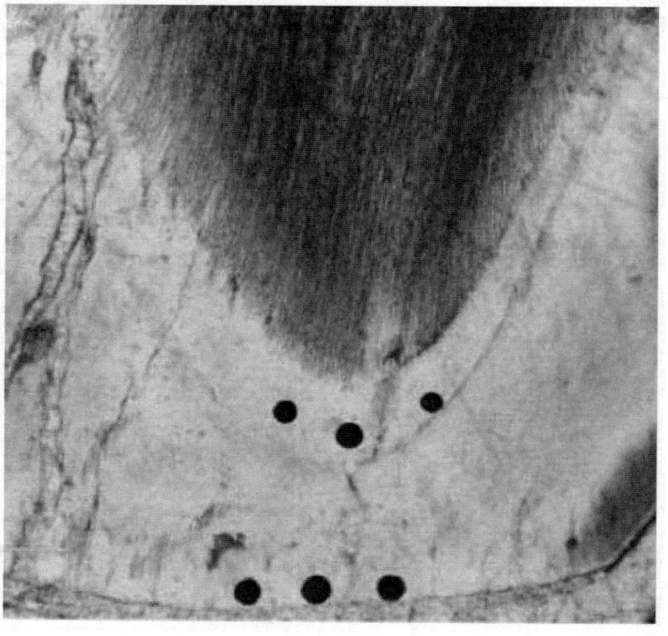

Figure 7. Points of measuring inner and outer enamel roughness.

Image roughness, which measures the regularity of the decalcified matrix, was significantly, 3-5 times, higher in DS teeth than in controls ($P<0.01$) in both inner and outer enamel (Table 4). Moreover in the control teeth, image roughness adjacent to the dentin was 37-50% greater than that measured in the outer enamel, while in DS teeth the differences between inner and outer enamel aspects were minimal, 5-16% (Table 5). These results show increased solubility of DS enamel coupled with greater irregularity of the organic matrix when compared with control teeth. They substantiate the results of the chemical analysis indicating a higher concentration of calcium salts, other than hydroxyapatite, in the DS deciduous molars coupled with a more irregular organic substrate. These findings suggest that enamel matrix apposition is impaired in DS second deciduous molars and not just the later stages of enamel maturation.

Conclusions

At least two of the studies reported here, that by Bell *et al.* (2001) and that of Zilberman *et al.* (2004), compared enamel thickness in permanent and deciduous teeth of the same tooth type. In both studies the later developing permanent tooth was more severely affected than the deciduous tooth of the same tooth type, indicating that that time of development rather than location of tooth in the jaw was the main factor involved.

The measurements taken on ground sections of exfoliated upper deciduous canines (Keinan *et al.* 2007), indicate advanced crown formation at birth in DS relative to controls. In contrast, the histological and chemical studies carried out on the second deciduous molar indicates that the reduced size characteristic of this tooth in DS children is due to growth insults affecting prenatal as well as postnatal development.

Table 4. Roughness parameters (mean for 3 points and range) measured on the inner and outer enamel of the normal and DS deciduous second molars. Each group is comprised of 4 teeth

		Inner enamel			Outer enamel	
	Rq	**Z**	**%SA**	**Rq**	**Z**	**%SA**
Control	**39.04** (23-52.1)	**283.11** (224-351)	**7.79** (3.37-13.5)	**29.70** (13.3-58.4)	**229.22** (103-367)	**10.20** (2.7-23.2)
DS	**196.44*** (140-235)	**1190.44*** (822-1467)	**18.81*** (6.8-30.7)	**189.2*** (143-271)	**1242.1*** (1020-1882)	**26.13*** (7.26-70.3)

Note: Rq - Image roughness - Root mean square average of height deviations taken from the mean image data plans.

Z - Maximum vertical distance between the highest and lowest data points in the image prior to the plane fit.

%SA - Image surface area difference - Difference between the image's three-dimensional surface area and two dimensional projected surface areas.

*= $P<0.05$ compared to control group.

Table 5. Ratios of the different roughness parameters (mean and range) calculated in the outer and inner enamel aspects for normal and DS deciduous second molars

	Rq inner /outer	**Z inner /outer**	**%SA inner /outer**
Normal (n=4)	**1.50** (0.89-2.95)	**1.37** (0.89-2.42)	**1.39** (0.26-3.74)
DS (n=4)	**1.11** (0.72-3.68	**1.16** (0.78-1.57)	**1.05** (0.29-3.74)

Crown formation at birth in DS second deciduous molars is less advanced at birth than in controls and the enamel is poorly mineralized in contrast with the enamel formed in DS canines during the same period (Keinan *et al.* 2006, 2007). It suggests that the developmental trajectories of these teeth were determined in the early stages of their embryogenesis and presumably reflects chronological differences in their initiation.

The studies reported here on the deciduous dentition were carried out on children karyotyped as possessing some variant of Trisomy 21, without reference to phenotypic differences expressed in the severity of associated growth insults. The fact that all studies reported a similar pattern of change in the deciduous teeth of DS children, may indicate that they reflect an underlying sequence of disruptive development expressed in the characteristic cranio-facial dysmorphia of DS infants. As we have attempted to show here, comparison of analysis of the deciduous teeth after they have been shed is one way of reconstructing successive stages of development in this and other conditions associated with impaired development.

Summary of Developmental Defects in the Deciduous Teeth of DS Children

In DS children the deciduous teeth show a consistent pattern of change. The incisors, canines and first molars tend to be larger than normal, while the second deciduous molars are smaller than normal.

The upper deciduous canines of DS children show a more advanced stage of crown formation at birth than controls

The second deciduous molars in DS children show a less advanced stage of crown formation at birth than controls

Morphogenesis is affected in the second deciduous molars, with the second deciduous molars showing reduced crown size and shape and taurodont roots.

The chemical composition of the enamel formed postnatally in DS deciduous canines and second deciduous molars differs. This may reflect chronological differences in their initiation. It suggests that the developmental trajectories of these teeth were determined in the early stages of their embryogenesis (Table 6).

Table 6. Summary of the effects of DS on tooth components of deciduous second molars

Tissue	Tooth component	Cell division (proliferation)	Function (apposition)	Function (mineralization)
Ectodermal	Enamel	Reduced in DS	Reduced in DS	Affected in Mesial cusps
Ecto-mesenchymal	Dentin-Pulp complex	Reduced in DS	Reduced in DS	Better in Distal cusps

References

Angelopoulou N, Souftas V, Sakadamis A, Mandroukas K, (1999). Bone mineral density in adults with Down's syndrome. *Eur. Radiol* .9:648-651.

Angelopoulou N, Matziari C, Tsimaras V, Sakadamis A, Souftas V, Mandroukas K, (2000). Bone mineral density and muscle strength in young men with mental retardation (with and without Down syndrome). *Calcif. Tissue Int* .66:176-180.

Baptista F, Varela A, Sardinha LB, (2005). Bone mineral mass in males and females with and without Down syndrome. *Osteoporosis. Int.* 16:380-388.

Barden HS, (1980). Mesiodistal crown size dimensions of permanent and deciduous teeth in Down syndrome. *Hum. Biol.* 52:247-253.

Barden HS, (1983). Growth and development of selected hard tissues in Down syndrome. A review. *Hum .Biol.* 55:359-376.

Benacerraf BR, Frigoletto FD, Green MF, (1986). Abnormal facial features and extremities in human trisomy syndromes: prenatal US appearance. *Radiology* 159: 243-246.

Bell E, Townsend G, Wilson D, Keiser J, Hughes T, (2001). Effect of Down syndrome on the dimensions of dental crowns and tissues. *Am. .J Hum. Biol.* 13:690-698.

Bimstein E, Wignall W, Cohen D, Katz J, (2008). Root surface characteristics of children with periodontal diseases. *J. Clin. Pediatr. Dent* .32:101-104.

Brabant H, (1975). Quelques observations anthropologiques sur la denture des infants mongoliens (syndrome de Down). *Cahiers de la Société Française d'Anthropologie Dento-facial*. 1:61-80.

Brown T, Townsend GC, (1984). Size and shape of mandibular first molars in Down syndrome. *Ann. Hum. Biol.* 11:281-290.

Cohen MM, Blitzer FJ, Arvystas MG, Bonneau RH., (1970). Abnormalities of the permanent dentition in trisomy G. *J. Dent. Res.* 49: Suppl:1386-93.

Cogulu D, Sabah E, Uzel A, Ozkinay F, (2006). Genotyping of *Streptococcus mutans* by using arbitrarily primed polymerase chain reaction in children with Down Syndrome. *Arch. Oral. Biol* .51: 177-182.

Coughlin JW, Christensen GJ, (1966). Growth and calcification in the prenatal human primary molars. *J. Dent. Res*. 45:1541-1547.

Deutsch D, Gedalia I, (1980). Chemically distinct stages in developing human fetal enamel. *Arch. Oral Biol.* 25:635-639.

Deutsch D, Pe'er E, (1982). Development of enamel in human fetal teeth. *J. Dent. Res.* Dec. Spec No. 1543-1551.

Deutsch D, Pe'er E, Gedalia I, (1985). Changes in size, morphology and weight of human anterior teeth during the fetal period. Growth. 48:74-85.

Deutsch D, Shapira L, (1987). Pattern of mineral uptake in the developing human deciduous enamel. *J. Craniofa.c Genet. Dev. Biol.* 7:137-143.

Garcia-Ramirez M, Toran N, Carrascosa A, Audi L, (1998). Down's syndrome: altered chondrogenesis in fetal rib. *Pediatr Res* 44:93-98.

Jaspers MT (1981). Taurodontism in Down's syndrome. *Oral Surg.. Oral Med. Oral. Path.*51:632-636.

Keinan D, Smith P, Zilberman U, (2006): Microstructure and chemical composition of primary teeth in children with Down syndrome and cerebral palsy. *Arch. Oral Biol.* 51:836-843.

Keinan D, Smith P, Zilberman U, (2007): Prenatal growth acceleration in maxilla deciduous canines of children with Down syndrome: Histological and chemical composition study. *Arch. Oral Biol.* 52:961-966.

Keinan D, Radku A, Smith P, Zilberman U, (2009). Acid resistance of the enamel in primary second molars from children with Down syndrome and Cerebral Palsy. *Open Dental J.* In press.

Kraus BS, Jordan RE (1965). *The human dentition before birth.* Lea and Febiger, Philadelphia. pp 136-138.

Lee SR, Kwon HK, Song KB, Choi YH, (2004). Dental caries and salivary immunoglobulin A in Down syndrome children. *J Pediatric Child Health.* 40:530-533.

Lomholt JF, Russell BG, Stoltze K, Kjaer I, (2002). Third molar agenesis in Down syndrome. *Acta Odontol. Scand.* 60:151-154.

Malago, W., Sommer, CA, Del Cistia Andrade C., Soares-Costa A., Possik PA, Cassago A, Santejo Silveira HC, Henrique-Silva F, (2005). Gene expression Profile of human Down Syndrome leukocytes. *Croat Med J* 46:647-656.

McMillan RS, Kashgarian J, (1961). Relation of human abnormalities of structure and function to abnormalities of dentition. II. Mongolism. *J. Am. Dent Assoc.* 63:368-373.

Moore CS, Roper RJ, (2007). The power of comparative and developmental studies for mouse models of Down syndrome. *Mamm. Genome* 18(6):431-443.

Patja K, Pukkala E, Sund R, Iivanaien M, Kaski M, (2006). Cancer incidence of persons with Down syndrome in Finland: A population based study. *Int J. Cancer*. 118:1769-1772.

Peretz B, Shapira J, Farbstein H, Arieli E, Smith P, (1998). Modified cusp relationships of mandibular molar teeth in children with Down's syndrome. *J. Anat.* 193:529-533.

Peretz B, Katzenel V, Shapira J, (1999). Morphometric variables of the primary second molar in children with Down syndrome. *Clin. Pediatr. Dent*. 23:333-336.

Prefumo F, Sethna F, Sairam S, Bhide A, Thilaganathan B, (2005). First-trimester ductus venosus, nasal bones, and Down syndrome in a high-risk population. *Obstet. Gynecol.* 105:1348-1354.

Robinson C, Connell S, Kirkham J, Brookes SJ, Shore RC, Smith AM, (2004). The effect of fluoride on the developing tooth. *Caries Res.* 38:268-276.

Sepulveda D, Allison DB, Gomez JE, Kreibich K, Brown RA, Pierson RN, Heymsfield SB, (1995). Low spinal and pelvic bone mineral density among individuals with Down syndrome. *Am. J. Ment .Retard* 100:109-114.

Shapiro BL, Gorlin RJ, Redman RS, Bruhl HH (1967). The palate and Down's syndrome. *N Engl. J. Med.* 276:1460-1463.

Skinner M, Dupras T, (1993). Variation in birth timing and location of the neonatal line in human enamel. *J. Forensic. Sci.* 38:1383-1390.

Skrinjaric T, Glavina D, Judic J, (2004). Palatal and dental arch morphology in Down syndrome. *Coll. Antropol* .28:841-847.

Ten Cate AR. *Oral Histology. Development, Structure and Function.* 5th ed. St. Louis. The CV Mosby Co. 1998. pp. 73-102.

Townsend GC, (1983). Tooth size in children and adults with Trisomy 21 "Down's Syndrome". *Arch Oral Biol* 28:159-166.

Townsend GC, (1987). A correlative analysis of dental crown dimensions in individuals with Down syndrome. *Hum. Biol* .59: 537-548.

Weijerman ME, van Furth AM, Noordegraaf AV,*van Wouwe JP, Chantal Broers JM, Gemke RJBJ, (2008). Prevalence, Neonatal Characteristics, and First-Year Mortality of Down Syndrome: A National Study. *J. Pediatrics* 152:15-19.

Zilberman U, Smith P, Kupietzky A, Mass E, (2004). The effect of hereditary disorders on tooth components: a radiographic morphometric study of two syndromes. *Arch. Oral. Biol.* 49:621-629.

In: Handbook of Down Syndrome Research
Editors: Dominicus Jelinek and Gijs Dvorak

ISBN 978-1-60741- 690-6

Chapter 19

Dealing with Down Syndrome Occurrence Risk

***Pietro Cavalli*[2], *Sara Tedoldi*[2], *Alberto Bottini*[1], and *Daniele Generali*[1]**
[1]Centro di Medicina Molecolare, Istituti Ospitalieri di Cremona, Cremona, Italy
[2]Servizio di Genetica, Istituti Ospitalieri di Cremona, Cremona, Italy

Abstract

Down syndrome (DS) represents both the most common trisomy in newborns and the most frequent genetic cause of mental retardation. It is mainly due to the presence of all or a part of a complete extra-chromosome 21 that approximately in 95% of cases is caused by an abnormal segregation during meiosis. Maternal non-disjunction is responsible of about 90% of those cases. A risk of 0,5-1% is generally given after a DS affected pregnancy. Thus, the chromosomal type of DS must be extensively studied, as the assessment of the recurrence risk depends on different cytogenetic causes. James et al. suggested a link between impaired folate metabolism and the risk of DS as the primary biological function of folate is to provide co-factors that carry one-carbon groups that play a pivotal role in DNA synthesis and methylation. Folate deficiency has been associated with abnormal chromosome segregation, supporting the possibility that low maternal folate status might be associated with the risk of non-disjunction. It is reported a significant association between frequency of C→T mutation at nucleotide 677 in the enzyme methylenetetrahydrofolate reductased and the risk of DS. Also the methionine synthase reductase A66G mutation was associated with DS risk. Both genes code for enzymes that control crucial key points in the folate pathway. In 2003 Barkai et al. noted a significantly high frequency of DS in pregnancies with risk for neural tube defects, a condition often associated with impaired folate metabolism, enforcing a link between those two pathological conditions on the common base of abnormal folate status. A periconceptional folic acid supplementation at 5 mg/die was suggested to reduce both the occurrence and recurrence risk of DS pregnancies and of neural tube defects. Moreover, maternal plasma homocysteine/methionine ratio level was higher in DS related-mothers than in controls, suggesting that folic acid supplementation could reduce the risk of trisomy 21 conceptuses. However, the cause on non-disjunction in trisomy 21 is still almost entirely unknown. Given the link between impaired folate metabolism DS occurrence and recurrence risk, those considerations further support the need of more extensive research on the use of folic acid to prevent non-disjunction events leading to free trisomy 21.

Introduction

Down Syndrome

Down Syndrome (DS) is a genetic disorder that delays in physical and intellectual development. The DS phenotype is caused in the great majority (about 95%) to a simple triple amount of chromosome 21. Around 90% reflects a maternal meiotic error [1]. Three-quarters of these maternal error occurs at meiosis I and one-quarter apparently at meiosis II [2].

Unbalanced translocation between chromosome 21 and a different acrocentric chromosome can be found in 3-4% of DS affected individuals. Approximately three fourths of these unbalanced translocation are *de novo*, and approximately one fourth are the result of familial translocations. In 1-2% of DS cases is caused by a mosaicism condition due to the co-esistance within the same individual of two cell lines, one normal and one trisomic. This condition is associated with a variable phenotype, more often less severe than homogenous trisomy 21.

The overall occurrence risk for DS corresponds to its birth prevalence, that has been estimated in 1/600-1/750 live births. However, as most of DS conceptuses are miscarried, it is estimated that the overall occurrence of DS is about 1/150 pregnancies [3, 4].

It is well known that the birth prevalence of DS is directly related to maternal age, increasing from 1/1500 at the age of 25 to 1/100 at age 40. As well as women have children at later ages, the overall population DS risk is increasing [5]. However, it should be reminded that most of DS live births are born to mothers under 35 years of age.

Down Syndrome Recurrence Risk

Recurrence of trisomy 21 in the same couple or in the same family could depend on different reasons: chance alone due to the maternal age-associated risk, parental mosaicism involving gonadal tissues, other causes of non-disjunction during meiosis[6]. A risk of 0,5-1% is generally given after a DS affected pregnancy [7]. More precisely, the woman excess risk should be calculate adding the excess risk (3.45 % at mid trimester) to the woman age risk. As an example, a 25 years old woman has a DS recurrence risk of 0.42%, while the same risk in a 40 years old woman is threefold (1.25%) [5].

Limiting the counselling process to the communication of those risk estimates represents an unsatisfactory and incomplete approach. The chromosomal type of DS must be extensively studied, as the assessment of the recurrence risk depends on different cytogenetic causes of DS [8].

Moreover, a significant increased recurrence risk must be considered even after a spontaneous abortion caused by a non viable trisomy, suggesting that prenatal diagnosis or screening should be recommended to younger women after a spontaneous trisomic abortion, underscoring the necessity to karyotype fetal tissues [6].

Comparing the observed number of homotrisomies at prenatal diagnosis with the expected number, Warburton and colleagues found that an higher DS recurrence risk should be expected for some women younger than 30 years in a North American population [6]. The same results has been obtained in the European populations [9], likely suggesting that, at least in those women, gonadal mosaicism in one of the parents could be responsible of free trisomy 21 recurrence. In addition, the presence of more than 2 cases of DS conceptuses in the same family, either regular and translocation trisomy, could be caused by gonadal mosaicism [10]. However, in the majority of cases, when the aberrant cell line is supposed to be confined to the gonads (parental germline mosaicism), the risk of subsequent trisomy 21 pregnancies can not be precisely estabilished nor predicted, and the DS recurrence as a consequence of mosaicism in germ cells is mainly made as a "bona fide" assertion.

Parental trisomy 21 low grade mosaic can be associated with a normal phenotype, hence the necessity to analyze a greater number of peripheral lymphocytes than usual. When parental mosaicism is suspected to be either in the germinal line and in the somatic cells, recurrence risk should be considered in a high range. As cytogenetic studies in skin fibroblasts do not seem to be superior over blood lymphocytes analysis [11], it is suggested that after a diagnosis of trisomy 21 to always perform extensive blood karyotyping on an appropriate numbers of metaphases.

Down Syndrome and Folate

The primary biological function of folate is to provide co-factors that carry one-carbon groups that play a pivotal role in DNA synthesis and methylation. Folate deficiency has been associated with aberrant chromosome segregation [12, 13], altered chromosome recombination [14] and abnormal DNA methylation [15].

In 1999, James et al. suggested a link between impaired folate metabolism and the risk of DS [16]. Evidence of a link between impaired maternal folate metabolism and the risk of DS pregnancies has been recently suggested in Indian population [17], in Turkish women [18], in Brazil [19], and in China [20] even these results has not been supported in all the studied population [16, 18, 21-33].

However, comparing mothers of individuals with DS and age-matched control females, James et al. found a significant association between frequency of C→T mutation at nucleotide 677 in the enzyme methylenetetrahydrofolate reductase (MTHFR [MIM 236250]) and the risk of DS [16]. Similar observations has been extended to another gene implicated in the folate metabolism, the methionine synthase reductase (MTRR, [MIM*602568]) in which A66G mutation was further associated with DS risk in Irish population [25].

Furthermore the combined presence of both MTRR A66G and MTHFR C667T polymorphisms has been associated with a higher risk of DS (OR = 4.08 95%CI 1.94-8.56) (22).

Both genes code for enzymes that control crucial key points in the folate pathway (one-carbon and homocysteine-methionine metabolism). More precisely they are involved in re-methylation and trans-sulfuration pathways, leading to DNA synthesis, epigenetic DNA modifications (methylation of CpG sequences), and regulating homocysteine plasma levels.

In particular, the C677T transition in MTHFR gene is associated with a thermolabile and less active enzyme, leading to abnormal DNA methylation and likely affecting gene expression and chromosome segregation [12, 13, 34]. DS risk in women carrying the same MTHFR polymorphisms in homozygous state have been assessed to be much higher than controls, up to a 7 fold increased risk (17). Mothers with these mutations were found to have a 2.6-fold higher risk for having a child with DS, compared with controls. A more recent study in 157 mothers of children with DS and 144 control mothers has found a 1.91-fold higher frequency of the 677C→T- MTHFR mutation among mothers of children with Down syndrome, compared with controls. The homozygous state for another mutation in FA metabolism, i.e. MTRR 66A→G was independently associated with a 2.57-fold increase in estimated risk for DS. The combined presence of the two polymorphism was associated with a four fold higher risk for DS. Moreover, the combination of different polymorphisms in the same gene (namely MTHFR C677T and 1298C) has been associate with an increased risk of DS [31],[35].

Recently, a common polymorphism (A80G) in the reduced folate carrier gene (RFC1 [MIM 600424]) has recently associated to increase DS occurrence risk. Its functions is to code for a human folate transporter in mammalian cells and tissues, since mammalian cells can not synthetize folate *de novo* [29, 31].

It has been suggested that even the viability and survival of trisomic conceptuses might be associated with particular combinations of polymorphisms in genes involved in the folate pathway [36, 37].

In 2003, Barkai et al. noted a significantly high frequency of DS in pregnancies at risk for neural tube defects, a condition often associated with impaired folate metabolism: they suggested a link between those two pathological conditions on the common base of abnormal folate status. A periconceptional folic acid supplementation at 5 mg/die was suggested to reduce both the occurrence and recurrence risk of DS pregnancies, and the risk of neural tube defects [38].

Children with DS often have reduced folate levels but the cause remains elusive [22, 39, 40]. Folate deficiency might depend on reduced folate absorbtion, that has been shown to be associated with inflammatory bowel disease (IBD): patients with IBD have higher homocysteine blood levels than controls, and lower plasma folate and vitamin B12 levels [41], depending on folate malabsorbtion, and altered folate metabolism [42]. At least a case report has been published in which aneuploidy recurrence in the same family was associated to folate deficiency likely caused by the coexistence of IBD and MTHFR C677T homozygous state in the mother [43]. Other causes of folate deficiency driven by impaired folate absorption and reduced folate transport across the intestinal wall are celiac disease, achlorhydria, the use of some antiepileptic drugs (phenytoin), zinc deficiency, intestinal diverticula, small bowel resection, and other conditions leading to intestine bacterial overgrowth. Impaired folate metabolism might be caused by other clinical conditions: the use of drugs that antagonize folate and/or inhibit dihydrofolate reductase (methotrexate and trimethoprim), alcoholism. Based on the causes possibly related to impared folate metabolism, the genetic counselling for DS should carefully take them in considerations with an extensive medical history and a correct clinical approach in order to determin any clinical/pathological cause of folate deficiency.

From a clinical point of view, the association between abnormal folate metabolism in mothers and their risk for free trisomy 21 might be assessed by genotyping polymorphism of enzymes involved in the one-carbon metabolic cycle such as the C677T polymorphism of the MTHFR gene [16, 22, 25] and the A66G polymorphism in the MTRR gene [22, 25].

Moreover, maternal plasma homocysteine levels, and its ratio to methionine, can be used as indicators of functional folate status [16, 22].

Furthermore, it has been postulated that folic acid supplementation could reduce the risk of trisomy 21 conceptuses, apart from neural tube defects. However, the benefit obtained from those fortification seems to be modest in reducing the prevalence of DS livebirths [44].

Under these circumstances, folate fortification is different from high doses of periconceptionl folic acid supplementation (up to 6 mg/die). That dosage should be strongly recommended during the first gestational month, in association to iron (150-300 mg/d of ferrous sulfate), as it could have a preventive effect against DS [45].

Maybe the expected reduction of DS risk associated with high periconceptional folate intake might have a modest effect, as nondisjunction leading to non mosaic trisomy 21 is mainly caused by an abnormal chromosome segregation during meiosis I, that takes place during the embryogenesis [3].

In the same way, maternal folate supplementation would affect mainly nondisjunction errors at meiosis II, that represent a less frequent event in DS pathogenesis. The cause on nondisjunction in trisomy 21 is still almost entirely unknown, and no etiogical factor has been clearly associated with human nondisjunction as a whole, except for the well-established link between advanced maternal age and trisomy. It has been suggested that nondisjunction leading to DS phenotype might be also associated with the age of the grandmother, and that maternal age plus maternal grandmother age should be taken in account as risk factors for the occurrence (and recurrence) of free trisomy 21 and DS phenotype [46].

Overall, conflicting results in assessing a relationship between genotypes likely causing impaired folate metabolism and DS occurrence risk might be in part explained by considering that different populations have different genetic backgrounds and differences in dietary habits. For example, a case control study from Italy found no differences in MTHFR C677T distribution in DS mother compared to control mothers. However the C677T polymorphism do not completely inactivate the enzyme function, but only reduces its efficiency. An enriched diet of folates, typical of mediterranean area can overcome this functional defect.

Folate deficiency, and not only the presence of polymorphisms in genes involved in the folate pathway, should be responsible of an increased risk of trisomy 21. French, Italian and Greek people usually have higher folate intakes than population from north Europe, in part explaining conflicting results in assessing an association between impaired folate metabolism and DS risk.

Altogether, those results suggest a likely association between impaired folate metabolism DS occurrence risk, and those considerations further support the need of more extensive studies on the use of folic acid to prevent nondisjunction events leading to free trisomy 21.

Furthermore if nondisjunction leading to DS occurrence could be somewhat linked to impaired folate metabolism and/or folate deficiency, cases of recurrence of the same condition need a more precised clinical definition.

Conclusion

Folic acid physiology, genetics, and clinical applications are subject to intensive basic and clinical research over the past decade. The proven efficacy in prevention of devastating and quite frequent congenital anomalies, i.e. DS or NTDs, gave rise to national health policies aimed at increasing the intake of folic acid in the general population of women of child-bearing age. A future direction in folic acid research is addressing genetic polymorphism of folic acid -dependent enzymes, identifying women who are at particularly high risk for maternity complications and congenital anomalies and targeting them with higher doses of folic acid, on an individual basis.

References

[1] Yoon, PW, Freeman, SB, Sherman, SL, *et al.* Advanced maternal age and the risk of Down syndrome characterized by the meiotic stage of chromosomal error: a population-based study. *Am. J. Hum. Genet.*, 1996; *58*(3): 628-633.

[2] Brown, AS, Feingold, E, Broman, KW, and Sherman, SL Genome-wide variation in recombination in female meiosis: a risk factor for non-disjunction of chromosome 21. *Hum. Mol. Genet.*, 2000; *9*(4): 515-523.

[3] Antonarakis, SE, Petersen, MB, McInnis, MG, *et al.* The meiotic stage of nondisjunction in trisomy 21: determination by using DNA polymorphisms. *Am. J. Hum. Genet.*, 1992; *50*(3): 544-550.

[4] Sherman, SL, Petersen, MB, Freeman, SB, *et al.* Non-disjunction of chromosome 21 in maternal meiosis I: evidence for a maternal age-dependent mechanism involving reduced recombination. *Hum. Mol. Genet.*, 1994; *3*(9): 1529-1535.

[5] Noble, J Natural history of Down's syndrome: a brief review for those involved in antenatal screening. *J. Med. Screen.*, 1998; *5*(4): 172-177.

[6] Warburton, D, Dallaire, L, Thangavelu, M, Ross, L, Levin, B, and Kline, J Trisomy recurrence: a reconsideration based on North American data. *Am. J. Hum. Genet.*, 2004; *75*(3): 376-385.

[7] Berini, RKE *Clinical Genetics Handbook*; 1987.

[8] Selikowitz, M Down syndrome: *The facts;* 1997.

[9] Stene, J, Stene, E, and Mikkelsen, M Risk for chromosome abnormality at amniocentesis following a child with a non-inherited chromosome aberration. A European Collaborative Study on Prenatal Diagnoses 1981. *Prenat. Diagn.*, 1984; *4 Spec No*(81-95.

[10] Sachs, ES, Jahoda, MG, Los, FJ, Pijpers, L, and Wladimiroff, JW Trisomy 21 mosaicism in gonads with unexpectedly high recurrence risks. *Am. J. Med. Genet. Suppl,* 1990; *7*(186-188.

[11] Harris, DJ, Begleiter, ML, Chamberlin, J, Hankins, L, and Magenis, RE Parental trisomy 21 mosaicism. *Am. J. Hum. Genet*., 1982; *34*(1): 125-133.

[12] Libbus, BL, Borman, LS, Ventrone, CH, and Branda, RF Nutritional folate-deficiency in Chinese hamster ovary cells. Chromosomal abnormalities associated with perturbations in nucleic acid precursors. *Cancer Genet. Cytogenet*., 1990; *46*(2): 231-242.

[13] Leyton, C, Mergudich, D, de la Torre, C, and Sans, J Impaired chromosome segregation in plant anaphase after moderate hypomethylation of DNA. *Cell Prolif.*, 1995; *28*(9): 481-496.

[14] MacGregor, JT, Wehr, CM, Hiatt, RA, *et al.* 'Spontaneous' genetic damage in man: evaluation of interindividual variability, relationship among markers of damage, and influence of nutritional status. *Mutat. Res.*, 1997; *377*(1): 125-135.

[15] Balaghi, M and Wagner, C DNA methylation in folate deficiency: use of CpG methylase. *Biochem. Biophys. Res. Commun*., 1993; *193*(3): 1184-1190.

[16] James, SJ, Pogribna, M, Pogribny, IP, *et al.* Abnormal folate metabolism and mutation in the methylenetetrahydrofolate reductase gene may be maternal risk factors for Down syndrome. *Am. J. Clin. Nutr.*, 1999; *70*(4): 495-501.

[17] Rai, AK, Singh, S, Mehta, S, Kumar, A, Pandey, LK, and Raman, R MTHFR C677T and A1298C polymorphisms are risk factors for Down's syndrome in Indian mothers. *J. Hum. Genet.*, 2006; *51*(4): 278-283.

[18] Boduroglu, K, Alanay, Y, Koldan, B, and Tuncbilek, E Methylenetetrahydrofolate reductase enzyme polymorphisms as maternal risk for Down syndrome among Turkish women. *Am. J. Med. Genet*. A, 2004; *127A*(1): 5-10.

[19] Biselli, JM, Goloni-Bertollo, EM, Zampieri, BL, Haddad, R, Eberlin, MN, and Pavarino-Bertelli, EC Genetic polymorphisms involved in folate metabolism and elevated plasma concentrations of homocysteine: maternal risk factors for Down syndrome in Brazil. *Genet. Mol.Res.*, 2008; *7*(1): 33-42.

[20] Wang, SS, Qiao, FY, Feng, L, and Lv, JJ Polymorphisms in genes involved in folate metabolism as maternal risk factors for Down syndrome in China. *J. Zhejiang. Univ. Sci*. B, 2008; *9*(2): 93-99.

[21] Botto, LD and Yang, Q 5,10-Methylenetetrahydrofolate reductase gene variants and congenital anomalies: a HuGE review. *Am. J. Epidemiol.,* 2000; *151*(9): 862-877.

[22] Hobbs, CA, Sherman, SL, Yi, P, *et al.* Polymorphisms in genes involved in folate metabolism as maternal risk factors for Down syndrome. *Am. J. Hum. Genet.,* 2000; *67*(3): 623-630.

[23] Isotalo, PA, Wells, GA, and Donnelly, JG Neonatal and fetal methylenetetrahydrofolate reductase genetic polymorphisms: an examination of C677T and A1298C mutations. *Am. J. Hum. Genet.,* 2000; *67*(4): 986-990.

[24] Chadefaux-Vekemans, B, Coude, M, Muller, F, *et al.* Methylenetetrahydrofolate reductase polymorphism in the etiology of Down syndrome. *Pediatr Res.,* 2002; *51*(6): 766-767.

[25] O'Leary, VB, Parle-McDermott, A, Molloy, AM, *et al.* MTRR and MTHFR polymorphism: link to Down syndrome? Am .J. Med. Genet., 2002; *107*(2): 151-155.

[26] Stuppia, L, Gatta, V, Gaspari, AR, *et al.* C677T mutation in the 5,10-MTHFR gene and risk of Down syndrome in Italy. *Eur.J. Hum. Genet.*, 2002; *10*(6): 388-390.

[27] Bosco, P, Gueant-Rodriguez, RM, Anello, G, *et al.* Methionine synthase (MTR) 2756 (A --> G) polymorphism, double heterozygosity methionine synthase 2756 AG/methionine synthase reductase (MTRR) 66 AG, and elevated homocysteinemia are three risk factors for having a child with Down syndrome. *Am. J. Med. Genet.* A, 2003; *121A*(3): 219-224.

[28] Botto, LD, Mulinare, J, Yang, Q, Liu, Y, and Erickson, JD Autosomal trisomy and maternal use of multivitamin supplements. *Am. J. Med. Genet. A*, 2004; *125A*(2): 113-116.

[29] Coppede, F, Marini, G, Bargagna, S, *et al.* Folate gene polymorphisms and the risk of Down syndrome pregnancies in young Italian women. *Am. J. Med. Genet.* A, 2006; *140*(10): 1083-1091.

[30] Eskes, TK Abnormal folate metabolism in mothers with Down syndrome offspring: review of the literature. Eur J Obstet Gynecol Reprod Biol, 2006; *124*(2): 130-133.

[31] Scala, I, Granese, B, Sellitto, M, *et al.* Analysis of seven maternal polymorphisms of genes involved in homocysteine/folate metabolism and risk of Down syndrome offspring. *Genet. Med.,* 2006; *8*(7): 409-416.

[32] Rosenblatt, DS Folate and homocysteine metabolism and gene polymorphisms in the etiology of Down syndrome. *Am. J. Clin. Nutr.,* 1999; *70*(4): 429-430.

[33] Takamura, N, Kondoh, T, Ohgi, S, *et al.* Abnormal folic acid-homocysteine metabolism as maternal risk factors for Down syndrome in Japan. *Eur. J. Nutr.*, 2004; *43*(5): 285-287.

[34] Titenko-Holland, N, Jacob, RA, Shang, N, Balaraman, A, and Smith, MT Micronuclei in lymphocytes and exfoliated buccal cells of postmenopausal women with dietary changes in folate. *Mutat Res*., 1998; *417*(2-3): 101-114.

[35] Acacio, GL, Barini, R, Bertuzzo, CS, Couto, EC, Annichino-Bizzacchi, JM, and Junior, WP Methylenetetrahydrofolate reductase gene polymorphisms and their association with trisomy 21. *Prenat. Diagn*., 2005; *25*(13): 1196-1199.

[36] Martinez-Frias, ML, Perez, B, Desviat, LR, *et al.* Maternal polymorphisms 677C-T and 1298A-C of MTHFR, and 66A-G MTRR genes: is there any relationship between polymorphisms of the folate pathway, maternal homocysteine levels, and the risk for having a child with Down syndrome? *Am. J. Med. Genet* .A, 2006; *140*(9): 987-997.

[37] Martinez-Frias, ML The biochemical structure and function of methylenetetrahydrofolate reductase provide the rationale to interpret the epidemiological results on the risk for infants with Down syndrome. *Am. J. Med. Genet.* A, 2008; *146A*(11): 1477-1482.

[38] Barkai, G, Arbuzova, S, Berkenstadt, M, Heifetz, S, and Cuckle, H Frequency of Down's syndrome and neural-tube defects in the same family. *Lancet*, 2003; *361*(9366): 1331-1335.

[39] Pogribna, M, Melnyk, S, Pogribny, I, Chango, A, Yi, P, and James, SJ Homocysteine metabolism in children with Down syndrome: in vitro modulation. *Am. J. Hum. Genet*., 2001; *69*(1): 88-95.

[40] Al-Gazali, LI, Padmanabhan, R, Melnyk, S, *et al.* Abnormal folate metabolism and genetic polymorphism of the folate pathway in a child with Down syndrome and neural tube defect. *Am. J. Med. Genet.*, 2001; *103*(2): 128-132.

[41] Mahmud, N, Molloy, A, McPartlin, J, *et al.* Increased prevalence of methylenetetrahydrofolate reductase C677T variant in patients with inflammatory bowel disease, and its clinical implications. *Gut,* 1999; *45*(3): 389-394.

[42] Morgenstern, I, Raijmakers, MT, Peters, WH, Hoensch, H, and Kirch, W Homocysteine, cysteine, and glutathione in human colonic mucosa: elevated levels of homocysteine in patients with inflammatory bowel disease. *Dig. Dis. Sci.*, 2003; *48*(10): 2083-2090.

[43] Cavalli, P and Luongo, R Multiple aneuploidy recurrence. *Am. J. Med. Genet* A, 2005; *137*(1): 104-105.

[44] Canfield, MA, Collins, JS, Botto, LD, *et al.* Changes in the birth prevalence of selected birth defects after grain fortification with folic acid in the United States: findings from a multi-state population-based study. Birth Defects Res A Clin. *Mol .Teratol.,* 2005; *73*(10): 679-689.

[45] Czeizel, AE and Puho, E Maternal use of nutritional supplements during the first month of pregnancy and decreased risk of Down's syndrome: case-control study. *Nutrition,* 2005; *21*(6): 698-704; discussion 774.

[46] Malini, SS and Ramachandra, NB Influence of advanced age of maternal grandmothers on Down syndrome. *BMC Med. Genet.,* 2006; *7*(4.)

In: Handbook of Down Syndrome Research
Editors: Dominicus Jelinek and Gijs Dvorak

ISBN 978-1-60741- 690-6

Chapter 20

DYRK1A Kinase and Neuronal Cytoskeleton: A New Look at Pathogenesis of Alzheimer's Disease Dementia from the Perspective of Down Syndrome

Karol Dowjat
Department of Developmental Neurobiology
New York State Institute for Basic Research in Developmental Disabilities, Staten Island, USA

Abstract

DYRK1A kinase, the gene located within triplicated region on chromosome 21 in Down syndrome (DS), has been found to be associated with neuronal cytoskeleton. In pathological brains of DS and Alzheimer's disease (AD) patients the levels of major cytoskeleton proteins forming complexes with DYRK1A were greatly reduced. The changes were specific for AD dementia and present in young DS individuals whose brains were free of pathological burden, suggesting that early dysfunction of cytoskeleton may be at the root of neurodegenerative processes responsible for AD. Any malfunction of cytoskeleton during brain development may result in sculpting of the memory system with significantly reduced memory capacity, which late in life can become saturated incapacitating brain to acquire a constant input of new epigenetic information. This triggers a compensatory response, which up-regulates neuronal plasticity and through activation of dedifferentiation program forces post-mitotic neurons back into the cell cycle. Re-entering the cell cycle and high plasticity burden imposed on neurons of the memory system lead to its gradual degeneration resulting in dementia. Down syndrome patients with their developmentally impaired neuronal networking, caused by abnormal expression of DYRK1A and other genes from the region critical for DS, lend a lot of support for the proposed cascade of events leading to dementia.

Alzheimer's disease (AD) is a progressive neurodegenerative disorder associated with memory loss that leads to dementia and death in late middle-aged and elderly individuals. The disease is characterized by the deposition of amyloid plaques, neurofibrillary tangles, dystrophic neurites and neuropil threads in the cortex and hippocampus, accompanied by neuronal and synaptic loss. Down syndrome (DS) patients are unusually susceptible to the disease developing Alzheimer's type dementia by the fourth decade of life, with the clinical and neuropathological features indistinguishable from the classical AD. The cause of the disease is still unknown and remains the primary focus of intensive research worldwide. DS patients who are easily identifiable at birth and whose AD fate is highly predictable, offer a unique opportunity to extend this research into very early stages that precede the appearance of AD-like neuropathology and onset of symptoms. As logic as the choice of DS individuals for modeling processes leading to AD might be, the ultimate justification for its applicability must come from the proof of common physiopathology underlying DS and AD dementia. Such proof is still missing unless we accept the"amyloid cascade hypothesis", a leading concept in the field of AD research, to be correct. According to this concept, accumulation and deposition of insoluble ß-amyloid (Aß) into AD plaques is the primary cause of AD-related neuronal death, cytoskeletal pathology and synaptic loss. ß-amyloid is the product of processing of amyloid precursor protein (APP), which gene is located on chromosome 21 close to the so-called Down syndrome critical region (DSCR) containing a subset of genes obligatory for Down syndrome. Whether trisomy-driven overexpression of APP gene in DS is at the root of AD dementia is still a matter of heated debate, but we shifted our attention to another gene from this region, which contribution to the impairment of cognitive functions and dementia of DS/AD individuals might be far greater than APP. The gene called DYRK1A is over-expressed in DS in gene-dosage dependent manner (Dowjat et al., 2007) and encodes a dual specificity serine/treonine kinase, which play a role as important regulator of neuronal networks and their complexity, both in developing and mature CNS. The well-documented role of DYRK1A in the maturation of CNS (reviewed in Benavides-Piccione et al., 2004), prompted us to focus our attention to possible association of this kinase with cytoskeleton proteins. Using immunoprecipitation techniques and brain tissue of control, DS and AD subjects, we have found that all major cytoskeleton proteins i.e. actin, tubulin, vimentin and neurofilaments are co-immunoprecipitating with DYRK1A.

As shown in figure 1, which depicts a representative Western blot analysis of DYRK1A immunoprecipitates from pooled frontal cortex tissue of six controls, twelve DS and four AD subjects, the levels of all four major cytoskeleton protein, except vimentin, were dramatically reduced in DS/AD brains.

These data, not only show for a first time the association of DYRK1A with neuronal cytoskeleton, but also, an extensive abnormalities in this association occurring in pathological brains of DS/AD patients. The changes seem to be specific for DS/AD, since they were not present in three unrelated mental retardation cases. Importantly, the patterns of those changes in DS and AD brains were quite similar, which in view of almost indistinguishable presentation of AD type dementia in both groups, strongly support the idea of common pathological mechanism being at the root of the disease.

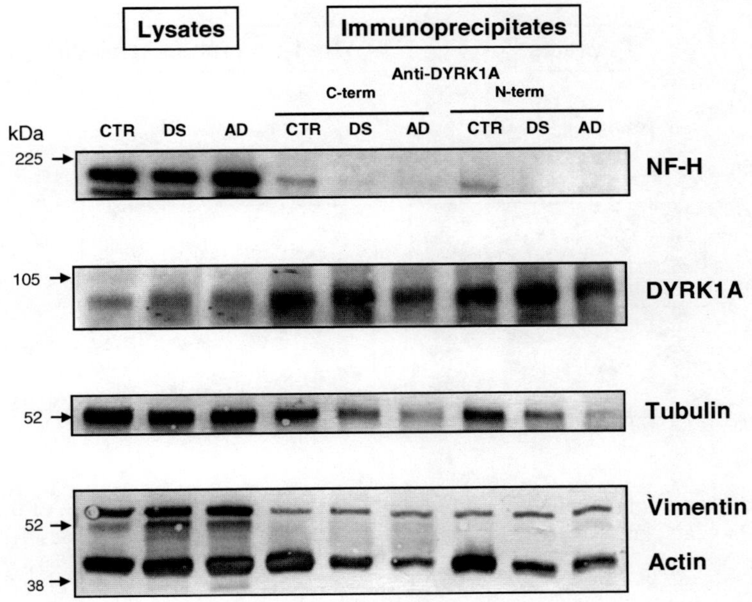

Figure 1. Co-immunoprecipitation of NF-H, tubulin, vimentin and actin with DYRK1A in frontal cortex of control, DS and AD subjects. For immunoprecipitation two anti-DYRK1A polyclonal antibodies from Santa Cruz directed against N- (G19) and C-terminus (H143,) of DYRK1A polypeptide were used. For DYRK1A detection on blots home-made monoclonal 8D9 antibody was used. NF-H subunit of neurofilaments, tubulin and actin were detected with monoclonal antibodies from Sigma. The immunoreactive bands were visualized by chemiluminescence using CDP star detection reagent from New England Biolabs.

Based on this similarity and the fact that DS patients develop AD-type neuropathology by the fourth decade of life, we attempted to determine whether those disease-specific abnormalities can be detected in the brains of young DS individuals, that is before development of neuropathology and the onset of symptoms. Accordingly, we examined pooled frontal cortex tissue of young (13-23 years) and old (48-65 years) control and DS subjects.

As shown in figure 2, which depicts immunoblotting profiles of DYRK1A immunoprecipitates for DYRK1A, vimentin and actin, in both young and old DS pools, the levels of actin were greatly reduced. This exactly reproduces our results obtained for DS and AD cases with the full-blown onset of symptoms. That the brains of young DS subjects used in this study are free of pathological burden, can be deduced from the low levels of vimentin, the marker of astrocytic reaction, one of the prevalent sign of AD-type neuropathology.

These findings clearly show that cytoskeleton abnormalities in DS and AD precede the development of neuritic plaques and neurofibrillary tangles, the hallmarks of Alzheimer's disease, suggesting that early dysfunction of cytoskeleton may be one of neurodegenerative processes responsible for AD.

Thus, it seems to be justified perceiving DS individuals as early diagnosed prospective AD patients who are carrying a specific set of changes involving complexes of DYRK1A and cytoskeleton proteins.

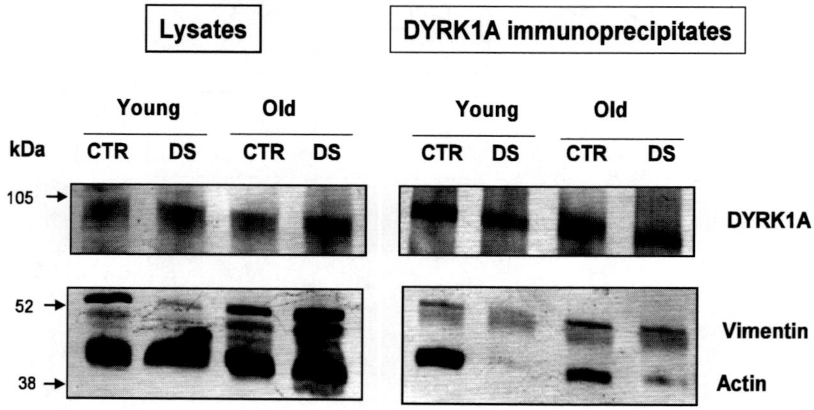

Figure 2. Comparison of immunoblotting profiles of DYRK1A immunoprecipitates of frontal cortex of young (13 and 23 years) and old (48-65 years) control and DS subjects. All details as described in the legend of figure 1.

Those changes, as well as, mutations in presenilins, APP, gelsolin and apoE isotype in familial AD, very likely contribute to abnormal development of brain neuronal circuitry affecting structures responsible for learning and memory. In fact, such abnormal development by all means applies to DS patients whose brains are smaller, displaying decreased neuronal density, diminished dendritic arborization and markedly reduced spines and synapse density with the regional distribution corresponding to affected structures in AD (reviewed in Dierssen and Ramakers, 2006). Abnormal development and plasticity of structural neuronal network connectivity may result in sculpting of the memory system with reduced capacity, which late in life may become overloaded creating "all circuits are busy" situation, incapacitating the brain to acquire a constant input of new epigenetic information. This triggers a compensatory response, which up-regulates neuronal plasticity and through activation of dedifferentiation programs forces neurons of the memory system to re-enter the cell cycle. Pushing post-mitotic, terminally differentiated neurons back into the cell cycle creates dysregulation of the balance between gatekeepers of the differentiated state and signal transduction pathways that transmit mitogenic signals and ultimately leads to death of the nerve cell. Impaired neuritogenesis and synaptogenesis caused by cytoskeletal abnormalities also contribute to ineffective plasticity responses and exacerbate the plasticity burden of AD. Aberrant sprouting, cytoskeleton abnormalities, secretion of ß-amyloid, hyperphosphorylation of tau protein, accumulation of growth-associated proteins, and the presence of cell cycle markers, are all manifestation of this aborted attempt of neurons to expand the brain memory capacity.

Hyperactive, aberrant neuroplasticity and neurogenesis are very prominent and well documented features in affected structures of AD brain. (see extensive reviews by Arendt, 2001; Teter and Ashford , 2002). Based on those features "the neuroplasticity" (Arendt, 2003) and "the cell cycle" (Nagy, 2005) theories were put forward. Although they provide a very plausible explanation of how the AD pathology develops, but they fail short in explaining what may be that "key" event that triggers the disease. Our concept, by pointing at compensatory response to reaching limits of memory capacity as an initiator of cascade of pathological processes leading to dementia, seems to fill this gap. Those limits are decided during development under genetic program of each individual. The memory size can be increased by experience i.e. learning and participation in the tasks requiring use of intellect, but the general range of connections for most nerve cells is undoubtedly specified by genes, such as those linked to familial AD, which were all found to be important regulators of neuronal network connectivity. Therefore, AD type dementia should be viewed as a late life consequence of genetically determined events occurring during brain development, however how late in life, if ever, it develops, greatly depends on lifestyles of those being at risk. Education and intellectual activity, through targeting mechanisms of memory cognitive reserve, or heavy input of data in information rich area, may greatly influence the timing and the outcome of the disease. Because of the need and complexity of interaction of genetic and environmental factors to produce the illness, proving a genetic predisposition to AD and finding responsible genes by applying conventional genetic linkage analysis, seems to be hardly achievable task.

Memory overload, first conceptualized by Clark (Clark, 2000), cannot be directly detected, but its occurrence can be deduced from behavioral changes of AD patients, mainly their inability to form new memories. The selective vulnerability of large pyramidal cells of the hippocampus is because of their primary role in the processing and storage of new memories. Subjects with mild cognitive impairment (MCI), condition that precedes AD dementia, produced much stronger MRI scan signals during the encoding of novel information, which could be a reflection of greater number of neuronal circuits sending a "busy signal" (Sperling and Albert, 2003). Memory overload seems to be a plausible explanation for higher incidence of AD dementia in developed countries (reviewed in Kaltzman, 2001) where people are exposed to higher input of new information..

The concept provides straightforward explanation for two major features of AD: age dependence and selectivity of pathology toward brain structures responsible for cognitive memory. It also links formation of neurofibryllary tangles and deposition of amyloid in one pathological cascade fueled by misguided attempt of terminally differentiated neurons to divide. The unique susceptibility of human brain to AD, yet another important feature of the disease, may stem from enormous complexity of environment created by humans imposing heavy burden on the memory system to deal with the high load of information during the long life spam.

The hypothesis predicts that limiting input of novel information combined with memory rehabilitation aiming at increasing cognitive reserve and therapeutic interventions targeted at attenuation of neuronal plasticity, should be beneficial for patients in less advanced stages of dementia.

The main purpose of this article, besides showing disease-specific cytoskeleton abnormalities involving DYRK1A kinase in the brain tissue of DS/AD subjects, was to encourage many field masters to go beyond "the amyloid cascade hypothesis", which for so long has been a driving force of AD research. Despite an unprecedented amount of research activity into the causative role of ß-amyloid in pathogenesis of AD, its translation into development of diagnostic tests and effective therapeutic approaches, has been disappointing. Thus, there is a need for new" there is life beyond Aß" theories, which can inspire more insightful and fruitful directions of research. Hopefully, the concept shortly outlined in this article, would provide such inspiration.

Acknowledgments

I would like to thank Dr. Tatyana Adayev for her excellent work on this project. The work was supported by funds from the New York State Office of Mental Retardation and Developmental Disabilities.

References

Dowjat, WK; Adayev, T; Kuchna, I.; Nowicki, K; Palminello, S.; Hwang, YW; Wegiel, JW. Trisomy-driven overexpression of DYRK1A kinase in the brain of subjects with Down syndrome. *Neurosci. Lett.*, 2007 413, 77-81

Benavides-Piccione, R; Ballesteros-Yáñez, M; Martinez de Lagrán, M; Elston, G; Estivill, X; Fillat, C; DeFelipe, J; Dierssen, M. On dendrites in Down syndrome and DS murine models; a spiny way to learn. *Prog. Neurobiol.* 2004 74, 111-126

Dierssen, M; Ramakers, GJA. Dendritic pathology in mental retardation: from molecular genetics to neurobiology. *Genes Brain and Behavior* 2006 5 (Suppl.2), 48-60

Arendt, T. Alzheimer's disease as a disorder of mechanisms underlying structural brain self-organization. *Neuroscience* 2001 102, 723-765

Teter, B; Ashford, JW. Neuroplasticity in Alzheimer's disease. *J. Neurosci. Res.* 2002 70, 402-437

Arendt, T. Synaptic plasticity and cell cycle activation in neurons are alternative effector pathways: the "Dr. Jekyll and Mr. Hyde concept" of Alzheimer's disease or the yin and yang of neuroplasticity. *Prog. Neurobiol.* 2003 71, 83-248

Nagy, Z. The last neuronal division: a unifying hypothesis for the pathogenesis of Alzheimer's disease. *J. Cell. Mol. Med.* 2005 9, 531-541

Clark, RP. Does longer-term memory storage never become overloaded, and would such overload cause Alzhemer's disease and other dementia? *Med. Hypotheses* 2000 55, 419-428

Sperling, RA; Albert MS. Functional MRI studies of episodic memory encoding in early Alzheimer's disease. In: Iqbal K., Winblad B editors. *Alzheimer's Disease and Related Disorders: Research Advances.* Bucharest, Ana Aslan Intl. Acad. of Aging, 2003, 225-235

Katzman, R. Epidemiology of Alzheimer's disease and dementia: Advances and challenges. In: Iqbal K, Sisodia S, Winblad B editors. *Alzheimer's Disease: Advances in Etiology, Pathogenesis and Therapeutics*. New York; John Wiley and Sons, Ltd; 2001; 11-21

Recommended Additional Readings

Agnati, LF; Zoli, M; Biagini, G; Fuxe, K. Neuronal plasticity and ageing process in the frame of the "Red Qeen Theory" *Acta Physiol. Scand.* 1992 145, 301-309

Neill, D. Alzheimer's disease: Maladaptive synaptoplasticity hypothesis. *Neurodegeneration* 1995 4, 217-232

Mesulam, MM. Neuroplasticity failure in Alzheimer's disease: Bridging the gap between plaques and tangles. *Neuron,* 1999 24, 521-529

Index

A

B

C

D

E

F

G

H

N

O

P

Q

R

S

T

X

Z